Nephrology

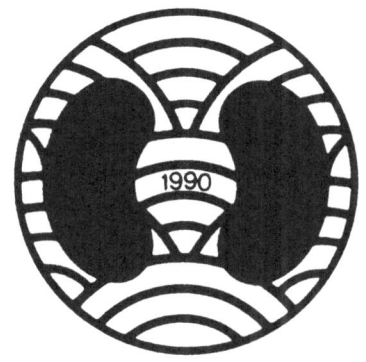

1990

Nephrology VOLUME **II**

PROCEEDINGS OF THE
XITH INTERNATIONAL CONGRESS OF NEPHROLOGY

Editor
Michinobu Hatano

Associate Editors
Nishio Honda · Hyoe Ishikawa · Kenkichi Koiso
Kiyoshi Kurokawa · Tadao Niijima
Nobuhiro Sugino · Susumu Takahashi

With 239 Figures

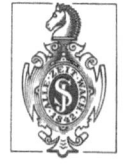

Springer Japan KK

Editor

MICHINOBU HATANO, M.D., Professor of Medicine, Director, Department of Internal Medicine, Nihon University School of Medicine, Tokyo, Japan

Associate Editors

NISHIO HONDA, Tokyo Senbai Hospital, Tokyo
HYOE ISHIKAWA, Nara Medical University, Nara
KENKICHI KOISO, The University of Tsukuba, Ibaraki
KIYOSHI KUROKAWA, University of Tokyo, Tokyo
TADAO NIIJIMA, Tokyo Seamen's Medical College, Tokyo
NOBUHIRO SUGINO, Tokyo Women's Medical College, Tokyo
SUSUMU TAKAHASHI, Nihon University, Tokyo

ISBN 978-3-540-70074-6

Library of Congress Cataloging-in-Publication Data
International Congress on Nephrology (11th: 1990: Tokyo, Japan); Nephrology: proceedings of the XIth International Congress of Nephrology/editors, Michinobu Hatano: associate editors, Nishio Honda...[et al.].
p. cm. Congress held in Tokyo, Japan, July 15-20, 1990. Includes bibliographical references. Includes index.
ISBN 978-3-540-70074-6   ISBN 978-3-662-35158-1 (eBook)
DOI 10.1007/978-3-662-35158-1

1. Kidneys – Diseases – Congresses.
2. Nephrology – Congresses. 3. Kidney Diseases – congresses. 4. Nephrology – congresses. I. Hatano, Michinobu, 1926-   . II. Honda, Nishio. III. Title. [DNLM: WJ 300 I59n 1990]. RC902.A2I56 1990. 616.6'1 –dc20. DNLM/DLC. for Library of Congress 91-4651

Typesetting: Publishers Service of Montana, Bozeman, Montana

Foreword

The proceedings of the XIth International Congress of Nephrology held in Tokyo in 1990, form the most international and complete document of the present state of basic and clinical science in nephrology. In addition, they document the progress made in this field during the 3 years since the London Congress. The result is nothing short of impressive. The material presented by the invited lecturers and the participants of the symposia all show a remarkable pattern; not only the "height" of the science, but also the depth of the specialized knowledge, both prerequisites of excellency in science, which do not necessarily imply narrowness of outlook. On the contrary, this written document of the Tokyo Congress is a witness to the enormous progress made over the last few years in communication between basic scientists and clinical scientists.

The International Society of Nephrology is a fine example of how fruitful and productive this interaction can be, if it is conducted with the desire to understand each other. The members of the Scientific Program Committee of the Tokyo Congress are to be congratulated, not only for a thoughtful and well designed program, but also for carefully selecting those speakers who, besides their own contribution to nephrological science, also have the talent of being able to communicate with a large, international audience. In particular, I would like to express my deep appreciation to the editors of the Proceedings for their commitment and industriousness which made it possible for this publication to appear so soon after the Congress.

Since the first Congress of the International Society of Nephrology in Evian in 1960, nephrologists have witnessed a phenomenal increase in knowledge, a progress which still continues and will do so in the future. The present proceedings are a snapshot of this process. The counterpoint to the intellectual challenge of acquiring deeper understanding is the duty and promise to utilize that understanding for the benefit of our patients.

KLAUS THURAU, M.D.
President,
International Society of Nephrology
(1987–1990)

v

Preface

The XIth International Congress of Nephrology was held in Tokyo, Japan from July 15–20, 1990.

Since the first congress in Evian, France in 1960, this is the first time that this prestigious congress has been held in Asia. Therefore, enthusiastic expectations were held by nephrologists not only in Japan but also throughout the world.

In organizing the congress under the estimable guidance of Prof. Klaus Thurau, President of the International Society of Nephrology, the ISN Executive Committee and the International Advisory Committee, Prof. Michinobu Hatano, Chairman of the local organizing committee as well as the organizing committee made every effort to make the congress a success.

Over three thousand participants from 71 countries attended the congress. These included 1,470 participants from Japan, 472 from the United States, 150 from France, and 128 from Italy. We were particularly pleased to welcome eight representatives from Czechoslovakia as well as an increased participation from other eastern European countries, the Soviet Union, and China. Forty-nine delegates from Taiwan were also in attendance.

The opening ceremony was held at the New Takanawa Prince Hotel in the presence of the Crown Prince, whose address noted that progress in nephrology would contribute greatly to the welfare of patients worldwide.

The scientific program consisted of 15 state-of-the-art lectures, 36 symposia, 11 workshops, 256 oral and 1,778 poster presentations. Following the advice of the ISN Executive Committee, the Scientific Program Committee encouraged the presentation of clinical and research papers at the same time in each session. This ensured that throughout the scientific program, discussions were constructive, and this helped to make the congress both stimulating and fruitful.

A total of 12 ISN satellite symposia, 4 overseas and 8 in Japan, were also held. The specific topics discussed at each symposium, combined with sightseeing tours at each site, contributed greatly to exchanges of both friendship and information.

Finally, we would like to express our sincere thanks and appreciation to the ISN Committee and all the participants of the congress.

KENZO OSHIMA, M.D.
President

YAWARA YOSHITOSHI, M.D.
Vice-President

YASUSHI UEDA, M.D.
Vice-President

HIROSHI ABE, M.D.
Vice-President

XIth International Congress of Nephrology

ORGANIZED BY: The Organizing Committee of the XIth International
                         Congress of Nephrology

UNDER THE AUSPICES OF: International Society of Nephrology

SPONSORED BY: Japanese Society of Nephrology
                         The Kidney Foundation, Japan

IN COOPERATION WITH: The Japanese Association of Medical Science
                         Japan Medical Association
                         The Japanese Urological Association
                         The Japan Society for Transplantation
                         Japanese Society for Artificial Organs
                         Japanese Society for Dialysis Therapy
                         The Japanese Society of Pediatric Nephrology
                         Japan Incorporated Medical Association for Dialysis

SUPPORTED BY: Ministry of Education, Science and Culture
                         Ministry of Health and Welfare
                         Science Council of Japan
                         Tokyo Metropolitan Government

The International Society of Nephrology

Management Committee

Klaus Thurau	FRG	President
Roscoe R. Robinson	USA	President Elect
Claude Amiel	France	Secretary-General
Robert W. Schrier	USA	Treasurer
Thomas E. Andreoli	USA	Editor, Kidney International
Saulo Klahr	USA	Councillor
D. Keith Peters	UK	Councillor

Council

Stephen Angielski	Poland
Robert C. Atkins	Australia
Knut Auklund	Norway
Vittorio Bonomini	Italy
Barry M. Brenner	USA
Giuseppe D'Amico	Italy
Vincent W. Dennis	USA
John H. Dirks	Canada
Evert J. Dorhout Mees	The Netherlands
Carl W. Gottschalk	USA
Jean-Pierre Grünfeld	France
Jean Hamburger	France
Klaus Hierholzer	FRG
David N.S. Kerr	UK
Saulo Klahr	USA
Robert T. McCluskey	USA
Gerhard Malnic	Brazil
D. Keith Peters	UK
Hidekazu Shigematsu	Japan
Jay Stein	USA
Nobuhiro Sugino	Japan
Guillermo Whittembury	Venezuela

XIth International Congress Officers

President	Kenzo Oshima
Vice Presidents	Yawara Yoshitoshi
	Yasushi Ueda
	Hiroshi Abe

ORGANIZING COMMITTEE

Chairman	Michinobu Hatano
Secretary-General	Susumu Takahashi

Members

Yoshio Aso	Tadashi Miyahara
Toshiyuki Furukawa	Toshihiko Nagasawa
Kohei Hara	Mitsuharu Narita
Nishio Honda	Hiromi Nihira
Takeshi Hoshi	Tadao Niijima
Kazunari Iidaka	Teruo Omae
Hyoe Ishikawa	Zensuke Ota
Chuichi Kawai	Fuminori Sakai
Teruo Kitagawa	Takao Sonoda
Kenkichi Koiso	Nobuhiro Sugino
Kiyoshi Kurokawa	Shizuo Tojo
Sunao Maki	

SCIENTIFIC PROGRAM COMMITTEE

Chairmen   Nobuhiro Sugino
                              Nishio Honda

Executive Secretary   Kiyoshi Kurokawa

Members
Akitoshi Ando   Koichi Matsumoto
Kikuo Arakawa   Toshihiko Nagasawa
Masaaki Arakawa   Mitsumasa Nagase
Hitoshi Endou   Yasushi Nakamoto
Mamoru Fujimoto   Hiroshi Nihei
Gerhard Giebisch   Michio Odaka
Takashi Harada   Hiroyuki Ohi
Eiji Higashihara   Yoshimasa Orita
Kazunari Iidaka   Kazuo Ota
Masashi Imai   Hideto Sakai
Hiroshi Kida   Osamu Sakai
Hikaru Koide   Tadasu Sakai
Kenkichi Koiso   Takao Saruta
Shozo Koshikawa   Hidekazu Shigematsu
Akio Koyama   Kenjiro Yamamoto
Kenji Maeda   Nobuyuki Yoshizawa
Sunao Maki

FUND RAISING COMMITTEE

Chairmen   Tadao Niijima
                              Hyoe Ishikawa

Members
Keishi Abe   Joichi Kumazawa
Yoshio Aso   Yuji Nagura
Tohru Azuma   Zensuke Ota
Kohei Hara   Tsutomu Sanaka
Yoshihei Hirasawa   Takao Sonoda
Hiroshi Kida   Naohiko Ueda

FINANCE COMMITTEE

Chairman   Kenkichi Koiso

Members
Hiroshi Kawamura   Gengo Osawa

Contents of Volume II

Symposia

Cytokines, Mitogens and Their Receptors on Glomerular Cells

Frontiers of Research on Natriuretic Peptides

Glomerular Cells and Extracellular Matrix

Renal Tubular Acidosis

Endothelin and the Kidney

Transplantation

Optical Techniques for Studying Kidney Cell Function

Management of Childhood Nephrotic Syndrome

Ca, Pi, PTH, and Vitamin D

Contents of Volume I

State of the Art Lectures

Symposia

Cyclosporine Nephrotoxicity: From Experimental Animal to Clinical Practice

Cell Volume Regulation in Health and Disease

Mechanisms of Renal Cell Injury of Acute Renal Failure

List of Contributors

For contributors' addresses see chapter opening pages

Symposia

Cytokines, Mitogens and Their Receptors on Glomerular Cells

Chair: Gary E. Striker (USA)
Itaru Kihara (Japan)

The Terminal Complement Complex C5b-9: A Possible Mediator of Acute and Chronic Glomerulonephritis

GERTRUD MARIA HÄNSCH, MATTHIAS SCHÖNERMARK, CHRISTOF WAGNER, GISELA SCHIEREN, and BERNHARD JAHN[1]

SUMMARY. Incubation of cultivated glomerular cells with the activated terminal complement components C5b-9 results in binding of C5b-9, but not in the killing of cells. One mechanism of cellular defense is the expression of a surface protein, C8 binding protein (C8bp), which was initially identified on human erythrocytes as an inhibitor of the terminal complement reaction. C8bp was also found on mesangial cells and glomerular epithelial cells. Its expression was enhanced upon complement attack. Even though C5b-9 is not lytic on glomerular cells it nevertheless stimulates the mesangial cells to release prostaglandin E, interleukin 1, tumor necrosis factor, and epithelial cells to synthesize collagen type IV. We propose that by releasing mediators from mesangial cells, C5b-9 contributes to the perpetuation of an acute inflammatory response and, by stimulating collagen synthesis, to the development of sclerosis.

The role of complement in the development of acute inflammation and also in glomerulonephritis is well established. With complement activation, e.g., by antigen-antibody complexes, the chemotactic peptide C5a is generated, which elicits leukocyte infiltration. C5a, as well as C3b, the latter when bound to surfaces, activate leukocytes, e.g., to release proteolytic or collagenolytic enzymes, oxygen radicals or eicosanoids, thus promoting tissue destruction as well as the infiltration of more leukocytes [1–4].

In recent years, another activity of the complement system has also gained increasing interest, namely the action of the terminal complement component C5b-9, known as the lytic entity of the complement cascade. By either classical or alternative pathway activation of complement, a C5b6 complex is generated, which inserts, after binding of C7, C8, and C9, into membrane lipid bilayer to form a transmembrane pore (Fig. 1) (for review see [5,6]). C56 complexes are generated also by complement-independent pathways. Lowering the pH [7], cleavage by proteolytic

---

[1]Institut für Immunologie der Universität Heidelberg, 6900 Heidelberg 1, Federal Republic of Germany

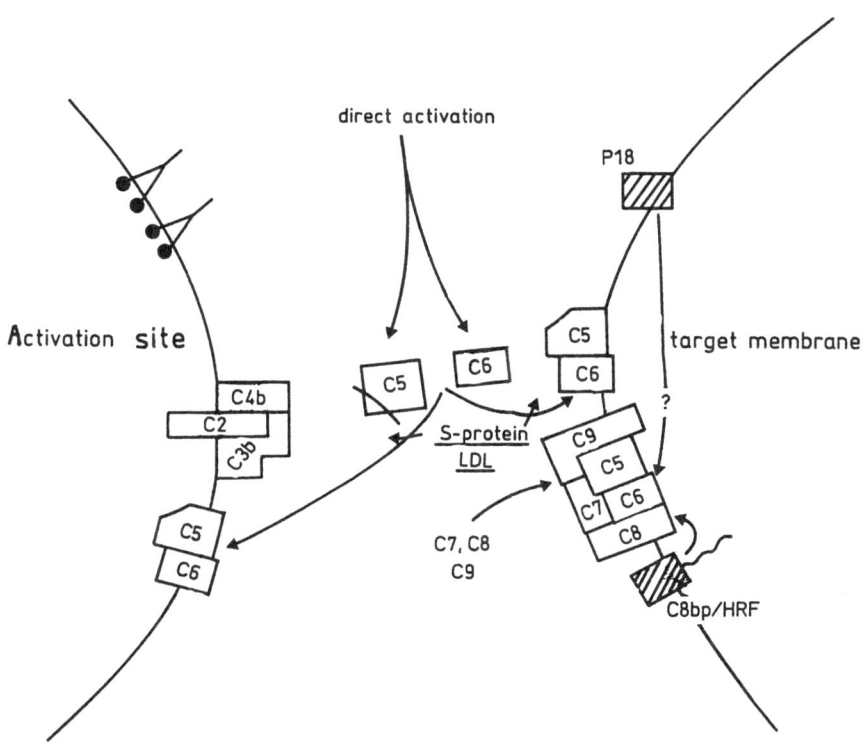

Fig. 1. Control of complement activation: By complement activation, a C5 cleaving enzyme (*C4b2a*) is generated. The cleaved C5, C5b, binds C6 and the ensuing C5b6 complex attaches reversibly to the membrane. Together with C7, C8, and C9 it inserts into the lipid bilayer. Binding of C5b6 can be prevented by fluid phase proteins, e.g., S-protein or low density lipoprotein (*LDL*), and by the efficient formation of C5b-9 by the intrinsic membrane protein C8 binding proteins, C8bp and P18

enzymes [8], or reactive oxygen species [9] are able to directly generate C56 complexes, which, together with C7, C8, and C9, form lytic complexes on membranes.

The C5b6 complex, once generated, does not necessarily bind at the site of activation, but might—for a short period of time—also bind to membranes in the vicinity; the complement reaction up to C9 will then proceed at the "innocent bystander" membrane [10,11].

The activation pathways and the complement attack phase are well regulated (Fig. 1), thus minimizing bystander lysis. S-protein or vitronectin, a serum protein, interferes with the binding of C5b6 and consequently with the formation of membrane-bound C5b-9. Among the inhibitory molecules, cell surface associated proteins, restricting the complement attack in a species-specific manner, are of special interest. With regard to regulation of the terminal complement components, an intrinsic 65kD membrane protein with high affinity for the complement protein C8, and to a minor extent for C9, has been identified, first on human erythrocytes [12],

Table 1. Cell functions elicited by sublytic doses of C5b-9[a]

Release of eicosanoids from
  monocytes (human, mouse, rat)
  macrophages (rat)
  granulocytes (human)
  platelets (human)
  Kupffer cells (rat)
  glomerular mesangial cells (rat, human)
  glomerular epithelial cells (rat)
  synovial fibroblasts (human)
  oligodendrocytes (rat)

Release of interleukin 1 from
  glomerular mesangial cells (rat, human)
  monocytes (human)

Release of oxygen radicals from
  glomerular mesangial cells (rat, human)
  granulocytes (human)

Release of collagen type IV from
  glomerular epithelial cells (rat, human)

Release of collagenase from
  synovial fibroblasts (human)

[a](From [5,6,26])

and later also on other peripheral blood cells [13]. This so-called C8 binding protein, most probably identical to the "homologous restriction factor" [14], interferes with the assembly of the C5b-9 complex by inhibiting the reaction of C8 with C9 [15]. Lack of C8bp, as seen in patients suffering from paroxysmal nocturnal hemoglobinuria, results in an extreme sensitivity of the afflicted erythrocytes to lysis by the terminal complement proteins, which can be fully overcome by incorporating isolated C8bp [16,17]. More recently, a further membrane protein (P18/CD59) with apparent complement-inhibiting activity has been described [18,19]; its mode of action and its relationship to C8bp have, however, not yet been clarified.

In erythrocytes, one single functional channel is enough to cause lysis, due to colloid osmotic swelling. In contrast, nucleated cells survive a limited number of channels [20], most probably due to repair processes, such as shedding or internalization of the complexes [21,22]. When studying these repair mechanisms, we and others found that in response to C5b-9, cells reacted with an enhanced lipid turnover, with liberation of free arachidonic acid, and eventually, with release of prostanoids [23–25]. This observation led to the hypothesis that C5b-9 might not only function

Table 2. Mediator release from cultivated mesangial cells[a]

Eicosanoids
Interleukin 1
Tumor necrosis factor
GM-colony-stimulating factor
Oxygen radicals

[a](From [28,29])

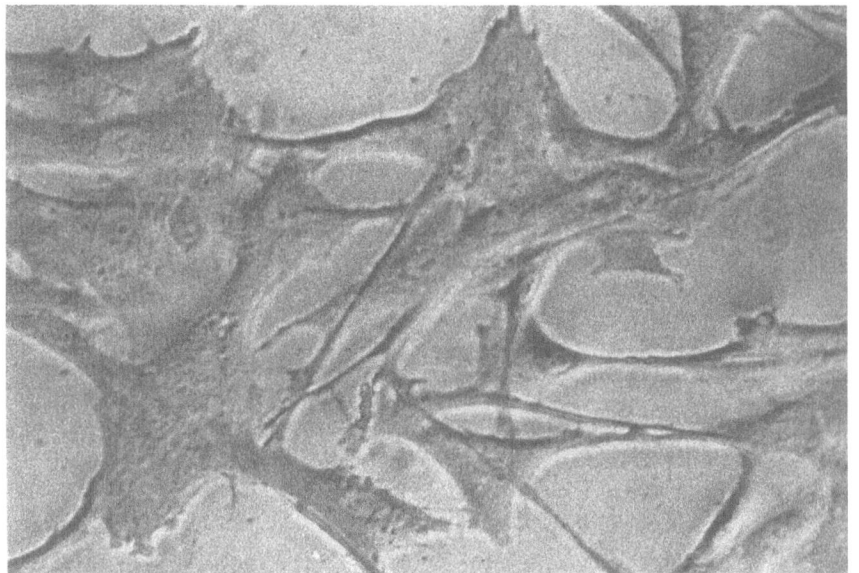

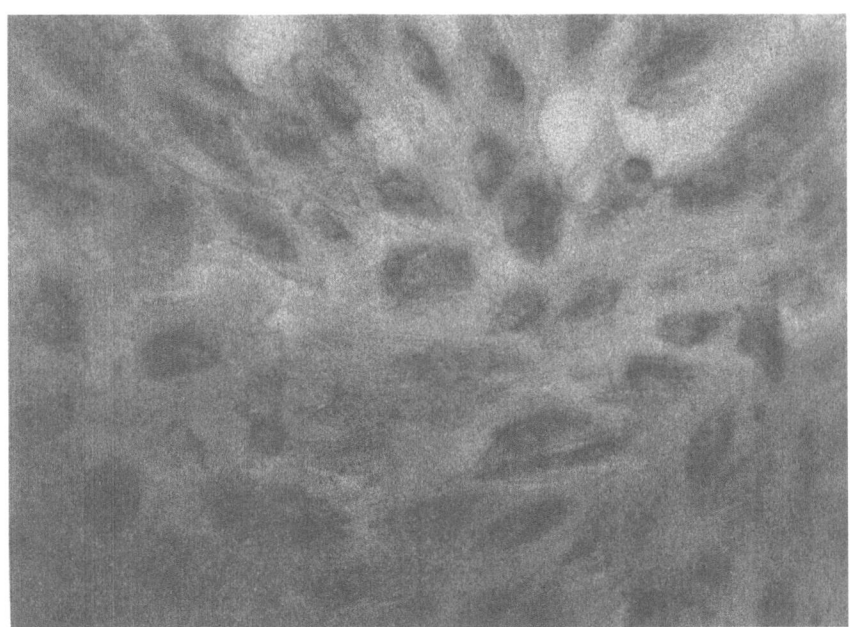

Fig. 2. Presence of C8-binding protein on cultured glomerular epithelial cells (*left*) and mesangial cells (*right*), shown by binding of a specific antibody and a peroxidase-coupled second antibody

as a lytic complex, but might, in sublytic doses, stimulate mediator release. Indeed, stimulation of various cells was found in response to C5b-9, resulting in release of lipid mediators and stimulation of protein synthesis (Table 1). How the C5b-9 stimulated cells is not yet known; increase in intracellular Ca^{2+} has been described, as well as activation of proteinkinase C, and enhanced lipid turnover (for review see [6]).

The question then arose whether the stimulatory function of C5b-9 might be relevant to physiological or pathophysiological events. Looking at glomerulonephritis, several lines of evidence suggested a role of C5b-9. Deposits of C5b-9 complexes are found in various forms of glomerulonephritis and experimental glomerulonephritis. Moreover, evidence for C5b-9 participation has been derived from experimental glomerulonephritis in complement-deficient animals. From these data the conclusion was drawn that proteinuria or the onset of sclerosis was critically dependent on the activity of the terminal complement components. This conclusion was further supported by studies with isolated perfused kidneys (for review see [26,27].

To analyze a possible role of C5b-9 in glomerulonephritis, we studied its interaction with glomerular cells. Since, in recent years, methods of growing cells from isolated glomeruli have been increasingly successful, it has become possible to study the functions of these cells independently of other cells [28,29]. During these studies it became quite obvious that mesangial cells are not only mere bystanders of inflammatory reactions, but that these cells can produce inflammatory mediators (summarized in Table 2). Mesangial cells also release collagenase, which might also contribute to tissue destruction [30]. The release of these proinflammatory mediators can be trig-

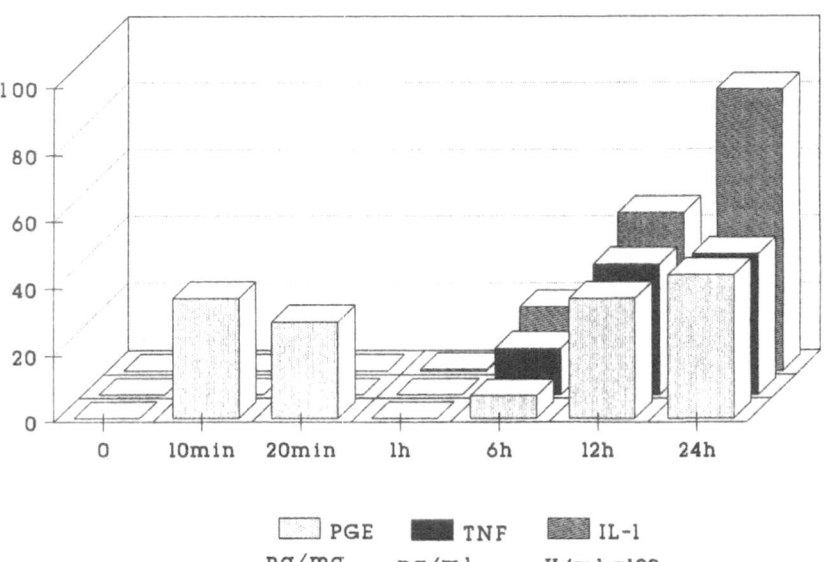

Fig. 3. Mediator release from cultured mesangial cells: The cells were incubated with sublytic doses of preactivated C5b6, C7, C8, and C9. After various times, release of prostaglandin E (*PGE*), interleukin 1 (*IL-1*), and tumor-necrosis factor (*TNF*) was tested by radioimmunoassay

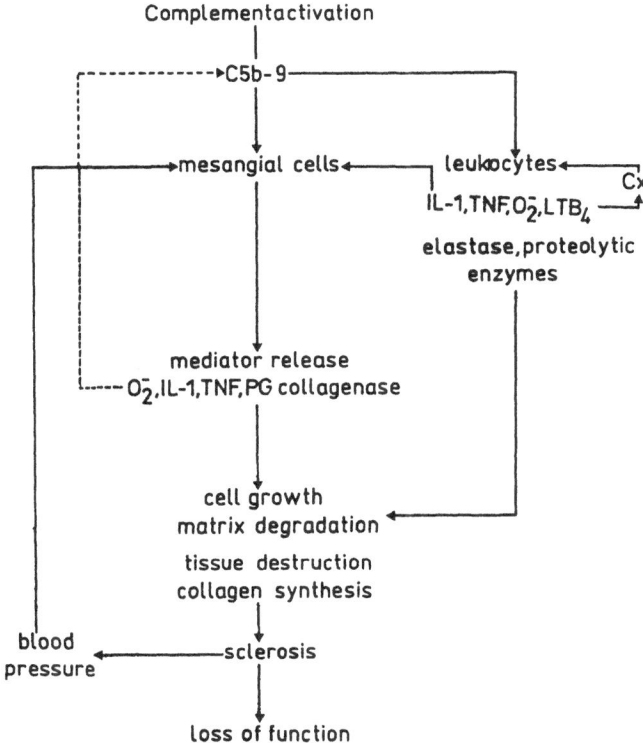

Fig. 4. Role of C5b-9 in acute and chronic inflammation: Activated C5b-9 directly releases inflammatory mediators from mesangial cells, which might promote inflammation. Concomitantly, C5b-9 also activates mediator release from leukocytes. The leukocyte mediators can stimulate other leukocytes, e.g., by causing chemotaxis (*Cx*), but can also affect mesangial cells. Interleukin-I (*IL-1*) might induce proliferation, release of tumor necrosis factor (*TNF*) and of collagenase, leading to tissue destruction. In addition to releasing mediators of acute inflammation, C5b-9 also affects collagen synthesis, thus contributing to the development of sclerosis. PG, prostaglandin; LTB$_4$, leukotriene B4

gered by other inflammatory mediators, e.g., by interleukin-I (Il-1), but also – and that will presented in more detail here – by the terminal complement components.

When cultured mesangial cells are incubated with purified human C5b6, C7, C8, and C9, rapid binding of C5b-9 is seen. The cells, however, survive the complement attack. On analyzing the molecular basis of complement resistance, we found that after prolonged incubation C5b-9 disappeared gradually from the cell membrane. Concomitantly with the C5b-9 binding, increasing amounts of the complement restricting membrane protein C8bp were expressed on the cell surface. In resident mesangial cells, C8bp is found on the membrane as well as in the cytoplasm (Fig. 2) [31]; by stimulation it is mobilized from the cytoplasmatic reservoirs, thus protecting against the formation of additional lytic complexes.

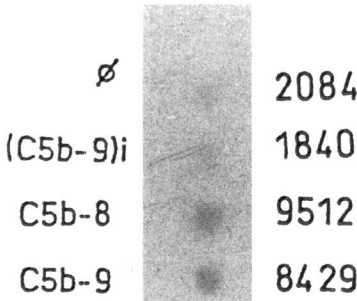

ø   2084

(C5b-9)i   1840

C5b-8   9512

C5b-9   8429

Fig. 5. Induction of collagen type IV synthesis in glomerular epithelial cells: The cells were incubated with sublytic doses of C5b-9, C5b-8, or inactivated C5b-9, respectively. After 2 h collagen type IV mRNA was detected by a cDNA probe (gift of Paul Killen, Ann Arbor, University of Michigan) by dot blot hybridization (*left*). After 24 h the collagen type IV synthesis was also enhanced; this was measured by adsorbing ^{3}H-proline containing protein to an antibody to collagen type IV (* cpm)

Even though mesangial cells are not killed by C5b-9, its interaction with the cell membrane nevertheless results in efficient stimulation of the cells. Rapid release of prostaglandin E is seen, followed by release of interleukin 1 and tumor necrosis factor, followed by a second rise in prostaglandin E (Fig. 3) [31].

By releasing mediators from mesangial cells, C5b-9 might, even in the absence of infiltrating leukocytes, promote an inflammatory reaction. Since C5b-9 also activates leukocytes to release mediators, which then in turn might trigger mesangial cells, other leukocytes, or even platelets, an ongoing inflammatory reaction will be even more enhanced. Considering the fact that complement is readily activated in inflamed tissue, e.g., not only by immune complexes, but also by destroyed cells [32], by exposed basement membrane [33], or by oxygen radicals [9], it is conceivable that even in the absence of the initial triggering event, the acute inflammation turns into a self-perpetuating process (shown schematically in Fig. 4).

One consequence of tissue destruction is tissue repair. By enhanced cell growth, as well as by enhanced matrix production, scar tissue is formed. After extensive destruction, tissue might also be replaced by less differentiated cells, by collagen or mesenchymal matrix, a phenomenon known as sclerosis [34,35].

Sclerosis is a hallmark of chronic glomerulonephritis; many causes for sclerosis have been discussed, especially mechanical stress due to high blood pressure. Alternatively, we tested whether inflammatory mediators might promote sclerosis by directly affecting the synthesis of extracellular matrix proteins.

Collagen type IV is a normal constituent of the basement membrane and it is produced by glomerular epithelial cells. In many forms of chronic glomerulonephritis, however, collagen deposits are also found in the mesangium, most probably due to enhanced synthesis by local cells [36,28].

Glomerular epithelial cells produce some collagen type IV under culture conditions. After incubation with sublytic doses of C5b-9, an increase in collage type IV specific mRNA was seen, 2–4 h after addition of C5b-9 (Fig. 5). After 12–24 h, extracellular collagen type IV was also enhanced; this was measured by biosynthetic labelling with ^{3}H-proline (Fig. 5). With C5b-9, collagen type IV specific mRNA was enhanced about 4–8-fold and protein synthesis was enhanced 5–10-fold, this being in the same range as the enhancement seen after stimulation with interleukin 1 [37].

Mesangial cells also respond to C5b-9 with enhanced collagen synthesis, again, this was tested by enhanced incorporation of radiolabelled proline into collagenase-digestible proteins.

Conclusions

Our data suggest a dual role of C5b-9. Firstly, by triggering the release of proinflammatory mediators such as Il-1 or prostanoids, C5b-9 might enhance the acute inflammatory response. Secondly, by inducing collagen synthesis, C5b-9 might contribute to sclerosis, and thereby to the progression of acute inflammation to chronicity, and finally, to renal failure.

Acknowledgment. This work has been supported by Deutsche Forschungsgemeinschaft Ha 1129/4-2 and Ha 1129/5-1.

References

1. Rother K, Rother U, Hänsch GM (1985) The role of complement in inflammation. Pathol Res Pract 180:117–124
2. Fligiel SEG, Johnson KJ, Ward PA (1988) The role of complement in immune complex induced tissue injury. In: Rother K, Till G (eds) The complement system. Springer, Berlin, pp 487–504
3. Cochrane CG, Unanue ER, Dixon FJ (1965) A role of polymorphonuclear leukocytes and complement in nephrotoxic nephritis. J Exp Med 122:99–116
4. Cochrane CG (1969) Mediation of immunologic glomerular injury. Transplant Proc 1:949–958
5. Hänsch GM (1988) The complement attack phase. In: Rother K, Till G (eds) The complement system. Springer, Berlin, pp 202–230
6. Shin ML, Carney DF (1988) Cytotoxic action and other metabolic consequences of the terminal complement proteins. In: Shin ML (ed) Cytotoxic mediators of inflammation and host defense. Progress in Allergy 40:44–48
7. Rother U, Hänsch GM, Rauterberg EW, Jungfer H, Rother K (1978) Deviated lysis. Lysis of unsensitized cells by complement. V Generation of the activity by low pH and low ionic strength. Z Immun Forsch 155:118–129
8. Wetsel RA, Kolb WP (1982) Complement-independent activation of the fifth component (C5) of human complement. Limited trypsin digestion resulting in the expression of biologic activity. J Immunol 128:2209–2216
9. Vogt W, von Zabern I, Hesse D, Nolte R, Haller Y (1986/87) Generation of an activated form of human C5 (C5b like C5) by oxygen radicals. Immunol Lett 14:209–215
10. Rother U, Hänsch GM, Menzel J, Rother K (1974) Deviated lysis: transfer of complement lytic activity to unsensitized cells. I Generation of the transferable activity on the surface of complement resistant bacteria. Z Immun Forsch 148:172–186
11. Götze O, Müller-Eberhard HJ (1970) Lysis of erythrocytes by complement in the absence of antibody. J Exp Med 132:898–915

12. Schönermark S, Rauterberg EW, Shin ML, Löke S, Roelcke D, Hänsch GM, (1986) Homologous species restriction in lysis of human erythrocytes. A membrane-derived protein with C8-binding capacity functions as an inhibitor. J Immunol 136:1772–1776

13. Blaas P, Berger B, Weber S, Peter HH, Hänsch GM (1988) Paroxysmal nocturnal hemoglobinuria (PNH Type III): enhanced stimulation of platelets by the terminal complement components is related to the lack of C8bp in the membrane. J Immunol 140:4045–4051

14. Zalman LS, Wood LM, Müller-Eberhard HJ (1987) Isolation of a human erythrocyte membrane protein capable of inhibiting expression of homologous complement channels. Proc Natl Acad Sci USA 83:6975–6979

15. Schönermark S, Filsinger S, Berger B, Hänsch GM (1988) A C8 binding protein of the human erythrocyte: interaction with the components of the complement attack phase. Immunology 63:585–590

16. Hänsch GM, Schönermark S, Roelcke D (1987) Paroxysmal nocturnal hemoglobinuria type III: lack of an erythrocytes membrane protein restricting the lysis by C5b-9. J Clin Invest 80:7–12

17. Zalman LS, Wood LM, Frank MM, Müller-Eberhard HJ (1987) Deficiency of the homologous restriction factor in paroxysmal nocturnal hemoglobinuria. J Exp Med 165:572–577

18. Sugita Y, Nakano Y, Tomita M (1988) Isolation of a new membrane protein from human erythrocytes which inhibits the formation of complement transmembrane channels. J Biochem (Tokyo) 104:633–637

19. Davies A, Simmons DL, Lale C, Harrison RA, Tighs H, Lachmann PI, Waldmann H (1989) CD59, an Ly-6-like protein expressed in human lymphoid cells, regulates the action of the complement membrane attack complex on homologous cells. J Exp Med 170:637–654

20. Koski CL, Ramm LE, Hammer CH, Mayer MM, Shin ML (1983) Cytolysis of nucleated cells by complement: cell death displays multi-hit characteristics. Proc Natl Acad Sci USA 80:3816–3820

21. Carney D, Hammer C, Shin ML (1986) Elimination of the terminal complement intermediates from the plasma membrane of nucleated cells: the rate of disappearance differs for cells carrying C5b-7 or C5b-8 or a mixture of C5b-8 and a limited number of C5b-9. J Immunol 134:1804–1809

22. Morgan PB, Dankert JR, Esser AF (1986) Recovery of human neutrophils from complement attack: removal of the membrane attack complex by endocytosis and exocytosis. J Immunol 138:246–253

23. Imagawa D, Osifchin NE, Paznekas WA, Shin ML, Mayer MM (1983) Consequence of cell membrane attack by complement: release of arachidonate and formation of inflammatory derivatives. Proc Natl Acad Sci USA 80:6647–6651

24. Betz M, Hänsch GM (1984) Release of arachidonic acid: a new function of the late complement components. Immunobiology 166:473–479

25. Hänsch GM, Seitz M, Martinotti G, Betz M, Rauterberg EW, Gemsa D (1984) Macrophages release arachidonic acid, prostaglandin E2 and thromboxane in response to the late complement components. J Immunol 133:2145–2150

26. Couser WG, Baker PJ, Adler S (1985) Complement and the direct mediation of glomerular injury: a new perspective. Kidney Int 2:879–890

27. Rauterberg EW (1987) Demonstration of complement deposits in tissue. In: Rother K, Till G (eds) The complement system. Springer, Berlin, pp 287–326

28. Striker GE, Striker LJ (1985) Biology of disease: glomerular cell culture. Lab Invest 53(2):122–131

29. Lovett DH, Sterzel RB (1986) Cell culture approaches to the analysis of glomerular inflammation. Kidney Int 30:246–254

30. Lovett DH, Sterzel RB, Kashgarian M, Ryan JL (1983) Neutral proteinase activity produced in vitro by cells of the glomerular mesangium. Kidney Int 23:342–348
31. Lovett D, Hänsch, GM, Goppelt M, Resch K (1987) Activation of glomerular mesangial cells by the terminal membrane attack complex of complement. J Immunol 138:2473–2480
32. Baker PJ, Osofsky SG (1980) Activation of human complement by heat-killed human kidney cells grown in culture. J Immunol 124:81–86
33. Williams JD, Czop JK, Abrahamson DR, Davies M, Austin KF (1984) Activation of the alternative complement pathway by isolated human glomerular basement membrane. J Immunol 133:394–399
34. Klahr S, Schreiner G, Ichikawa I (1988) The progression of renal disease. N Engl J Med 318:1657–1666
35. Bruijn JA, Hogendorn PCW, Hoedemaker PJ, Fleuren GL (1988) The extracellular matrix in pathology. J Lab Clin Med 111:140–149
36. Striker LM, Killen PD, Chi E, Striker GE (1984) The composition of glomerulosclerosis and membranoproliferative glomerulonephritis. Lab Invest 51:181–196
37. Torbohm I, Berger B, Schönermark M, von Kempis J, Rother K, Hänsch GM (1989) Modulation of collagen synthesis in human glomerular epithelial cells by interleukin 1. Clin Exp Immunol 75:427–431

The Biosynthesis and Action of Tumor Necrosis Factor α in the Kidney

Laurent Baud, Bruno Fouqueray, Carole Philippe, and Hélène Affres[1]

Summary. Like other cytokines, tumor necrosis factor alpha (TNF_α) belongs to a network of mediators of cell-to-cell communication. Both monocytes/macrophages and resident glomerular and tubular cells are apparently the cellular source of TNF_α in the kidney. In the glomerulus its cell surface expression and secretion are regulated by the local production of prostaglandins and reactive oxygen species; its secretion is enhanced in experimental models of immune complex glomerulonephritis. Following its synthesis, TNF_α binding to specific cell surface membrane receptors of glomerular mesangial cells and monocytes/macrophages is modulated by the local production of reactive oxygen species. In mesangial cells, this binding is associated with increased prostaglandin synthesis, cyclic AMP accumulation, expression of MHC antigens and of 5'-nucleotidase, and release of procoagulant activity, reactive oxygen species, and proteoglycans. Thus TNF_α appears to promote coagulation, inflammatory response, and sclerosis in the glomerulus.

Cytokines regulate the growth, differentiation, and functions of cells involved in immunity and inflammation. They belong to a network of mediators of cell-to-cell communication, which includes also arachidonic acid metabolites, reactive oxygen species (ROS), and polypeptide hormones. Cytokines were initially named according to their biological effects, and then, after their aminoacid sequence was established, by the term "interleukin" followed by a number [1]. Some of them have retained their original names, such as tumor necrosis factor (TNF) and lymphotoxin (LT), two factors recognized because of their cytotoxic and anti-tumor properties.

TNF was first described by Carswell et al. in the serum of BCG-primed, endotoxin-treated animals. This factor, produced mainly by monocytes/macrophages, has been shown to induce hemorrhagic necrosis of tumors in recipient animals, and to lyse tumor cells in vitro (reviewed in [2]). It was purified to homogeneity and its primary structure was eventually established. This was found to be similar to that of cachectin, a macrophage-derived protein which is able to

---

[1]INSERM U64, Hôpital Tenon, 4 rue de la Chine, 75020 Paris Cedex 20, France

suppress lipoprotein lipase activity in isolated adipocytes. Lymphocyte-derived LT has been also cloned. Although this factor has cytotoxic properties similar to those of TNF, it exhibits only 30% aminoacid homology. A nomenclature has been adopted that employs the term TNF α for TNF/cachectin, and TNF_β for LT. It is now evident that both TNF_α and TNF_β serve as general mediators of inflammatory processes. The present review will be centered on TNF_α since it has several unique properties which implicate it as an endogenous mediator of renal injury in human and experimental renal diseases.

TNF Gene Expression

The TNF_α gene is located on chromosome 6 in man and is closely linked to the major histocompatibility complex [2,3]. Monocytes/macrophages contain detectable levels of TNF_α messenger RNA (mRNA), prior to induction by bacterial lipopolysaccharide (LPS). Upon exposure to LPS, the transcription of the TNF_α gene is increased approximately threefold; thereafter, its half-life is controlled chiefly by the presence of a highly conserved AU-rich sequence located in the 3' untranslated region [2]. Such a sequence, which is also found in the mRNA encoding other cytokines, confers instability on messages that contain it. LPS induces a concomitant increase in the production of prostaglandin E_2 (PGE_2) which, in turn, limits the level of transcription of TNF_α mRNA by elevating intracellular cyclic AMP [4]. In addition to LPS, a variety of stimuli are capable of causing TNF_α mRNA expression, including toxic shock syndrome toxin 1, viruses, parasites, cytokines (interferon $_\gamma$: INF_γ; interleukin 2: IL_2), neuropeptides, and immune complexes.

Not only monocytes/macrophages, but also lymphocytes, endothelial and vascular smooth muscle cells, glial cells in the central nervous system, Kupffer cells in the liver, Paneth cells of the intestinal epithelium, and several epithelial tumor cells have been found to exhibit TNF_α mRNA expression upon exposure to these stimuli. Kidney cells express TNF_α mRNA under physiologic conditions, as detected by Northern blotting [5]. After injection of LPS, this expression increases to a greater extent than in other tissues. The precise localization of TNF_α mRNA in the kidney is still unknown, but recent reports suggest that both glomerular mesangial cells [6] and proximal tubular epithelial cells [7] could be responsible for this expression. In LPS-activated rat mesangial cells, TNF_α gene expression is characterized by two hybridizing bands: one strongly hybridizing band and a second weaker band of higher molecular weight which could represent a precursor to the main TNF_α mRNA (6).

Molecular Forms of TNF_α

TNF_α bears a secretory protein signal sequence, and thus, unlike IL_1, is synthesized by the classical secretory pathway through the endoplasmic reticulum and Golgi apparatus. Its synthesis starts with the elaboration of a precursor or prohormone, which is subsequently cleaved during processing to yield the mature protein. The mature human 17 kDa TNF_α consists of 157 aminoacids. The uncleaved precursor of

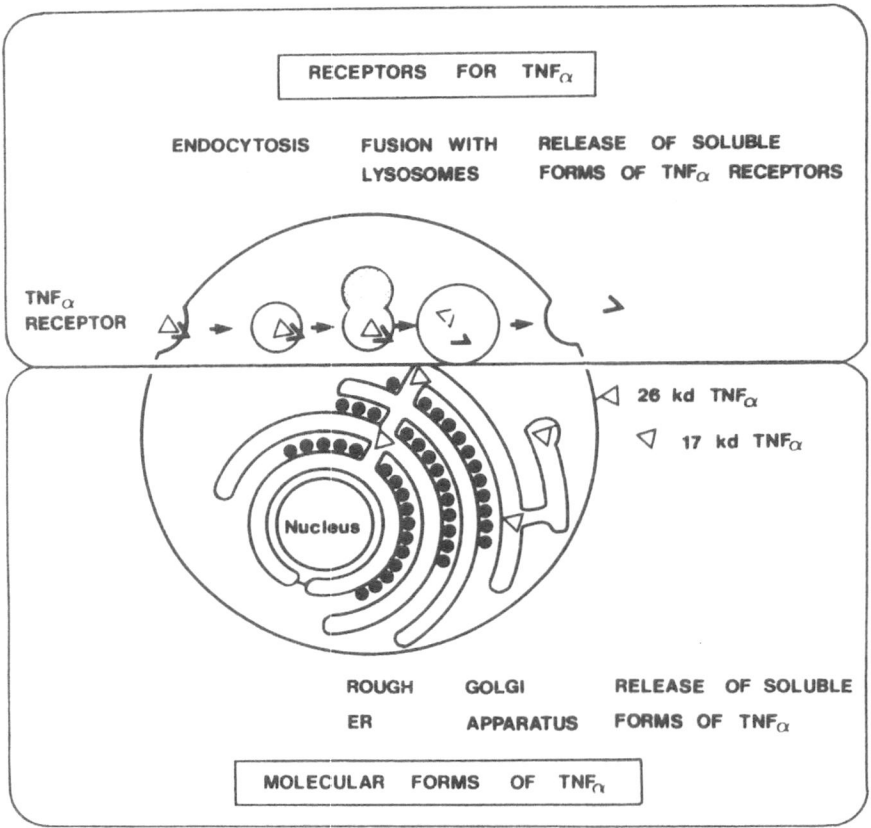

Fig. 1. Schematic view of how TNF_α is synthesized and released and how TNF_α binding to its receptor is followed by rapid internalization and degradation

26 kDa contains 76 supplementary residues, including a long hydrophobic region of 26 aminoacids, allowing it to be expressed as an integral transmembrane protein [8]. How 26 kDa integral transmembrane TNF_α is processed to the 17 kDa secretory component is unknown. But it has been shown that both molecules are active and exhibit possibly different tissue specificities and different biological activities (Fig. 1).

TNF_α molecule is functionally defined as promoting both lysis of the TNF_α-sensitive L929 murine fibroblast cell line, and suppression of lipoprotein lipase activity in adipocytes [6]. In cultured rat mesangial cells [9] as in macrophages [10], cell associated TNF_α activity is demonstrable after less than 1 h exposure to LPS, peaks at 2 h, and decreases progressively thereafter, while TNF_α activity increases in the medium. The progressive rise of TNF_α activity in the medium is followed after 9 h by evident decay. Flow cytometry experiments and immunohistochemical studies reveal that two thirds of LPS-activated macrophages [10] and LPS-activated mesangial cells [9] exhibit TNF_α expression at their surface. The greatest part of these cell-associated TNF_α molecules persists after low pH treatment, indicating that they are integral membrane proteins and not molecules attached to cell surface receptors. Proximal tubular cells, transformed by SV_{40}, which express TNF mRNA upon LPS challenge, do not release TNF_α activity into the medium, whereas they produce membrane-bound TNF_α [11].

The mechanisms whereby cell surface expression and secretion of TNF_α are regulated have been extensively studied, in both macrophages and mesangial cells. Low PGE_2 concentrations enhance, whereas high concentrations (> 10 ng/ml) suppress TNF_α release [12]. This complex effect results from the activation of biochemical pathways that have conflicting effects on TNF_α production. Indeed cyclic GMP, which is preferentially increased by low concentrations of PGE_2, stimulates TNF_α release, whereas cyclic AMP, which is increased by high concentrations of PGE_2 [6,12] or by various pharmacologic agents, suppresses it. Because TNF_α is a potent inducer of PGE_2 and cyclic AMP production [13], the inhibition of TNF_α production by PGE_2 is considered as the negative arm of a regulatory circuit which can be blocked by nonsteroidal antiinflammatory drugs. In contrast, the production of TNF_α is positively regulated in macrophages by platelet-activating factor (PAF). Interaction with a specific receptor and subsequent synthesis of 5-lipoxygenase byproducts, including leukotriene B_4 (LTB_4) are required for this effect. The finding that TNF_α induces the release of PAF from macrophages suggests [14], in this case, the existence of a powerful amplification loop.

There is also in vitro evidence of bidirectional interaction between TNF_α and ROS, which are both generated by monocytes/macrophages and mesangial cells. TNF_α is capable of stimulating ROS production by these cells [15], and ROS, in turn, may enhance the release of TNF_α [9,16]. Desferrioxamine (DFX), an iron chelator which prevents the generation of hydroxyl radical via the Haber-Weiss reaction, has been shown to reduce the concentration of TNF_α in culture media of macrophages [16], and mesangial cells [9] through decrease of its release and acceleration of its inactivation [9]. There are at least two different ways in which DFX might decrease the release of TNF_α from LPS-activated mesangial cells. First, DFX could limit TNF_α synthesis at the transcriptional and post-transcriptional levels. Second, DFX could indirectly interfere with the generation of TNF_α when its 26 kDa precursor form is processed to yield a 17 kDa molecule. Because DFX inhibits the release of TNF_α into the medium, but enhances its cell surface expression, it is tempting to speculate that this drug prevents occurrence of the mechanism whereby TNF_α detaches from the membrane. Indeed, hydroxyl radical or its metabolites might induce the cleavage of membrane-associated TNF_α through the activation of latent metalloproteinases and/or the inactivation of proteinase inhibitors [9].

Additionally, different drugs have been shown to affect TNF_α production by monocytes/macrophages and mesangial cells. For instance, corticosteroids and cyclosporine A both reduce TNF_α production by LPS-activated monocytes. Cyclosporine A inhibits the release of TNF_α without modifying its cell-associated form [17]. Antibiotics have similar inhibitory effects. For example, quinolones [18] and aminoglycosides (L. Baud, unpublished observations) decrease extracellular TNF_α production by LPS-activated monocytes in a dose-dependent manner. Collectively, these results may have implications in transplant therapy.

Renal Production of TNF$_\alpha$ in Pathological Processes

Preliminary reports indicate that TNF$_\alpha$ is produced by glomeruli isolated from rats with an accelerated autologous form of nephrotoxic serum nephritis [19]. This is associated with infiltration of the glomeruli by monocytes/macrophages. In support of their contributing role, these cells have been shown to release TNF$_\alpha$ when incubated in vitro with glomerular basement membrane-containing immune complexes [20].

Interestingly, enhanced gene expression for TNF$_\alpha$ has been demonstrated in the renal cortex of two models of spontaneous lupus nephritis, the MRL-1pr [21] and (NZB × NZW)F1 mice [22]. In addition, TNF$_\alpha$ bioactivity has been found in the medium of glomeruli isolated from MRL-1pr mice but not in that from normal congenic MRL++ mice [21]. Again, invading macrophages are the likely source of TNF$_\alpha$ production in the glomerulus. This is in contrast with the observation that peritoneal macrophages from (NZB × NZW)F1 mice express a weak TNF$_\alpha$ bioactivity [23], and with the observation that, in patients with systemic lupus erythematosus, the serum levels of TNF$_\alpha$ are unaltered [24]. The implications of these reports, as well as of other studies on serum TNF$_\alpha$ [25], for the diagnosis and management of renal diseases are still unknown.

Characterization of Receptors for TNF$_\alpha$ and Their Regulation

Studies of the tissue distribution of label after injection of radioiodinated TNF$_\alpha$ demonstrate that 8% of the dose is recovered from the kidneys [26]. This represents a specific binding since reduction of labeling is observed when unlabeled TNF$_\alpha$ is injected together with the tracer. In fact, virtually all somatic tissues, with the exception of erythrocytes, express a receptor for TNF$_\alpha$. Receptor numbers are highly variable, ranging from 200 to 50,000 sites per cell with a high affinity for TNF$_\alpha$ (Kd of 0.1–3.0 nM). But the biological effects of TNF$_\alpha$ are maximally expressed at receptor occupancies of 5–10%. After binding of TNF$_\alpha$ to its receptor, the TNF$_\alpha$ receptor complex is internalized, without further recycling of the receptor (Fig. 1). Experimental support has accumulated for the upregulation of TNF$_\alpha$ receptors by INF γ and agents that stimulate protein kinase A (PKA) and for their downregulation by corticosteroids, and agents that stimulate protein kinase C (PKC). The mechanisms whereby downregulation by PKC occurs include decreased affinity, reduced density, and increased internalization of TNF$_\alpha$ binding sites. Ding et al. [27] have demonstrated that LPS also promotes the internalization of TNF$_\alpha$ receptors on the surface of macrophages. More recently, we have obtained data indicating that ROS downregulate TNF$_\alpha$ binding, but only slightly increase the degree of internalization of TNF$_\alpha$ receptors [28]. Indeed, exposure of mesangial cells, blood monocytes, or TNF$_\alpha$-sensitized murine L929 fibroblasts to hydrogen peroxide (H$_2$O$_2$) promotes a loss of about 50% in the density of cell membrane TNF$_\alpha$ receptors. This is associated, in L 929 cells, with a decrease in the cytotoxic activity of TNF$_\alpha$ [28]. Conversely, the treatment of blood monocytes with antioxidant drugs such as DFX causes the upregulation of TNF$_\alpha$ receptors through a decrease of their turnover rate (L. Baud, unpublished observations). This further suggests a particular susceptibility of TNF_α receptors to the oxidative damage. It should be noted that the presence of cystein repeats in the extracellular domain of the 55 kDa TNF_α receptor may account for this observation [29].

Soluble forms of the receptors for TNF_α are released from target cells into the plasma and may represent a mechanism by which TNF_α molecules are inactivated [29] (Fig. 1). Such TNF_α binding proteins are found in the urine as well. Uromodulin or Tamm-Horsfall protein, a polypeptide which binds TNF_α with a high affinity via carbohydrate chains, has also been isolated from human urine. However, it does not inhibit the cytotoxic activity of this cytokine. An alternative cause of the inactivation of TNF_α is its degradation by either neutrophil proteolytic enzymes or by hypochlorous acid. In summary, there are several observations in the literature showing that TNF_α efficiency may be modulated at the receptor level. In contrast, to date, there are only few data regarding the intracellular pathways of TNF_α signal transduction and their regulation.

TNF_α Action on Kidney Cells

Only a few of the studies on renal TNF_α action have been performed in vivo. The first to be published described the pattern of lesions induced in suckling mice by daily subcutaneous injections of TNF_α. The kidneys of these mice showed no abnormalities in the glomeruli, but had some cytoplasmic granules in the proximal tubules [30], which probably represented reabsorption of proteins from the lumen. Thereafter, T. Bertani et al. [31] studied glomerular functional and structural changes induced by intravenous infusion of TNF_α to the rabbit. The main finding was the presence of endothelial cell swelling, polymorphonuclear leukocyte accumulation, and fibrin formation in the capillaries. Glomeruli from rats injected with TNF_α also showed a transient influx of neutrophils into capillaries, but no formation of thrombi [32]. Nevertheless, TNF_α administration to rats with antiglomerular basement membrane antibody-mediated nephritis caused a substantial amplification of the glomerular injury, characterized by intra-capillary thrombi and endothelial cell swelling [32]. These structural abnormalities were associated with functional changes, including a dose-dependent increase of proteinuria. Similarly, chronic administration of TNF_α in low doses to mice with spontaneous lupus nephritis increased proteinuria and worsened renal disease and mortality [22], whereas higher doses were protective [23]. This latter event could be the result of changes in cell-mediated immunity more than changes in humoral immunity [33].

There are a number of different ways in which TNF_α might affect the structure and function of both glomerular and tubular cells. They have been identified in in vitro studies.

Prostaglandin Synthesis

TNF_α, either alone or synergistically with IL_1, increases prostaglandin synthesis by glomerular mesangial cells [13, 34–36]. This effect can be measured in vitro as an increased accumulation of PGE_2, $PGF_{2\alpha}$ and 6 keto $PGF_{1\alpha}$, which is the stable breakdown product of PGI_2 [13], in mesangial cell culture medium. This requires a long incubation period, and is inhibited by both actinomycin D and cycloheximide, which is consistent with an increase of transcription and translation. Additionally, TNF_α increases the release of phospholipase A_2 activity [34] together with arachidonic acid [36], and induces cyclooxygenase activity, suggesting possible regulation at two distinct levels.

TNF_α also stimulates cyclic AMP accumulation in the mesangial cell culture medium [13]. Because indomethacin suppresses the effect of TNF_α on prostaglandins but only reduces the effect on cyclic AMP, it is likely that TNF_α stimulates cyclic AMP levels in part independently of its effect on prostaglandin production. Through its effect on prostaglandins and cyclic nucleotides, TNF_α may affect both proliferation and activation of mesangial cells.

Cell Proliferation

There have been reports published both of TNF_α-mediated enhancement and of TNF_α-mediated inhibition of mesangial cell proliferation. Many laboratories have found that TNF_α causes a significant increase of DNA synthesis by rat [37,38] and human [39] mesangial cells, when cultured in serum-free media. This effect has been reported to be not associated with phospholipase C activation and phosphatidic acid production [38]. In contrast, TNF_α does not affect [13] or even inhibits growth of proliferating rat mesangial cells [40]. The origin of this discrepancy is not clear. It is possible that, in serum-enriched media, the endogenous prostaglandin production simultaneously induced by TNF_α antagonizes its growth-promoting effect. Indeed, coincubation of proliferating mesangial cells with TNF_α and indomethacin is associated with an increase of DNA synthesis [37]. Alternatively, because TNF_α-stimulated synthesis of platelet-derived growth factor (PDGF) may be responsible for mesangial cell growth [39], the addition of serum and, hence, of PDGF in excess might mask TNF_α-induced cell proliferation.

Cell Activation

Upon exposure to TNF_α, glomerular and tubular cells may acquire new functions without growth modification. Indeed, in addition to increased production, by glomerular epithelial cells, of a chemotactic factor for polymorphonuclear leukocytes [41], TNF_α may stimulate mesangial cells to express MHC class I and class II antigens [40] and 5'-nucleotidase [42], and to synthesize procoagulant activity [43], ROS [15], and proteoglycans [44]. Thus TNF_α appears to promote coagulation, inflammatory response, and sclerosis in the glomerulus. TNF_α also induces the synthesis of different lipid molecules, including prostaglandins and PAF, which could act as mediators of mesangial cell contraction. It should be noted that this phenomenon might be offset in vivo by the increased synthesis of the potent vasodilatator nitric oxide.

Finally, TNF_α, like IL_1, promotes a marked increase in sodium-dependent uptake of solutes by proximal tubule cells [45]. The TNF_α expression in these cells [11] raises the possibility that, in the absence of inflammatory cells, they may modulate the functions of the proximal nephron.

In conclusion, it is now clear that TNF_α may exert a wide range of action on the kidney. Apparently both monocytes/macrophages and resident kidney cells are sources of this cytokine in pathological and possibly in physiological reaction. Availability of specific TNF_α agonists or antagonists should help to extend our knowledge in this field and could open new and interesting methods in therapeutics.

Acknowledgments. Portions of this work were supported by the "Institut National de la Santé et de la Recherche Médicale" and the "Faculté de Médecine Saint-Antoine." The authors thank Mrs Miranda and Mrs Knobloch for secretarial assistance.

References

1. Dinarello CA, Mier JW (1987) Lymphokines. N Engl J Med 317:940–945
2. Beutler B, Cerami A (1986) Cachectin and tumour necrosis factor as two sides of the same biological coin. Nature 320:584–588
3. Beutler B, Cerami A (1988) The common mediator of shock, cachexia, and tumor necrosis. Adv Immunol 42:213–231
4. Kunkel SL, Spengler M, May MA et al. (1988) Prostaglandin E_2 regulates macrophage-derived tumor necrosis factor gene expression. J Biol Chem 263:5380–5384
5. Ulich TR, Guo K, Del Castillo J (1989) Endotoxin-induced cytokine gene expression in vivo. 1. Expression of tumor necrosis factor mRNA in visceral organs under physiologic conditions and during endotoxemia. Am J Pathol 134:11–14
6. Baud L, Oudinet J-P, Bens M et al. (1989) Production of tumor necrosis factor by rat mesangial cells in response to bacterial lipopolysaccharide. Kidney Int 35:1111–1118
7. Wuthrich RP, Glimcher LH, Yui MA et al. (1990) MHC class II, antigen presentation and tumor necrosis factor in renal tubular epithelial cells. Kidney Int 37:783–792
8. Kriegler M, Perez C, de Fay K et al. (1988) A novel form of TNF/cachectin is a cell surface cytotoxic transmembrane protein: Ramifications for the complex physiology of TNF. Cell 53:45–53
9. Affres H, Perez J, Hagege J et al. (to be published) Cell surface expression and release of tumor necrosis factor by lipopolysaccharide-stimulated mesangial cells: effect of desferrioxamine. Kidney Int
10. Chensue SW, Remick DG, Shmyr-Forsch C et al. (1988) Immunohistochemical demonstration of cytoplasmic and membrane-associated tumor necrosis factor in murine macrophages. Am J Pathol 133:564–572
11. Jevnikar AM, Wuthrich RP, Glimcher LH et al. (1990) LPS and $IL-_{1\alpha}$ stimulated proximal tubular cells produce tumor necrosis factor in vitro (abstract). Kidney Int 37:417
12. Renz H, Gong J-H, Schmidt A et al. (1988) Release of tumor necrosis factor-α from macrophages. Enhancement and suppression are dose-dependently regulated by prostaglandin E_2 and cyclic nucleotides. J Immunol 141:2388–2393
13. Baud L, Perez J, Friedlander G et al. (1988) Tumor necrosis factor stimulates prostaglandin production and cyclic AMP levels in rat cultured mesangial cells. FEBS Lett 239:50–54
14. Camussi G, Bussolino F, Salvidia G et al. (1987) Tumor necrosis factor/cachectin stimulates peritoneal macrophages, polymorphonuclear neutrophils, and vascular endothelial cells to synthesize and release platelet-activating factor. J Exp Med 166:1390–1404
15. Radeke HH, Meier B, Topley N et al. (1990) Interleukin 1-α and tumor necrosis factor-α induce oxygen radical production in mesangial cells. Kidney Int 37:767–775
16. Chaudhri G, Clark IA (1989) Reactive oxygen species facilitate the in vitro and in vivo lipopolysaccharide-induced release of tumor necrosis factor. J Immunol 143:1290–1294
17. Remick DG, Nguyen DT, Eskandari MK et al. (1989) Cyclosporine A inhibits TNF production without decreasing TNF mRNA levels. Biochem Biophys Res Commun 161:551–555

18. Bailly S, Fay M, Gougerot-Pocidalo M-A (1990) Effects of quinolones on TNF production by human monocytes. Pathol Biol Paris 38:267–271
19. Wiggins RC, Eldredge C, Kunkel S (1987) Monokine production by glomeruli at different stages of crescent formation in the rabbit. Proc 4th Int Congress Nephrology, 368 p
20. Vissers MCM, Fantone JC, Wiggins R et al. (1989) Glomerular basement membrane-containing immune complexes stimulate tumor necrosis factor and interleukin-1 production by human monocytes. Am J Pathol 134:1–6
21. Boswell JM, Yui MA, Burt DW et al. (1988) Increased tumor necrosis factor and IL-1$_\beta$ gene expression in the kidneys of mice with lupus nephritis. J Immunol 141:3050–3054
22. Brennan DC, Yui MA, Wuthrich RP et al. (1989) Tumor necrosis factor and IL-1 in New Zealand black/white mice. Enhanced gene expression and acceleration of renal injury. J Immunol 143:3470–3475
23. Jacob CO, McDevitt HO (1988) Tumour necrosis factor-α in murine autoimmune lupus nephritis. Nature 331:356–358
24. Maury CPJ, Teppo AM (1989) Tumor necrosis factor in the serum of patients with systemic lupus erythematosus. Arthritis Rheum 32:146–151
25. Maury CPJ, Teppo AM (1987) Raised serum levels of cachectin/tumor necrosis factor in renal allograft rejection. J Exp Med 166:1132–1137
26. Beutler BA, Milsark IW, Cerami A (1985) Cachectin/tumor necrosis factor: production, distribution, and metabolic fate in vivo. J Immunol 135:3972–3977
27. Ding AH, Sanchez E, Srimal S et al. (1989) Macrophages rapidly internalize their tumor necrosis factor receptors in response to bacterial lipopolysaccharide. J Biol Chem 264:3924–3929
28. Baud L, Affres H, Perez J et al. (1990) Reduction in tumor necrosis factor binding and cytotoxicity by hydrogen peroxide. J Immunol 145:556–560
29. Schall TJ, Lewis M, Koller KJ et al. (1990) Molecular cloning and expression of a receptor for human tumor necrosis factor. Cell 61:361–370
30. Gresser I, Woodrow D, Moss J et al. (1987) Toxic effects of recombinant tumor necrosis factor in suckling mice. Comparisons with interferon α/β. Am J Pathol 128:13–18
31. Bertani T, Abbate M, Zoja C et al. (1989) Tumor necrosis factor induces glomerular damage in the rabbit. Am J Pathol 134:419–430
32. Tomosugi NI, Cashman SJ, Hay H et al. (1989) Modulation of antibody-mediated glomerular injury in vivo by bacterial lipopolysaccharide, tumor necrosis factor, and Il-1. J Immunol 142:3083–3090
33. Gordon C, Wofsy D (1990) Effect of recombinant murine tumor necrosis factor-α on immune function. J Immunol 144:1753–1758
34. Pfeilschifter J, Pignat W, Vosbeck K et al. (1989) Interleukin 1 and tumor necrosis factor synergistically stimulate prostaglandin synthesis and phospholipase A2 release from rat renal mesangial cells. Biochem Biophys Res Commun 159:385–394
35. Floege J, Topley N, Wessel K et al. (1990) Monokines and platelet-derived growth factor modulate prostanoid production in growth arrested, human mesangial cells. Kidney Int 37:859–869
36. Topley N, Floege J, Wessel K et al. (1989) Prostaglandin E$_2$ production is synergistically increased in cultured human glomerular mesangial cells by combinations of IL-1 and tumor necrosis factor-α. J Immunol 143:1989–1995
37. Perez J, Baud L, Ardaillou R (1989) Tumor necrosis factor stimulates prostaglandin, cyclic AMP, and DNA synthesis by cultured rat mesangial cells (abstract). Kidney Int 35: 318
38. Nakazato Y, Kester M, Mene P et al. (1989) Tumor necrosis factor stimulates mesangial cell proliferation independent of polyphosphoinositide turnover or phosphatidic acid formation (abstract). Kidney Int 35:179
39. Silver BJ, Jaffer FE, Abboud HE (1989) Platelet-derived growth factor synthesis in mesangial cells: induction by multiple peptide mitogens. Proc Natl Acad Sci USA 86:1056–1060

40. Martin M, Schwinzer R, Schellekens H et al. (1989) Glomerular mesangial cells in local inflammation. Induction of the expression of MHC class II antigens by IFN-γ. J Immunol 142:1887–1894

41. Watanabe K, Nakagawa H (1990) Cytokines enhance the production of a chemotactic factor for polymorphonuclear leukocytes by rat renal glomerular epithelioid cells. Nephron 54:169–175

42. Savic V, Stefanovic V, Ardaillou N et al. (to be published) Induction of ecto-5'-nucleotidase of rat cultured mesangial cells by interleukin-1 and tumour necrosis factor-α. Immunology

43. Wiggins RC, Njoku N, Sedor JR (1990) Tissue factor production by cultured rat mesangial cells. Stimulation by TNF and lipopolysaccharide. Kidney Int 37:1281–1285

44. Davies M, Shewring L, Thomas G et al. (1989) Stimulation of proteoglycan synthesis in rat mesangial cells in response to tumour necrosing factor (abstract) Kidney Int 35:344

45. Schreiner GF, Kohan DE (1990) Regulation of renal transport processes and hemodynamics by macrophages and lymphocytes. Am J Physiol 258:F761–F767

The Renal Biology of Endothelins

BARRY M. BRENNER[1,2] and ANDREW J. KING[1,2]

SUMMARY. Endothelin (ET) is distinguished from other endogenous vasoactive peptides by its biphasic pressure response and its sustained duration of action. There is marked regional variability in the sensitivity to either the vasodilatory or the vasoconstrictor effects of ET. The renal vascular bed is exquisitely sensitive and may be an important target organ for ET. The extent to which ET functions as an autocrine, paracrine, or circulating mediator is as yet unclear. Evidence suggests that ET may play a role as a mediator of chronic volume and blood pressure regulation and contribute to sustained renal ischemia in pathophysiological states. Eventual development of effective blockers of ET action will aid in understanding the in vivo effects of ET.

Introduction

It is now well recognized that the endothelium lining the vasculature is capable of transducing hemodynamic and humoral signals into appropriate changes in vascular smooth muscle tone [1]. The effector branch of the endothelial cell response to these mechanical and chemical signals is mediated, at least in part, by auto-production of soluble vasodilating and vasoconstricting factors [2]. Two such vasorelaxants are prostacyclin and endothelium-derived relaxing factor (EDRF). EDRF activity stems in part from nitric oxide (NO), derived from the guanido nitrogen(s) of L-arginine [3], as well as nitrosothiols [4]. Recently, vascular endothelium has also been shown to synthesize endothelin (ET), a 21 amino acid polypeptide with potent vasocon-

[1]Renal Division and Department of Medicine, Brigham and Women's Hospital, Boston, MA 02115, USA
[2]The Harvard Center for the Study of Kidney Diseases, Harvard Medical School, Boston, MA 02115, USA

strictor properties [5]. This review focuses primarily on the role of ET in the modulation of glomerular function.

The original discovery of ET by Yanagisawa et al. [5] stimulated a burst of investigation into the role of this family of peptides in the modulation of regional and systemic hemodynamics. First isolated and purified from porcine aortic endothelial cells, ET-1 is a 21 amino acid peptide encoded by a single gene [5]. Three isoforms have been identified (ET-1,2,3), and are present in all species examined [6]. Isolated vascular rings and muscle strips respond to ET with a sustained contractile response accompanied by a rise in intracellular free calcium and an increase in inositol trisphosphate [5,7]. Intravenous bolus ET leads to a biphasic systemic pressor response, which results from transient systemic vasodilation followed by sustained vasoconstriction [5,6]. The initial vasodilation appears to be due to ET-induced EDRF release in that L-NMMA, an analog of L-arginine (L-Arg) which competitively inhibits the conversion of L-Arg to NO, markedly attenuates the hypotensive effects of ET-1 in anesthetized rats.

Renal Endothelin Receptors

Autoradiographic studies using ^{125}I ET-1 reveal high affinity binding to glomeruli, vasa recta bundles, and the inner medulla, a distribution of binding which is similar to that of atrial natriuretic peptide (ANP) and angiotensin II (AII) [9,10]. High affinity binding sites are also present on cultured glomerular mesangial cells [11–13]. Cross-linking of [125]ET-1 to intact rat mesangial cells reveals two binding proteins of 60kDa and 73kDa [12]. Both ET-1 and ET-2 bind to the higher molecular weight receptor, whereas all 3 ET isoforms bind to the smaller protein. An increase in mesangial cytosolic free calcium occurs in response to ET, implying that these binding sites represent true receptors (see below) [7,14,15].

Synthesis of Endothelin

Expression of preproendothelin-1 mRNA in porcine aortic endothelium is increased by a variety of chemical and mechanical stimuli, including the calcium ionophore A23187, thrombin, epinephrine [5], transforming growth factor β (TGF β) [16] and enhanced shear stress [17]. Expression of a 2.3 kb preproendothelin-1 mRNA in cultured bovine glomerular endothelial cells has been shown by Northern analysis using a full length preproendothelin-1 cDNA [18]. This expression is enhanced by co-incubation with agonists known to increase glomerular endothelial cytosolic free calcium, including bradykinin, thrombin, ATP and platelet activating factor [18]. In addition, under basal conditions, glomerular endothelial cells release ET in a time-dependent fashion, a response markedly enhanced by co-incubation with bradykinin [18]. Finally, several renal epithelial cell lines (MDCK, LLCPK$_1$) release ET-1 in a time-dependent fashion [19,20]. Taken together, the evidence for glomerular and renal epithelial cell ET biosynthetic capabilities and the widespread renal ET binding sites strongly suggest a local role for ET in the modulation of renal hemodynamics.

Whole Kidney Responses

When administered intravenously or directly into the renal artery of intact animals, ET induces dose-dependent renal vasoconstriction [11,21,22]. As a renal vasoconstrictor, ET-1 is up to 30 times more potent than AII [21]. As with the systemic response, transient renal vasodilation precedes vasoconstriction.

In anesthetized rats, intravenous boluses of ET-1 result in dose-dependent and sustained reductions of renal plasma flow (RPF) with variable effects on glomerular filtration rate (GFR) [22]. Moderate doses of ET lead to a proportionately greater reduction in RPF than GFR; thus, filtration fraction increases. Higher doses lead to parallel reduction in RPF and GFR [22]. Others have noted parallel reduction of GFR and RPF when ET is infused into the renal artery of rats, or with intravenous infusion in dogs [23]. A similar pattern is seen in isolated perfused kidneys, indicating that the renal response is independent of the systemic effects [21].

Co-infusion of dihydropyridine Ca^{2+} channel blockers with ET into rat renal arteries markedly blunts the vasoconstrictor response, suggesting that renal vasoconstriction is, at least in part, due to the activation of voltage-sensitive Ca^{2+} channels [23]. Co-infusion of pharmacologic doses of ANP, which stimulates particulate guanylate cyclase, also blunts the systemic and renal effects of endothelin [23,24]. Although ET is a potent secretagogue of ANP [25], it is unclear whether ANP exerts a counter-regulatory influence on ET in vivo [23].

Intravenous ET administration, in doses which do not severely compromise filtration, induces a modest natriuresis in rats [22]. When renal perfusion pressure is maintained constant with an aortic snare, the natriuresis is attenuated, suggesting that this effect is, at least in part, pressure-related [22]. In suspensions of rabbit inner medullary collecting duct cells, ET also reduces ouabain-sensitive O_2 consumption, an effect not seen in proximal tubule cells [26]. A reduction of the initial rate of Rb^+ uptake by ET implies decreased Na^+/K^+ ATPase activity. This response is blocked by the cyclooxygenase inhibitor, ibuprofen, suggesting that inhibition of transport is mediated by prostanoids. Indeed, in collecting duct cells, ET stimulates release of PGE_2, a known inhibitor of Na^+/K^+ ATPase in these cells [26]. Autoradiographic labeling of renal parenchyma by ^{125}I ET reveals intense staining of the inner medulla [9,10]. In addition, as noted above, several renal epithelial cell lines synthesize and release ET [19,20] raising the possibility that locally generated ET modulates renal medullary transport functions independent of its renal hemodynamic effects.

Effects of Endothelin on Glomerular Hemodynamics

Afferent and efferent arterioles, the primary resistance vessels of the kidney, are highly sensitive to the vasoconstrictive effects of ET; thus, ET has marked effects on the determinants of glomerular ultrafiltration [14,22,24,27,28]. Studies to date have shown differing sensitivity of the pre- and post-glomerular arterioles, depending primarily on the dose and route of administration. Intravenous infusion of mildly pressor doses of ET (0.63 pmol/min) into anesthetized rats leads to a proportionately greater increase in efferent than in afferent arteriolar resistance, hence an increase in mean glomerular capillary hydraulic pressure ($\bar{P}_{GC}$) [22]. Offsetting this pro-filtration force is a fall in the glomerular capillary plasma flow rate (Q_A); thus at this low dose, single nephron glomerular filtration rate (SNGFR) remains relatively constant [22]. Higher doses of ET-1 (10 pmol/min) also lead to a proportionately greater increase in efferent than in afferent arteriolar tone [14]. This dose causes more intense renal vasoconstriction, leading to a fall in Q_A. This, in conjunction with a marked reduction in K_f, leads to a fall in SNGFR [14]. In keeping with these findings, studies of isolated perfused glomerular arterioles demonstrate that half-maximal contraction of efferent arterioles ($3.2 \pm 4.0 \times 10^{-12}M$) is achieved with doses 3 orders of magnitude less than for afferent arterioles ($1.4 \pm 2.5 \times 10^{-9}M$) [28]. This vasoconstriction is unaffected by co-infusion of saralasin, an AII receptor antagonist [28]. By contrast, direct infusion of ET (0.16 pmol/min) into a branch of the renal artery leads to predominant afferent arteriolar constriction, a reduction in $\bar{P}_{GC}$, and no significant effect on K_f [29]. A similar pattern of constriction is also noted in isolated perfused hydronephrotic kidneys [27]. Overall, these studies highlight the sensitivity of the glomerular microvasculature to exogenous ET, with nearly all of the determinants of glomerular ultrafiltration being affected.

Effects of Endothelin on Mesangial Cells

Angiotensin II, norepinephrine and arginine vasopressin are each capable of inducing a contractile response in mesangial cells, thereby contributing to the fall in the K_f seen with these agents. Similarly, ET induces dose-dependent contractile effects on cultured mesangial cells [14,30,31]. In these cells ET led to rearrangements of F actin microfilament bundles, consistent with a motile response [31]. As with other vasoconstrictors the contractile effects of ET on mesangial cells may be dampened by concurrent stimulation of prostanoids. Phospholipase A_2 activity is stimulated by ET, leading to increased arachidonate release from mesangial cells as well as release of $PGE_2 > PGI_2 > TXA_2$ [31]. Furthermore, ET-induced PGE_2 production significantly potentiates β agonist-induced cAMP production, which also serves to dampen mesangial contraction [31]. These results suggest that the reduction in K_f by ET is, at least in part, due to mesangial cell contraction.

Mesangial cells respond to low dose (10 pM) ET-1 infusion with a slow rise in cytosolic free calcium, an effect blocked by EGTA but not by nifedipine [15]. Higher doses lead to a brisk increase in intracellular free calcium, followed by a slow return toward baseline. EGTA has no effect on the early rise in Ca^{2+} but abrogates the tonic phase of calcium elevation. These results suggest that, as with the vascular smooth muscle cells, the rapid phase is associated with the release of calcium from intracellular stores, whereas entry of external calcium contributes to the delayed phase. The rise in intracellular Ca^{2+} is paralleled by an increase in inositol phosphate turnover, indicating activation of phospholipase C. Finally, ET is a potent co-mitogen in quiescent mesangial cells, but not in Swiss 3T3 fibroblasts [14,15]. This response may relate to ET-induced activation of Na^+/H^+ exchange. In addition, ET significantly stimulates expression of the proto-oncogenes *c-fos* in mesangial cells and *c-myc/c-fos* in vascular smooth muscle cells, suggesting a possible role for ET in vascular and glomerular hypertrophy [15,32].

Potential Role of Endothelin in Acute Renal Failure

Cyclosporine (CyA) therapy in humans and animals induces marked renal vasocon-striction with a reduction of GFR [33]. Several studies have recently implicated ET in this renal vasoconstrictor response [34,35]. CyA-induced vasoconstriction in iso-lated perfused rat kidneys is largely overcome by co-infusion of anti-ET antibody, but not by non-immune serum [34]. Studies of intravenous CyA with simultaneous intrarenal artery infusion of anti-ET in rats corroborate these findings in vivo [35]. These studies suggest a role for ET in acute CyA-induced renal vasoconstriction. Whether ET is an important mediator in chronic cyclosporine toxicity awaits further investigation. In addition to augmented ET production, endothelium-dependent vasodilatory responses may also be impaired, since isolated perfused kidneys from CyA-treated rats exhibit shifts of the vasodilatory dose response curves to acetylcho-line [36].

Despite an impaired ability of the ischemic kidney to respond to endothelium-dependent vasodilators, there is recent evidence to suggest that ischemia augments ET production. Infusion of anti-ET antibody into a branch of a rat renal artery sig-nificantly ameliorates renal vasoconstriction induced by 25 minutes of ischemia [29]. Whether this reflects an increase in local production of ET and/or a change in receptor number or binding is as yet unclear. Of interest, however, ET binding site density of rat cardiac membranes is markedly increased by ischemia [37]. Small changes in affinity occur with ischemia of > 30 minutes duration. Increased binding site density is further enhanced by reperfusion, and is prevented by hypothermic per-fusion [37]. Whether similar changes take place in the kidney is not yet known. Taken together, the effects of ischemia on ET receptor density and the stimulation of ET production by CyA may have important implications in the pathogenesis of early renal allograft dysfunction.

Finally, acute infusion of endotoxin in rats is well known to induce renal vasocon-striction [38]. Rats and sheep infused with endotoxin have marked increases in plasma ET concentrations which may contribute to this vasoconstriction [39,40]. Endotoxin also induces NO production from vascular smooth muscle cells [41], which may counterbalance the effects of ET. Plasma levels of ET are elevated in patients with acute renal failure from a variety of causes, and fall with improvement of renal function [42]. Accordingly, future studies are required to determine whether blockade of ET production and/or binding will prove beneficial in the treatment of acute renal failure.

Acknowledgments. Andrew J. King is the recipient of an Individual National Research Service Award of the NIH (1F32DK08003). Studies were supported in part by NIH grant DK35930.

References

1. Brenner BM, Troy JL, Ballermann BJ (1989) Endothelium-dependent vascular responses. Mediators and Mechanisms. J Clin Invest 84:1373–1378
2. Davies PF, Oleson SP, Clapham DE, Morrel EM, Schoen FJ (1988) Endothelial Communi-cation. State of the art lecture. Hypertension 11:563–572

3. Palmer RMJ, Ferrige AG, Moncada S (1987) Nitric oxide release accounts for the biological activity of endothelium-derived relaxing factor. Nature 327:524–526
4. Myers PR, Minor RLJ, Guerra RJ, Bates JN, Harrison DG (1990) Vasorelaxant properties of the endothelium-derived relaxing factor more closely resemble S-nitrocysteine than nitric oxide. Nature 345:161–163
5. Yanagisawa M, Kurihara H, Kimura S, Tomobe Y, Kobayashi M, Mitsui Y, Yazaki Y, Goto K, Masaki T (1988) A novel potent vasoconstrictor peptide produced by vascular endothelial cells. Nature 332:411–415
6. Inoue A, Yanagisawa M, Kimura S, Kasuya Y, Miyauchi T, Goto K, Masaki T (1989) The human endothelin family: three structurally and pharmacologically distinct isopeptides predicted by three separate genes. Proc Natl Acad Sci USA 86:2863–2867
7. Marsden PA, Danthuluri NR, Brenner BM, Ballermann BJ, Brock TA (1989) Endothelin action on vascular smooth muscle involves inositol trisphosphate and calcium mobilization. Biochem Biophys Res Commun 158:86–93
8. Whittle BJR, Lopez-Belmonte J, Rees DD (1989) Modulation of the vasodepressor actions of acetylcholine, bradykinin, substance P and endothelin in the rat by a specific inhibitor of nitric oxide formation. Br J Pharmacol 98:646–652
9. Kohzuki MC, Johnston CI, Chai SY, Casley DJ, Mendelsohn FAO (1989) Localization of endothelin receptors in rat kidney. Eur J Pharmacol 160:193–194
10. Koseki C, Imai M, Hirata Y, Yanagisawa M, Masaki T (1989) Autoradiographic distribution in rat tissues of binding sites for endothelin: a neuropeptide? Am J Physiol 256:R858–R866
11. Badr KF, Munger KA, Sugiura M, Snajdar RM, Schwartzberg M, Inagami T (1989) High and low affinity binding sites for endothelin on cultured rat glomerular mesangial cells. Biochem Biophys Res Commun 161:776–781
12. Martin ER, Brenner BM, Ballermann BJ (to be published) Heterogeneity of cell surface endothelin receptors. J Biol Chem
13. Sugiura M, Snajdar RM, Schwartzberg M, Badr KF, Inagami T (1989) Identification of two types of specific endothelin receptors in rat mesangial cells. Biochem Biophys Res Commun 162:1396–1401
14. Badr KF, Murray JJ, Breyer MD, Takahashi K, Inagami T, Harris RC (1989) Mesangial cell, glomerular and renal vascular responses to endothelin in the rat kidney. J Clin Invest 83:336–342
15. Simonson MS, Wann S, Mene P, Dubyak GR, Kester M, Nakazato Y, Sedor JR, Dunn MJ (1989) Endothelin stimulates phospholipase C, Na/H exchange, c-fos expression, and mitogenesis in rat mesangial cells. J Clin Invest 83:708–712
16. Kurihara H, Yoshizumi M, Takaku M, Yanagisawa M, Masaki T, Hamaoki M, Kato H, Yazaki Y (1989) Transforming growth factor β stimulates the expression of endothelin mRNA by vascular endothelial cells. Biochem Biophys Res Commun 159:1435–1440
17. Yoshizumi M, Kurihara H, Sugiyama T, Takaku F, Yanagisawa M, Masaki T, Yazaki Y (1989) Hemodynamic shear stress stimulates endothelin production by cultured endothelial cells. Biochem Biophys Res Commun 161:859–864
18. Marsden PA, Dorfman DM, Brenner BM, Orkin BJ, Ballermann BJ (1989) Endothelin: gene expression, release and action in cultured cells of the renal glomerulus. Am J Hypertens 2(2):49A
19. Kosaka T, Suzuki N, Matsumoto H, Itoh Y, Yasuhara T, Onda H, Fujino M (1989) Synthesis of the vasoconstrictor peptide endothelin in kidney cells. FEBS Lett 249:42–46
20. Shichiri M, Hirata Y, Emori T, Ohta K, Nakajima T, Sato K, Sato A, Marumo F (1989) Secretion of endothelin and related peptides from renal epithelial cell lines. FEBS Lett 253:203–206
21. Cairns HS, Rogerson ME, Fairbanks LD, Neild GH, Westwick J (1989) Endothelin induces

an increase in renal vascular resistance and a fall in glomerular filtration rate in the rabbit isolated perfused kidney. Br J Pharmacol 98:155-160

22. King AJ, Brenner BM, Anderson S (1989) Endothelin: a potent renal and systemic vasoconstrictor peptide. Am J Physiol 256:F1051-F1058

23. Katoh T, Chang H, Uchida S, Okuda T, Kurakawa K (1990) Direct effects of endothelin in the rat kidney. Am J Physiol 258:F397-F402

24. Hirata Y, Matsuoka H, Kimura K, Fukui K, Hayakawa H, Suzuki E, Sugimoto T, Yanagisawa M, Masaki T (1989) Renal vasoconstriction by the endothelial cell-derived peptide endothelin in spontaneously hypertensive rats. Circ Res 65:1370-1379

25. Mantymaa P, Leppaluoto J, Ruskoaho H (1990) Endothelin stimulates basal stretch-induced atrial natriuretic peptide secretion from the perfused rat heart. Endocrinology 126:587-595

26. Zeidel ML, Brady HR, Kone BC, Gullans SR, Brenner BM (1989) Endothelin, a peptide inhibitor of Na/K ATPase in intact renal tubular epithelial cells. Am J Physiol 257: C1101-C1107

27. Loutzenhiser R, Epstein M, Hayashi K, Horton C (1990) Direct visualization of effects of endothelin on the renal microvasculature. Am J Physiol 258:F61-F68

28. Yuan BH, McMurtry IF, Conger JD (1989) Effect of endothelin on isolated perfused rat afferent and efferent arterioles. Clin Res 37:586A

29. Kon V, Yoshioka T, Fogo A, Ichikawa I (1989) Glomerular actions of endothelin in vivo. J Clin Invest 83:1762-1767

30. Culebras M, Montanes I, Lopez-Farre A, Millas I, Lopez-Novoa JM (1989) Effect of endothelin on renal function and on the contraction of cultured rat mesangial cells. Med Sci Res 17:245-246

31. Sinmonson MS, Dunn MJ (1990) Endothelin-1 stimulates contraction of rat glomerular mesangial cells and potentiates β-adrenergic-mediated cyclic adenosine monophosphate accumulation. J Clin Invest 85:790-797

32. Komuro I, Kurihara H, Sugiyama T, Yoshizumi M, Takaku F, Yazaki Y (1988) Endothelin stimulates c-fos and c-myc expression and proliferation of vascular smooth muscle cells. FEBS Lett. 238:249-252

33. Myers B (1986) Cyclosporine nephrotoxicity. Kidney Int 30:964-974

34. Dedan J, Perico N, Remuzzi G (1990) Role of endothelin in cyclosporine-induced renal vasoconstriction. Kidney Int 37:479A

35. Kon V, Sugiura M, Inagami T, Harvie BR, Ichikawa I, Hoover RL (1990) Role of endothelin in cyclosporin-induced glomerular dysfunction. Kidney Int 37:1487-1491

36. Gerkins JF (1989) Cyclosporine treatment of normal rats produces a rise in blood pressure and decreased renal vascular responses to nerve stimulated, vasoconstrictors and endothelium-dependent dilators. J Pharmacol Exp Ther 250:1105-1112

37. Liu J, Chen R, Casley DJ, Nayler WG. Ischemia and reperfusion increase ^{125}I-labeled endothelin-1 binding in rat cardiac membranes. Am J Physiol 258:H829-H835

38. Badr KF, Kelley VE, Rennke HG, Brenner BM (1986) Roles for thromboxane A and leukotrienes in endotoxin-induced acute renal failure. Kidney Int 30:474-480

39. Morel DR, Lacroix JS, Hemsen A, Steinig A, Pittet JF, Lundberg JM (1989) Increased plasma and pulmonary lymph levels of endothelin during endotoxin shock. Eur J Pharmacol 167:427-428

40. Sugiura M, Inagami T, Kon V (1989) Endotoxin stimulates endothelin-release in vivo and in vitro as determined by radioimmunoassay. Biochem Biophys Res Commun 161:1220-1227

41. Beasley D, Brenner BM, Schwartz JH (1990) Interleukin-1 activates guanylate cyclase in rat vascular smooth muscle cells by inducing nitric oxide. FASEB J 4:685A

42. Tomita K, Ujiie K, Nakanishi T, Tomura S, Matsuda O, Ando K, Shichiri M, Hirata Y, Marumo F (1990) Plasma endothelin levels in patients with acute renal failure (letter). N Engl J Med 321:1127

Effect of Insulin-Like Growth Factor-I on Glomerular Cells in Vitro

LILIANE J. STRIKER[1]

SUMMARY. Since mesangial proliferation is the hallmark of many human glomerular diseases we investigated whether glomerular cells have receptors for insulin-like growth factor-I (IGF-I), a growth peptide. All three glomerular cell types; mesangial, epithelial, and endothelial cells were found to have surface receptors for IGF-I. This peptide was a potent mitogen for mesangial cells in vitro and acted as a progression factor. In addition, IGF-I-like molecules may play an important role in glomerular disease.

Introduction

The insulin-growth factors are a family of peptides that were originally discovered in the late 1950s. The early work was performed by Salmon and Daughaday [1], who established that one of the major effects of growth hormone was mediated through the production of a liver factor which stimulated the incorporation of labeled SO_4 into cartilage, which was therefore called "sulfation-factor." This soluble factor was further characterized and was shown to exert multiple effects on cell mitogenesis and differentiation. The term "Somatomedin," coined in 1972, was further completely replaced by that of Insulin-like growth factor (IGF-I). In 1978, Rinkerknecht and Humbel [2], isolated two peptides, with a molecular weight of 7500, from human plasma. One of these peptides, which contained 70 amino-acids, was basic (pI 8.1–8.5) and had a 48% structural homology with proinsulin. Because of this homology, and because this peptide had some effects comparable to those known for insulin in vivo, these investigators proposed the name of IGF-I for this molecule.

Whereas it was initially assumed that IGF-I was exclusively synthesized in the liver and acted as a hormone on the target organs, it was subsequently shown that this pep-

[1]NIDDK, MDB, National Institute of Health, Building 10, Room 3 N 110, Bethesda, MD 20892, USA

tide was produced locally by multiple tissues [3]. The production of IGF-I was also found to be regulated not only by growth hormone (GH), but also by multiple other factors. In the plasma, IGF-I binds to carrier proteins called IGF-1 binding proteins (IGF-BP) [4,5].

Several lines of evidence support a role for IGF-I in the kidney [6]. The administration of this peptide to intact animals is accompanied by an increase in glomerular filtration rate [7]. In addition, following a unilateral nephrectomy, there is an increase in the level of extractable IGF-I in the remaining kidney, suggesting that this peptide is a growth factor for the kidney [6,8]. We have examined whether glomerular cells had receptors for IGF-I. We found that this peptide was a mitogen for mesangial cells [9,10]. These cells produced IGF-I and IGF-I binding proteins in a coordinate fashion, suggesting that the glomerulus is an important target for this peptide [11]. The present paper reviews the evidence gathered in our laboratory that IGF-I plays a role in the physiology of mouse and human glomerular cells in vitro.

Receptors for IGF-I on Mesangial Cells

Mouse Mesangial Cells

Material and Methods

Mesangial cells were isolated and propagated, according to methods previously published, from a strain of mice which is devoid of glomerular disease [12]. The cells were characterized and subcultured as described [9]. These elongated cells contained long parallel actin filaments, but no cytokeratin or von-Willebrand antigen; these two features characterizing epithelial or endothelial cells, respectively.

All studies were performed on cells between passages 8 and 20. To ensure that these were a representative mesangial population, experiments were repeated on a second cell line, isolated independently from the initial glomerular outgrowth.

All experiments were performed on confluent cells. These were incubated in serum-free medium for 15 hours. The binding studies were performed on monolayers, as reported by Conti et al. [9]. The conditions were optimized for temperature, time, and pH dependency. The specificity of IGF-I binding was determined using unlabeled recombinant IGF-I, porcine insulin, and MSA (rat IGF-II). At the end of the incubation period the monolayers were washed and solubilized in order to measure the cell-associated radioactivity. The radioactivity bound in the presence of an excess of unlabeled IGF-I represented the non-specific binding, which was subtracted from the total to calculate the specific binding.

To assess the mitogenic effect of IGF-I, mesangial cells were plated in medium containing 20% serum. Twenty-four hours later the medium was removed and the cells were repeatedly washed; the medium was then changed to serum-free medium supplemented with 0.1% of bovine serum albumin (BSA). After a period varying from 24 to 72 hours, the cells were incubated in fresh serum-free medium containing IGF-I. Sixteen hours later, ³H thymidine was added for a total of 4 hours. The cell layer was solubilized with NaOH and counted.

Table 1. Analysis according to scatchard

Cell type	Kd	Number of receptors/cell
Human mesangial cells	1.35×10^{-9}	1.04×10^5
Mouse mesangial cells	1.27×10^{-9}	0.64×10^5
Mouse endothelial cells	2.25×10^{-9}	1.62×10^5
Mouse epithelial cells	$1.5 \ \times 10^{-9}$	2.45×10^5

Results

Radiolabeled IGF-I bound specifically to the mesangial cell surface. The binding was dependent on time and temperature. The pH-dependence of the binding was comparable to that found for other cell types. Non-specific binding accounted for only 10% of total binding. Degradation of the tracer appeared to be minimal. The optimal conditions selected for competition experiments were 150 minutes, 15°C, and a pH of 7.8. A type I receptor was identified in competition studies utilizing unlabeled IGF-I, insulin, and IGF-II. The estimated kd was 1.27×10^{-9}. The number of receptors was calculated to be 64×10^4 per cell. (Tables 1 and 2). This receptor was further characterized using solubilized cell fractions and wheat-germ agglutinin eluates (WGA). The kd obtained from the receptor preparation and from WGA eluates were, respectively, 2.3×10^{-9} and 3.7×10^{-10}.

The peak of mitogenesis, as detected by thymidine incorporation, occurred 18 hours after the addition of IGF-1. As shown in Table 2, there was a 2.6-fold increase above the levels found for unstimulated cells.

Human Mesangial Cells

Material and Methods

Normal human glomeruli were obtained from the non affected areas of kidneys removed for cancer or from organs not used for transplantation. The initial outgrowth appeared within one week after the initial plating. Patches of elongated cells were selected with cloning rings and were dilute-plated until we obtained homogenous cells which were further identified as mesangial populations. Mesangial cells appeared initially stellate before they reached confluence, after which they formed a multilayer of parallel arrays. The cells contained long filaments of actin, and also contained desmin, myosin, and vimentin intermediate filaments. There was

Table 2. Mitogenesis

Cell type	Dose of IGF-I	Exposure (hours)	Increase over control
Human mesangial cells	10 ng/ml	14	2.1
Mouse mesangial cells	10 ng/ml	18	2.5
Mouse endothelial cells	10 ng/ml	18	1.10
Mouse epithelial cells	10 ng/ml	18	1.47

specific angiotensin-II binding on the surface of the cells, as reported by Doi et al. [10]. All the studies were performed between passages 4 and 9.

The binding experiments were performed using the same method as those described above for mouse mesangial cells. In addition, we examined the effect of various concentrations of a monoclonal antibody directed against the IGF-I receptor (αIR-3) on the IGF-I binding to the receptor. The presence of IGF-I receptors was also examined on the surface of the cells by immunofluorescence microscopy, using the same antibody.

SDS-polyacrylamide gel electrophoresis and autoradiographic studies were performed on immunoprecipitates obtained by incubating αIGF-3 with receptor-enriched preparations obtained by WGA chromatography.

Studies of mitogenesis were completed by an analysis of the labeling index. Briefly, cells were plated on plastic chamber-slides. They were stimulated for optimal periods by the various ligands of interest, in the presence of ^{3}H thymidine. Autoradiography was performed on the slides. The labeling index was expressed as the percentage of nuclei labeled [10].

Results

The binding of radiolabeled IGF-I was measured on cells that had been starved for 0–48 hours. The maximal binding was reached at 12 hours and was 27.2% + 2.6% per 10^6 cells after an incubation period of 150 minutes, with a non-specific binding of 3.8%. Analysis of the data by Scatchard's method indicated that the cells had a single type of receptor with a kd of 1.35×10^{-9}. The estimated number of receptors per cell was 1.04×10^5.

The antibody to the receptor inhibited the IGF-I binding in a dose-dependent manner. By immunofluorescence, this antibody stained a large number of small dots over the cell surface, presumably representing coated pits present on the cell membranes. The identification of the receptor revealed two major bands, of 130 k and 90 k, which are thought to correspond to the α and β subunits of the receptor. A minor band of 150 kd also found in the precipitate was presumed to represent partially reduced α and β fragments.

The mitogenesis was measured by thymidine incorporation after the addition of either IGF-I or insulin. Following the addition of recombinant IGF-I, there was a dose-dependent increase in mitogenesis (Table 1). In contrast, there was only a minor increase in response to high doses of insulin, suggesting that the observed effect was mediated through the IGF-I receptor. The labeling index, which was used to deter-

Table 3. Labeling index

Ligands	Labeling index (% labeled nuclei)
Control	1.06
PDGF	2.01
IGF-I	3.35
PDGF + IGF-I	5.19
PDGF + IGF-I (sequentially)	5.27

mine the number of cells entering S phase, showed that IGF-I was much more efficient if the cells were initially exposed to a competence factor, such as platelet-derived growth factor (PDGF). These data confirm that the effect of IGF-I is that of a progression factor. (Table 3) [10,13,14].

Receptors for IGF-I on Mouse Endothelial and Epithelial Cells

Materials and Methods

Glomerular endothelial and epithelial cells from normal mice were established, maintained, and identified in culture, as previously described [12]. All experiments were performed on cells between passages 14 and 25. Endothelial or epithelial cells were plated in 35mm dishes or 24 well dishes in their respective complete media. Experiments were performed on confluent cells, following a 16 hour preincubation in serum-free medium, as described above for mesangial cells.

To perform IGF-I receptor crosslinking, cells were grown to confluence in 100mm dishes and were incubated with [125I]IGF-I, in the presence or absence of excess cold IGF-I or insulin, under standard binding conditions. The [125I]IGF-I bound to its receptor was cross-linked by the addition of DSS [10]. The cells were solubilized, collected, and concentrated. The sample was then electrophoresed, under reducing conditions, on an SDS-polyacrylamide gel and was exposed for autoradiography.

Results

Specific [125I]IGF-I binding to glomerular endothelial and epithelial cells was time and temperature dependent, and the optimal pH was found to be 7.8. In both cell types non-specific binding accounted for less than 10% of the total binding and it did not increase over time. The kd was 2.25×10^{-9} for endothelial cells and 1.5×10^{-9} for epithelial cells.

A single radioactive band was obtained in both endothelial and epithelial cell extracts. The apparent molecular weight under reducing conditions was 145k and 142k, respectively. This band was no longer detectable when cells were incubated in the presence of unlabeled IGF-I, and its intensity decreased when cells were incubated with insulin [15].

Endothelial and epithelial cells failed to show any mitogenic activity following exposure to IGF-I, using conditions under which this peptide could stimulate mesangial cell mitogenesis (Table 1).

Release of Insulin-Like Growth Factor I by Mesangial Cells in Culture

Materials and Methods

Mesangial cells were grown to approximately 80% confluence, washed with basal medium, and incubated in serum-free medium containing 0.1% BSA. This medium was discarded and the cells were incubated for up to 72 hours in fresh basal medium which was collected for further analysis.

The culture medium was centrifuged and acidified as previously described [11], in order to dissociate free IGF from binding proteins. After concentration, the samples were treated by manual reverse-phase chromatography with Sep-pak c18 cartridges. After extraction, it was found that the recovery of IGF-I was as high as 80%–90%.

IGF-I activity was detected by two methods: a radioimmunoassay, using a polyclonal antibody to human IGF-I (UBK 487) generated by L.E. Underwood, and provided by the NIDDK and the National hormone and pituitary program (University of Maryland, School of Medicine). The antibody was used at a dilution of 1:18 000. Human recombinant IGF-I was used as a standard and [^{125}I]IGF-I was used as the tracer.

In addition, IGF-I was measured by the ability of the cell culture medium to inhibit IGF-I binding to mouse mesangial cell culture in the radioreceptor assay, as described above.

Results

The supernatant of glomerular mesangial cells contained an immunoreactive IGF-I-like molecule. In contrast, supernatants from either endothelial or epithelial cells did not contain immunoreactive IGF-I. These results were confirmed independently, using a radioreceptor assay. The concentration of IGF-I was much higher (tenfold) using this method, as compared to the radioimmunoassay, presumably because the antibody used was directed against human, rather than mouse, IGF-I.

Finally, using reverse-phase chromatography, it was established that samples of supernatants from mesangial cells contained a single peak of IGF-I activity.

In addition, we examined the amount of IGF-I released by mesangial cells and found that it was regulated by cell density. Sparse cells released greater amounts of IGF-I-like molecules than did confluent cells. In parallel, mesangial cells released an IGF-I binding protein.

Discussion

The presence of specific receptors on all three glomerular cell types supports the hypothesis that IGF-I plays a role in glomerular cell physiology. Furthermore, IGF-I acted as a progression factor for mesangial cells when these were made competent after exposure to PDGF. In contrast, endothelial and epithelial cells did not exhibit any mitogenesis after exposure to IGF-I.

Other investigators have reported the presence of receptors for IGF-I in glomerular mesangial cells from other species [16–18]. The significance of these findings in vivo is not yet elucidated. A dysregulation of mesangial cell mitogenesis in vivo may be one of the pathological events leading to glomerular diseases which progress to sclerosis. This would be envisaged in diseases as diverse as diabetes mellitus, IgA disease, light chain systemic disease, and membranoproliferative glomerulonephritis. In this group of disorders, proliferation of resident cells from the mesangial areas constitutes the initial event, which is further followed by increased matrix formation [19,20].

Mesangial cells respond to multiple combinations of growth-related peptides in vitro [21]. Normally, their growth in vivo is tightly regulated and appears minimal, as shown by autoradiographic studies performed in rats and mice [22,23]. These cells are capable not only of responding to IGF-I, but also of releasing an immunoreactive IGF-I molecule.

Furthermore, we found that mesangial cells produced IGF-I binding proteins [24]. In mouse mesangial cells, the release of IGF-BP was coordinately regulated with that of IGF-I molecules. These observations suggest that the IGF-I axis is quite important in the biology of mesangial cells. The normal regulation of IGF-I and IGF-I binding protein release is not yet elucidated. Our preliminary findings suggest, however, that cells which are confluent produce much less IGF-I and IGF-BP than do sparse cells. These observations favor a role for IGF-I in the control of mesangial cell proliferation and suggest that alterations of this regulation could be an important factor in progressive glomerular disease.

The role of IGF-I in vivo is not yet elucidated. In mice transgenic for IGF-I, we have observed an increase in the size of the glomeruli and a mild mesangial proliferation, contrasting with lesions that occur in growth-hormone transgenic mice [25]. Further analysis will be required to establish the role of IGF-I in disease states.

References

1. Salmon WD, Daughaday WH (1957) A hormonally controlled serum factor which stimulates sulfate incorporation by cartilage in vitro. J Lab Clin Med 49:825–836
2. Rinderknecht E, Humbel RE (1978) The amino acid sequence of human insulin-like growth factor-I and its structural homology with proinsulin. J Biol Chem 253:2769–2776
3. D'Ercole AJ, Stiles AD, Underwood LE (1984) Tissue concentrations of somatomedin-C: further evidence for multiple sites of synthesis and paracrine or autocrine mechanisms of action. Proc Natl Acad Sci USA 81:935–939
4. Froesch ER, Schmid C, Schwander J, Zapp J (1985) Actions of insulin-like growth factors. Annu Rev Physiol 47:443–467
5. Rechler MM, Nissley SP (1985) The nature and regulation of the receptors for insulin-like growth factors. Annu Rev Physiol 47:425–442
6. Hammerman MR (1989) The growth hormone-insulin-like growth factor axis in kidney. Am J Physiol 257:F503–F514
7. Hirschberg R, Kopple JD (1989) Evidence that insulin-like growth factor I increases renal plasma flow and glomerular filtration rate in fasted rats. J Clin Invest 83:326–330
8. Fagin JA, Melmed S (1987) Relative increase in insulin-like growth factor I messenger ribonucleic acid levels in compensatory renal hypertrophy. Endocrinology 120:718–724
9. Conti FG, Striker LJ, Lesniak MA, MacKay K, Roth J, Striker GE (1988) Studies on binding and mitogenic effect of insulin and insulin-like growth factor I in glomerular mesangial cells. Endocrinology 122:2788–2795
10. Doi T, Striker LJ, Elliot SJ, Conti FG, Striker GE (1989) Insulin-like growth factor-1 is a progression factor for human mesangial cells. Am J Pathol 134:395–404
11. Conti FG, Striker LJ, Elliot SJ, Andreani D, Striker GE (1988) Synthesis and release of insulin-like growth factor I by mesangial cells in culture. Am J Physiol 255:F1214–F1219
12. MacKay K, Striker LJ, Elliot S, Pinkert CA, Brinster RL, Striker GE (1980) Glomerular epithelial, mesangial, and endothelial cell lines from transgenic mice. Kidney Int 33:677–684
13. Pfeifle B, Boeder H, Ditschuneit H (1987) Interaction of receptors for insulin-like growth factor I, platelet-derived growth factor, and fibroblast growth factor in rat aortic cells. Endocrinology 120:2251–2258

14. Stiles CD, Capone GT, Scher CD, Antoniades HN, Van Wyk JJ, Pledger WJ (1979) Dual control of cell growth by somatomedins and platelet-derived growth factor. Proc Natl Acad Sci USA 76:1279-1283

15. Conti FG, Elliot S, Striker LJ, Striker GE (1989) Binding of insulin-like growth factor-I by glomerular endothelial and epithelial cells: Further evidence for IGF-I action in the renal glomerulus. Biochem Biophys Res Commun 163:952-958

16. Aron DC, Rosenzweig JL, Abboud HE (1989) Synthesis and binding of insulin-like growth factor I by human glomerular mesangial cells. J Clin Endocrinol Metab 68:585-591

17. Arnqvist HJ, Ballerman BJ, King GL (1988) Receptor for and effects of insulin and IGF-1 in rat glomerular mesangial cells. Am J Physiol 23:C411-C416

18. Abrass CK, Raugi GJ, Gabourel LS, Lovett DH (1988) Insulin and insulin-like growth factor I binding to cultured rat glomerular mesangial cells. Endocrinology 13:2432-2439

19. Striker LJ, Doi T, Elliot S, Striker GE (1989) The contribution of mesangial cells to progressive glomerulosclerosis. In: Klahr S (ed) Seminars in nephrology, vol 9. WB Saunders, Philadelphia, pp 318-329

20. Fogo A, Ichikawa I (1989) Evidence for the central role of glomerular growth promoters in the development of sclerosis. In: Klahr S (ed) Seminars in nephrology, vol 9. WB Saunders, Philadelphia, pp 329-343

21. Jaffer F, Saunders C, Shultz P, Throckmorton D, Weinshell E, Abboud HE (1989) Regulation of mesangial cell growth by polypeptide mitogens. Am J Pathol 135:261-269

22. Pabst R, Sterzel RB (1983) Cell renewal of glomerular cell types in normal rats. An autoradiographic analysis. Kidney Int 24:626-631

23. Vancura P, Miller WL, Little JW, Malt RA (1970) Contribution of glomerular and tubular RNA synthesis to compensatory renal growth. Am J Physiol 219:78-88

24. Perfetti R, Conti FG, Elliot S, Striker LJ, Striker GE (1989) Mouse glomerular mesangial cells in culture produce IGF-I binding proteins. 71st annual meeting of Endocrinology, 1989. Seattle, United States

25. Doi T, Striker LJ, Quaife CJ, Conti FG, Palmiter RD, Behringer RR, Brinster RL, Striker GE (1988) Progressive glomerulosclerosis develops in transgenic mice chronically expressing growth hormone and growth hormone releasing factor but not in those expressing insulin-like growth factor-1. Am J Pathol 131:398-403

Frontiers of Research on Natriuretic Peptides

Chair: Thomas Maack (USA)
Fumiaki Marumo (Japan)

Brain Natriuretic Peptide is a Novel Cardiac Hormone Secreted from the Ventricle in Humans

MASASHI MUKOYAMA, KAZUWA NAKAO, YOSHIHIKO SAITO,
YOSHIHIRO OGAWA, KIMINORI HOSODA, SHIN-ICHI SUGA,
GOTARO SHIRAKAMI, HIROO IMURA[1], MICHIHISA JOUGASAKI,
KENJI OBATA, and HIROFUMI YASUE[2]

SUMMARY. Using a specific radioimmunoassay for human brain natriuretic peptide (hBNP), with a monoclonal antibody against hBNP, we investigated the secretion of this peptide in comparison with that of atrial natriuretic peptide (ANP), in normal and failing human hearts. The plasma BNP-like immunoreactivity (BNP-LI) level in normal subjects was 0.90 ± 0.07 fmol/ml, which was 16% of the ANP-LI level. In contrast, the plasma BNP-LI level increased markedly in patients with congestive heart failure (CHF), with a progressive rise in proportion to the severity of CHF. The plasma BNP-LI level surpassed the ANP-LI level in cases with severe CHF, and the percentage increment of the plasma BNP-LI level in severe cases was one order of magnitude greater than that of the plasma ANP-LI level. There was a significant step-up of the plasma BNP-LI level in the coronary sinus, compared with that in the aortic root, and the difference in plasma BNP-LI levels between the coronary sinus and the aorta, $\Delta_{(CS-Ao)}BNP$, increased with the severity of CHF. In addition, the difference in BNP-LI levels between the anterior interventricular vein and the aorta ($\Delta_{(AIV-Ao)}BNP$) was comparable to $\Delta_{(CS-Ao)}BNP$, indicating that BNP is secreted predominantly from the ventricle. From these results, we conclude that BNP, a novel cardiac hormone, is secreted predominantly from the ventricle in humans, in striking contrast with ANP, which is secreted mainly from the atrium. We further conclude that as the plasma level of hBNP in CHF is more markedly augmented than that of ANP, this suggests a discrete pathophysiological role of BNP in a dual natriuretic peptide system.

[1]Second Division, Department of Medicine, Kyoto University School of Medicine, Kyoto, 606 Japan
[2]Division of Cardiology, Kumamoto University Medical School, Kumamoto, 860 Japan

Introduction

Since the discovery of atrial natriuretic peptide (ANP) in the heart, and subsequently in the brain, ANP has been implicated in body fluid homeostasis and blood pressure control, both as a hormone and as a neuropeptide [1-3]. We and others have demonstrated previously that the synthesis and secretion of ANP in the heart are increased in patients with congestive heart failure (CHF), in a manner related to the severity of CHF [4-8].

More recently, brain natriuretic peptide (BNP) was isolated from the porcine brain [9]; this peptide shows a remarkable sequence homology to ANP and has peripheral and central actions similar to those of ANP [9-12]. We demonstrated that BNP is also synthesized in, and secreted into the circulation from, the porcine heart [13]. Subsequently, we isolated BNP from the rat heart [14]. To date, however, little is known about BNP in humans, since antisera against porcine or rat BNP have failed to detect any BNP-like immunoreactivity (BNP-LI) in human tissues, suggesting a structural diversity of BNP among species.

Recently, we have isolated human BNP (hBNP) from the atrium, and determined its amino acid sequence [15]. Human BNP is composed of 32 amino acid residues, whose sequence is identical to the sequence, [77-108], of the hBNP precursor deduced from the cDNA sequence [16]. In the present study, with a monoclonal antibody against hBNP, we established a specific radioimmunoassay (RIA) for hBNP. Using the RIA, we investigated the secretion of hBNP, in comparison with that of ANP, in normal subjects and in patients with CHF.

Methods

Subjects

Eleven healthy male subjects (aged 25-33 years, mean 29.6 years) and 48 patients with heart disease (33 men and 15 women, aged 16-78 years, mean 55.0 years) were studied. They included 17 patients with coronary artery disease, 13 with valvular heart disease, 7 with dilated cardiomyopathy, 7 with hypertensive heart disease, 2 with congenital heart disease, 1 with hypertrophic obstructive cardiomyopathy, and 1 with myocarditis. According to the functional classification of the New York Heart Association (NYHA) [17], 10 patients, with no limitation of physical activity, were classified as class I, 16 patients were classified as class II, 17 as class III, and 5 as class IV, in the order of increasing cardiovascular disability. None of the patients had evidence of renal failure. Informed consent was obtained from the patients and the study was approved by the ethical committee on human research of Kyoto University (No. 61-9).

Plasma Samples

Blood for peripheral plasma samples was obtained from the antecubital vein while subjects were in a recumbent position. This procedure was performed at 9:00 A.M. after an overnight fast. The blood was transferred to chilled glass tubes containing Na_2EDTA (1 mg/ml) and aprotinin (1000 KIU/ml, Ohkura, Kyoto, Japan); plasma

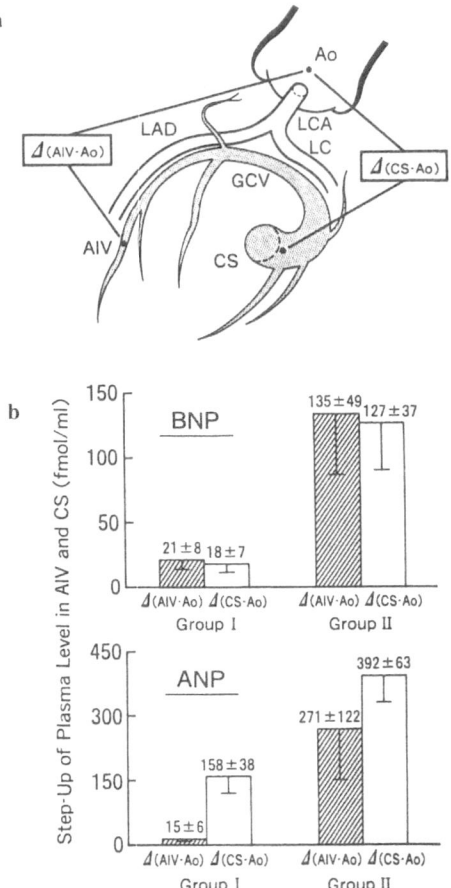

Fig. 1a. Schematic representation of the coronary venous system and three sampling points (*indicated as dots*). AIV, anterior interventricular vein; GCV, great cardiac vein; CS, coronary sinus; Ao, aortic root; LCA, left coronary artery; LAD, left anterior descending artery; LC, left circumflex artery; $\Delta_{(AIV-Ao)}$, the difference in the plasma level between the AIV and the Ao; $\Delta_{(CS-Ao)}$, the difference in the plasma level between the CS and the Ao. **b** Step-ups of BNP (*top*) and ANP (*bottom*) levels in the AIV (*hatched columns*) and in the CS (*open columns*). Patients are classified into Group I and Group II according to the level of $\Delta_{(AIV-Ao)}$ANP, as described in the text

was immediately frozen and stored at $-20\,^\circ$C until assay. In 11 patients undergoing diagnostic cardiac catheterization (8 men and 3 women, aged 21–69 years), plasma samples were obtained from various sites, including the coronary sinus (CS), the anterior interventricular vein (AIV), and the aortic root (Ao) (see Fig. 1a). The difference in plasma ANP levels between the AIV and the Ao ($\Delta_{(AIV-Ao)}$ANP), which reflects the amount of ANP released from the ventricle, was calculated according to methods used in our previous study [8], and the patients were classified into two groups, those with normal (Group I), and those with increased ventricular secretion of ANP (Group II). Among the 6 patients in Group I, 2 were in NYHA class I and 4 were in class II, while of the 5 patients in Group II, 4 were in NYHA class II and 1 was in class III.

RIA for hBNP

Using a monoclonal antibody, we performed an RIA for hBNP, following the RIA method for ANP previously reported [18]. A monoclonal antibody, KY-hBNP-I, raised against hBNP[83–108] conjugated to bovine thyroglobulin, recognized the ring structure of hBNP. The antibody was incubated, either with standard hBNP or with plasma samples (25 μl), in 0.2 ml assay buffer for 24 hours at 4°C, after which 0.05 ml [^{125}I] [Tyr^{82}]-hBNP[83–108] (10000 cpm) was added; the mixture was then further incubated for 24 hours at 4°C. Bound and free ligands were separated by the dextran-coated charcoal method [18]. For the measurement of plasma BNP-LI levels in normal subjects, BNP was extracted from 5–10 ml plasma, using a Sep-Pak C$_{18}$ cartridge (Waters, Milford, Mass.) [13]. The mean recovery of 3–15 fmol/ml standard hBNP added to plasma was 70%. The minimal detectable concentrations of BNP-LI in plasma with and without extraction were 0.4 and 10 fmol/ml, respectively. The intra- and interassay coefficients of variation were 8.4% ($n=8$) and 6.4% ($n=8$), respectively. The cross-reactivity with α-hANP in this RIA was less than 0.005% on a molar basis.

RIA for ANP

The RIA for ANP was performed as previously described [18]. The cross-reactivity with hBNP was less than 0.01% on a molar basis.

Statistical Analysis

Data were expressed as means ± SE. Statistical analysis was performed using Student's t-test or Duncan's multiple range test.

Results

Peripheral Plasma BNP-LI Level

Serial dilution curves of plasma samples, with and without extraction, were parallel to the standard curve of hBNP. The plasma BNP-LI level in 11 normal subjects was 0.90 ± 0.07 fmol/ml, which was only 16% ± 2% of their ANP-LI level (6.4 ± 0.9 fmol/ml).

In contrast, the plasma BNP-LI level increased significantly in patients with heart disease (Fig. 2). In patients with mild CHF, the elevation was moderate (NYHA class I, 13 ± 3.1 fmol/ml; class II, 56 ± 24 fmol/ml). However, plasma BNP-LI levels were markedly elevated in patients with severe CHF (NYHA class III, 148 ± 37 fmol/ml; class IV, 267 ± 80 fmol/ml). Thus, a progressive rise in the plasma BNP-LI level, in accordance with the severity of CHF, was observed. The plasma ANP-LI

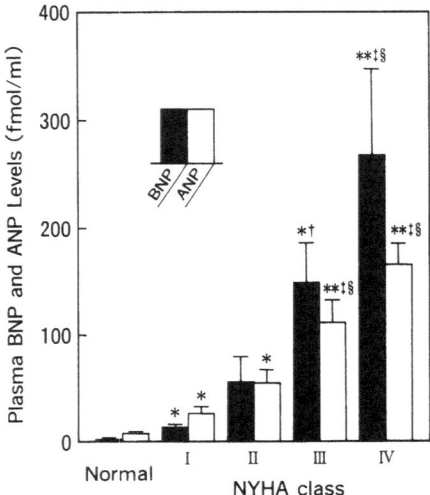

Fig. 2. Plasma BNP (*closed columns*) and ANP (*open columns*) levels in normal subjects and in patients with heart disease. NYHA class, the functional classification of the New York Heart Association. *$P < 0.01$, **$P < 0.001$ compared with values in normal group. †$P < 0.05$, ‡$P < 0.01$ compared with values in NYHA class I group. §$P < 0.01$ compared with values in NYHA class II group

level also increased according to the severity of the disease (Fig. 2), but the increase of ANP-LI was less marked than that of BNP-LI. In patients with severe CHF (NYHA classes III and IV), mean plasma BNP-LI levels surpassed mean ANP-LI levels (Fig. 2). When compared with normal levels, the percentage increment of plasma BNP-LI in severe CHF was much more prominent (200–300 times) than that of ANP-LI (20–30 times).

BNP-LI in Plasma Obtained During Cardiac Catheterization

In order to elucidate the source of plasma BNP, BNP-LI levels in plasma taken from various sites during cardiac catheterization were measured in 11 patients (Fig. 1a). Plasma BNP-LI levels in the CS (132 ± 53 fmol/ml) were 2–3 times higher than those in the Ao near the coronary ostium (66 ± 33 fmol/ml) in all cases, demonstrating that BNP-LI is secreted from the heart into the circulation through the CS.

In order to further investigate the secretion of hBNP from the heart, we measured the plasma BNP-LI level in the AIV, and analyzed $\Delta_{(AIV-Ao)}$BNP and $\Delta_{(CS-Ao)}$BNP (Fig. 1a) in comparison with $\Delta_{(AIV-Ao)}$ANP and $\Delta_{(CS-Ao)}$ANP in two groups of patients. Plasma BNP-LI and ANP-LI levels from the peripheral vein in Group I were 22 ± 10 fmol/ml and 47 ± 16 fmol/ml, respectively, while those in Group II were 99 ± 51 fmol/ml and 108 ± 27 fmol/ml, respectively. The value for $\Delta_{(AIV-Ao)}$ANP of Group I was less than 50 fmol/ml, indicating that ANP secretion from the ventricle was minimal in these patients. In contrast, $\Delta_{(AIV-Ao)}$ANP of Group II ranged from 72 to 747 fmol/ml, showing that a significant amount of ANP was secreted from the ventricle in Group II. As shown in Fig. 1b, in Group I patients, $\Delta_{(CS-Ao)}$ANP was 10 times greater than $\Delta_{(AIV-Ao)}$ANP. This pattern of ANP secretion in the coronary circulation clearly shows that ANP is secreted predominantly from the atrium. The secretory pattern of hBNP, however, showed a striking contrast with that of ANP. A significant step-up of the BNP-LI level was observed in the AIV, and $\Delta_{(AIV-Ao)}$BNP was comparable to $\Delta_{(CS-Ao)}$BNP, indicating that hBNP is secreted predominantly from the ventricle in these patients. In Group II, $\Delta_{(AIV-Ao)}$BNP, as well as $\Delta_{(CS-Ao)}$BNP, increased significantly compared with those of Group I, and there was also no difference between $\Delta_{(AIV-Ao)}$BNP and $\Delta_{(CS-Ao)}$BNP. Both $\Delta_{(AIV-Ao)}$ANP and $\Delta_{(CS-Ao)}$ANP increased in these patients, and an increase of $\Delta_{(AIV-Ao)}$ANP was evident.

Discussion

The present study demonstrates that hBNP is a novel cardiac hormone, secreted predominantly from the ventricle in humans. The step-up of hBNP concentration in plasma taken at the CS clearly indicates that the major source of circulating hBNP is the heart. Furthermore, a significant step-up in the plasma hBNP level between the Ao and the AIV, which drains the left ventricle but not the atrium [8] (Fig. 1a), clearly demonstrates that hBNP is secreted from the ventricle. Moreover, there was no significant difference between the plasma hBNP levels of the AIV and the CS, suggesting that hBNP secreted from the atrium constitutes a minor portion of hBNP in the CS plasma in these patients. In contrast with hBNP secretion, ANP is secreted predominantly from the atrium, as clearly shown in patients of Group I (Fig. 1b). Although the exact share of the ventricle in hBNP secretion from the whole heart is not clear, it is highly likely that hBNP is secreted predominantly from the ventricle and that the atrial contribution to hBNP secretion is much smaller than its contribution to ANP secretion. These findings in the human heart are consistent with our recent observations of BNP secretion from the rat heart, which showed that approximately 60% of secreted rat BNP was derived from the ventricle [19].

The present study demonstrates that the plasma hBNP level is markedly augmented in patients with CHF, in proportion to the severity of CHF (Fig. 2). The plasma hBNP level reached as high as 500 fmol/ml in the severest cases, although its normal level was 0.90 ± 0.07 fmol/ml. Thus, the percentage increment in the plasma level of hBNP is much greater (one order of magnitude or more) than that of ANP in severe CHF. Furthermore, the present study demonstrates the marked augmentation of $\Delta_{(AIV-Ao)}$BNP in Group II patients (Fig. 1b), showing augmented secretion of hBNP from the ventricle of the failing heart. In addition to the augmented secretion from the heart, the marked increase in the plasma level of hBNP, out of proportion to that of ANP in CHF, could, at least in part, be due to a decreased clearance of hBNP from the circulation, compared to the clearance of ANP. This decreased clearance could be due to a renal or an extra-renal mechanism. Further studies are needed in order to clarify the regulatory mechanism of hBNP secretion from the heart, the clearance of hBNP from the circulation, and the functional role of the markedly increased plasma hBNP in the setting of CHF.

In conclusion, the present study demonstrates that BNP is a novel cardiac hormone, secreted predominantly from the ventricle in humans, and that, in patients with CHF, the plasma level of hBNP is much more augmented than that of ANP.

Combined with the recent discovery of a biologically active receptor relatively specific for BNP [20], these findings suggest a possible pathophysiological role of BNP, distinct from that of ANP, in cardiovascular control, and, furthermore, the findings suggest the presence of an exquisite dual natriuretic peptide system.

Acknowledgments. We thank Drs. H. Matsuo, N. Minamino (National Cardiovascular Center, Suita, Japan), and K. Kangawa (Miyazaki Medical College, Miyazaki, Japan) for kindly providing synthetic peptides. We also thank Drs. Y. Kambayashi, K. Inouye, and N. Yoshida (Shionogi Research Laboratories, Osaka, Japan) for valuable discussion. The excellent secretarial work of Ms. H. Kato, Ms. A. Kibune, and Ms. Y. Kawabata is also gratefully acknowledged.

References

1. De Bold AJ (1985) Atrial natriuretic factor: a hormone produced by the heart. Science 230:767–770
2. Kangawa K, Matsuo H (1984) Purification and complete amino acid sequence of α-human atrial natriuretic polypeptide. Biochem Biophys Res Commun 118:131–139
3. Nakao K, Morii N, Itoh H, Yamada T, Shiono S, Sugawara A, Saito Y, Mukoyama M, Arai H, Sakamoto M, Imura H (1986) Atrial natriuretic polypeptide in brain – implication of central cardiovascular control – J Hyperten 4(Suppl 6):S492–S496
4. Tikkanen I, Fyhrquist F, Metsarinne K, Leidenius R (1985) Plasma atrial natriuretic peptide in cardiac disease and during infusion in healthy volunteers. Lancet II:66–69
5. Burnett JC Jr, Kao PC, Fu DC, Heser DW, Heublein D, Granger JP, Opgenorth TJ, Reeder GS (1986) Atrial natriuretic peptide elevation in congestive heart failure in the human. Science 231:1145–1147
6. Sugawara A, Nakao K, Morii N, Yamada T, Itoh H, Shiono S, Saito Y, Mukoyama M, Arai H, Nishimura K, Obata K, Yasue H, Ban T, Imura H (1988) Synthesis of atrial natriuretic polypeptide (ANP) in human failing hearts – evidence for altered processing of ANP precursor and augmented synthesis of β-human ANP–. J Clin Invest 81: 1962–1970
7. Saito Y, Nakao K, Arai H, Nishimura K, Okumura K, Obata K, Takemura G, Fujiwara H, Sugawara A, Yamada T, Itoh H, Mukoyama M, Hosoda K, Kawai C, Ban T, Yasue H, Imura H (1989) Augmented expression of atrial natriuretic polypeptide gene in ventricle of human failing heart. J Clin Invest 83:298–305
8. Yasue H, Obata K, Okumura K, Kurose M, Ogawa H, Matsuyama K, Jougasaki M, Saito Y, Nakao K, Imura H (1989) Increased secretion of atrial natriuretic polypeptide (ANP) from the left ventricle in patients with dilated cardiomyopathy. J Clin Invest 83:46–51
9. Sudoh T, Kangawa K, Minamino N, Matsuo H (1988) A new natriuretic peptide in porcine brain. Nature 332:78–81
10. Itoh H, Nakao K, Yamada T, Shirakami G, Kangawa K, Minamino N, Matsuo H, Imura H (1988) Antidipsogenic action of a novel peptide "brain natriuretic peptide" in rats. Eur J Pharmacol 150:193–196
11. Shirakami G, Nakao K, Yamada T, Itoh H, Mori K, Kangawa K, Minamino N, Matsuo H, Imura H (1988) Inhibitory effect of brain natriuretic peptide on central angiotensin II-stimulated pressor response in conscious rats. Neurosci Lett 91:77–83
12. Yamada T, Nakao K, Itoh H, Shirakami G, Kangawa K, Minamino N, Matsuo H, Imura H (1988) Intracerebroventricular injection of brain natriuretic peptide inhibits vasopressin secretion in conscious rats. Neurosci Lett 95:223–228

13. Saito Y, Nakao K, Itoh H, Yamada T, Mukoyama M, Arai H, Hosoda K, Shirakami G, Suga S, Minamino N, Kangawa K, Matsuo H, Imura H (1989) Brain natriuretic peptide is a novel cardiac hormone. Biochem Biophys Res Commun 158:360–368
14. Kambayashi Y, Nakao K, Itoh H, Hosoda K, Saito Y, Yamada T, Mukoyama M, Arai H, Shirakami G, Suga S, Ogawa Y, Jougasaki M, Minamino N, Kangawa K, Matsuo H, Inouye K, Imura H (1989) Isolation and sequence determination of rat cardiac natriuretic peptide. Biochem Biophys Res Commun 163:233–240
15. Kambayashi Y, Nakao K, Mukoyama M, Saito Y, Ogawa Y, Shiono S, Inouye K, Yoshida N, Imura H (1990) Isolation and sequence determination of human brain natriuretic peptide in human atrium. FEBS Lett 259:341–345
16. Sudoh T, Maekawa K, Kojima M, Minamino N, Kangawa K, Matsuo H (1989) Cloning and sequence analysis of cDNA encoding a precursor for human brain natriuretic peptide. Biochem Biophys Res Commun 159:1427–1434
17. The Criteria Committee of the New York Heart Association (1964) Diseases of the heart and blood vessels; nomenclature and criteria for diagnosis, 6th edn. Little, Brown, Boston
18. Nakao K, Sugawara A, Morii N, Sakamoto M, Suda M, Soneda J, Ban T, Kihara M, Yamori Y, Shimokura M, Kiso Y, Imura H (1984) Radioimmunoassay for α-human and rat atrial natriuretic polypeptide. Biochem Biophys Res Commun 124:815–821
19. Ogawa Y, Nakao K, Mukoyama M, Shirakami G, Itoh H, Hosoda K, Saito Y, Arai H, Suga S, Jougasaki M, Yamada T, Kambayashi Y, Inouye K, Imura H (1990) Rat brain natriuretic peptide – tissue distribution and molecular form –. Endocrinology 126:2225–2227
20. Chang MS, Lowe DG, Lewis M, Hellmiss R, Chen E, Goeddel DV (1989) Differential activation by atrial and brain natriuretic peptides of two different receptor guanylate cyclases. Nature 341:68–72

Structural and Functional Relationships of Atrial Peptide Receptor Subtypes

J. Gordon Porter, Forrest H. Fuller, Judith A. Miller, Lisa C. Gregory, and John A. Lewicki[1]

SUMMARY. The atrial natriuretic peptides (ANP) elicit numerous biological effects by interacting with multiple ANP receptors. At least three receptors have been characterized. The ANP A-receptor, and a related receptor, the ANP B-receptor, contain an ANP binding domain and guanylate cyclase catalytic activity in a single polypeptide chain. These receptors promote increases in intracellular cyclic guanosine monophosphate (GMP) which then mediate many of the direct biological actions of the atrial natriuretic peptides. A third receptor, the ANP C-receptor, is not a guanylate cyclase. Rather, this receptor mediates the sequestration and metabolic clearance of ANP from the circulation. A cDNA encoding the human ANP C-receptor was cloned from a human kidney cDNA library. The deduced amino acid sequence is 95% identical to that of the bovine ANP C-receptor. In addition, the extracellular binding domain of the human ANP C-receptor is 33% identical with the human ANP A-receptor. The localization of ANP C-receptor mRNA in human adult and fetal kidney and fetal heart provides further evidence that this receptor is operative in mediating the metabolic clearance of ANP in man.

Introduction

The family of atrial natriuretic peptides elicits a number of biological effects directed at the maintenance of blood pressure and extracellular fluid volume [1]. These effects are mediated by the specific binding of the peptides to cell surface receptors that have been characterized in a variety of target tissues, including vasculature, kidney, adrenal, and brain [2]. Pharmacological and molecular cloning studies have demonstrated heterogeneity of the atrial natriuretic peptide receptors, and at least three forms of atrial natriuretic peptide receptors have been identified [3–6]. The dynamic physiological actions of the atrial peptides are regulated by interactions of the peptides with these multiple receptor subtypes.

---

[1]California Biotechnology Inc., 2450 Bayshore Parkway, Mountain View, CA 94043, USA

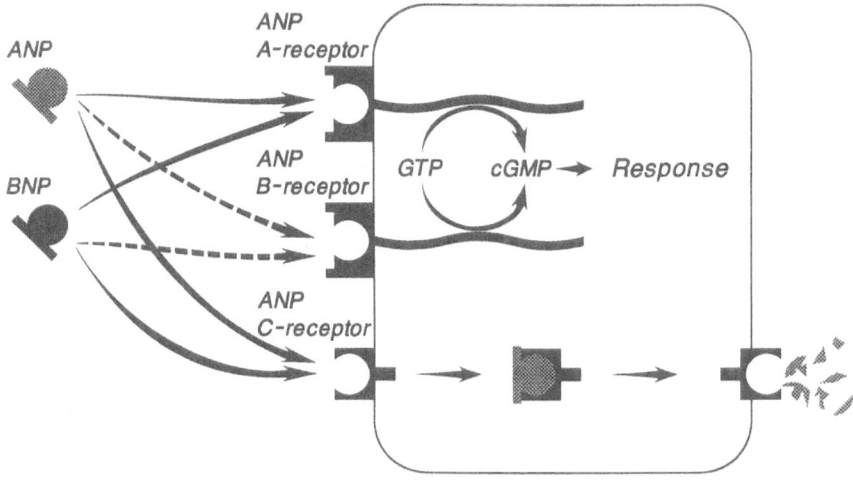

Fig. 1. A model depicting the atrial natriuretic receptor subtypes. GTP, guanosine triphosphate

Our current understanding of the intracellular role and ligand specificity of the ANP receptors is depicted in Fig. 1. The ANP A-receptor has been cloned based on its unique association with particulate guanylate cyclase. The early observations that ANP stimulates particulate guanylate cyclase activity and that ANP binding activity copurifies with particulate guanylate cyclase provided the initial clues for an association between these two molecular entities [7–8]. By screening mammalian cDNA libraries with probes derived from the DNA sequence encoding sea urchin sperm guanylate cyclase, Chinkers et al. were able to identify clones encoding a protein that contains specific ANP binding and guanylate cyclase activity within a single polypeptide chain [5]. This ANP A-receptor is thus characterized by an extracellular ANP binding domain, a single transmembrane region, and an intracellular guanylate cyclase domain. Binding of ANP to this receptor elicits a rise in intracellular levels of cyclic GMP, which presumably then mediates many of the direct biological responses of the peptide. The ANP A-receptor binds both ANP and BNP with high affinity. However, carboxyl terminal truncated ANP analogs interact only weakly with this site.

A related receptor, the ANP B-receptor is similarly comprised of an external ligand binding domain, a single transmembrane domain, and an internal guanylate cyclase region. ANP A- and B- receptors also display several regions of amino acid sequence conservation, particularly in the guanylate cyclase domain. Upon expression in mammalian cells, the ANP B-receptor binds ANP and BNP quite weakly (Kda = 25 μM and 6 μM) and this has led to speculation that an as yet unidentified hormone may be the natural ligand for this site [6].

A third ANP receptor, the ANP C-receptor, mediates the metabolic clearance of ANP [9]. This receptor does not contain a guanylate cyclase domain and is not coupled to the prominent renal, adrenal or hemodynamic actions of these peptides, as specific ANP C-receptor ligands do not have any functional activity in isolated preparations of these tissues. However, this receptor features prominently in the dynamic in vivo actions of the atrial peptides, by regulating the clearance of the hormone, thus affecting circulating ANP levels [10]. This contention is supported by studies in which ANP C-receptor specific ligands are infused into intact animals. By saturating C-receptors, and thus inhibiting clearance of native ANP, these ligands elicit 2–5 fold increases in steady state plasma ANP concentrations, leading to profound natriuresis, diuresis, and suppression of renin and aldosterone [9,11]. The ANP C-receptor is comprised of an external ligand binding domain, a single transmembrane domain, and a short cytoplasmic sequence of 37 amino acids. The C-receptor binds ANP and BNP with high affinity ($^\sim$1 nM) and also avidly binds small truncated analogs of these peptides, including a linear octapeptide fragment derived from within the 17-membered ring of ANP [12].

The atrial peptide receptors have been cloned from several species. However, the ANP C-receptor has not been well characterized in man. We have now cloned the human ANP C-receptor, and are now able to make a detailed comparison of this protein to the previously described bovine C-receptor and to the human ANP A-receptor.

Materials and Methods

Library Screening

An oligo dT primed human kidney library, propagated in bacteriophage λ gt 11 vector, was plated onto E. coli host strain cf 1600, and transferred in duplicate onto nitrocellulose filters using standard techniques. Approximately 10^6 recombinant phage were screened using nick-translated bovine ANP C-receptor cDNA (ANPRc1/4) (Fuller et al., 1988 [4]) as a hybridization probe, as discussed below. The DNA bound to the nitrocellulose filters was denatured, the filters were baked at 80°C for 2h and prehybridized in a solution containing 50% formamide, 5 × Denhardt's solution, 6X SSC (1X SSC is 0.16 M NaCl, 0.016 M Na Citrate), 50 mM NaPO$_4$, and 10 μg/ml sheared salmon sperm DNA at 42°C. Hybridization was performed in the same solution plus 1.0×10^6 cpm ^{32}P-labelled probe per filter at 42°C. After hybridization, the filters were washed in 6X SSC, 0.1% SDS two times at room temperature, and once each in 6X SSC, 55°C for 15 min and 1X SSC, 55°C for 15 min. Filters were exposed to X-ray film for 1–3 days. Of 11 original hybridizing plaques, 3 were followed through subsequent rounds of purification. DNA inserts from these phage were isolated and subcloned into M13 for sequence determination as described below. One of these clones (clone 1) was used to screen a human placental cDNA library; subsequently a second human kidney library from which clones corresponding to the 5′ half of the cDNA were isolated.

Northern Blot Analysis

Poly(A)$^+$ RNA was isolated from human fetal lung and kidney tissue by the guanidinium isothiocyanate method as described by Chirgwin et al. [13], followed by oligo(dT)-cellulose chromatography. RNA was first denatured in formamide and formaldehyde at 50°C and was then fractionated on a 1.4% agarose gel containing 40 mM morpholinopropanesulfonic acid (pH 7.0), 10 mM sodium acetate, 1 mM

EDTA, and 2.2 M formaldehyde, and was transferred to nitrocellulose. Mobilities of RNA size standards (BRL) were determined by ethidium bromide staining prior to transfer. RNA was attached to nitrocellulose by baking the filters at 80°C for 2 h. The filters were hybridized in 50% formamide, 5X SSC, using, as probe, purified insert DNA from a cDNA clone (clone 1) encoding a portion of the human ANP C-receptor. DNA was radiolabelled with ^{32}P-nucleotide triphosphates by nick-translation. Filters were washed in 6X SSC, 0.1% SDS at room temperature for 20 min, and then in 1X SSC, 0.1% SDS at 65°C for 20 min and were analyzed by autoradiography.

DNA Sequencing

All DNA sequences were determined using the enzymatic method [14] by subcloning into M13 [15] and were confirmed from overlapping DNA strands. Sequences were analyzed using the Gel and Seq programs (Intellicorp, Inc., Mountain View, Calif.).

Results and Discussion

Several partial length cDNA clones encoding the human ANP C-receptor were isolated from human kidney cDNA libraries (see Materials and Methods). An analysis of overlapping sequences and comparison with bovine ANP C-receptor sequences allowed construction of a complete cDNA encompassing the complete coding region. A schematic of the human ANP C-receptor is shown in Fig. 2.

The open reading frame of 1626 nucleotides, deduced by homology with the bovine ANP C-receptor, defines a 541 amino acid sequence containing a signal peptide sequence and a pro-receptor domain. The predicted length of the mature human ANP C-receptor is 496 amino acids. The receptor is highly conserved (95%) and differs from the bovine C-receptor at only 27 of 496 amino acids which are scattered throughout the molecule. The five cysteines within the extracellular domain are conserved in both species and are likely to be important for receptor conformation. Four consensus sequences for N-linked glycosylation sites are completely conserved, although glycosylation of the human C-receptor has not yet been demonstrated.

A schematic of the human A-receptor, derived from the sequence of Lowe et al. [16], is also shown in Fig. 2. The extracellular domains of these two proteins are 33% homologous, but the protein sequence diverges completely in the cytoplasmic region. The ANP C-receptor contains only 37 cytoplasmic amino acids, while the ANP A-receptor is comprised of 568 amino acids within the cell. It is noteworthy that if the ANP C-receptor has a function in addition to clearance, the signalling mechanism would have to be contained in this abbreviated intracellular region. An analysis of the two proteins reveals that the cysteine residues of the C-receptor are conserved in the A-receptor. However, the extracellular domain of the A-receptor contains two additional cysteines. Thus, the tertiary structure of the two proteins may differ. This would not be surprising in view of the differential ligand specificity of the two receptors.

With respect to potential ligand binding domains, it is interesting to note that a 28 amino stretch of the ANP A-receptor and the ANP C-receptor (amino acid residues 132–159) is more than 75% conserved between these receptors [16]. It seems quite significant that this 28 amino acid region is completely identical in the human and bovine

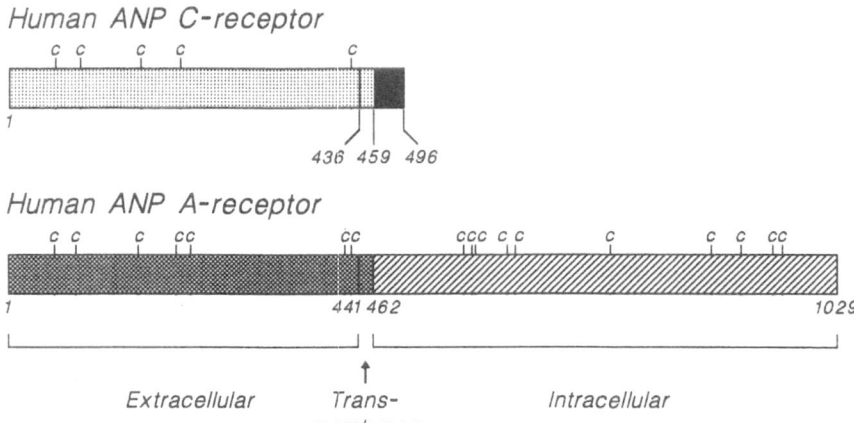

Fig. 2. Schematic representations of the human ANP A-receptor and human ANP C-receptor. *C* denotes cysteine residues. The *numbers below* each receptor represent amino acid positions beginning with the first Met of the predicted open reading frame

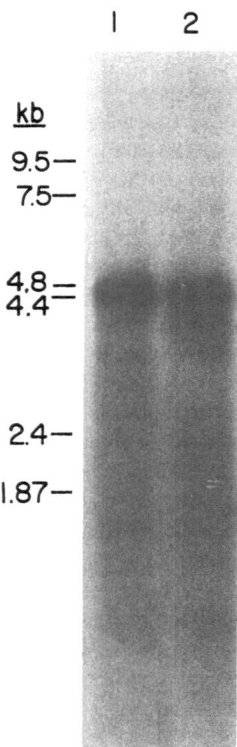

Fig. 3. Northern blots of human ANP C-receptor mRNA from human fetal lung (*lane 1*) or fetal heart (*lane 2*). Northern blots were performed as described in Materials and Methods

ANP C-receptors. Competition binding experiments with $125_{I\text{-}ANP}$ following transient expression of the human and bovine ANP C-receptors in mammalian cells demonstrated comparable high affinity for ANP (6×10^{-9}M), suggesting that this conserved extracellular region may be important in ligand recognition. Further studies are necessary to define the potential significance of this region of the molecule.

The functional significance of the ANP C-receptor in man is supported by its presence in several human tissues. Northern blots of poly A^+ mRNA from human fetal heart and kidney are shown in Fig. 3. Unlike the mRNA for the bovine C-receptor, which exhibits size heterogeneity in a number of tissues and cell lines [4], the human receptor is encoded by a single 5.4 kb mRNA in these tissues. Similar hybridization intensity is observed in both tissues, suggesting a comparable abundance of ANP C-receptor mRNA in each tissue. While the clearance function of the C-receptor has been well characterized in kidney, its possible role in the heart is unclear. While it has been suggested recently that the C-receptor may also be coupled to signal transduction [13], further data is needed to validate this proposal. Nevertheless, it is interesting to speculate on a possible role for the ANP C-receptor in regulating cardiac function, or perhaps in the release of ANP in man.

In summary, molecular cloning studies have afforded a detailed understanding of the structural relationships between the ANP receptor subtypes. It is anticipated that similar studies may uncover additional atrial peptide receptors in the upcoming months. When coupled with our current understanding of the functional role of these receptors, this information provides an appreciation of the complex and dynamic manner in which the natriuretic peptides regulate cardiovascular and renal homeostasis.

References

1. Baxter JD, Lewicki JA, Gardner DG (1988) Atrial natriuretic peptide. Bio/Technology 6:529–546
2. Leitman DC, Andresen JW, Kuno T, Kamisaki Y, Chang JK, Murad F (1986) Identification of multiple binding sites for atrial natriuretic factor by affinity cross-linking in cultured endothelial cells. J Biol Chem 261:11650–11655
3. Scarborough RM, Schenk DB, McEnroe G, Arfsten A, Kang L-L, Schwartz K, Lewicki JA (1986) Truncated atrial natriuretic peptide (ANP) analogs: comparison between receptor binding affinity and cyclic GMP stimulation in cultured aortic smooth muscle cells. J Biol Chem 261:12960–12964
4. Fuller F, Porter G, Arfsten A, Miller J, Schilling J, Scarborough RM, Lewicki JA, Schenk D (1988) Atrial natriuretic peptide clearance receptor: complete sequence and functional expression of cDNA clones. J Biol Chem 263:9395–9401
5. Chinkers M, Garbers DD, Chang M-S, Lowe DG, Chin H, Goeddel DV, Schulz S (1989) A membrane form of guanylate cyclase is an atrial natriuretic peptide receptor. Nature 338:78–83
6. Chang M-S, Lowe DG, Lewis M, Hellmin R, Chen E, Goeddel DV (1989) Differential activation by atrial and brain natriuretic peptides of two different receptor guanylate cyclases. Nature 341:68–71
7. Waldman S, Rapoport RM, Murad F (1984) Atrial natriuretic factor selectively activates particulate guanylate cyclase and elevates cyclic GMP in rat tissues. J Biol Chem 259:14322–14344

8. Kuno T, Andresen JW, Kamisaki Y, Waldman SA, Chang LY, Saheki S, Leitman DC, Nakane M, Murad F (1986) Co-purification of an atrial natriuretic factor receptor and particulate guanylate cyclase from rat lung. J Biol Chem 261:5817-5823

9. Maack T, Suzuki M, Almeida FA, Nussenzveig D, Scarborough RM, McEnroe GA, Lewicki JA (1987) Physiological role of silent receptors of atrial natriuretic factor. Science 238:675-678

10. Almeida FA, Suzuki M, Scarborough RM, Lewicki JA, Maack T (1989) Clearance function of type C receptors of atrial natriuretic factor in rats. Am J Physiol 256:R469-R475

11. Gregory LC, Scarborough RM, Metzler CH, McEnroe GA, Maack T, Lewicki JA (1988) Effects of acute infusion of a C-ANP receptor specific compound in conscious dog. J Cell Biochem [Suppl] 12A:23

12. Scarborough RM, Arfsten A, Kang L-L, Schwartz K, McEnroe GA, Porter JG, Suzuki M, Maack T, Lewicki JA (1988) Linear fragments of ANPs bind to C-ANP receptors with high affinity. J Cell Biochem [Suppl] 12A:20

13. Chirgwin JM, Pryzbyla AE, MacDonald RJ, Rutter NJ (1979) Isolation of biologically active ribonucleic acid from sources enriched in ribonuclease. Biochemistry 18:5294-5299

14. Sanger F, Nicklen S, Coulsen AR (1977) DNA sequencing with chain-terminating inhibitors. Proc Natl Acad Sci USA 74:5463-69

15. Messing J (1983) New M13 vectors for cloning. In: Grossman L, Moldave K (eds) Methods enzymology 101. Academic, New York, pp 20-78

16. Lowe DG, Chang M-S, Hellmin R, Chen E, Singh S, Garbers DL, Goeddel DV (1989) Human atrial natriuretic peptide receptor defines a new paradigm for second messenger signal transduction. EMBO J 8:1377-1384

17. Anand-Srivastava MB, Sairam MR, Cantin M (1990) Ring-deleted analogs of atrial natriuretic factor inhibit adenylate cyclase/cAMP system. J Biol Chem 265:8566-8572

Functional Properties and Cell Biology of Renal and Vascular Receptors of Atrial Natriuretic Factor

DANIEL R. NUSSENZVEIG, BEATRIZ M.A. FONTOURA, JURAJ OKOLICANY, AKIRA OWADA, and THOMAS MAACK[1]

Introduction

Atrial natriuretic factor (ANF) is secreted mainly by the heart atria in response to volume expansion and increases in atrial pressure or stretch. The hormone has important effects in several tissues, resulting in modulation of plasma volume, extracellular fluid volume, and blood pressure (for review, see [1,2]). There are two general classes of ANF receptors in peripheral tissues. Biological receptors proper (B-ANF receptors) mediate the ANF-induced increase in cGMP and many, if not all, of the physiological effects of the hormone [3]. These receptors were shown to contain guanylate cyclase in the cytoplasmic domain of their molecules [4]. This is a first example of a biological receptor which directly catalyzes the formation of a small second messenger upon hormone binding [4]. The other class of ANF receptors is widely distributed, at orders of magnitude larger in density than B-ANF receptors, in several tissues and cells, including kidney cortex, endothelial and vascular smooth muscle cells, and fibroblasts. The functional and biochemical nature of this receptor (named C-ANF receptor) has been fully characterized [5,6]. C-ANF receptors do not mediate any of the known effects of the hormone, but have an important role in the removal of ANF from the circulation [5]. This is a first example of a separate class of clearance receptors for a circulating polypeptide hormone. The extracellular domains of B-ANF receptors and C-ANF receptors have considerable homology [4], explaining the finding that both receptors have a similar very high affinity for native ANF_{1-28} [3,7].

In this overview, we will briefly consider some of the work done by our laboratory on the distribution and function of renal and vascular receptors of ANF.

[1]Department of Physiology and Cardiovascular Center, Cornell University Medical College, New York, NY 10021, USA

Renal Receptors of ANF

Renal Effects of ANF

ANF has complex renal vascular, hemodynamic, and tubular effects [1,2,8-20]. ANF increases glomerular filtration without necessarily increasing renal blood flow [8-14]. This is due to an efferent vasoconstrictive effect of ANF that may or may not be accompanied by an afferent dilation [8,10,11,13,14]. As a result, glomerular capillary hydrostatic pressure rises, increasing glomerular filtration rate (GFR) [10,13]. In addition, ANF is a potent antagonist of renal vasoconstriction induced by hormonal or non-hormonal agents [8,11]. ANF may also increase the glomerular ultrafiltration coefficient, which further contributes to the increase in GFR [13]. Consistent with these effects are the autoradiographic findings showing that ANF receptors are distributed in glomerular and vascular structures of the kidney cortex [21,22].

More controversial is whether or not ANF has direct or even indirect proximal tubular actions. Attempts to detect such effects by micropuncture or isolated perfused tubule techniques were, in general, negative [14]. Nevertheless, the increase in fractional lithium clearance and the increase in phosphate excretion have been interpreted to suggest a proximal tubular action of the hormone [12]. However, up to the present, investigators have been unable to detect ANF receptors or ANF-induced increase in cGMP in proximal tubule preparations [23]. Recently, however, it has been shown that ANF is able to antagonize angiotensin II-induced increase in proximal tubule sodium and water reabsorption [19].

ANF has marked effects on the renal papilla, decreasing the hypertonicity of its interstitium [1,2,9] and directly or indirectly impairing load-reabsorption balance of sodium in papillary collecting ducts [15]. In view of the close apposition of vascular, interstitial, and epithelial structures in the renal papilla, autoradiographic studies on the localization of ANF receptors in this kidney region are inconclusive [21,22]. ANF specific binding and generation of cGMP was detected in isolated papillary collecting duct, but not in outer medullary segments of collecting ducts, and only to a very small extent in thick ascending limb of Henle's loop and cortical collecting ducts [24]. Accordingly, specific binding, generation of cGMP, and inhibition of sodium uptake occur in purified suspensions of cells from papillary collecting duct but not in those from medullary collecting duct or Henle's loop [16,17]. Patch clamp experiments in cultured inner papillary collecting duct cells indicate that ANF is able to block an amiloride-sensitive cation channel in these cells [25]. Furthermore, ANF directly inhibits NaCl cotransport in isolated perfused cortical collecting ducts of the rat [22]. Finally, we recently detected major specific binding of ANF and generation of cGMP in cultured renomedullary interstitial cells from the rat (see below).

ANF Receptors in the Rat Kidney

Studies in the isolated perfused rat kidney show that the kidney cortex contains more than 95% of the total renal population of ANF receptors. Cortical receptors of ANF have a very high density (Bmax = 7 pmoles/g tissue) and affinity (Kd = 50 pM). On the other hand, the renal papilla contains fewer than 2% of the renal binding sites of ANF, but the density of these sites is fairly high (Bmax = 3 pmoles/g tissue) [26].

In the isolated rat kidney there is an almost perfect identity between the binding curves of ANF_{1-28} in the kidney cortex and the dose-response curves of renal vascular (relaxation of pre-constricted renal vasculature), hemodynamic (increase in GFR and filtration fraction (FF)) and excretory (increase in excretion of fluid and electrolytes) effects of ANF [26]. Specific binding and renal effects of ANF are detectable at ANF perfusate concentrations of 10–100 pM, which are near normal plasma levels of ANF in the rat. Furthermore, the ED_{50} of ANF effects is very close to its Kd of binding (50–100 pM), and maximal effects are observed at ANF concentrations that lead to saturation of its specific binding sites (1–10 nM). The very high affinity of cortical binding sites, together with the low ED_{50} of ANF effects, is further evidence that this hormone is an important endogenous modulator of renal vascular resistance, glomerular filtration rate, and fluid and electrolyte excretion.

Clearance Receptors of ANF in the Kidney

The overwhelming majority of renal receptors of ANF is constituted by C-ANF receptors that, in contrast to B-ANF receptors, do not mediate any of the known renal effects of the hormone. Binding and effects of ring-C terminal deleted analogues of ANF such as Des[Gln^{18}, Ser^{19}, Gly^{20}, Leu^{21}, Gly^{22}]rANF4-23-NH_2 (henceforth referred to as C-ANF)$_{4-23}$ were tested in the isolated perfused rat kidney preparation [5]. $C-ANF_{4-23}$, similarly to ANF_{1-28}, displaced more than 95% of [^{125}I]-ANF_{1-28} from its binding sites in whole kidney and kidney cortex at a perfusate concentration of 100 nM. On the other hand, in the renal papilla $C-ANF_{4-23}$ displaced only 50% of [^{125}I]-ANF_{1-28} from its binding sites. Competition binding studies further demonstrated that the apparent affinity of $C-ANF_{4-23}$ for ANF receptors was very high, only 5–10 times lower than that of native ANF_{1-28}. These experiments demonstrated that $C-ANF_{4-23}$ binds with high affinity to the overwhelming majority of ANF receptors in whole kidney and kidney cortex.

Excess prefusate concentration of $C-ANF_{4-23}$ (1 μM) had no effects on its own in any of the measured renal function parameters in the isolated perfused rat kidney, including GFR, FF, renal vascular resistance, and fluid and electrolyte excretion. Furthermore, this excess concentration also did not alter the dose-response curves of ANF_{1-28} on the above mentioned parameters. Thus, $C-ANF_{4-23}$ had no agonist or antagonist action, in spite of occupying more than 95% of the total ANF receptor population in the isolated rat kidney [5]. On the basis of these results, we concluded that the overwhelming majority of renal receptors of ANF is biologically silent, in the sense that they did not mediate any of the known renal effects of the hormone. We further postulated that these receptors, which we named C-ANF receptors, may serve as peripheral storage/clearance binding sites for ANF and that in this manner they play an important role in the removal of ANF from the circulation and in the plasma homeostasis of the hormone [5]. Conclusive evidence that this is indeed the case is summarized below.

The Clearance Role of C-ANF Receptors in the Rat

$C-ANF_{4-23}$ was administered to intact conscious and/or anesthetized rats to determine whether blockage of C-ANF receptors increased plasma levels of endogenous immunoreactive (ir)ANF, induced renal and systemic effects, and altered the metabolism of ANF.

Constant infusion of $C\text{-}ANF_{4\text{-}23}$ practically doubled plasma levels of endogenous irANF [5,7]. The increase in plasma irANF induced by blockage of C-ANF receptors in anesthetized rats was accompanied by expected renal and systemic effects [5,7]. Mean blood pressure decreased slightly, but significantly, by approximately 10 mmHg and GFR, urine volume, and sodium excretion were significantly increased. The quantitative effects of the infusion of $1\mu g/kg$ per min of $C\text{-}ANF_{4\text{-}23}$ corresponded to those obtained by an infusion of native $ANF_{1\text{-}28}$ (0.02–0.03 µg/min per Kg body wt) that increased plasma irANF to the same extent as that obtained by the infusion of $C\text{-}ANF_{4\text{-}23}$. The results of these studies indicate that blockage of C-ANF receptors increases plasma levels of endogenous ANF, which in turn leads to natriuretic and blood pressure lowering effects. The results of these experiments also show that relatively modest increases in plasma ANF are biologically effective, which further attests to the significance of this hormone as a modulator of plasma volume and blood pressure.

Administration of $C\text{-}ANF_{4\text{-}23}$ (1 µg/min per Kg body wt) markedly altered the pharmacokinetics of a single bolus injection of $[^{125}I]\text{-}ANF_{1\text{-}28}$ in intact anesthetized rats [27]. Thus, $C\text{-}ANF_{4\text{-}23}$ reduced the apparent volume of distribution at steady state (Vss) and metabolic clearance rate (MCR) to half of the control value, consistent with the doubling of the plasma levels of endogenous irANF by this dose of the C-ANF receptor ligand. Saturating doses of $C\text{-}ANF_{4\text{-}23}$ (10 µg/min per Kg body wt) led to further reduction of Vss to one-third, and of MCR to one-quarter of control values. With the higher dose there was a significant increase in plasma half-life of administered $[^{125}I]\text{-}ANF_{1\text{-}28}$. These results demonstrate that binding to C-ANF receptors is responsible for the very large apparent volume of distribution of ANF and that these receptors are importantly involved in the removal of the hormone from the circulation. Correspondingly, blockage of C-ANF receptors also led to a marked delay in the appearance of $[^{125}I]\text{-}ANF_{1\text{-}28}$ hydrolytic products in plasma. This further demonstrates that a major fraction of ANF metabolism in the rat is due to C-ANF receptor-mediated hydrolysis of the peptide.

In our laboratory we have recently shown that small linear peptide analogues of ANF, containing 5 amino acids of the ring structure of native $ANF_{1\text{-}28}$, bind to C-ANF but not to B-ANF receptors. The effects of these small linear peptide analogues on plasma levels, volume of distribution, and metabolic clearance rate of ANF were similar to those described above for $C\text{-}ANF_{4\text{-}23}$ [28]. These findings raise hopes for the future development and use of orally active ligands of C-ANF receptors.

ANF Receptor Subtypes in Isolated Glomeruli

Glomeruli are a major site for ANF action and also receive a large fraction of the cardiac output. Accordingly, isolated glomeruli were shown to contain a high density of ANF receptors and to generate cGMP in a dose-dependent manner when incubated with biologically active atrial peptides [29]. Studies in our laboratory have demonstrated that the majority (approximately 80%) of the total ANF receptor population in isolated glomeruli is constituted by C-ANF receptors [30].

ANF Receptor Subtypes in Cultured Glomerular Mesangial Cells

Saturation binding studies using $[^{125}I]$-ANF_{1-28} showed that the density of total ANF receptors in cultured mesangial cells was 28 fmoles/million cells with a Kd of 77 pM [30,31]. Saturation binding studies with $[^{125}I]$-(Y^3)-C-ANF_{3-23}, a specific ligand of C-ANF receptors, show a similar affinity (Kd = 83 pM) but a lower density of binding sites (Bmax = 9.6 fmoles/million cells) than that obtained for the total ANF receptor population [32]. Saturation binding studies with $[^{125}I]$-ANF_{1-28} in the presence of 0.1 μM C-ANF_{4-23}, a concentration that occupies all C-ANF receptors available, showed a receptor density of 20.0 fmoles/million cells with a Kd of 241 pM. Thus, C-ANF receptors constitute approximately 30% of the total ANF receptor population in mesangial cells. This value is much lower than the proportion of C-ANF receptors in whole isolated glomeruli (80%). Different passages of cultured glomerular mesangial cells express the proportion of surface ANF receptors variably. Thus in later passages (after the 20th passage) of cloned cultured glomerular mesangial cells we found that surface C-ANF receptor became undetectable, whereas there was no change or even an increase in density of surface B-ANF receptors compared to the earlier passages.

ANF_{1-28} generates a dose-related increase in cGMP in cultured mesangial cells, with a maximal generation of 106 ± 9 pmoles of cGMP/2 min per million cells and an ED_{50} of 5 nM. C-ANF_{4-23} (1 μM) did not generate cGMP and did not potentiate or antagonize the cGMP generating effect of ANF_{1-28} [31]. Thus, cultured glomerular mesangial cells have functionally distinct B-ANF and C-ANF receptors with a similar very high affinity for native ANF_{1-28}. Furthermore, it is apparent that B-ANF and C-ANF receptors do not interact as far as generation of the second messenger (cGMP) is concerned.

ANF Receptor Subtypes in Cultured Renomedullary Interstitial Cells (RMIC)

Binding studies in the isolated perfused rat kidney preparation have revealed that the renal papilla contains B-ANF and C-ANF receptors at fairly high densities and in almost identical proportions [26]. Freshly prepared suspensions of inner medullary collecting duct cells were shown to contain guanylate cyclase-coupled B-ANF receptors [16,17], but their receptor density is too low to account for the whole receptor density that we observed in the papilla. Since renomedullary interstitial cells are a prevalent cell type of the renal medulla, we developed a culture of renomedullary interstitial cells (RMIC) from the rat to determine ANF receptor subpopulations in these cells [32]. Electron microscopy of the cultured cells showed the typical features of RMIC in vivo, including prominent lipid droplets. Equilibrium saturation and competition binding studies showed a very high density of high affinity binding sites for the native form of the hormone, ANF_{1-28} (Bmax = 23,000 sites/cell; Kd = 50 pM). There was only minimal binding of C-ANF_{4-23}, a specific ligand of C-ANF receptors. ANF_{1-28} markedly increased cGMP from 1.3 ± 0.3 to 106 ± 22 pmoles cGMP/2 min per million cells, with an ED_{50} of 1.2 nM. The effect of ANF_{1-28} on cGMP was nearly additive to that of sodium nitroprusside and was not potentiated or antagonized by C-ANF_{4-23}. The results demonstrate that in contrast to the whole kidney tissue, the overwhelming majority of ANF receptors in RMIC are guanylate cyclase coupled B-ANF receptors. The density of B-ANF receptors in RMIC is the highest reported to date in the literature for any cell type. The maximal ANF-induced generation of cGMP is equivalent to that found in glomerular mesangial cells in our laboratory and is also one of the highest reported to date in other cells. The results indicate that RMIC are an important target cell for ANF in the renal papilla. This suggests that RMIC may mediate some of the known effects of ANF in this kidney region and/or may influence the secretion of an anti-hypertensive substance(s) by these cells. Further work is needed to clarify the exact role of the effects of ANF in renomedullary interstitial cells.

Cellular Mechanisms of C-ANF Receptor-Mediated Hydrolysis of ANF

Specific receptor-mediated endocytosis and lysosomal hydrolysis is a common mechanism by which peptide hormones, as well as non-hormonal proteins, are disposed of by cells [33]. Lysosomotropic weak bases, such as NH_4Cl or chloroquine, by virtue of increasing the normally low pH of lysosomes, are universal and specific inhibitors of lysosomal hydrolysis of peptidic substances. Therefore, in order to test whether lysosomal hydrolysis is implicated in the metabolism of ANF mediated by C-ANF receptors we first determined the effects of NH_4Cl on the hydrolysis of ANF in the isolated perfused rat kidney [34]. In this preparation, NH_4Cl as well as chloroquine practically abolished the renal hydrolysis of $[^{125}I]$-ANF$_{1-28}$, demonstrating that lysosomal hydrolysis is the major mode of renal metabolism of ANF. Since binding to C-ANF receptors accounts for > 95% of the total accumulation of ANF in the kidney, these results are consistent with the interpretation that renal metabolism of ANF is due to C-ANF receptor-mediated endocytosis with subsequent delivery of ANF to lysosomes where it undergoes complete hydrolysis to amino acids. To gain further insights into this process we used cultured cells with an absolute predominance and high density of C-ANF receptors. Results of these studies are briefly summarized below.

Metabolism of ANF Mediated by C-ANF Receptors in 3T3 Swiss Albino Mouse Fibroblasts

Binding studies in cultured 3T3 Swiss albino mouse fibroblasts have shown that these cells have high affinity C-ANF receptors with a density of approximately 20000 receptors/cell, but no detectable B-ANF receptors [35]. Experiments of cell internalization and metabolism of $[^{125}I]$-ANF$_{1-28}$ have shown that radioiodinated ANF$_{1-28}$ is internalized in a temperature-dependent manner: there is no receptor internalization at 4°C, receptors are internalized at an initial rate of 4% of occupied C-ANF receptors/min at 22°C and 12% of occupied C-ANF receptors/min at 37°C. Of the internalized peptide, 51% and 74% is released as $[^{125}I]$-monoiodotyrosine to the medium by 15 min of incubation at 22°C and 37°C, respectively. NH_4Cl had no effect on the rate of internalization of $[^{125}I]$-ANF$_{1-28}$, but markedly reduced the appearance of $[^{125}I]$-monoiodotyrosine in the medium to 4% and 40% of the internalized peptide by 15 min of incubation at 22°C and 37°C, respectively. Blockage of C-ANF receptors by C-ANF$_{4-23}$ or ANF$_{1-28}$ practically abolished the internalization and hydrolysis of [^{125}I]ANF$_{1-28}$ [35]. These results demonstrate that C-ANF receptor-mediated endocytosis and delivery of the ligand to lysosomes is the basic mechanism of ANF removal from the circulation.

C-ANF Receptor-Mediated Internalization of ^{125}I-ANF$_{1-28}$ and Receptor Recycling in Cultured Aorta Smooth Muscle Cells

To further study the cell physiology of C-ANF receptor-mediated clearance of ANF, we determined internalization and recycling, as well as retroendocytosis and lysosomal hydrolysis, of atrial peptides in cultured bovine vascular smooth muscle cells [36,38]. These cells have the highest density of C-ANF receptors (200000–500000 sites/cell) reported to date in the literature [30]. At 37°C, C-ANF receptors internalized at a rate of 4.7% of occupied receptors/min. After 30 min incubation, 50% of [^{125}I]-ANF$_{1-28}$ initially bound to C-ANF receptors was hydrolysed and the product of hydrolysis ([^{125}I]-monoiodotyrosine) was released to the medium. Hydrolysis of [^{125}I]-ANF$_{1-28}$ was practically abolished when cells were incubated in the presence of NH$_4$Cl (10 mM) or excess (0.1 µM) C-ANF$_{4-23}$ or ANF$_{1-28}$. Retroendocytosis of intact [^{125}I]-ANF$_{1-28}$ was also detected when intracellular accumulation of the intact labeled peptide was maximized by previous incubation with NH$_4$Cl. Experiments designed to study the fate of internalized C-ANF receptors revealed that these receptors recycle back to the cell surface after dissociation from their ligand in endosomes. In this manner, surface C-ANF receptor density decreased to 56% and then returned to 93% of its initial value by incubation with saturating concentrations of [^{125}I]-ANF$_{1-28}$, for 15 and 60 min, respectively. At 60 min, the amount of labeled peptide which was hydrolyzed corresponded to one complete cycle of the total population of surface C-ANF receptors [36,38]. Similar results were obtained with [^{125}I](Y^3)-C-ANF$_{3-23}$, a labeled specific ligand of C-ANF receptors [37]. Cycloheximide, a potent protein synthesis inhibitor, does not interfere with cell surface C-ANF receptor replenishment. Detergent solubilization and cell surface receptor trypsinization have shown that the intracellular C-ANF receptor pool is small and cannot account for the cell surface C-ANF receptor replenishment. Consequently, these results demonstrate that cell surface C-ANF receptor replenishment is due to receptor reutilization [38]. Furthermore, experiments showed that C-ANF receptor internalization and recycling did not depend on the presence of the ligand.

In summary, the results of this study demonstrate that ANF molecules bound to C-ANF receptors are rapidly internalized. After dissociation from their receptors in endosomes, ANF molecules are delivered to lysosomes, where they undergo complete hydrolysis. There is some retroendocytosis of receptor-ligand complexes, but the actual degree and physiological role of this process remain to be elucidated. Internalized C-ANF receptors are rapidly recycled to the cell membrane, thus becoming available to mediate another cycle of internalization and lysosomal hydrolysis of ANF. This process is independent of the presence of the ligand. From the data it can be calculated that in cultured vascular smooth muscle cells, the entire population of C-ANF receptors is internalized and recycled every hour. Finally, due to rapid and complete recycling, there is no short-term down regulation of C-ANF receptors by ANF.

The effectiveness of C-ANF receptors in the exercise of their clearance function is due to the combination of a very high affinity for ANF, wide distribution in strategic organs and tissues, rapid internalization, and constant availability due to rapid recycling.

Conclusions

In this brief review of recent studies in our laboratory we have summarized the evidence showing that there are two functionally distinct classes of ANF receptors. B-ANF receptors mediate the ANF-induced increase in cGMP and the known renal and systemic effects of the hormone; these receptors are found in many tissues and cells including adrenal, vascular smooth muscle, and endothelial cells. They are also prevalent kidney structures, particularly in glomerular mesangial cells and renomedullary interstitial cells. C-ANF receptors do not mediate increases in cCMP or any of the known renal or systemic effects of ANF, but have a major role in the removal of ANF from the circulation. However, it cannot be ruled out at present that C-ANF receptors may also mediate some unknown effect of ANF. C-ANF receptors constitute the overwhelming majority of the total ANF receptor population in several tissues, including the kidney cortex. They are strategically located for their clearance function, with prevalent localization in vascular smooth muscle cells, glomeruli, endothelial cells, and fibroblasts. The cellular mechanisms of the clearance function of C-ANF receptors were recently elucidated in our laboratory. ANF binds with high affinity to these receptors and the receptor-ligand complex is rapidly internalized. The internalized hormone is delivered to lysosomes, where it undergoes complete hydrolysis to amino acids, whereas the internalized C-ANF receptors are rapidly recycled to the cell surface. In this manner, the location, high density, high affinity, and rapid recycling of C-ANF receptors make them ideally suited to remove ANF from the circulation.

The results of our studies provide the first evidence of a separate class of clearance receptors for a polypeptide hormone. The full physiological implications of this finding remain to be elucidated, but it is likely that C-ANF receptors contribute importantly to the plasma homeostasis of ANF by acting as a hormonal buffer system. In addition, specific ligands of C-ANF receptors may be therapeutically useful since, by blocking the clearance function of this receptor, they increase the plasma levels of endogenous ANF and, consequently, increase desirable natriuretic and blood pressure lowering effects.

Acknowledgment. Research was supported by NIH Grant DK 14241.

References

1. Maack T (1986) Atrial natriuretic factor: a physiological link between the heart and the kidney. In: Bromm B, Luggers DW (eds) Physiologie Aktuell, vol 2. Gustav Fisher, Stuttgart, pp 59–85
2. Atlas SA, Maack T (1987) Effects of atrial natriuretic factor on the kidney and the renin-angiotensin-aldosterone system. Endocrinol Metab Clin North Am 16:107–143
3. Leitman DC, Murad F (1987) Atrial natriuretic factor receptor heterogeneity and stimulation of particulate guanylate cyclase and cyclic GMP accumulation. Endocrinol Metab Clin North Am 16:79–105

4. Chinkers M, Garbers DL, Chang MS, Lowe DG, Chin HM, Goeddel DV, Schulz S (1989) A membrane form of guanylate cyclase is an atrial natriuretic peptide receptor. Nature 338:78–83
5. Maack T, Suzuki M, Almeida FA, Nussenzveig D, Scarborough RM, McEnroe GA, Lewicki JA (1987) Physiological role of silent receptors of atrial natriuretic factor. Science 238:675–678
6. Fuller F, Porter JG, Arfsten AE, Miller J, Schilling JW, Scarborough RM, Lewicki JA, Schenk DB (1988) Atrial natriuretic peptide clearance receptor. Complete sequence and functional expression of cDNA clones. J Biol Chem 263:9395–9401
7. Maack T, Suzuki M, Nussenzveig DR, Owada A, Scarborough RM, Lewicki JA, Almeida FA (1988) Clearance receptors of atrial natriuretic factor. In: Needleman P (ed) UCLA symposia on molecular and cellular biology new series. Alan R. Liss, New York, pp 57–76 (Biological and molecular aspects of atrial factors, vol 81)
8. Camargo MJ, Kleinert HD, Atlas SA, Sealey JE, Laragh JH, Maack T (1984) Ca-dependent hemodynamic and natriuretic effects of atrial extract in isolated rat kidney. Am J Physiol 246: 2)-P F447–F455
9. Maack T, Marion DN, Camargo MJ, Kleinert HD, Laragh JH, Vaughan ED Jr, Atlas SA (1984) Effects of auriculin (atrial natriuretic factor) on blood pressure, renal function, and the renin-aldosterone system in dogs. Am J Med 77:1069–1075
10. Dunn BR, Ichikawa I, Pfeffer JM, Troy JL, Brenner BM (1986) Renal and systemic hemodynamic effects of synthetic atrial natriuretic peptide in the anesthetized rat. Circ Res 59:237–246
11. Maack T, Camargo MJ, Kleinert HD, Laragh JH, Atlas SA (1985) Atrial natriuretic factor: structure and functional properties. Kidney Int. 27:607–615
12. Burnett JC Jr, Granger JP, Opgenorth TJ (1984) Effects of synthetic atrial natriuretic factor on renal function and renin release. Am J Physiol 247: 2)-P F863–F866
13. Fried TA, McCoy RN, Osgood RW, Stein JH (1986) Effect of atriopeptin II on determinants of glomerular filtration rate in the in vitro perfused dog glomerulus. Am J Physiol 250: 2)-P F1119–F1122
14. Huang CL, Lewicki J, Johnson LK, Cogan MG (1985) Renal mechanism of action of rat atrial natriuretic factor. J Clin Invest 75:769–773
15. Sonenberg H, Honrath U, Chong CK, Wilson DR (1986) Atrial natriuretic factor inhibits sodium transport in medullary collecting duct. Am J Physiol 250: 2)-P F963–F966
16. Zeidel ML, Silva P, Brenner BM, Seifter JL (1987) cGMP mediates effects of atrial peptides on medullary collecting duct cells. Am J Physiol 252: 2)-P F551–F559
17. Zeidel ML (1988) In: Davidson AM (ed) Nephrology: V1. Balliere Tindall, London, pp 145–154
18. Maack T (1988) In: Davidson AM (ed) Nephrology: V1. Balliere Tindall, London, pp 123–136
19. Harris PJ, Thomas D, Morgan TO (1987) Atrial natriuretic peptide inhibits angiotensin-stimulated proximal tubular sodium and water reabsorption. Nature 326:697–698
20. Nonoguchi H, Sands JM, Knepper MA (1989) ANF inhibits NaCl and fluid absorption in cortical collecting duct of rat kidney. Am J Physiol 256: 2)-P F179–F188
21. Bianchi C, Gutkowska J, Thibault G, Garcia R, Genest J, Cantin M (1985 Radioautographic localization of 125I-atrial natriuretic factor (ANF) in rat tissues. Histochemistry 82: 441–452
22. Koseki C, Hayashi Y, Torikai S, Furuya M, Ohnuma N, Imai M (1986) Localization of binding sites for alpha-rat atrial natriuretic polypeptide in rat kidney. Am J Physiol 250: 2)-P F210–F216
23. Stokes TJ Jr, McConkey CL Jr, Martin KJ (1986) Atriopeptin III increases cGMP in glomeruli but not in proximal tubules of dog kidney. Am J Physiol 250: 2)-P F27–F31

24. Nonoguchi H, Knepper MA, Manganiello VC (1987) Effects of atrial natriuretic factor on cyclic guanosine monophosphate and cyclic adenosine monophosphate accumulation in microdissected nephron segments from rats. J Clin Invest 79:500–507

25. Light DB, Schweibert EM, Karlson KH, Stanton BA (1989) Atrial natriuretic peptide inhibits a cation channel in renal inner medullary collecting duct cells. Science 243: 383–385

26. Suzuki M, Almeida FA, Nussenzveig DR, Sawyer D, Maack T (1987) Binding and functional effects of atrial natriuretic factor in isolated rat kidney. Am J Physiol 253: 2)-P F917–F922

27. Almeida FA, Suzuki M, Scarborough RM, Lewicki JA, Maack T (1989) Clearance function of type C receptors of atrial natriuretic factor in rats. Am J Physiol 256: 2)-P R469–R477

28. Okolicany J, Scarborough B, McEnroe G, Kang L-L, Lewicki J, Maack T (1990) Specific blockage of C-ANF receptors by small linear peptide analogues causes natriuresis in the rat (abstract). Kidney Int 37:342

29. Ballermann BJ, Hoover RL, Karnovsky MJ, Brenner BM (1985) Physiologic regulation of atrial natriuretic peptide receptors in rat renal glomeruli. J Clin Invest 76:2049–2056

30. Nussenzveig DR, Scarborough R, Lewicki J, Maack T (1988) Clearance receptors of atrial natriuretic factor (C-ANF receptors) in isolated glomeruli and mesangial cells in culture (abstract). Kidney Int 33:279

31. Nussenzveig DR, Owada A, Scarborough R, Arfsten A, Maack T (1988) Biological (B) and clearance (C) receptors of ANF in cultured mesangial cells and fibroblasts (abstract). Am J Hypertens 1:121A

32. Fontoura BMA, Nussenzveig DR, Pelgon KA, Maack T (1990) Atrial natriuretic factor receptors in cultured renomedullary interstitial cells. Am J Physiol 258:C692–C699

33. Wall DA, Maack T (1985) Endocytic uptake, transport, and catabolism of proteins by epithelial cells. Am J Physiol. 248:C12–C20

34. Owada A, Nussenzveig DR, Maack T (1988) Receptor-mediated hydrolysis of atrial natriuretic factor (ANF) in isolated perfused rat kidney (IK) (abstract). Am J Hypertens 1:121A

35. Nussenzveig DR, Fontoura BMA, Scarborough R, Lewicki J, Maack T (1989) Clearance (C) receptors mediate internalization and lysosomal hydrolysis of ANF in fibroblasts (abstract). Kidney Int 35:285

36. Nussenzveig DR, Lewicki JA, Maack T (1989) Internalization, recycling and function of clearance receptors of atrial natriuretic factor (ANF) in vascular smooth muscle cells (abstract). In: Proceedings of the 71st annual meeting of the endocrine society. Seattle, United States. p 1113

37. Nussenzveig DR, Lewicki JA, Maack T (1990) Cellular mechanisms of the clearance function of C-ANF receptors (abstract). Kidney Int 37:341

38. Nussenzveig DR, Lewicki JA, Maack T (1990) Cellular mechanisms of the clearance function of type C receptors of atrial natriuretic factor. J Biol Chem 265:(in press)

Polarity of Tubular Epithelia

Chair: Eberhard Frömter (FRG)
Gerhard Malnic (Brazil)

Comparison Between Apical and Basolateral Transporters in Tubular Epithelia: A Dual Location of Na$^+$/H$^+$-Exchange with Different Properties

VALERIA CASAVOLA, CORINNA HELMLE-KOLB, and HEINI MURER[1]

SUMMARY. Na$^+$/H$^+$-exchange located in the plasma membrane of epithelial cells may fulfill a dual role: i) epithelial transport functions, such as in bicarbonate reabsorption and ii) cell homeostatic functions ("housekeeping"). A dual location of the Na$^+$/H$^+$-exchange has been documented for renal tubular epithelia, such as rabbit proximal tubule S$_3$ segment [1,2]. By microspectrofluorometry, we have analyzed for the polarized expression of the Na$^+$/H$^+$-exchange in an established renal cell line LLC-PK$_1$/PKE$_{20}$. In agreement with previous data on tracer flux measurements [3,4], we observed Na$^+$/H$^+$-exchange activities on both cell surfaces; we found that apical Na$^+$/H$^+$-exchange is less sensitive to ethylisopropyl-amiloride inhibition than basolateral activity. Forskolin and 8 Br-cAMP (i.e., activation of kinase A) lead to inhibition of apical and basolateral Na$^+$/H$^+$-exchange; phorbolester (i.e., activation of kinase C) leads to inhibition of apical and stimulation of basolateral Na$^+$/H$^+$-exchange activities. Vasopressin and calcitonin lead to inhibition of apical Na$^+$/H$^+$-exchange and stimulation of basolateral Na$^+$/H$^+$-exchange activity. Thus, renal epithelial cells may contain two different Na$^+$/H$^+$-exchange activities which show different pharmacological and regulatory properties and may serve different functions.

Introduction

Vectorial epithelial transport of solutes requires different transport properties of plasma membrane domains facing the apical and serosal (basolateral) compartments, respectively. For example, in absorptive secondary active transport functions, e.g., Na$^+$-coupled glucose absorption, Na$^+$-solute cotransport systems can mediate uphill influx at the apical cell side and Na$^+$-independent efflux at the basolateral cell pole will complete transcellular solute movement [5]. It should be noted, however, that

---

[1]Department of Physiology, University of Zürich, CH - 8057 Zürich, Switzerland

epithelial polarity with respect to transport functions can also be based on more subtile differences in transport properties. For amino acid reabsorption in the proximal tubule, Na^+-dependent transport pathways can be found on both cell surfaces; vectorial flux will then be determined by differences either in their capacities and/or kinetics or in their mode of energetization (e.g., Na^+/solute coupling coefficients, [5]).

For bicarbonate absorbing epithelia, the proton-secretory mechanism is usually on the apical cell surface; in renal proximal tubule this is a Na^+/H^+-exchange mechanism [6]. Besides this "epithelial" apical Na^+/H^+-exchange activity, basolateral Na^+/H^+-exchange activity may coexist in epithelial cells. This has been shown for small intestinal epithelial cells [7] as well as for rabbit S_3 proximal tubular epithelia [1,2].

LLC-PK_1/PKE_{20}, a renal epithelial cell line, was selected on the basis of its amiloride-resistance in a selection protocol and was found to have high Na^+/H^+-exchange activities in the apical as well as in the basolateral cell surface [3,4]. We have used this tissue culture model system to ask questions related to differences in the basic properties, as well as differences in regulatory characteristics, between apical and basolateral Na^+/H^+-exchange activities. Interestingly, we have observed that apical and basolateral Na^+/H^+-exchange activities are not only different with respect to their sensitivity to amiloride inhibition, but also with respect to hormonal regulatory phenomena [8,9,10].

Methods

For the studies to be summarized in this report we have used LLC-PK_1/PKE_{20}-cells grown on collagen coated teflon filters to confluent monolayers [8,9,10]; PKE_{20}-cells were obtained from Dr. C.W. Slayman (New Haven, Conn., USA, [3,4]). After mounting confluent monolayers on permeant support in a specially constructed "sandwich" chamber [11] and separate perfusion of the apical and basolateral compartment, intracellular pH (pH_i) was recorded by using the intracellular pH-indicator BCECF (Molecular Probes) [11,12,13]. Na^+/H^+-exchange was defined as Na^+-dependent recovery from a NH_4Cl-preload induced intracellular acidification; this Na^+-dependent recovery mechanism was competitively inhibited by ethylisopropylamiloride [8,9,10,14].

Results and Discussion

In agreement with trace flux studies [3,4], we have found Na^+/H^+-exchange activities on the apical as well as on the basolateral cell surface of LLC-PK_1/PKE_{20}-cell monolayers; the capacity of the apical Na^+/H^+-exchange activity was 20%–30% higher than basolateral activity [9,10]. Na^+-saturation kinetics revealed an apparent K_m-value of 25 mM and no difference between apical and basolateral activity [8,9,10]. Similar experiments performed previously in our laboratory with the same technique showed only apical Na^+/H^+-exchange activity in an established renal cell line derived from opossum kidney (OK-cells) [12,13] and only basolateral activity in wild type LLC-PK_1-cells [11] as well as in LLC-PK_1/$Clone_4$-cells, the parent cell line of LLC-PK$_1$/PKE$_{20}$ [8,9,10]. These initial experiments clearly document a dual location of Na$^+$/H$^+$ exchange in the cultured renal epithelial cell line LLC-PK$_1$/PKE$_{20}$.

Inhibition of Apical and Basolateral Na$^+$/H$^+$-Exchange in LLC-PK$_1$/PKE$_{20}$ Monolayers by Ethylisopropylamiloride (EIPA)

The amiloride analogue EIPA is known to be a competitive inhibitor of Na$^+$/H$^+$-exchange activities [14]. Na$^+$-dependent pH$_i$-recovery from an acid load due to superfusion with 20 mM Na was inhibited by 94% $\pm$ 2% at the basolateral cell surface but only by 31% $\pm$ 4% at the apical cell surface; in the presence of 140 mM Na$^+$ in the perfusate, inhibition at the basolateral cell surface was 66% $\pm$ 15% and at the apical surface was 16% $\pm$ 9%. These results [8,9,10] are clear evidence for a relative resistance to inhibition by EIPA of apical Na$^+$/H$^+$-exchange in LLC-PK$_1$/PKE$_{20}$ as compared to Na$^+$/H$^+$-exchange at the basolateral cell surface of the same cell and evidence for a competitive interaction between Na$^+$ and EIPA. Thus, two Na$^+$/H$^+$-exchange activities with different inhibitory properties seem to be expressed at the two different cell surfaces of LLC-PK$_1$/PKE$_{20}$-cells.

Effect of Pharmacological Activation of Proteinkinase A and Proteinkinase C on Apical and Basolateral Na$^+$/H$^+$-Exchange Activities in LLC-PK$_1$/PKE$_{20}$

Plasma membrane Na$^+$/H$^+$-exchange is usually inhibited by cAMP/kinase A mediated pathways and stimulated by diacylglycerol/kinase C mediated pathways [13,14]. In a recent study on OK-cells we found parathyroid hormone-dependent inhibition of apical Na$^+$/H$^+$-exchange; this hormone-dependent inhibition of Na$^+$/H$^+$-exchange could be mimicked by 8 Br-cAMP and by forskolin — both leading to activation of proteinkinase A — as well as by phorbolester leading to activation of kinase C [17,18]. The LLC-PK$_1$/PKE$_{20}$-cell system offers the possibility of looking for regulation of two differently located Na$^+$/H$^+$-exchange activities within the same cell (single cell microspectrofluorometry). Apical Na$^+$/H$^+$-exchange activity in LLC-PK$_1$/PKE$_{20}$-cells was inhibited within minutes by 8 Br-cAMP (2.5×10^{-4} M; 42% $\pm$ 8%), forskolin (10 μM; 65% $\pm$ 7%), phorbolester (TPA, 0.1 μM; 56% $\pm$ 5%) and phorbolester plus forskolin (above concentrations; 40% $\pm$ 1%). Basolateral Na$^+$/H$^+$-exchange activity was inhibited by 8 Br-cAMP (2.5×10^{-4} M; 42% $\pm$ 8%) and forskolin (10 μM; 48% $\pm$ 5%); it was stimulated by phorbolester (TPA, 0.1 μM; 37% $\pm$ 3%) and by phorbolester plus forskolin (above concentrations (40% $\pm$ 8%). These data document separate regulatory control of apically and basolaterally located Na$^+$/H$^+$-exchange activities and, further, suggest the coexistence of two separately controlled Na$^+$/H$^+$-exchange activities in LLC-PK$_1$/PKE$_{20}$-cells [8,9,10].

Effect of Vasopressin and Calcitonin on Apical and Basolateral Na$^+$/H$^+$-Exchange Activities in LLC-PK$_1$/PKE$_{20}$

LLC-PK$_1$-cells are known to express V$_1$-receptors (coupled to phospholipase C) as well as V$_2$-receptors coupled to adenylatecyclase [19]; receptors for calcitonin have also been described [19]. Thus, it was of interest to analyze for the relative importance of proteinkinase A and proteinkinase C mediation in vasopressin or in calcitonin mediated control of apical or basolateral Na^+/H^+-exchange in LLC-PK_1/PKE_{20}-cells. Vasopressin leads, within minutes, to inhibition of apical Na^+/H^+-exchange (2×10^{-6} M; 26% $\pm$ 1%); basolateral Na^+/H^+-exchange activity was stimulated by the same vasopressin treatment (17% $\pm$ 2%) [8,9,10].

This result suggests that either the kinase A and the kinase C regulatory pathways are activated together or that only the kinase C regulatory pathway is activated by vasopressin. Additional experiments indicated that the same treatment leads to a cellular accumulation of cAMP [10]. Thus, vasopressin exerts a dual effect on the two differently located Na^+/H^+-exchangers; this is best explained by vasopressin's actions via V_1 (cAMP-independent)- and via V_2 (cAMP-dependent)-receptor events.

Similar effects are observed for calcitonin. Calcitonin treatment leads, within minutes, to inhibition of apical Na^+/H^+-exchange (3×10^{-7} M; 25% $\pm$ 2%) and to stimulation of basolateral Na^+/H^+-exchange activities (27% $\pm$ 8%). These data, together with a measured increase in cAMP, again suggest that calcitonin effects must be mediated by two pathways, cAMP-dependent and cAMP-independent regulatory cascades.

Conclusions

Epithelial cells may contain two Na^+/H^+-exchange activities which are under different hormonal control and which can also be distinguished by their sensitivity to amiloride inhibition. Figure 1 summarizes the main observations obtained in our study on LLC-PK_1/PKE_{20}-monolayers, a tissue culture model for (proximal) tubular epithelia [3,4,8,9,10,19]. It should be noted that a similar dual location of Na^+/H^+-exchange activity might also be present in native proximal tubular epithelia [1,2], although regulatory hormones in the proximal tubule would not include vasopressin and calcintonin, but could be related to other agonists. In LLC-PK_1/PKE_{20}-cell monlayers, apical Na^+/H^+-exchange, as compared to basolateral activity, is resistant to EIPA inhibition. Proteinkinase A activation (by cAMP) leads to inhibition of apically and basolaterally located Na^+/H^+-exchange activities; proteinkinase C activation by diacylglycerol (DAG) leads to inhibition of apical, but

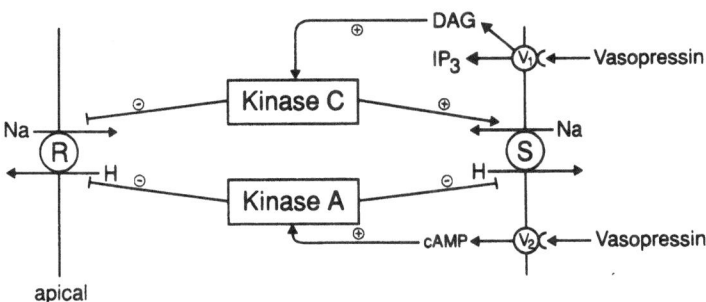

Fig. 1. Dual location of Na^+/H^+-exchange in LLC-PK_1/PKE_{20} monolayers and vasopressin-induced regulatory control. R, amiloride-resistant; S, amiloride-sensitive; DAG, diacylglycerol; IP_3, inositoltrisphosphate

stimulation of basolateral Na^+/H^+-exchange activity. As illustrated in Fig. 1 vasopressin exerts contrasting effects on apical and basolateral Na^+/H^+-exchange activities: apical activity is inhibited and this can be mediated by both kinase A and kinase C; basolateral activity is stimulated, and inhibition can be mediated only by activation of kinase C.

Acknowledgments. The financial support of the Swiss National Science Foundation (Grant Nr. 3.851.088), the "Stiftung für wissenschaftliche Forschung an der Universität Zürich," the "Hartman Müller Stiftung," the "Geigy-Jubiläumsstiftung," and the "Sandoz Stiftung" are gratefully acknowledged. We are grateful to Dr. C.F. Slayman for giving us access to LLC-PK$_1$/PKE$_{20}$- and LLC-PK$_1$/Clone$_4$-cells.

References

1. Kurtz I (1989) Basolateral membrane Na^+/H^+ antiport, Na^+/base cotransport, and Na^+-independent Cl^-/base exchange in the rabbit S_3 proximal tubule. J Clin Invest 83:616–622
2. Kurtz I (1987) Apical Na^+/H^+ antiporter and glycolysis-dependent H^+-ATPase regulate intracellular pH in the rabbit S_3 proximal tubule. J Clin Invest 80:928–935
3. Haggerty JG, Agarwal N, Reilly RF, Adelberg EA, Slayman CW (1988) Pharmacologically different Na^+/H^+-antiporters on the apical and basolateral surfaces of cultured kidney cells (LLC-PK$_1$). Proc Natl Acad Sci USA 85:6797–6801
4. Haggerty JG, Agarwal N, Cragoe EJ, Adelberg EA, Slayman CW (1988) LLC-PK$_1$ mutant with increased Na^+/H^+-exchange and decreased sensitivity to amiloride. Am J Physiol 255:C495–C501
5. Kinne R (1986) Epithelial transport: The interplay between ionic gradients and cell polarity. In: Alvarado F, van Os C (eds) Ion gradient-coupled transport (INSERM symposium 26). Elsevier, Amsterdam, pp 255–273
6. Alpern RJ (1990) Cell mechanisms of proximal tubule acidificiation. Physiol Rev 70:79–114
7. Barros F, Dominguez P, Velasco G, Lazo PS (1986) Na^+/H^+-exchange is present in basolateral membranes from rabbit small intestine. Biochem Biophys Res Commun 134:827–834
8. Casavola V, Helmle-Kolb C, Murer H (1989) Separate regulatory control of apical and basolateral Na^+/H^+-exchange in renal epithelial cells. Biochem Biophys Res Commun 165:833–837
9. Casavola V, Helmle-Kolb C, Montrose MH, Murer H (1990) Polarized expression of Na^+/H^+-exchange activities in clonal LLC-PK$_1$ cells (Clone$_4$ and PKE$_{20}$): 1. Basic characterization (in preparation)
10. Casavola V, Helmle-Kolb C, Montrose MH, Murer H (1990) Polarized expression of Na^+/H^+-exchange activities in clonal LLC-PK$_1$ cells (Clone$_4$ and PKE$_{20}$):2. Hormonal regulation (in preparation)
11. Montrose MH, Friedrich T, Murer H (1987) Measurements of intracellular pH in single LLC-PK$_1$ cells: Recovery from acid load via basolateral Na^+/H^+-exchange. J Membr Biol 97:63–78
12. Montrose MH, Murer H (to be published) Regulation of intracellular pH by cultured opossum kidney (OK) cells. Am J Physiol
13. Montrose MH, Murer H (to be published) Polarity and kinetics of Na^+/H^+-exchange in cultured opossum kidney (OK) cells. Am J Physiol
14. Vigne P, Frelin C, Cragoe EJ, Lazdunski M (1983) Ethylisopropylamiloride: a new and highly potent derivative of amiloride for the inhibition of the Na^+/H^+-exchange system in various cell types. Biochem Biophys Res Commun 116:86–90

15. Grinstein S, Rothstein A (1986) Mechanisms of regulation of the Na^+/H^+-exchanger. J Membr Biol 90:1-12
16. Frelin C, Vigne P, Ladoux A, Lazdunski M (1988) The regulation of the intracellular pH in cells from vertebrates. Eur J Biochem 174:3-14
17. Helmle-Kolb C, Montrose MH, Stange G, Murer H (1990) Regulation of Na^+/H^+-exchange in opossum kidney cells by parathyroid hormone, cyclic AMP and phorbol esters. Pflugers Arch 415:461-470
18. Helmle-Kolb C, Montrose MH, Murer H (to be published) PTH-Regulation of Na^+/H^+-exchange in opossum kidney cells: Polarity and mechanisms. Pflugers Arch
19. Gstraunthaler GJA (1988) Epithelial cells in tissue culture. Renal Physiol Biochem 11:1-42

Electrophysiological Localization of Transporters in the Distal Nephron Segments

KOJI YOSHITOMI, MASASHI IMAI[1], TOSHIKATSU SHIMIZU[2],
JUNICHI TANIGUCHI[3], and FUMIAKI YAMASAKI[4]

SUMMARY. The distal convoluted tubule (DCT) and the connecting tubule (CNT) from the rabbit kidney were investigated by electrophysiological techniques, isotopic flux measurement, and microfluorometry, in order to characterize the ion transport properties of cell membranes. When the DCT and the CNT were perfused in vitro, the transepithelial voltage (V_T) displayed lumen negative, and the transepithelial resistances (R_T) were relatively low, as in the category of leaky epithelia. Random cellular impalement revealed that the basolateral membrane voltage (V_B) of the DCT showed Gaussian distribution, whereas the CNT consisted of two cell populations, having different V_B and different fractional resistance of the apical membrane (fR_A). The CNT cell had a high V_B and lower fR_A and the intercalated (IC) cell in the CNT had a low V_B and higher fR_A. Using ion substitution and channel inhibitors, the conductive properties of DCT cells and CNT cells revealed that the luminal membrane had both Na^+ and K^+ conductances and that the basolateral membrane had both K^+ and Cl^- conductances. Intercalated cells of CNT had only a Cl^- conductance in the basolateral membrane. Besides Na^+ conductance in the luminal membrane of CNT cells, two other modes of Na^+ entry process were observed. One pathway was the Na/Cl cotransporter, revealed by isotopic ion flux studies, which was inhibitable with thiazide diuretics, and the other was a non-selective cation conductance, which was not sensitive to amiloride and was opened by parathyroid hormone (PTH). From intracellular calcium measurement and calcium flux studies, it was found that the latter mode serves as a route for calcium entry pathway in CNT cells.

[1]Department of Pharmacology, Jichi Medical School, Minamikawachi 3311-1, Tochigi, 329-04 Japan
[2]Shionogi Research Laboratories, Shionogi and Co., Ltd., Fukushima, Osaka, 553 Japan
[3]Research Institute, National Cardiovascular Center, Suita, Osaka, 565 Japan
[4]Fuji Central Research Lab., Mochida Pharmaceutical Co. Ltd., Gotenba, Shizuoka, 412 Japan

Introduction

It has generally been accepted that the function of the distal convoluted tubule (DCT) is reabsorption of NaCl and Ca^{2+} and secretion of K^+. This knowledge is based mainly on micropuncture studies on rat in vivo. However, the transitions from DCT to connecting tubule (CNT), or from CNT to cortical collecting duct (CCD), are gradual and several cell types are mixed within the transitional portion. In vitro microperfusion of DCT (and CNT) isolated from rabbit kidney has an advantage over the in vivo micropuncture studies of rat distal nephron, since the transition from DCT to CNT is clear. The DCT is characterized by its special location and shape, together with its calcitonin sensitivity in the distal nephron segments. For years, the exact mechanism of ion transport has been unknown, because of the difficulty of isolating the tubule. However, we have succeeded in identifying several membrane characteristics by elecctrophysiological means [1–5]. In the first step we found the exact location and appearance of DCT from collagenase-treated kidney, since microdissection from the collagenase-treated kidney was very easy. Eventually we used intact tubules for macroconductance measurements, together with patch clamp studies in collagenase-treated tubules. Thus far we have found that the DCT plays a significant role in the reabsorption of NaCl and Ca^{2+} and the secretion of potassium. We also found that DCT had an ability to increase the reabsorption rate of NaCl when dietary intake of NaCl was increased [3].

The connecting tubule (CNT) is a nephron segment located between the distal convoluted tubule (DCT) and the cortical collecting duct (CCD). The functional significance of this segment had been neglected for a long time, until Morel and his associates [6] reported that the CNT was a unique segment with respect to adenylate cyclase response to hormones. Subsequently, Imai [7] confirmed this view by observing that the changes in transmural voltage $(_1)$ in response to hormones are distinct from those observed in the DCT and in the CCD. Limited numbers of studies [2,8–10] suggest that the CNT plays a significant role in the renal tubular transport of Na^+, K^+, Cl^-, HCO_3^- and Ca^{2+}. According to these studies, the CNT is assumed to be one of the target sites of isoproterenol, parathyroid hormone (PTH), and thiazide diuretics.

Material and Methods

In Vitro Microperfusion of Isolated DCT and CNT

Isolated nephron segments were perfused in vitro according to the method of Burg et al. [11]. With slight modification [2,12]. Male Japanese white rabbits weighing 2.0–2.5 kg were maintained on standard rabbit chow and tap water ad libitum. The animals were anesthetized with pentobarbital (35 mg/kg,i.v.). The kidneys were removed and coronal slices were placed in ice-cold intracellular-fluid-like solution of the following composition (mM): 14 KCl, 44 K_2HPO_4, 14 KH_2PO_4, 9 $NaHCO_3$, and 160 sucrose. The connecting tubule was isolated by free hand dissection under a stereo microscope, according to the criteria reported previously [7,10]. A tubular segment was transferred to a bath chamber mounted on an inverted microscope (Olympus, IMT-2) and was perfused with in vitro microperfusion equipment developed by Narishige (Tokyo, Japan). The bathing fluid was supplied through a heating water jacket and was allowed to flow at a rate of 6–9 ml/min. The temperature of the bathing solution was maintained at 37°C. The tubular lumen was perfused under gravity at a rate of 10–20 nl/min.

Electrical Measurement

The transepithelial voltage (V_t) and voltage deflection (dV_o) were measured through the lumen of the perfusion pipette, which was connected to one channel of a dual electrometer (Duo 773, WP Instruments, New Haven, Conn., USA) with 1 mol/l agar bridge and calomel half cell. A flowing boundary 1 mol/l KCl electrode or 1 mol/l KCl agar bridge, which was connected to a calomel half cell, was placed at the outflow of the bath and served as a system ground. In the case of cable analysis, the tubules were cannulated with double barrelled perfusion pipettes (theta borosilicate glass, no. 1402401, Hilgenberg, Malsfeld, FRG) as reported previously [2,12]. Through one barrel of the perfusion pipette, current (I_o) was passed into the tubular lumen via an Ag-AgCl wire, then the transepithelial resistance (R_t) and the fractional resistance of the apical membrane (fR_A) were measured. The current was passed from a stimulator (SEN-7103, Nihon Kohden, Tokyo, Japan) with a stimulus isolator (S-1540, Nihon Kohden, Tokyo, Japan), which served as a constant current source. The voltage deflection at the distal end of the tubule (dV_t) was measured by a 1 mol/l KCl agar bridge cannulated into the collecting pipette, which was connected to the other channel of the dual electrometer. The cable parameters were determined using cable equations was reported previously [2,12], assuming that both ends of the cable were closed.

The basolateral membrane voltage (V_B) was measured with conventional microelectrodes, which were pulled from borosilicate glass tubing of 1.5 mm OD and 0.87 mmID (Hilgenberg, no. 14033521, Malsfeld, FRG) on a vertical puller (PE-2, Narishige, Tokyo, Japan). They were filled with 1 mol/l KCl solution and had a resistance of 150–200 megaohm and negligible tip potentials (< 5 mV). They were fixed to a microelectrode holder containing a Ag-AgCl pellet and were connected to an electrometer (8100, Single electrode system, Dagan, Minneapolis, USA). To impale a tubular cell, a microelectrode was positioned against the basolateral membrane with a hydraulic micromanipulator (MO-102N, Narishige, Tokyo, Japan) which was mounted in another micromanipulator (MN-1, Narishige, Tokyo, Japan) fixed to the stage of a microscope (IMT-2, Olympus, Tokyo, Japan). The microelectrode advanced into the cell by using current oscillations ("Buzz").

All the voltages were monitored by a digital storage oscilloscope (VC-6050, HITACHI, Tokyo, Japan) and stored on an FM-tape recorder (XR-30, TEAC, Tokyo, Japan).

Solutions

The artificial solution used in this study contained in mmol/l; NaCl 110, KCl 5, Na_2HPO_4 0.8, $CaCl_2$ 1.5, $MgCl_2$ 1.0, D-glucose 8.3. L-alanine 5, L-glutamate 3.5, and $NHCO_3$ 25. The solution was gassed with 5% CO_2/95% O_2. In the experiment with Na^+ removal from the control solution, NaCl and $NaHCO_3$ were replaced by equimolar choline Cl and choline HCO_3. In the case of increasing K^+ concentration, 45 mmol/l NaCl was replaced by KCl (50 mmol/l K^+ solution). In the experiment with Cl⁻ reduction, NaCl was replaced by Na gluconate, and $CaCl_2$ was increased around 6.0 mmol/l, in order to keep ionic Ca^{2+} activity constant (19 mmol/l Cl⁻ solution). Amiloride HCl was purchased from Sigma Chemicals (St. Louis, Mo., USA).

Statistical Analysis

All the values were expressed as the means $\pm$ SEM. Comparison between two groups was made using either a paired or non-paired Student t-test when appropriate. P values less than 0.05 were considered to be significant.

Results

Mechanism of Ion Transport in DCT

Basic Electrical Properties

When the DCT was perfused with symmetrical solution, the transepithelial voltage displayed lumen negative, indicating the presence of Na⁺ channel [1–5]. The transepithelial resistance was 21.8 ohm·cm², indicating that DCT is in the category of leaky epithelia [2]. It is of interest that the magnitude of V_l is dependent on the luminal flow rate, as described by Imai [1,7] and Shimizu et al. [10]. As the flow rate becomes higher, V_l shows lower lumen negativity. Whether this phenomenon is explained by flow rate or by luminal pressure is presently unknown. The distribution of the basolateral membrane voltage (V_B) is nearly Gaussian, with an average V_B of −77.8 mV. The fractional resistance of the luminal membrane was 0.78, indicating the ionic conductive pathway(s) in the luminal membrane [2].

The Luminal Membrane

Amiloride decreased the V_l and the luminal membrane was hyperpolarized by 5 mV. Na⁺ removal from the lumen also hyperpolarized the luminal membrane by 8 mV. Addition of Ba^{2+}, or luminal perfusion with high K⁺ solution, depolarized the luminal membrane, by 42.6 mV and 37.5 mV, respectively, indicating the presence of K⁺ channel [2]. Decrease in luminal Cl⁻ concentration did not change the luminal membrane voltage, suggesting the absence of Cl⁻ conductance.

The Basolateral Membrane

When the K⁺ concentration in the bathing fluid was increased, or when Ba^{2+} was added to the bath, the basolateral membrane was depolarized by 45.8 mV and 18.3 mV, respectively [2]. Using the patch clamp technique, Taniguchi et al. [4] were able to observe two kinds of K⁺ channel in the basolateral membrane. One type was a Ba^{2+} sensitive K⁺ channel of 50–60 pS single channel conductance, and the other was a flickering and Ba^{2+} insensitive K⁺ channel of 77 pS. Reduction of Cl⁻ concentration in the bath caused only by a small positive deflection of V_B; however, 14 mV depolarization was observed in the presence of Ba^{2+} with the same maneuver. These data indicate that a small Cl⁻ conductance exists in the basolateral membrane.

Effect of Calcitonin on Ca^{2+} Transport

Net Ca^{2+} flux was measured by using Fura-2 in the perfusate [5]. This revealed that significant Ca^{2+} reabsorption, which is stimulated by calcitonin and cyclic AMP, takes place in DCT. Furthermore, Ca^{2+} reabsorption was decreased in the presence of ouabain, or when Na^+ was removed from the bath, indicating the existence of secondary active Ca^{2+} transport which is coupled to Na^+, namely the Na/Ca exchanger. In order to transport Ca^{2+} from lumen to bath, there must be an entry step in the luminal membrane. However, with respect to the entry pathway for Ca^{2+} in the luminal membrane, we have no data at present.

Mechanism of Ion Transport in the Connecting Tubule

Electrical Properties of CNT

When the tubule was perfused with symmetrical solutions, the transepithelial voltage (V_T) displayed -3.0 ± 0.4 mV ($n=49$), lumen being negative. This observation was consistent with the finding which was reported previously from our laboratory [5,7-10,13]. Cable analysis of the CNT revealed that the transepithelial resistance (R_T) was 28.9 ± 2.5 ohm·cm² ($n=19$), indicating that the CNT is also in the category of leaky epithelia.

Evidence for Two Cell Populations; CNT and IC Cells

Although morphological studies have disclosed that the CNT has a cellular heterogeneity, namely CNT cells and IC cells, no report is available at present with respect to the conductive nature of the CNT cell. Therefore we impaled the cells of the CNT with conventional microelectrodes in order to investigate the electrical properties of the cell membranes [13]. Random impalement of the CNT revealed that there were two groups of cells having different basolateral membrane voltage. One group had a V_B of -73.1 ± 1.1 mV ($n=77$) and the other group had a V_B of (-28.1 ± 1.8 mV) ($n=39$). The low V_B cell, by analogy with the cortical collecting duct or the medullary collecting duct, is assumed to be an intercalated cell. In 19 cases of cable analysis with cellular impalement of electrodes, the fractional resistance of the luminal membrane (fR_A) was also divided into two groups. In all cases, the low fR_A group (0.50 $\pm$ 0.05, $n=22$) corresponded to high V_B cells and the converse held for the high fR_A group (0.96 $\pm$ 0.01, $n=9$). Thus, the low V_B and high fR_A cells in the CNT are analogous to the IC cells in the collecting duct. By exclusion, the other type of cell must be the CNT cell.

The Luminal Membrane of the CNT Cell

Since the transepithelial voltage always displayed lumen negative, suggesting the existence of Na^+ channel in the luminal membrane, we applied amiloride to the tubular lumen. When the tubular lumen was perfused with 10^{-5} mol/l amiloride, the transepithelial voltage was decreased from -14.3 ± 2.1 to -0.1 ± 0.2 mV ($n=4$, $P<0.01$) and the basolateral membrane in the CNT cell was hyperpolarized slightly, by 2.8 ± 1.4 mV ($n=4$, NS). No change of V_B was observed in the IC cell (0.3 ± 0.3 mV, $n=4$, NS) upon amiloride application. In order to confirm that the changes of V_l and V_B in response to amiloride were driven by the changes in luminal membrane conductance of the CNT cell, the fractional resistance of the apical membrane (fR_A) was monitored by current injection. Indeed this was true, since the transepithelial resistance (R_l) was increased from 36.1 ± 6.4 to 42.8 ± 7.6 ohm·cm² ($n=4$, $P<0.05$) and the fR_A of the CNT cell was increased from 0.49 ± 0.06 to 0.66 ± 0.05 ($n=4$, $P<0.001$). The fR_A of the IC cell did not change at all (0.97 ± 0.01 vs. 0.97 ± 0.01, $n=4$). These results indicate that the luminal membrane of the CNT cell has a Na⁺ conductance which is inhibitable with amiloride.

When the luminal concentration of K⁺ was changed from 5 to 50 mmol/l, V_l increased from -2.4 ± 0.5 to -7.9 ± 1.7 mV ($n=14$, $P<0.05$) and the basolateral membrane of the CNT cell was depolarized by 35.6 ± 1.1 mV ($n=14$, $P<0.001$). To further confirm this result, the lumen was perfused with Ba²⁺ (2 mmol/l). The transepithelial voltage increased from -6.3 ± 1.3 to -11.1 ± 1.1 mV ($n=4$, $P<0.05$) and the basolateral membrane was depolarized by 18.8 ± 3.1 mV ($n=4$, $P<0.01$). These results indicate that K⁺ conductance is also present in the luminal membrane of the CNT cells.

The Basolateral Membrane of the CNT Cell

In order to examine the conductive properties of the basolateral membranes in the CNT cells, concentration changes of K⁺ or Cl⁻ in the bathing solution were applied. In the CNT cells, an increase in K⁺ concentration from 5 to 50 mmol/l in the bathing solution depolarized the basolateral membrane from -78.3 to -34.8 mV. Further, a reduction in Cl− concentration from 120 to 19 mM in the bath depolarized the basolateral membrane by 13.7 mV.

To examine the barium sensitivity of K⁺ conductance, 2 mmol/l of BaCl₂ was added to the bathing solution. The basolateral membrane of the CNT cell was depolarized by 35.3 ± 2.1 mV ($n=9$), on average. When a sudden reduction in Cl⁻ concentration was applied in the presence of Ba²⁺ in the bath, CNT cells displayed a sharp depolarization of the basolateral membrane (24.3 ± 2.6 mV, $n=8$) which was larger than in the absence of Ba²⁺.

Effect of PTH on Ca²⁺ Transport and V_T

When PTH was applied to CNT from the bath, net Ca²⁺ flux was markedly increased and the transepithelial voltage (V_l) displayed a biphasic response: initial increase in lumen negativity, followed by gradual and sustained decrease in V_l [14]. This phenomenon was mimicked by cyclic AMP. In the presence of amiloride in the lumen, we could observe only the initial phase, indicating that the second phase could be attributed to the inhibition of Na⁺ conductance. The same disappearance of second phase was observed when the lumen was made Ca²⁺ free, suggesting that the increase in cell Ca²⁺ in response to PTH might be related to the inhibition of the Na⁺ channel. The first phase of increase in V_l was abolished only when the lumen was perfused with Na⁺ free solution, indicating that PTH has a role in opening the amiloride-insensitive cation conductance, which can carry Ca^{2+} together with Na^+. This was confirmed by cell Ca^{2+} measurement using Fura-2 [15]. PTH caused a sustained increase in cell Ca^{2+}, and gradual decrease, under the baseline level of cell Ca^{2+}, was observed after PTH withdrawal, indicating the dual effects of PTH: stimulating both the entry process and the extrusion mechanism.

In the basolateral membrane, there must be a Ca^{2+} extrusion mechanism. PTH-stimulated increase in Ca^{2+} flux was abolished in the presence of ouabain or in the absence of Na^+ ion in the bath. These results indicated the existence of a secondary active Ca^{2+} transport which is coupled to Na^+, namely the Na/Ca exchanger. Cell Ca^{2+} measurement confirmed the view that Na^+ removal from the bath caused an exaggerated increase in cell Ca^{2+} in CNT cells.

Discussion

General Transport Properties of DCT and CNT

Morphological study shows that the distal convoluted tubule (DCT) consists of a homogeneous cell type (the DCT cell), whereas the connecting tubule (CNT) consists of heterogeneous cell types (CNT cells and intercalated cells). Morel et al. [6] were the first to report that, among distal nephron segments, the DCT and CNT were unique with regard to response of adenylate cyclase activity to various hormones, such as calcitonin, isoproterenol, vasopressin, and PTH. Subsequently, Imai [7] confirmed this view by observing that the voltage responses to these hormones in the DCT, CNT, and CCD were distinct. He also reported that the water permeabilities of the DCT and CNT were very low, compared with that of the cortical collecting duct. Recently, we have examined other aspects of these segments, using electrophysiological studies and ion flux measurement of Ca^{2+}, Na^+, K^+, and cell Ca^{2+} movement in response to the above mentioned hormones and in response to changes in dietary intake of NaCl.

Distribution of Transporters in DCT and CNT

Almeida and Burg [8] reported that the transepithelial resistance of the CNT was low (31 ohm·cm²). In the present study, we also confirmed this value (28.9 ohm·cm²). It is of interest to note that all distal tubules, including the distal straight tubule (DST), distal convoluted tubule (DCT), and CNT, are leaky segments. The transepithelial resistances found so far are very low in all these segments. However, there is a tendency for the resistance to increase along the axis of the nephron. In contrast, the transepithelial resistance of the collecting duct is very high.

In the present study, we confirmed previous observations [1–5,7–10,13] that both DCT and CNT generate lumen negative voltage. Shimizu et al. [3,10] reported that addition of 10^{-5} M amiloride to the lumen abolished the lumen negative V_t, suggesting that Na^+ conductance in the luminal membrane is critical for negative V_t. This notion has become definite since the finding that amiloride in the lumen increased transepithelial resistance and fractional apical resistance, together with hyperpolarizing the luminal membrane [2]. The luminal membrane in the DCT and CNT also has K^+ channels which are inhibitable with Ba^{2+}. Therefore, the conductive properties of the luminal membrane are very similar to those of the collecting duct cell. However, particularly in the CNT cell, we observed other modes of Na^+ transport in the luminal membrane: namely the Na/Cl cotransporter, which is inhibitable with thiazide [10], and a non-selective cation conductance, which is able to carry Na^+ and Ca^{2+} [14]. The significance of the latter transport will be discussed later.

Both DCT and CNT cells were characterized by high V_H and fR_A, of $0.50 - 0.78$. An fR_A lower than unity may be accounted for by the existence of both Na^+ and K^+ conductances in the luminal membranes of both cells, conductances which were inhibitable with amiloride and Ba^{2+}, respectively. The basolateral membrane of the CNT had a large K^+ conductance and a small Cl^- conductance. The apparent transference numbers for K^+ and Cl^- were calculated to be 0.75 and 0.16 in DCT cells, and 0.71 and 0.28 in CNT cells, respectively. Thus, almost 90%–99% of the ionic conductance in the basolateral membrane is accounted for by K^+ and Cl^- conductances, with K^+ conductance being preferential.

Physiological Significance of DCT and CNT

The major task of the DCT and the CNT is considered to be the reabsorption of NaCl. Secretion of K^+ [16] and absorption of Ca^{2+} [1,9] would be considered as phenomena secondary to active Na^+ transport, since K^+ secretion takes place as a backleak from the cell, via luminal K^+ conductance, and Ca^{2+} reabsorption has recently been shown to be related to the Na^+/Ca^{2+} exchanger in the basolateral membrane [5,14,15,17]. Ca^{2+} transport is specifically stimulated by calcitonin and PTH in the DCT and the CNT, respectively.

The DCT cell has a special ability to reabsorb NaCl, in that the rate of NaCl reabsorption and K^+ secretion changes depending on the volume of dietary NaCl intake. When animals were given an increased NaCl intake, DCT cells became large and both net Na^+ reabsorption and net K^+ secretion were increased. It was demonstrated that the sizes of the Na^+ and K^+ conductances were increased together with increased Na-K-ATPase activity [3].

Among the distal nephron segments, the net Na^+ reabsorption in CNT is the highest [8,10]. This corresponds to the activity of Na-K-ATPase. Na-K-ATPase activity is 6 times greater in the CNT than in the CCD. The net Na^+ flux across the CNT has been reported to be 20.3 $pmol·cm^{-1}·s^{-1}$ [8], whereas the net Na^+ fluxes of the DCT and the CCD were 13.7 [16] and $2.7 - 5.7$ $pmol·cm^{-1}·s^{-1}$, respectively. In CNT, trichlormethiazide, one of the potent thiazide diuretics, was shown to inhibit lumen-to-bath Na^+ flux by 32.3% and net Cl^- flux by 30.6%, by inhibiting the Na^+/Cl^- cotransporter in the luminal membrane [10]. In the present study, when amiloride (10^{-5} mol/l) was applied to the lumen, the magnitude of decrease in the equivalent short circuit current (V_t/R_t) was calculated to be 395 $\mu A/cm^2$, corresponding to 30.8 $pmol·cm^{-1}·s^{-1}$. This value is consistent with the magnitude of the decrease in lumen-to-bath Na^+ flux, 32.5 $pmol·cm^{-1}·s^{-1}$ (46.1%), found in our previous study [10]. Thus, in the CNT the sum of Na^+/Cl^- cotransport and amiloride-sensitive Na^+ conductance yields around 78% of the total transepithelial Na^+ flux. The remaining 22% could be mediated by the Na^+/H^+-Cl^-/HCO_3^- exchanger and by an amiloride-insensitive cationic conductance. It has recently been suggested, by Shimmizu et al. [14], that the latter mechanism is the entry pathway for Ca^{2+} at the luminal membrane.

References

1. Imai M, Nakamura R (1982) Function of distal convoluted and connecting tubules studied by isolated nephron fragments. Kidney Int 22:465–472
2. Yoshitomi K, Shimizu T, Taniguchi J, Imai M (1989) Electrophysiological characterization of rabbit distal convoluted tubule. Pflugers Arch 414L457–463
3. Shimizu T, Yoshitomi K, Taniguchi J, Imai M (1989) Effect of high NaCl intake on Na and K transport in rabbit distal convoluted tubule. Pflugers Arch 414:500–508
4. Taniguchi J, Yoshitomi K, Imai M (1989) K^+ channel currents in basolateral membrane of distal convoluted tubule of rabbit kidney. Am J Physiol 256:F246–F254
5. Shimizu, T, Yoshitomi K, Nakamura M, Imai M (1990) Effects of PTH, calcitonin, and cAMP on calcium transport in rabbit distal nephron segments. Am J Physiol 259:F408–F414
6. Morel F, Chabardes D, Imbert M (1976) Functional segmentation of the rabbit distal tubule by microdetermination of hormone-dependent adenylate cyclase activity. Kidney Int 9:264–277
7. Imai M (1979) The connecting tubule: A functional subdivision of the rabbit distal nephron segments. Kidney Int 15:346–356
8. Almeida AJ, Burg MB (1982) Sodium transport in the rabbit connecting tubule. Am J Physiol 243:F330–F334
9. Imai M (1981) Effect of parathyroid hormone and N',O'-dibutyryl cyclic AMP on Ca transport across the rabbit distal nephron segments perfused in vitro. Pflugers Arch 390:145–151
10. Shimizu T, Yoshitomi K, Nakamura M, Imai M (1988) Site and mechanism of action of trichlormethiazide in rabbit distal nephron segments perfused in vitro. J Clin Invest 82:721–730
11. Burg MB, Grantham J, Abramow M, Orloff J (1966) Preparation and study of fragments of single rabbit nephrons. Am J Physiol 210:1293–1298
12. Yoshitomi K, Koseki C, Taniguchi J, Imai M (1987) Functional heterogeneity in the hamster medullary thick ascending limb of Henle's loop. Pflugers Arch 408:600–608
13. Yoshitomi K, Shimizu T, Imai M (1988) Functional cellular heterogeneity in the rabbit connecting tubule. Kidney Int 33:430
14. Shimizu T, Yoshitomi K, Nakamura M, Imai M (1990) Effect of parathyroid hormone on the connecting tubule from the rabbit kidney; biphasic response of transmural voltage. Pflugers Arch 416:254–261
15. Shimizu T, Yamasaki F, Imai M, Yoshitomi K (1990) Regulation of calcium transport in the distal nephron segments. Kidney Int 37:461
16. Shareghi GR, Stoner LC (1978) Calcium transport across segments of the rabbit distal nephron in vitro. Am J Physiol 235:F367–F375
17. Bourdeau JE, Lau K (1989) Effects of parathyroid hormone on cytosolic free calcium concentration in individual rabbit connecting tubules. J Clin Invest 83:373–379

Vesicle Trafficking and Membrane Polarity in Epithelial Cells: Relationship to Intercalated Cell Function in Kidney Collecting Ducts

DENNIS BROWN[1]

SUMMARY. Many plasma membrane components are delivered to their appropriate membrane domain in membrane-bounded vesicles, and the control of vesicle targeting and fusion are, therefore, critical elements in epithelial cell function. This review discusses some current concepts of how the specificity of this targeting process may be determined, including protein structure, microtubule pathways, and GTP-binding proteins as fusion factors. These concepts of epithelial cell polarity generation and maintenance are of tremendous functional importance to the kidney, because epithelial cells lining the kidney collecting duct have developed highly-specialized, yet independent systems for the rapid modulation of the composition of their plasma membranes in response to different stimuli. In particular, the ability of subpopulations of collecting duct intercalated cells to insert a proton pumping ATPase into opposite plasma membrane domains is a remarkable cell biological feat that provides a unique opportunity for investigating mechanisms of protein targeting in epithelia.

Introduction

The plasma membrane composition of virtually all eucaryotic cells is established, maintained, and modified by the process of membrane recycling. Specific plasma membrane components are inserted by exocytosis of transport vesicles, and are removed by endocytosis of segments of the membrane in which particular proteins are concentrated. It is particularly important for kidney function that epithelial cells lining the urinary tubule can respond rapidly to changes in the composition of their environment; epithelial cells lining the kidney collecting duct have developed highly-specialized, yet independent systems for the rapid modulation of the composition of their plasma membranes in response to different stimuli [1]. Vasopressin induces the

[1]Renal Unit, Massachusetts General Hospital and Department of Pathology, Harvard Medical School, Boston, MA 02114, USA

cycling of vesicles that are thought to carry water channels to and from the apical plasma membrane of principal cells, thus rapidly modulating the water permeability of this membrane. In the intercalated cells of the collecting duct, hydrogen ion secretion is controlled by the recycling of vesicles carrying proton pumps to and from the plasma membrane. In both cell types, "coated" carrier vesicles are involved, but whereas clathrin-coated vesicles participate in water channel recycling, the vesicles in intercalated cells are coated with the cytoplasmic domains of proton pumps. In addition to these rapidly recycling membrane components, kidney epithelial cells are highly polarized with respect to many other membrane proteins that play an integral role in tubular function in all regions of the urinary tubule. These molecules have been localized using a variety of techniques from physiological measurements of tubular function to immunocytochemical detection at the light and/or electron microscopical level. This review will first examine some of the potential mechanisms by which integral membrane proteins may find their way to specific plasma membrane domains, and will then summarize studies related to the polarized distribution of a proton pumping ATPase in kidney epithelial cells.

Generation of Polarity in Epithelial Cells

Because epithelia function as selective barriers separating two different types of extracellular milieux, it is necessary for them to generate and maintain the polarity of a wide variety of plasma membrane proteins and lipids. Many plasma membrane components are delivered to the appropriate membrane domain in membrane-bounded vesicles, and so the control of vesicle targeting and fusion are critical elements in epithelial cell function. A considerable amount of work is now aimed at understanding the molecular mechanisms that determine the selectivity of vesicle movement and fusion, and some of the key areas of current investigation are:

The Role Played by Targeting Sequences that Form Part of the Structure of Individual Proteins

Some amino acid sequences allow proteins to be inserted into mitochondrial membranes [2], while others are required for clustering of proteins into clathrin-coated pits on the cell surface [3]. Other covalent modifications of proteins, such as the addition of mannose-6-phosphate groups to carbohydrate side chains, are required to direct lysosomal hydrolases to lysosomes [4]. Yet other amino acid sequences cause proteins to be retained in the rough endoplasmic reticulum, and prevent their transfer to the Golgi apparatus [5]. Recently, it has been proposed that a phosphatidylinositol-glycan anchor that links a special class of proteins to the lipid bilayer may be a signal for incorporation of these proteins into the apical plasma membrane of epithelial cells [6]. Based on these studies, and others examining the role of cytoplasmic domains of viral glycoproteins in the targeting process [7], it is generally believed that the amino acid sequence of a given protein will play a large part in determining its final destination in a cell. For this reason, our finding that subpopulations of intercalated cells in the kidney collecting duct can insert a proton pumping ATPase into the apical or basolateral plasma membrane domain is intriguing [8], since most plasma membrane proteins appear to be restricted to one pole of the cell or the other.

The Role of Cytoskeletal Elements in Directing Vesicular Traffic in Cells

Considerable data have accumulated showing that microtubule disruption by agents such as colchicine can interfere severely with intracellular membrane traffic, secretory processes, lysosomal distribution, and the processing and packaging of proteins at the level of the Golgi apparatus [9-14]. In an earlier study, we showed that colchicine interferes with the processing, packaging, and stimulated secretion of newly-synthesized amylase from the rat parotid gland, but that it does not affect secretion of pre-formed amylase that had already been packed into secretory granules [12]. In the same study, we also showed that colchicine severely disrupts the structure of the Golgi apparatus, causing the ordered cisternae to be replaced by swarms of small vesicles. Recently, it has been shown that following Golgi disruption by nocodazole, the reclustering of scattered Golgi elements occurs along microtubules [15].

Despite these dramatic effects on the secretory apparatus, whether microtubules are involved in the generation and maintenance of epithelial cell polarity is still an unresolved issue. Conflicting results [16,17] have been obtained in virally-infected cells concerning the importance of microtubules for the polarized insertion of membrane proteins (in this case, viral proteins). Much less work has been performed using endogenous proteins, but recent data indicate that nocodazole inhibits the normal insertion of an endogenous apical membrane protein in cultured cells [18], and microtubule disruption has a dramatic effect on cell polarity in intestinal epithelial cells, resulting in the formation of patches of brush-border microvilli and the appearance of normally apical proteins such as alkaline phosphatase on the basolateral plasma membrane [9,13,19]. How microtubules may influence the intracellular movement of organelles and transporting vesicles is emerging as a result of the discovery of so-called microtubule motors (kinesin and cytoplasmic dyneins); these proteins, isolated from cytosolic fractions of cells, have the capacity to induce ATP-dependent organelle movement along isolated microtubules in either an anterograde or retrograde direction [20]. Recent observations on the pH dependence of lysosomal distribution in fibroblasts have been suggested to result from the selective switching on or off of different microtubule motors at different cytoplasmic pH values [10]. The possibility that microtubules are involved in the movement of transporting vesicles to the apical pole of epithelial cells, and that this movement may be pH-dependent, is of clear relevance to the physiological response of collecting duct intercalated cells to different acid-base conditions. Indeed, in turtle bladder, acidification in response to CO_2 is inhibited by colchicine [21].

The actin-based microfilamentous system is also of importance to intracellular vesicle trafficking, although the effects of cytochalasins, which disrupt the structure and function of actin filaments, are less consistent than those of microtubule disrupting agents. For example, in some endocrine cells, cytochalasin B causes an increase in the initial secretory response [22], whereas in the toad urinary bladder it causes a decrease in the vasopressin-stimulated increase in transepithelial water permeability, a process which also involves exocytotic events [14,23]. It is apparent from our examination of 3-dimensional electron micrographs of freeze-dried, rotary shadowed epithelial cells, that cytoplasmic organelles and vesicles have a complex interaction

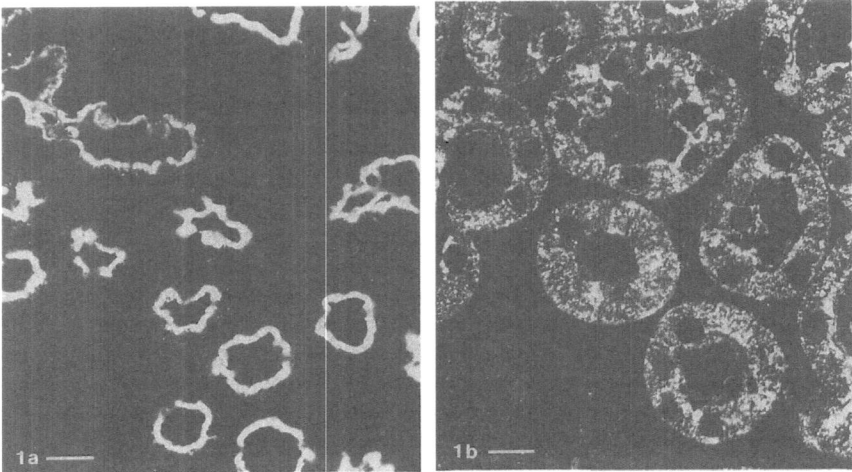

Fig. 1a,b. Frozen sections of control (**a**) and colchicine-treated (**b**) rat cortex stained with anti-bodies against gp330. In control kidney, gp330 is concentrated at the apical pole of proximal tubule cells, whereas after colchicine-induced disruption of microtubules, it is present on vesicles scattered throughout the cytoplasm (see [29]). Bar = 20 μm

with microfilaments, and in many cases appear to be almost entirely "cocooned" in the dense subapical network of actin filaments (Hartwig and Brown, unpublished results). Furthermore, there are reports in the literature that the charged surface of artificial liposomes can act as a surface that induces actin polymerization in vitro [24]. In addition, there is accumulating evidence that many transmembrane proteins are linked either directly or indirectly to the cytoskeleton [25,26]. Of particular interest to the mechanism of proton and bicarbonate transport in the kidney is the well-known interaction of band 3 with spectrin in the erythrocyte [25], and with non-erythrocyte spectrin (fodrin) in intercalated cells [27]; the sodium-potassium ATPase has also been found to be linked to cytoskeletal elements in MDCK cells [28]. These transmembrane linkages certainly play an important role in the maintenance of polarized membrane domains. Clearly, the potential interaction between microtubules, microfilaments and intracellular vesicles requires that the contributions of all three elements be considered in any scheme of vesicle trafficking and the generation and maintenance of cell polarity.

GTP-Binding Proteins and Vesicle Targeting

Once vesicles containing a specific cargo of protein and lipid have been formed and transported to the vicinity of their site of fusion in the cell cytoplasm, how is the final process of fusion with their target membrane controlled? Our recent studies using an apical membrane glycoprotein of the proximal tubule brush border, gp330, have shown that colchicine treatment of rats results in a dramatic redistribution of this glycoprotein in the cell (Fig. 1a,b). Instead of its usual exclusively apical localization, it is found on many vesicles scattered throughout the cytoplasm after drug treatment

[29]. However, despite the fact that many of these vesicles are found close to the basolateral plasma membrane, no evidence for a significant incorporation of gp330 into the basolateral membrane was found. This suggests that the mere proximity of a vesicle to a membrane is not sufficient to ensure fusion, and that most probably a second level of control is exerted that requires some specific recognition signal between the vesicle and the target membrane domain. The microtubules would, then, be required to direct vesicles to the apical pole of the cell, and thereby to increase the local concentration of fusion-competent vesicles beneath the apical plasma membrane. As discussed above, however, colchicine-treatment of intestinal epithelial cells *does* result in the appearance of apical markers on the basolateral membrane. One potential explanation for this is that these proteins are packaged into the "wrong" transporting vesicles after microtubule disruption. Thus, the targeting error in these cells is made at the level of sorting in the Golgi apparatus, not at the level of vesicle-plasma membrane interaction. In the proximal tubule, the vesicles containing gp330 that redistribute throughout the cell may be derived mainly from the apical plasma membrane, owing to the high rate of apical membrane recycling in this cell type. For this reason, they may not be able to fuse with the basolateral membrane. The contribution of newly-synthesized gp330 to the total, redistributed intracellular pool is unknown.

In view of the undoubted specificity of intracellular fusion events which is necessary to maintain the characteristic protein/lipid fingerprint of individual membranes, it is likely that some type of "ligand-receptor" interaction between donor and acceptor membranes is required, and one developing area of research concerns the role of guanine-nucleotide binding proteins (G-proteins) in this process. The G-proteins that are linked to signal transduction events at the cell surface, and also control the gating of a number of ion channels on the cell membrane, are heterotrimeric structures consisting of alpha, beta and gamma subunits [30]. These G-protein subunits combine with a receptor protein and an effector such as adenylyl cyclase to form a functional unit, and all these elements are associated in the same membrane microdomain to provide selectivity and amplification in the signalling pathway. The intrinsic GTPase activity of the alpha subunit that hydrolyses GTP to GDP to stop the transduction of the signal is an important "timer" element in the signal transduction cascade.

However, recent work has shown that GTP-binding proteins are also associated with some intracellular compartments, and that a distinct class of ras-like small molecular weight G-proteins (SMGs) [31, 32] may play a role in vesicle trafficking and fusion events [33]. These small molecular weight G-proteins appear to be widely distributed in both membranes and cytosol, and some are also substrates for ADP-ribosylation induced by bacterial toxins, particularly those from *Clostridium botulinum* [32], *Clostridium perfringens* [34], and cholera toxin [35].

While the analogy with heterotrimeric G-proteins has led to the assumption that each of these proteins participates in a signal transduction pathway, this assumption remains unproven. In particular, all of the SMGs studied to date lack one or more of the essential elements required for signal transduction. For example, while all, by definition, bind GTP, some have little (ras) [36] or no (ARF) [37] GTPase activity. However, this "timer" function can be served by a distinct cytosolic protein, GAP (GTPase activating protein), which enhances the GTPase activity of two of the SMGs, ras and rho [38]. In addition, another SMG, ARF [37], is able to stimulate the cholera-toxin induced ADP ribosylation of the alpha subunit of Gs, indicating that some degree of crosstalk may exist between SMGs and the heterotrimeric G-proteins.

This discussion leads to the idea that these SMGs are ideal candidates to be involved in vesicle targeting, because the sequential and selective interactions between these proteins and the other proteins necessary for them to function in "signal transduction" would ensure that only when a vesicle carrying a particular SMG met with a membrane carrying another necessary component to reconstitute function, would vesicle fusion ensue. According to a hypothesis proposed by Bourne [33], an integral membrane protein present on an intracellular vesicle would form a membrane-associated complex with a specific G-protein. A docking protein on a recipient (target) membrane would then recognize this G-protein complex on the vesicle, and thereby induce GTP hydrolysis, resulting in vesicle fusion. This hydrolysis of GTP to GDP should be blocked by non-hydrolyzable GTP analogues and should inhibit vesicle fusion; this is precisely what has been demonstrated in isolated vesicle fractions from the Golgi region [39]. Furthermore, secretory processes in mast cells and neutrophils have also been linked to G-proteins [40], and G-proteins have been localized on the membranes of secretory granules in yeast and chromaffin cells [41, 42]. Most recently, a soluble NEM-sensitive factor that resembles the SEC18 gene product of yeast [43], and a second soluble fusion factor found in cytosol have been proposed to interact with an integral membrane protein to control vesicle fusion at the level of the Golgi apparatus [44]; the same NEM-sensitive factor is also required for vesicle mediated transport between the RER and the Golgi [45], a known function of SEC18 in yeast [46]. Most recently, three integral membrane proteins that are necessary for vesicle fusion to occur have been isolated from Golgi membranes [47]. These data support the idea outlined above that multiple protein interactions may be required to reconstitute a functional complex that catalyses membrane fusion events.

Polarized Function in Kidney Intercalated Cells

Proton Pump Localization and Recycling in Intercalated Cells

The concepts of epithelial cell polarity outlined above are of tremendous functional importance to the kidney. Distinctive morphological alterations occur in intercalated cells during an increase in H^+ secretion by collecting ducts [48, 49]. Following induced acidosis in rats, an increase in the apical surface area of intercalated cells is accompanied by a decrease in the number of specialized cytoplasmic vesicles, known as tubulovesicles [48], presumably as a result of their exocytotic fusion with the apical plasma membrane. Previous studies in turtle bladder and the collecting duct had shown that vesicles containing proton pumps are inserted into the apical membrane of these carbonic anhydrase rich cells during acidosis [49, 50]. Tracer studies with horseradish peroxidase demonstrated that these specialized coated vesicles were also involved in endocytotic events [51]. Specific antibodies against different subunits of the proton pumping ATPase from bovine kidney medulla were used to show that the vesicle coating material contained defined subunits of the proton pump [8, 52]. The "coat" seen on the cytoplasmic side of the plasma membrane of some intercalated cells also contained the same pump subunits and the structure of the membrane coat was elucidated, using the rapid-freeze, deep-etch technique, in which high resolution

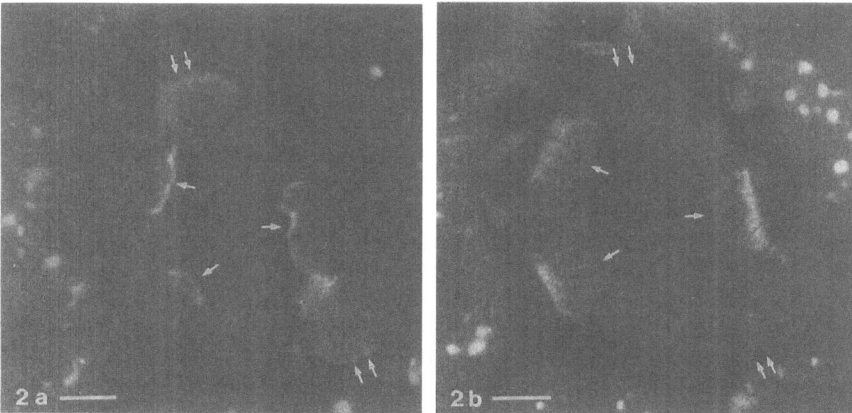

Fig. 2a,b. Consecutive semithin 1μm sections showing a cortical collecting duct stained with antibodies against a proton pumping ATPase (**a**) and a band 3-like anion exchanger (**b**). A-type intercalated cells show basolateral staining for band 3 and apical staining for the proton pump (*single arrows*). In contrast, B-type intercalated cells with basolateral or diffuse/bipolar proton pump staining (*double arrows*) are not labeled with anti band 3 antibodies. (See [57]). The brightly fluorescent spots in proximal tubules are autofluorescent lysosomes. Bar = 10 μm

microscopic images of proteins can be obtained. It was shown that the membrane-coating material had a structure that was identical to that of immunoaffinity-purified proton pumps, incorporated into phospholipid liposomes [52], thus confirming its identity as part of the proton pumping ATPase responsible for distal urinary acidification.

Opposite Polarity of Proton Pumps in A and B Intercalated Cells

This and other work suggested that tubulovesicles fuse with the apical plasma membrane during acidosis and incorporate their membrane into this plasma membrane domain. However, in the cortical collecting duct [48] and in the turtle urinary bladder [53], two morphological variants of "carbonic anhydrase-rich" cell have been described, which are believed to be proton-secreting (A-cells) or bicarbonate-secreting (B-cells). Both types co-exist in kidney cortical collecting ducts, in accord with the ability of this tubule segment to secrete either net acid or net base under different physiological conditions of acidosis or alkalosis. Using anti-proton pump antibodies, we demonstrated that while all medullary intercalated cells have proton pumps associated with their apical plasma membrane, cortical intercalated cells had three patterns of labeling (Fig. 2a): apical, basolateral, and diffuse cytoplasmic or bipolar [8]. This finding provided direct support for the idea that different intercalated cells in the cortex are responsible for either proton (apical pumps) or bicarbonate (basolateral pumps) secretion into the tubule lumen. It is possible that the cells with a diffuse staining might be an intermediate or transitional cell type. There was an inverse relationship between the number of cells stained diffusely or basolaterally, while the number of apically-stained cells was relatively constant among different animals.

Cellular Remodelling in Intercalated Cells

Provocative data by Schwartz et al. [54] suggested that A and B cells may be interconvertible, and may change their functional polarity by inserting proton pumps into either apical or basolateral plasma membranes, depending on prevailing acid-base conditions of the animal. However, more recent work reported that A and B cells do not interconvert during alterations in acid-base status [55]. While this question has not yet been clearly resolved, several observations are pertinent. The A cells have a basolateral band 3-like chloride-bicarbonate exchanger [27, 56], whereas no chloride-bicarbonate exchanger has yet been located by immunocytochemistry in type B cells, either in the apical or the basolateral plasma membrane. Double staining studies show that all B-type intercalated cells with basolateral or diffuse proton pump staining lack detectable band 3, while the vast majority of cells with apical proton pumps show strong basolateral band 3 staining (Fig. 2). However, we consistently found a small (1%) population of cortical intercalated cells with apical proton pumps but no basolateral band 3 [57]. Whether this cell type is a distinct population or a transitional type of intercalated cell is unknown. The absence of band 3-like antigenicity on the apical surface of all intercalated cells demonstrates that if a simple exchange of transporting molecules from apical to basolateral plasma membrane and vice-versa occurs in these cells during adaptation to acid-base loads, then the apical anion exchanger must be modified in some way that renders it undetectable by a range of anti-band 3 antibodies [27, 56, 57]. In acidotic animals, functionally-detectable apical anion exchangers appear to be internalized by B-intercalated cells [58], but whether or not proton pumps are subsequently inserted into the apical membrane of the same cells is still unclear. By immunofluorescence microscopy, a decrease in the number of basolaterally stained intercalated cells is found in the cortex of rats with metabolic acidosis; the number of cells with "apical" proton pumps increases both after acute (6h) gavage with NH_4Cl (D. Brown, I. Sabolic, and S. Gluck, unpublished), as well as after chronic 14 day NH_4Cl treatment [59]. Whether these "apical" pumps are associated with the plasma membrane or are present in subapical vesicles remains to be determined.

Role of Microtubules in Vesicle Trafficking in Intercalated Cells

Whether or not the same intercalated cell is able to transfer membrane transporters from one pole of the cell to the other, the observation that intercalated cell subpopulations can maintain an opposite polarity with respect to proton pumps remains a finding of great cell biological interest. One possibility that might explain differential targeting of proton pumps is that the apical and basolateral versions of the proton ATPase may not be identical in subunit composition; this difference could confer domain specificity on the targeting process. Another possibility is that the microtubular network is somehow different in cells with apical or basolateral proton pumps, and that vesicles containing the pumps move selectively to only one pole of the cell. As discussed above, it has been proposed that microtubule tracks are important for the delivery of apical proteins, but that basolateral proteins are routed to the

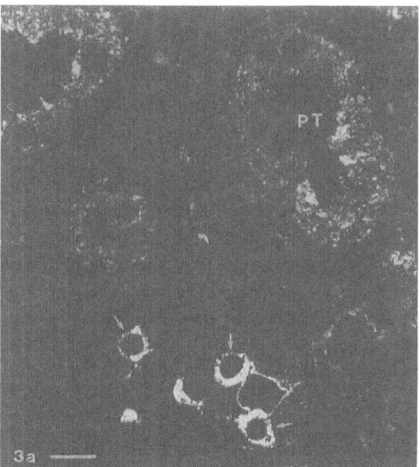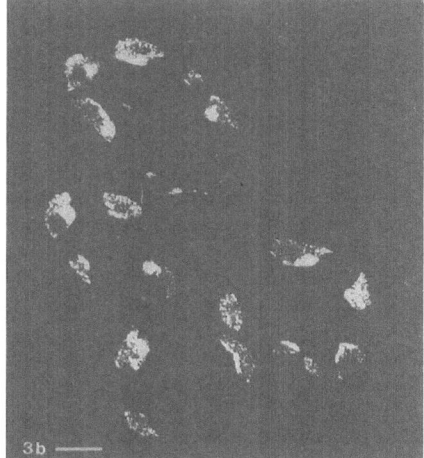

Fig. 3a,b. Part of the cortex (**a**) and inner stripe (**b**) of colchicine-treated rat kidney stained with antibodies against a proton pumping ATPase. In the cortex, proton pumps are distributed on vesicles scattered throughout the cytoplasm of both proximal tubule epithelial cells, and intercalated cells (*arrows*). In the inner stripe of the outer medulla, vesicles containing proton pumps are also distributed throughout the cytoplasm of heavily-labeled intercalated cells. This study was performed in collaboration with Dr. Ivan Sabolic (MGH, Boston) and Dr. Stephen Gluck (Washington University Jewish Hospital, St. Louis, Mo). Bar = 20 μm

base of the cell by a default pathway. In this way, microtubule depolymerization might be expected to result in basolateral, rather than apical insertion of proton pumps. This prediction assumes that vesicles carrying proton pumps are competent to fuse with either apical or basolateral plasma membranes, and that the specificity of the process lies exclusively in the delivery of the vesicles to the appropriate membrane domain. However, this is clearly not the case with another apical membrane protein, gp330, which is present in vesicles that do not fuse with the wrong (i.e., the basolateral) plasma membrane (see above).

This prediction was tested in animals treated for up to 24h with colchicine to induce microtubule depolymerization. In these animals, proton pumps were no longer polarized to one pole of the cell, but they were concentrated in numerous vesicles scattered throughout the cytoplasm (D. Brown, I. Sabolic and S. Gluck, submitted for publication). A similar scattered distribution was seen in A and B intercalated cells, as well as in epithelial cells of the proximal tubule (Fig. 3a). Of particular note is that A-type cells in the inner stripe of the outer medullar did not concentrate proton pumps in their basolateral plasma membranes (Fig. 3b). These results indicate that microtubule depolymerization alone is not sufficient to account for the final differences in the membrane distribution of proton pumps seen in A and B intercalated cells. As is also the case for gp330-containing vesicles in the proximal tubule, an additional level of control must govern the final fusion process between these re-routed vesicles and their target membrane region. The nature of this control process is unknown, but any of the factors discussed in the initial part of this review could be involved.

References

1. Brown D (1989) Membrane recycling and epithelial cell function. Am J Physiol 256: F1–F12
2. Verner K, Schatz G (1988) Protein translocation across membranes. Science 241:1307–1313
3. Davis CG, Lehrman MA, Russell DW, Anderson RGW, Brown MS, Goldstein JL (1986) The J. D. mutation in familial hypercholesterolemia: amino acid substitution in cytoplasmic domain impedes internalization of LDL receptors. Cell 45:15–24
4. Sly WS, Fisher HD (1982) The phosphomannosyl recognition system for intracellular and intercellular transport of lysosomal enzymes. J Cell Biochem 18:319–347
5. Rose JK, Doms RW (1988) Regulation of protein export from the endoplasmic reticulum. Ann Rev Cell Biol 4:257–288
6. Lisanti MP, Caras IW, Dovitz MA, Rodriguez-Boulan E (1989) A glycophospholipid membrane anchor serves as an apical targeting signal in polarized epithelial cells. J Cell Biol 109:2145–2156
7. Garoff H (1985) Using recombinant DNA techniques to study protein targeting in the eucaryotic cell. Ann Rev Cell Biol 1:403–445
8. Brown D, Hirsch S, Gluck S (1988) An H^+ ATPase is present in opposite plasma membrane domains in subpopulations of kidney epithelial cells. Nature 331:622–624
9. Achler C, Filmer D, Merte C, Drenckhahn D (1989) Role of microtubules in polarized delivery of apical membrane proteins to the brush border of the intestinal epithelium. J Cell Biol 109:179–189
10. Heuser J (1989) Changes in lysosome shape and distribution correlated with changes in cytoplasmic pH. J Cell Biol 108:855–864
11. Matteoni R, Kreis TE (1987) Translocation and clustering of endosomes and lysosomes depends on microtubules. J Cell Biol 105:1253–1265
12. Patzelt C, Brown D, Jeanrenaud B (1977) Inhibitory effect of colchicine on amylase secretion by rat parotid glands. Possible localization in the Golgi area. J Cell Biol 73:578–593
13. Pavelka M, Ellinger A, Gangl A (1983) Effect of colchicine on rat small intestinal adsorptive cells I. Formation of basolateral microvillus borders. J Ultrastruct Res 85:249–259
14. Taylor A (1977) Role of microtubules and microfilaments in the action of vasopressin. In: Andreoli TE, Grantham JJ, Rector FC (eds) Disturbances in Body Fluid Osmolality. Am Physiol Soc, Bethesda, pp 97–124
15. Kreis T (1989) Reclustering of scattered Golgi elements occurs along microtubules. Eur J Cell Biol 48:250–263
16. Salas P, Misek D, Vega-Salas D, Gundersen D, Cereijido M, Rodriguez-Boulan E (1986) Microtubules are not critically involved in the biogenesis of epithelial cell surface polarity. J Cell Biol 102:1853–1867
17. Rindler MJ, Ivanov IE, Sabatini DD (1987) Microtubule-acting drugs lead to the nonpolarized delivery of the influenza hemagglutinin to the cell surface of polarized Madin-Darby canine kidney cells. J Cell Biol 104:231–241
18. Eilers U, Klumperman J, Hauri HP (1989) Nocodazole, a microtubule-active drug, interferes with apical protein delivery in cultured intestinal epithelial cells. J Cell Biol 108:13–22
19. Hasegawa H, Watanabe K, Nakamura T, Nagura H (1987) Immunocytochemical localization of alkaline phosphatase in absorptive cells of rat small intestine after colchicine treatment. Cell Tiss Res 250:521–529
20. Vale RD (1987) Intracellular transport using microtubule-based motors. Ann Rev Cell Biol 3:347–378
21. Stetson DL, Steinmetz PR (1983) Role of membrane fusion in CO_2 stimulation of proton secretion by turtle bladder. Am J Physiol 245:C113–C120

22. Orci L, Gabbay KH, Malaisse WJ (1972) Pancreatic beta-cell web: its possible role in insulin secretion. Science 175:1128–1130
23. Muller J, Kachadorian WA, DiScala VA (1980) Evidence that ADH-stimulated intramembrane particle aggregates are transferred from cytoplasmic to luminal membranes in toad bladder epithelial cells. J Cell Biol 85:83–95
24. Laliberte A, Gicquad C (1988) Polymerization of actin by positively-charged liposomes. J Cell Biol 106:1221–1227
25. Bennett V (1985) The membrane skeleton of human erythrocytes and its implications for more complex cells. Annu Rev Biochem 54:273–304
26. Nelson WJ, Veshnock PJ (1986) Dynamics of membrane-skeleton (fodrin) organization during development of polarity in Madin-Darby kidney epithelial cells. J Cell Biol 103: 1751–1765
27. Drenkhahn D, Schluter K, Allen DP, Bennett V (1985) Co-localization of Band 3 with ankyrin and spectrin at the basal membrane of intercalated cells in the rat kidney. Science 230:1287–1289
28. Nelson WJ, Hammerton RW (1989) A membrane-cytoskeletal complex containing Na⁺, K⁺-ATPase, ankyrin, and fodrin in Madin-Darby canine kidney (MDCK) cells: implications for the biogenesis of epithelial cell polarity. J Cell Biol 108:893–902
29. Gutmann EJ, Niles JL, McCluskey RT, Brown D (1989) Colchicine-induced redistribution of an endogenous apical membrane glycoprotein (gp 330) in kidney proximal tubule epithelium. Am J Physiol 257:C397–C407
30. Gilman AG (1987) G-proteins: transducers of receptor-generated signals. Annu Rev Biochem 56:615–649
31. McGrath JP, Capon DJ, Goeddel DV, Levinson AD (1984) Comparative biochemical properties of normal and activated human ras p21 protein. Nature 310:644–649
32. Bokoch GM, Mumby SM (1988) Purification and characterization of the 22,000-Dalton GTP-binding protein substrate for ADP-ribosylation by botulinum toxin, G_{22K*}. J Biol Chem 263:16744–16749
33. Bourne HR (1988) Do GTPases direct membrane traffic in secretion? Cell 53:669–671
34. Aktories K, Weller U, Chhatwal GS (1987) Clostridium botulinum type C produced a novel ADP-ribosyltransferase distinct from botulinum C2 toxin. FEBS Lett 212:109–113
35. Heyworth CM, Whetton AD, Wong S, Martin RB, Houslay MD (1985) Insulin inhibits the cholera-toxin-catalysed ribosylation of a Mr-25,000 protein in rat liver plasma membranes. Biochem J 228:593–603
36. Barbacid MA (1987) Ras genes. Annu Rev Biochem 56:779–827
37. Kahn RA, Gilman AG (1986) The protein cofactor necessary for ADP-ribosylation of Gs by cholera toxin is itself a GTP binding protein. J Biol Chem 261:7906–7911
38. Trahey M, McCormick F (1987) A cytoplasmic protein stimulates normal N-ras p21 GTPase, but does not affect oncogenic mutants. Science 238:542–545
39. Melancon P, Glick BS, Malhotra V, Weidman PJ, Serafini T, Gleason ML, Orci L, Rothman JE (1987) Involvement of GTP-binding "G" proteins in transport through the Golgi stack. Cell 51:1053–1062
40. Nuße O, Lindau M (1988) The dynamics of exocytosis in human neutrophils. J Cell Biol 107:2117–2123
41. Toutant M, Aunis D, Bockaert J, Homburger V, Rouot B (1987) Presence of three pertussis toxin substrates and Go alpha immunoreactivity in both plasma and granule membranes of chromaffin cells. FEBS Lett 215:339–344
42. Goud B, Salminen A, Walworth NC, Novick PJ (1988) A GTP-binding protein required for secretion rapidly associates with secretory vesicles and the plasma membrane in yeast. Cell 53:753–768
43. Wilson DW, Wilcox CA, Flynn GC, Chen E, Huang WK, Henzel WJ, Block MR, Ullrich A, Rothman JE (1989) A fusion protein required for vesicle-mediated transport in both mammalian cells and yeast. Nature 339:355–359

44. Weidman PJ, Melancon P, Block MR, Rothman JE (1989) Binding of and N-ethylmale-imide-sensitive fusion protein to Golgi membranes requires both a soluble protein and an integral membrane receptor. J Cell Biol 108:1589–1596

45. Beckers CJM, Block MR, Glick BS, Rothman JE, Balch WE (1989) Vesicular transport between the endoplasmic reticulum and the Golgi stack requires the NEM-sensitive fusion protein. Nature 339:397–398

46. Novick P, Ferro S, Schekman R (1981) Order of events in the yeast secretory pathway. Cell 25:461–469

47. Clary D, Rothman JE (1990) Purification of three related peripheral membrane proteins needed for vesicular transport. J Biol Chem 265:10109–10117

48. Madsen KM, Tisher CC (1986) Structure-function relationships along the distal nephron. Am J Physiol 250:F1–F15

49. Schwartz GJ, Al-Awqati Q (1985) Carbon dioxide causes exocytosis of vesicles containing H^+ pumps in isolated perfused proximal and collecting tubules. J Clin Invest 75:1638–1644

50. Gluck S, Cannon C, Al-Awqati Q (1982) Exocytosis regulates urinary acidification in turtle bladder by rapid insertion of H^+ pumps into the luminal membrane. Proc Natl Acad Sci USA 79:4327–4331

51. Brown D, Weyer P, Orci L (1987) Non-clathrin coated vesicles are involved in endocytosis in kidney collecting duct intercalated cells. Anat Rec 218:237–242

52. Brown D, Gluck S, Hartwig J (1987) Structure of the novel membrane-coating material in proton-secreting epithelial cells and identification as an H^+ ATPase. J Cell Biol 105:1637–1648

53. Stetson DA, Steinmetz PR (1985) A and B types of carbonic anhydrase-rich cells in turtle bladder. Am J Physiol 249:F553–F565

54. Schwartz GJ, Barasch J, Al-Awqati Q (1985) Plasticity of functional epithelial polarity. Nature 318:368–371

55. Verlander JW, Madsen KM, Tisher CC (1988) Effect of acute respiratory acidosis on two populations of intercalated cells in rat cortical collecting duct. Am J Physiol 253:F1142–F1156

56. Schuster VL, Bonsib SM, Jennings ML (1986) Two types of collecting duct mitochondria-rich (intercalated) cells: lectin and band 3 cytochemistry. Am J Physiol 251:C347–C355

57. Alper SL, Natale J, Gluck S, Lodish HF, Brown D (1989) Subtypes of intercalated cells in rat kidney collecting duct defined by antibodies against erythroid band 3 and renal vacuolar H^+-ATPase. Proc Natl Acad Sci USA 86

58. Satlin LM, Schwartz GJ (1989) Cellular remodelling of HCO_3^- secreting cells in rabbit renal collecting duct in response to an acidic environment. J Cell Biol 109:1279–1288

59. Bastani B, Purcell H, Hemken P, Gluck S (1990) Adaptational changes in rat kidney H^+ ATPase after chronic acid (AC) or alkali (AL) loading. Kidney Int 37:532a

Sorting of Surface Proteins and Lipids in Epithelial Cells

KAI SIMONS[1]

SUMMARY. The sorting of newly synthesized apical and basolateral proteins in epithelial cells seems to follow three different scenarios. In Madin-Darby canine kidney (MDCK) cells, apical and basolateral proteins are sorted primarily on the exocytic route in the trans Golgi network. In hepatocytes they are sorted on the endocytic-transcytotic route. In intestinal Caco-2 cells both pathways are used. We have proposed that all the data can be accommodated by a model in which sorting to the apical domain is signal-mediated, while delivery to the basolateral domain represents a default pathway [1].

Introduction

Epithelial cells are polarized to carry out their vectorial functions in secretion, absorption, and ion transport. The plasma membrane of each epithelial cell is divided into two domains with distinct protein and lipid compositions [2,3]. An apical domain confronts the organism's exterior and a basolateral domain, attached to an underlying extracellular matrix, faces the interior. The proteins in the apical domain seem to vary according to epithelial cell type and function, whereas the basolateral domain is more like the plasma membrane of non-polarized cells and contains proteins responsible for nutrient uptake, for regulation of intracellular ionic environment, and for growth control, in addition to epithelial-specific junctional and adhesion proteins. The two plasma membrane domains are separated by circumferential tight junctions which form an occluding barrier between neighboring cells and simultaneously prevent intermixing of apical and basolateral components [4,5].

One central problem in the field of epithelial cell biology is how the polarized distribution of newly synthesized surface proteins and lipids is achieved. Three different

---

[1]European Molecular Biology Laboratory, Meyerhofstr. 1, Postfach 10.2209, D-6900 Heidelberg, Federal Republic of Germany

scenarios are now known. The first one is the best studied and derives from analysis of biosynthetic membrane traffic in filter-grown kidney MDCK cells. When epithelial cells are cultured on permeable supports, they form a tightly polarized cell layer that mimics the epithelial organization observed in vivo [2]. Both exogenous viral glycoproteins and endogenous surface proteins are sorted before they reach the plasma membrane, most likely in the trans-Golgi network (TGN) of the Golgi complex [2,3,1,6]. In the TGN of MDCK cells, apical and baso-lateral proteins are packaged into separate apical and basolateral carrier vesicles which transport the proteins to their surface destinations [7]. In addition to resident apical and basolateral proteins that carry out their functions in the apical or the basolateral membranes respectively, there is another class of epithelial surface proteins that function in transporting ligands from one surface domain to the other across the cell [8]. These transcytosing receptors include the polymeric immunoglobulin receptor (pIgR) which transports IgA and IgM from the basolateral to the apical side in a variety of epithelia [9]. This receptor is not present in MDCK cells, but when the cDNA encoding the rabbit pIgR is expressed in these cells, the newly synthesized receptor is routed from the Golgi complex to the basolateral side, and after endocytosis from the basolateral membrane, pIgR undergoes transcytosis to the apical side [10]. Such transcytosing proteins can therefore be present on both the basolateral and the apical membranes. Recent studies have confirmed that endogenous proteins present on both sides of MDCK cells are involved in transcytosis in both directions [11].

MDCK cells also secrete newly synthesized proteins into the apical and the basolateral media. Secretion is polarized, e.g., laminin and heparan proteoglycan are secreted in the basolateral direction, while glycoprotein (GP) 80 is predominantly secreted into the apical medium [12,13]. The mechanism responsible for the polarity of secretion is not yet known, but, most likely, secretory proteins bind to sorting receptors in the Golgi complex; the complexes are then sorted into apical and basolateral carrier vesicles in a way which is analogous to the mechanism by which mannose 6-phosphate containing enzymes are bound to mannose 6-phosphate receptors; these carrier vesicles are in turn sorted into clathrin-coated vesicles for delivery to the endocytic pathway [14]. If exogenous secretory proteins such as lysozyme are expressed in MDCK cells, they become secreted in an unpolarized fashion [15,16]. Since the cells presumably lack the appropriate sorting receptors for these exogenous proteins, they distribute passively into the luminal contents of both the apical and the basolateral carrier vesicles. In this way, they are delivered indiscriminately to both sides of the epithelium.

Not only are the proteins of the apical and basolateral plasma membrane domains different, but their lipid compositions also differ [17]. The lipid constituents of the apical membrane are unusual because of their high content of sphingolipids. This layer of glycolipids facing the exterior protects the cells from outside injuries. The basolateral membrane, on the other hand, has a lipid composition similar to that of the plasma membrane of non-polarized cells. Differences in lipid compositions of the epithelial membrane domains also seem to be generated during biosynthetic membrane traffic. Sphingolipid sorting has been studied in filter-grown MDCK cells [18]. The data suggest that glycosphingolipid sorting, like protein sorting, takes place in the TGN and that the sphingolipids are included in the same exocytic carrier vesicles as the membrane proteins.

The second scenario for sorting proteins to the epithelial cell surface is provided by studies with hepatocytes. Each hepatocyte has several apical poles, which line the bile canaliculi and are separated from the intervening basolateral membranes by tight junctions. Hubbard et al. have shown that both apical and basolateral membrane proteins are delivered from the Golgi complex to the basolateral membrane before sorting occurs [19]. The apical proteins are sorted after endocytosis to basolateral early endosomes and are then delivered by transcytosis to the apical side. The apical proteins that have been studied seem to follow the route taken by the transcytosing pIgR. They probably have no other alternative because the apical route from the TGN appears to be missing in hepatocytes. The massive amounts of albumin and other secretory proteins produced by hepatocytes are secreted constitutively from the basolateral (sinusoidal) membrane. Proteins found in the bile seem to be derived from the blood, either by transcytosis across the liver cell or by passage between the cells. The reason for the lack of a direct secretory route from the TGN to the apical side may be the need to avoid the loss of newly synthesized plasma proteins into the bile. If membrane traffic from the TGN to the hepatocyte cell surface were possible only by transport along the basolateral route, then sorting receptors would not be required for exocytosis. Constitutive secretion could occur simply by default.

The third scenario for epithelial protein sorting is derived from recent studies with intestinal CaCo-2 cells [20]. These cells seem to use features from both the MDCK and the hepatocyte sorting mechanisms. Some apical proteins (such as sucrase-isomaltase) are routed directly from the TGN, while other apical proteins (amino peptidase N and dipeptidyl peptidase IV) use both the direct route to the apical membrane and the transcytotic pathway via the basolateral membrane. Secretion of proteins in CaCo-2 cells occurs mainly in the basolateral direction [21,22]. Expression of exogenous immunoglobulin kappa light chains leads to secretion of 90% of the protein into the basolateral medium, while only 10% is secreted apically. The available data thus suggest that the apical route from the TGN exists but it may not have as high a capacity in CaCo-2 cells as in MDCK cells.

The simplest model for explaining these results is to postulate that only one of the two epithelial pathways for delivery of surface proteins operates by signal-recognition (Fig. 1). We have suggested that apical sorting from the TGN is the pathway that requires specific sorting signals, whereas the basolateral pathway from the TGN operates by default, as proposed for membrane traffic to the cell surface from the TGN in non-polarized cells [1,6,17]. The differences in routing from the TGN would be reduced to either the non-existence of an apical route from the TGN in hepatocytes, or to differences in the affinities of apical proteins for the sorting machinery in the TGN of CaCo-2 cells. Apical proteins not sorted into apical carrier vesicles would be included in the basolateral default vesicles for delivery to the basolateral side. The sorting of the apical proteins from the basolateral side requires an additional sorting step that probably takes place immediately after endocytosis from the basolateral plasma membrane into early endosomes from which the transcytotic carrier vesicles form [1,6] (Fig. 2).

This model for epithelial sorting specifies that apical membrane protein should have specific sorting signals whereas basolateral membrane proteins require none. Is this model compatible with what is known of epithelial sorting signals? Unfortunately, an affirmative answer is not possible from available data [12,23]. Despite numerous attempts, identification of the sorting signals for transmembrane proteins

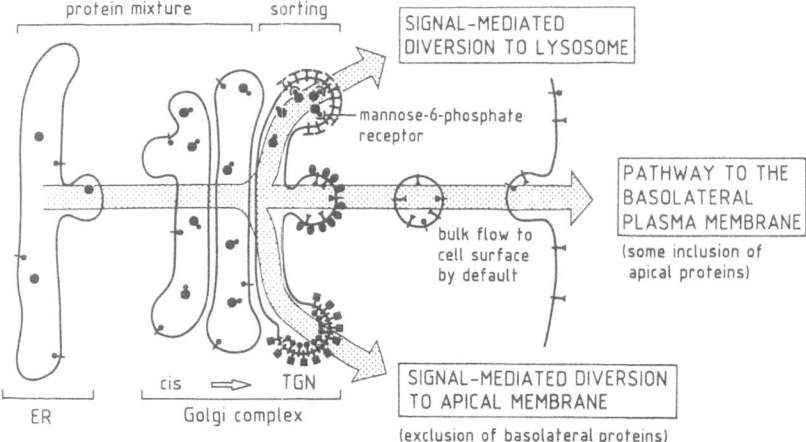

Fig. 1. Working model for sorting from the trans-Golgi network (*TGN*) in MDCK cells. Three possible exit routes from the trans-Golgi network are indicated; two of which lead to the plasma membrane and one which leads to lysosomes [14]. Inclusion in the apical transport vesicles requires specific signals and unrecognized proteins are specifically excluded. The basolateral transport vesicles represent the bulk flow route and carry those proteins to the surface which have not been segregated by selective sorting processes. Constitutive secretory proteins are not indicated, but their vectorial delivery is assumed to be dependent on binding to membrane-bound receptors. In the absence of recognition, soluble proteins would be free to be carried with the fluid phase to both membrane domains. (Model from [6])

has not been successful. Most studies would agree that the sorting information is in the extracytoplasmic domain of both apical and basolateral proteins. Expression of chimeric proteins are usually routed to the apical cell surface if they contain the extracytoplasmic part of an apical protein. However, several notable exceptions are known [24–26]. The observed results can, however, be accommodated by apical-specific sorting and delivery to basolateral membranes by default. Sorting into apical vesicles would have to depend on both signal-mediated inclusion and specific exclusion of both basolateral proteins and proteins which contain apical sorting signals, but have cytoplasmic domains with structures that are incompatible with the formation of the specific protein-protein interactions which are necessary for the assembly of the apical carrier vesicle [1]. It is possible that post-translational modifications, e.g., phosphorylation, can regulate whether exclusion occurs or not [24]. Another possibility is that the binding of an accessory protein to the cytosolic domain leads to exclusion.

The open question is whether glycolipid sorting operates in all epithelial cells [17] and whether or not transcytosis involves glycolipid sorting. Does basolateral to apical transcytosis involve the same machinery as that which is used for making apical carrier vesicles in the TGN? Or is it a different machinery with its own sorting specificity? Since the magnitude of transcytotic traffic is considerable [27], it is difficult to envisage transcytosis without both protein and lipid sorting. Otherwise, the two plasma membrane domains would slowly intermix. The sorting of sphingolipids in

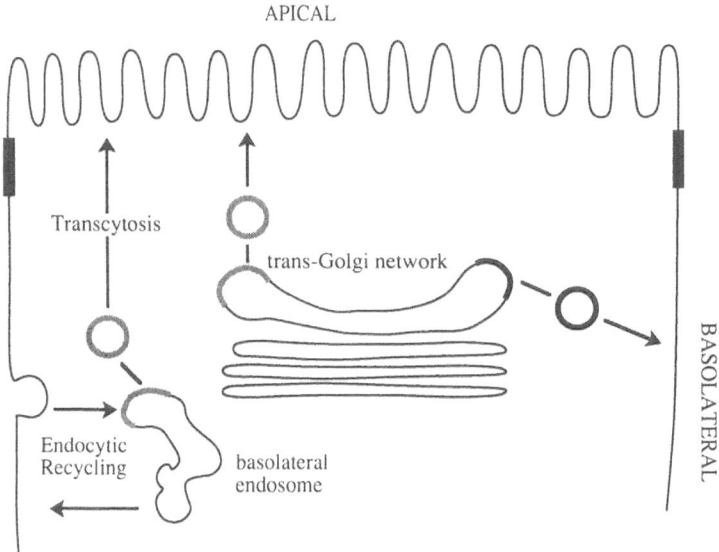

Fig. 2. Sorting pathways for newly synthesized apical and basolateral proteins in epithelial cells. Apical proteins that are not sorted in the apical direction in the trans-Golgi network (*TGN*) leave the Golgi by the postulated default pathway to the basolateral side. Here the apical proteins become internalized by endocytosis in the early endosomes (see [29] and [30]). The proteins can be recycled back to the basolateral domain or sorted into transcytosic vesicles that carry the proteins to the apical surface domain. One important difference between sorting from the trans-Golgi network and from the basolateral early endosomes is the time spent in the sorting compartment. Newly synthesized apical proteins reside only a short time in the Golgi complex before exiting, while apical proteins at the basolateral cell surface can recycle back and forth between the plasma membrane and the early endosome before being included into a transcytotic carrier vesicle. Proteins with a low affinity to the postulated sorting protein in the trans-Golgi network might leave the trans-Golgi network by the basolateral route before being sorted. These apical proteins can be slowly sorted to the apical side from the basolateral endosome by transcytosis [1]. ER, endoplasmic reticulum

the TGN of MDCK cells has been postulated to be coupled to protein sorting [17]. Apical proteins have been proposed to interact with sorting receptors, which in turn interact with glycosphingolipid clusters to form a subdomain in the TGN membrane which is induced to bud with putative accessory proteins into a carrier vesicle. Basolateral proteins and lipids would be excluded because they cannot participate in the cooperative bonding process. An interesting group of proteins are those with glycophospholipid anchors. In several epithelial cell types, these are predominantly localized to the apical membrane [28]. Recent studies have shown that the glycophospholipid anchors themselves contain the apical sorting signals. It is, therefore, possible that these proteins are sorted into the apical carrier vesicles in the same way as glycolipids are.

Concluding Remarks

The challenge in the field of epithelial protein and lipid sorting is the identification of the proteins which are responsible for apical and basolateral sorting and specific targeting to the correct membrane domain. The first steps in this direction have been taken by the isolation of apical and basolateral carrier vesicles, derived from the trans-Golgi network of MDCK cells [7]. It is now possible to study the individual proteins of these vesicles and to study their function in sorting and vesicle targeting.

References

1. Simons K, Wandinger-Ness A (1990) Polarized sorting in epithelia. Cell 62:207–210
2. Simons K, Fuller SD (1985) Cell surface polarity in epithelia. Annu Rev Cell Biol 1:243–288
3. Rodriguez-Boulan E, Nelson J (1989) Morphogenesis of the polarized epithelial cell phenotype. Science 245:718–725
4. Gumbiner B, Simons K (1987) The role of uvomorulin in the formation of epithelial occluding junctions. John Wiley and Sons, New York, pp 168–180
5. Simons K (1990) The epithelial tight junction: occluding barrier and fence. In: Edelman GM, Cunningham BA, Thiery J-P (eds) Morphoregulatory molecules, vol 2. John Wiley and Sons, New York 341–356
6. Wandinger-Ness A, Simons K (1991) The polarized transport of surface proteins and lipids in epithelial cells. In: Hanover J, Steer C (eds) Intracellular Trafficking of Proteins. Cambridge University Press, Cambridge 575–612
7. Wandinger-Ness A, Bennett MK, Antony C, Simons (1990) Distinct transport vesicles mediate the delivery of plasma membrane proteins to the apical and basolateral domains of MDCK Cells. J Cell Biol 111:987–1000
8. Van Deurs B, Petersen OW, Olsnes S, Sandvig K (1989) The ways of endocytosis. Int Rev Cytol 117:31–178
9. Mostov KE, Simister NE (1985) Transcytosis. Cell 43:389–390
10. Mostov KE, Deitcher DL (1986) Polymeric immunoglobulin receptor expressed in MDCK cells transcytoses IgA. Cell 46:613–621
11. Brändli AW, Parton RG, Simons K (1990) Transcytosis in MDCK cells: identification of glycoproteins transported bidirectionally between both plasma membrane domains. J Cell Biol, in press
12. Caplan M, Matlin KS (1989) Sorting of membrane and secretory proteins in polarized epithelial cells. Mod Cell Biol 8:71–127
13. Urban J, Parczyk K, Leutz A, Kayne M, Kondor-Koch C (1987) Constitutive apical secretion of an 80-kDa sulfated glycoprotein complex in the polarized epithelial Madin-Darby canine kidney cell line. J Cell Biol 105:2735–2743
14. Kornfeld S, Mellman I (1989) The biogenesis of lysosomes. Annu Rev Cell Biol 5:483–525
15. Gottlieb TA, Beaudry G, Rizzolo L, Colman M, Rindler M, Adesnik M, Sabatini DD (1986) Secretion of endogenous and exogenous proteins from polarized MDCK cell monolayers. Proc Natl Acad Sci USA 83:2100–2104
16. Kondor-Koch CB, Bravo R, Fuller SD, Cutler D, Garoff H (1985) Exocytic pathways exist to both the apical and the basolateral cell surface of the polarized epithelial cell MDCK. Cell 43:297–306
17. Simons K, van Meer G (1988) Lipid sorting in epithelial cells. Biochemistry 27:6197–6202

18. van Meer G, Stelzer EHK, Wijnaendts-van-Resandt R, Simons K (1987) Sorting of sphingolipids in epithelial (Madin-Darby canine kidney) cells. J Cell Biol 105:1623–1635
19. Hubbard AL, Stieger B, Bartles JR (1989) Biogenesis of endogenous plasma membrane proteins in epithelial cells. Annu Rev Physiol 51:735–770
20. Matter K, Brauchbar M, Bucher K, Hauri H-P (1990) Sorting of endogenous plasma membrane proteins occurs from two sites in cultured human intestinal epithelial cells. Cell 60:429–437
21. Traber MG, Kayden HJ, Rindler MJ (1987) Polarized secretion of newly synthesized lipoproteins by the Caco-2 human intestinal cell line. J Lipid Res 28:1350–1363
22. Hughson EJ, Cutler DF, Hopkins CR (1989) Basolateral secretion of kappa light chain in the polarized epithelial cell line, Caco-2. J Cell Sci 94:327–332
23. Roth MG (1989) Molecular Biological Approaches to Protein Sorting. Annu Rev Physiol 51:797–810
24. Casanova JE, Breitfeld PP, Ross SA, Mostov KE (1990) Phosphorylation of the polymeric immunoglobulin receptor required for its efficient transcytosis. Science 248:742–745
25. Roth MG, Ktistakis N, Shia S-P, Zwart D, Thomas D, Brewer C (1990) Recombinant glycoproteins as probes for sorting events occurring during intracellular transport (abstract). FASEB J 4:A2180
26. Hunziker W, Mellman I (1989) Expression of macrophage-lymphocyte receptors in MDCK cells: polarity and transcytosis differ for isoforms with or without coated pit localization domains. J Cell Biol 109:3291–3302
27. von Bonsdorff C-H, Fuller SD, Simons K (1985) Apical and basolateral endocytosis in MDCK cells grown on nitrocellulose filters. EMBO J 4:2781–2792
28. Lisanti MP, Rodriguez-Boulan E (1990) Glycophospholipid membrane anchoring provides clues to the mechanism of protein sorting in polarized epithelial cells. TIBS 15:113–118
29. Bomsel M, Prydz K, Parton RG, Gruenberg J, Simons K (1989) Endocytosis in filter-grown Madin-Darby canine kidney cells. J Cell Biol 109:3243–3258
30. Parton RG, Prydz K, Bomsel M, Simons K, Griffiths G (1989) Meeting of the apical and basolateral endocytic pathways of the Madin-Darby canine kidney cell in late endosomes. J Cell Biol 109:3259–3272

Masugi Memorial Symposium: Experimental Nephritis and Its Contribution to Nephrology

Chair: Hidekazu Shigematsu (Japan)
Curtis B. Wilson (USA)

Matazo Masugi and Nephrotoxic Nephritis

Yozo Masugi[1]

Matazo Masugi, the author's father and the discoverer of nephrotoxic serum nephritis, was born in Japan almost 100 years ago – in 1896 in Ohtsu, a city near Kyoto. The house where he was born still stands, and he lived there with his parents until 1917, at which time, having graduated from Senior high school in Kyoto, he went to Tokyo to enter the Medical School of Tokyo Imperial University.

In 1921, upon graduation, he entered the Department of Pathology of this university. After undergoing fundamental training in pathological anatomy for several years, in 1925 he was given an opportunity to further his studies in basic medical science in Europe.

At that time, the main overseas destination for medical scholars funded by the Japanese government was Germany. Possibly for this reason, he first went to the Institute of Pathology, known as Aschoff House, at Freiburg University. There, under the guidance of Professor Aschoff, he continued studies into the relationship between monocytes and histiocytes [1] that had been initiated by the late Professor Kiyono of Kyoto University.

In the following year, on completion of this work, he transferred to the Pathology Institute of Basel University in Switzerland. There, under Professor Rössle, he engaged in the study of specific anti-serum action on monocellular organisms such as paramecium, in order to develop prototypes of cytotoxic cellular damage. As a consequence of these studies, he concluded that the action of cytotoxin on paramecia caused an initial paralysis in the organisms that ultimately led to death [2]. Because of his involvement in this research, it can be assumed that his general interest in the actions of cytotoxin was thus developed.

In October 1927, he returned to Japan via the United States, and soon after, at the age of 32, he was appointed the Professor of Pathology at Chiba Medical School. During this period, maintaining his original interest in cytotoxic cells and tissue damage, he began to study kidney and liver changes in rats after respective adminis-

---

[1]Department of Pathology, Nippon Medical School, Tokyo, 113, Japan

trations of nephrotoxin or hepatotoxin. Each cytotoxin prepared for this purpose was made from immunized rabbits.

Two years later, in 1929, at a convention of the Japanese Pathological Society [3], he reported the first results of his investigations into cytotoxic organ changes, wherein he concluded that cytotoxin could produce damage in targeted parenchymal cells, such as the damage to urinary tubuli of the kidney produced by nephrotoxin, or the damage produced in hepatic cells by hepatotoxin administration. At the same time, however, he noted a generalized anaphylactic shock that occurred in some animals. Therefore, he also presented the associated evidence of a functional derangement of the vascular system that occurred through reversed anaphylaxis, due to antibody conjugation to the vascular tissues.

In retrospect, this observation appears to be the first step toward his later discovery of nephrotoxic serum nephritis. Still, he apparently did not focus much attention on glomerular changes in these experiments.

In any event he was not greatly satisfied with the results that he obtained regarding cytotoxic organ changes in these provisional experiments. Thus, during the next few years, he continued to experiment on rats, administering nephrotoxin or hepatotoxin, concentrating his search on the primary effect of cytotoxin on the targeted organ.

Finally, after many experiments, he came to realize that the primary target of the cytotoxin must be the vascular system of the target organ, such as the glomerular capillaries of the kidney in the case of nephrotoxin administration. Therefore, damage to the parenchymal cells, such as to the tubular epithelia, which hitherto had been generally thought to be the target, was secondary to the glomerular change. Using this same reasoning, the effect of the hepatotoxin on the liver was also interpreted as being due to vascular change, in this case, change in the periportal areas. In conclusion, he speculated that the changes produced by nephrotoxin in the kidney of rat were similar to the changes of human glomerulonephritis, and that the changes produced by hepatotoxin in the liver corresponded to the changes of human eclampsia.

In later years, he recalled how difficult it was to upset the previously unchallenged concept of the cytotoxin target, especially that of nephrotoxin. In any event, he reported these findings to the annual review of the Japanese Pathological Society in 1931 [4], and later he contributed an article to Ziegler's Beitrage zur path. Anatomie in 1933 [5], although this latter article had no accompanying microscopic pictures of the target organs.

Confident of his findings, he decided to use larger animals, such as rabbits, for successive experiments. For preparing the anti-rabbit kidney serum he used duck, the animal that was then usually used for the production of antisera to blood group-specific substances. Further, in pursuing his experiments, he not only studied each rabbit kidney histologically, but also followed the clinical and the laboratory data of each experimental animal given nephrotoxin.

In this manner, he concluded that the nephrotoxic serum nephritis of his experimental rabbits was similar, both pathologically and clinically, to human glomerulonephritis. Further, he was able to create many kinds of diffuse glomerulonephritis in his experimental animals. According to the anti-kidney antibody titer of the antiserum he used and by varying the amount of the administered volume, he was able to induce acute, subacute, or chronic, diffuse glomerulonephritis, as well as an acute variety that terminated in a diffuse, glomerular fibrin thrombus formation.

Based on this capability, he came to decide that this specific antigen-antibody reaction, i.e., the allergic reaction occurring at the glomerular capillaries, was the pathogenetic factor responsible for diffuse glomerulonephritis.

In 1932, he contributed this evidence to the annual review of the Japanese Pathological Society [6]. Two years later, he submitted his findings to Ziegler's Beitrage zur path. Anatomie, along with a series of histological pictures of his experimental animals and their pertinent clinical charts [7]. This latter article had a considerable impact on the medical world, and the existence of nephrotoxic serum nephritis gradually came to be accepted internationally, and was later verified through many other experimental reports.

Among the many studies of cytotoxic organ changes that he pursued, only nephrotoxic serum nephritis became accepted as having a pathogenetic significance. As I have mentioned previously, he also thought that the periportal vascular change that occurred in the liver of rats after hepatotoxin administration was similar to human eclamptic liver change, although this observation did not gain acceptance.

He also pursued studies of heart changes produced in rats after administration of an anti-heart serum, i.e., a cardiotoxin prepared from rabbits. However, he was unable to induce a rheumatoid heart, although he did report the finding of sporadic vascular changes in the interstitium of the heart that he felt were general manifestations of cytotoxic organ change [8]. Additionally, in 1938, in the field of human pathology, he is thought to have been the first person to describe the vascular changes of diffuse schlerodermia in the skin [9].

He would have continued to expand his research, but he began to suffer from persistent anemia of unknown origin, and in March 1939 he had to be hospitalized, thus making it impossible for him to pursue his studies independently.

His lecture on allergy and its pathologic significance [10], which he had been asked to give at the convention of the Japanese Pathological Society in April 1939, had to be read by someone else. This lecture covered not only nephrotoxic serum nephritis, but also multiple allergic disorders in experimental animals and in human diseases that he had studied.

In April 1942, his days as a professor officially ended, and in March 1944, he retired from Chiba Medical School due to illness. Shortly after, in August 1945, World War II in Asia ended. The following year, though his health was very poor, he took on professorial work in pathology at some private medical schools in Tokyo.

His post-war days, however, were numbered, and in September 1947, after being confined to bed for two weeks, he died at the age of 51. An autopsy disclosed a massive bilateral hemothorax and diffuse pericardial adhesions of an undetermined nature.

This briefly covers my father's career and the work that he accomplished. It is said that the administration of nephrotoxin in experimental animals was originated as a procedure by Lindemann in 1900 [11]. The achievement of Matazo Masugi, however, was that he altered a prevailing idea, proving that the target of nephrotoxin was not the tubular epithelia, but the glomeruli in the kidney. Moreover, he clarified the significance of the allergic reaction that occurs at the glomerular capillaries in the pathogenesis of diffuse glomerulonephritis.

Permit a final observation. Matazo Masugi speculated that the apparent period of latency in rabbit nephrotoxic nephritis, brought about by the administration of duck antiserum, was due to the necessary lag time for the nephrotoxin and the glomeruli to combine.

Retrospectively, I regret that he may not have read Kay's two phase theory, concerning the occurrence of nephrotoxic nephritis, that was published in November 1940 [12]. The world was at war, so that he may not have been able to read this paper, and thus we are deprived of his learned opinion.

References

1. Masugi M (1927) Über die Beziehungen zwischen Monozyten und Histiocyten. Beitr Path Anat 76:396–443
2. Masugi M (1927) Über die Wirkung des Normal- sowie des spezifischen Immunserums auf die Paramäzien. Über die Immunität derselben gegen die beiden Serumwirkungen. Krhtforschg 5:375–402
3. Masugi M (1929) Über die spezifisch zytotoxische Wirkung des Antinieren- und -leberserums sowie über die sog. umgekehrte Anaphylaxie. Trans Jpn Path Soc 19:132–137
4. Masugi M, Tomizuka Y (1931) Über die spezifisch zototoxischen Veränderungen der Niere und der Leber durch das spezifische Antiserum (Nephrotoxin und Hepatotoxin). Zugleich ein Beitrag zur Pathogenese der Glomerulonephritis. Trans Jpn Path Soc 21:329–341
5. Masugi M (1933) Über das Wesen der spezifischen Veränderungen der Niere und der Leber durch das Nephrotoxin bzw. das Hepatotoxin. Zugleich ein Beitrag zur Pathogenese der Glomerulonephritis und der eklamptischen Lebererkrankung. Beitr Path Anat 91:82–112
6. Masugi M, Sato Y, Murasawa S, Tomizuka Y (1932) Über die experimentelle Glomerulonephritis durch das spezifische Antinierenserum. Trans Jpn Path Soc 22:614–628
7. Masugi M (1934) Über die experimentelle Glomerulonephritis durch das spezifische Antinierenserum. Ein Beitrag zur Pathogenese der diffusen Glomerulonephritis. Beitr Path Anat 92:429–466
8. Masugi M, Sato Y, Todo S (1935) Über die Veränderungen des Herzens durch das spezifische Antiherzserum. Experimentelle Untersuchungen über die allergischen Gewebsschäden des Herzens. Trans Jpn Path Soc 25:211–216
9. Masugi M, Yä S (1938) Die difuse Sklerodermie und ihre Gefässveränderung. Virchows Arch [A] 302:39–62
10. Masugi M (1939) Die Allergie und ihre pathologische Bedeutung. Trans Jpn Path Soc 29:603–631
11. Lindemann W (1900) Sur le mode d'action de certains poisons renaux. Ann Inst Pasteur 13:49–59
12. Kay CF (1940) The mechanism by which experimental nephritis is produced injected with nephrotoxic duck serum. J Exp Med 72:559–572

In Situ Immune Complex Nephritis

Arnold Vogt[1]

Introduction

Until the beginning of the nineteen eighties it was generally believed that glomerulonephritis was a "soluble complex disease" [1–3], the exception being that induced by anti-GBM antibody. Glomerular injury was considered to be the result of antigen-antibody deposits, with inflammation-inducing properties, which had previously been formed within the circulation [4]. This way of looking at things – for a long time it almost had the status of a dogma – was eventually challenged by Couser and Salant [5], who pointed at observations in passive Heymann nephritis, where the disease is not the result of circulating immune complexes but arises from combinations of the anti Fx1A antibody with particular surface structures of the glomerular epithelial cells [6,7]. The main target molecule has been identified as a glycoprotein of 330 kD, known as gp 330 [8].

The target molecule in passive Heymann nephritis is an intrinsic structure of the glomerulus, as in Masugi nephritis. In human immune complex nephritis the putative nephritogenic antigens are more likely to be non-glomerular components, of exogenous – in the case of postinfectious glomerulonephritis (GN) – or autologous – in the case of an autoimmune associated GN like Lupus nephritis – origin.

Antigens Possessing Affinity for the Glomerular Basement Membrane (GBM)

Postulating that there is an in situ mechanism of immune complex formation with an exogenous antigen in most forms of human immune complex glomerulonephritis (ICGN), one readily hits on the idea that the nephritogenic antigen should possess a

[1]Institute of Medical Microbiology, D-78 Freiburg, Federal Republic of Germany

particular quality which is responsible for its binding to distinct structures in the glomerulus. Izui, prompted by in vitro findings, was the first to propose such an affinity for DNA in systemic lupus erythematosus (SLE) associated nephritis [9]. Though it turns out that DNA alone does not possess an affinity for the GBM in vivo [10], the idea of a "planted antigen" stimulated a body of interesting experimental work. In 1979 Golbus and Wilson showed that Concanavalin A can be planted in the GBM and can act as a target for subsequently injected antibody [11]. A number of lectins can bind to various structures in the kidney [12], but it is questionable whether lectins are included among nephritogenic antigens. In the beginning of the 1980s, three groups independently drew attention to cationic antigens and their potential role as planted antigens. Border's groups [13,14], working with the experimental model of chronic serum sickness, found cationized antigen to be far more effective in inducing nephritis than the native anionic molecule.

Gallo and co-workers, studying the fate of passively administered preformed immune complexes, observed a predominantly capillary localization when complexes were prepared from cationized antigen, in contrast to the mesangial deposition of complexes prepared from unmodified (anionic) antigen [15-17]. Our group studied the influence of the charge and size of protein molecules on their capability of acting as planted antigens for circulating antibodies [18-22]. All authors unanimously emphasized the ability of both cationic antigens and cationic immune complexes to form subepithelial deposits. Complexes prepared from unmodified (anionic) antigen localize predominantly within the mesangium or in the subendothelial space [23,24]. Only when complexes were prepared in high antigen excess, or when small complexes were obtained with low avidity antibody, have subepithelial deposits been noted [25].

Influence of Charge and Size on the Affinity of Proteins for the GBM

Polycations not only have more easy access to the glomerular filtration barrier, they also interact with the anionic structures of the GBM [21]. In contrast to unmodified proteins, circulating molecules will accumulate along the glomerular capillary wall when highly cationized, and they may persist in the GBM for a while. To interact with and persist in the GBM, the cationic molecule must fulfill certain requirements. In addition to having a high positive overall charge (pI greater than 8.5) the size is critical (>40 kD). Accumulation of cationic molecules in the GBM increases with increasing size. Small molecules like monomeric lysozyme (MW 14400, pI 11.3) are not retarded within the GBM even though they are highly positively charged. Intravenously injected ovalbumin (40 kD) only becomes detectable along the GBM when heavily cationized (pI > 10.0). Ferritin, on the other hand, will already fix to the GBM when its pI is about 9.0 [21]. The persistence of cationized proteins in the GBM is clearly governed by charge and size. While highly cationized ferritin can be detected in the glomeruli of rats up to 16h after intravenous injection of 5 to 10 mg per animal, highly cationized ovalbumin is demonstrable for less than 2 hours.

In Situ Immune Complex Formation

From the foregoing it is clear that for an injected antibody to reach a planted antigen the antibody has to be administered within a relatively short interval after antigen administration. With highly cationized HuIgG and ferritin, an interval of 15 minutes–2 hours between antigen and antibody administration will result in massive subepithelial immune deposits. From electronmicroscopic studies with ferritin we learned that the immune complexes were formed primarily on the endothelial site, and were transferred, with time, to the subepithelial region, where they persisted for weeks [21].

Though massive subepithelial immune complex formation occurs after intravenous injection of both antigen and antibody, nephritis can be induced only when the cationized antigen is perfused intrarenally, followed by intravenous injection of the specific antibody. This puzzling aspect of the experimental model of in situ immune complex nephritis is also seen in the active model, where the cationized antigen has to be injected intrarenally into the immunized animal [22]. The reason for this is not known. It may be connected with the influence of cationized proteins on the clotting and complement systems or it may be due to the fact that antibody binds less well to cationized antigens [26]. The latter reason, however, is less likely to be true because very small amounts, i.e., a few micrograms of cationized antigen and antibody, are sufficient to induce a fullblown, unilateral nephritis [20].

Polycations can Mediate the Glomerular Deposition of Polyanions

The glomerular deposition of highly anionic molecules can be mediated by polycations. Native ferritin (ESR 61 Å), which, due to its size (500 kD) and negative charge (pI 4.5–4.8), is not able to enter the GBM, accumulates massively within the lamina rara of an animal which has been previously injected with the polycation polethyleneimine [27,28]. We have explored this idea with polydisperse DNA fragments and the naturally occurring polycation histone. In contrast to the general assumption that DNA and anti-DNA-antibodies are essentially involved in the pathogenesis of SLE associated GN, we propose that binding of histones to the GBM is the initiating event in the development of Lupus nephritis. DNA alone does not possess any affinity for the GBM. After intravenous injection no significant deposition of DNA in the isolated glomeruli can be detected [10]; however, when histone, which like (PEI), possesses a high affinity for the GBM, has been injected previously then massive deposits of DNA fragments can be found along the glomerular capillary wall [29].

Our hypothesis that histones are one of the nephritogenic antigens involved in the pathogenesis of Lupus nephritis is supported by the finding that histones can frequently be detected by indirect immunofluorescence staining in glomerular deposits of Lupus nephritis. This holds true for kidneys of diseased NZB/NZW F_1 mice [30], graft versus host mice, and for kidney biopsies obtained from patients with Lupus nephritis (unpublished work). In this connection it is of interest that antibodies to histones can be found regularly in the sera of patients with Lupus nephritis [31].

Cationic Antigens Involved in the Pathogenesis of Postinfectious GN

Our efforts to identify nephritogenic cationic proteins from bacteria associated with postinfectious GN were at first less successful than the studies reported above. The expectation in 1982 that we had, for the first time, identified a nephritogenic antigen from an infectious agent, proved to be premature. The streptococcal antigen found in the glomerular deposits [32] was identified as a cationic streptococcal protease, which had been described and characterized earlier by Liu and Elliot [33] and which possessed, as we had to learn, no affinity for the GBM in its monomeric form. In fact, none of the three streptococcal antigens so far accused of being involved in the pathogenesis of acute post-streptococcal glomerulonephritis (APSGN) – the nephritis strain associated protein (NSAP) of Zabriskies' group [34], the endostreptosin of Lange's group [35] or our cationic streptococcal protease – fulfill the most important of Koch's postulates, that is, they are not capable of inducing nephritis in experimental models.

Outlook

The search for nephritogenic antigens in postinfectious GN has to continue. I believe that the model of in situ immune complex nephritis, as experience with Lupus nephritis has taught us, can lead us to a successful strategy for finding or identifying nephritogenic candidates from infectious agents.

The most important message from the experimental model is that nephritogenic antigens, most likely, will have an affinity for the GBM. Thus the logical first step is to screen for bacterial or viral proteins which reveal affinity for the GBM. Highly cationic proteins with a critical size do possess an affinity for the GBM. Our proposed strategy at the moment is to isolate fractions of cationic proteins from infectious agents which are known to cause postinfectious ICGN. After intravenous injection of the ^{125}I labelled fraction the glomeruli are isolated and the proteins bound to the glomeruli are separated on SDS-PAGE and detected by autoradiography. Comparison of the bands found in the isolated glomeruli with the injected fractions after SDS-PAGE-autoradiography enables one to identify and (hopefully) to isolate and to evaluate the nephritogenicity of the protein which possesses affinity for the GBM.

Using this procedure we were able to identify cationic proteins, both with strong affinity for the GBM, from two bacteria: *Yersinia enterocolitica* (pI > 10.0) [36] and *Staphylococcus aureus* (pI > 10.0) [37]. The Yersinia protein is composed of a 19 kD polypeptide, but occurs in dimeric and aggregated form with a size exceeding 65 kD (as judged from gel filtration). The staphylococcal protein migrates in SDS-PAGE as a 31 kD band. With the latter antigen we were able to induce proteinuria and kidney damage after a single intravenous injection into immunized rats. The nephritogenic potency of the Yersinia antigen is under study.

Thus, the model of in situ ICGN may lead us to a successful method for identifying cationic nephritogenic antigens involved in naturally occurring ICGN.

References

1. Cameron JS (1983) The pathogenesis of glomerulonephritis. In: Bertani T, Remuzzi G (eds) Glomerular injury. 300 years after Morgagni. Wichtig Edition, Milan, pp 11–30
2. Dixon FJ (1968) The pathogenesis of glomerulonephritis. Am J Med 44:493–498
3. Wilson CB, Dixon FJ (1981) The renal response to immunological injury. In: Brenner BM, Rector FC (eds) The kidney. WB Saunders, Philadelphia, p 1237
4. Cochrane CG, Koffler D (1973) Immune complex disease in experimental animals and in man. Adv Immunol 16:185–264
5. Couser WG, Salant DJ (1980) In situ immune complex formation and glomerular injury (editorial review). Kidney Int 17:1–13
6. Van Damme BJC, Fleuren GJ, Bakker WW, Vernier RL, Hoedemaeker PJ (1978) Experimental glomerulonephritis in the rat induced by antibodies directed against tubular antigens. IV. Fixed glomerular antigens in the pathogenesis of heterologous immune complex glomerulonephritis. Lab Invest 38:502–510
7. Couser WG, Steinmuller DR, Stilmant MM, Salant DJ, Lowenstein LM (1978) Experimental glomerulonephritis in the isolated perfused rat kidney. J Clin Invest 62:1275–1287
8. Kerjaschki D, Farquhar MG (1983) Immunocytochemical localization of the Heymann nephritis antigen (GP 330) in glomerular epithelial cells of normal Lewis rats. J Exp Med 157:667–685
9. Izui S, Schur PH, Kunkel HG (1967) Immunologic studies concerning the nephritis of systemic lupus erythematosus. J Exp Med 126:607–623
10. Stoeckl F, Schmiedeke T, Sugisaki Y, Mertz A, Batsford S, Vogt A (1990) DNA has no affinity for the GBM in vivo: binding is mediated by histone (abstract). Kidney Int 37:434
11. Golbus SM, Wilson CB (1979) Experimental glomerulonephritis induced by in situ formation of immune complexes in the glomerular capillary wall. Kidney Int 16:148–157
12. Holthofer H (1983) Lectin binding sites in kidney: A comparative study of 14 animal species. J Histochem Cytochem 31:431–537
13. Ward HJ, Cohen AH, Border WA (1984) In situ formation of subepithelial immune complexes in the rabbit glomerulus: requirement of a cationic antigen. Nephron 36:257–264
14. Border WA, Ward HJ, Kamil ES, Cohen AH (1982) Induction of membranous nephropathy in rabbits by administration of an exogenous cationic antigen: Demonstration of a pathogenic role for electrical charge. J Clin Invest 69:451–461
15. Gallo GR, Caulin-Glaser T, Lamm ME (1981) Charge of circulating immune complexes as a factor in glomerular basement membrane localization in mice. J Clin Invest 67:1305–1313
16. Caulin-Glaser T, Gallo GR, Lamm EM (1983) Nondissociating cationic immune complexes can deposit in glomerular basement membrane. J Exp Med 158:1561–1572
17. Gallo GR, Caulin-Glaser T, Emancipator SN, Lamm ME (1983) Nephritogenicity and differential distribution of glomerular immune complexes related to immunogen charge. Lab Invest 48:353–362
18. Batsford SR, Takamiya H, Vogt A (1980) A model of in situ immune complex glomerulonephritis in the rat induced by planted, cationized antigen. Clin Nephrol 14:211–216
19. Batsford SR, Oite T, Takamiya H, Vogt A (1980) Anionic binding sites in the glomerular basement membrane: possible role in the pathogenesis of immune complex glomerulonephritis. Renal Physiol 3:336–340
20. Oite T, Batsford SR, Mihatsch MJ, Takamiya H, Vogt A (1982) Quantitative studies of in situ immune complex glomerulonephritis in the rat induced by planted, cationic antigen. J Exp Med 155:460–474

21. Vogt A, Rohrbach R, Shimizu F, Takamiya H, Batsford S (1982) Interaction of cationized antigen with rat glomerular basement membrane: In situ immune complex formation. Kidney Int 22:27–35

22. Oite T, Shimizu F, Suzuki Y, Vogt A (1985) Ultramicroscopic localization of cationized antigen in the glomerular basement membrane in the course of active, in situ complex glomerulonephritis. Virchows Arch [Cell Pathol] 48:107–118

23. Koyama A, Niwa Y, Shigematsu H, Taniguchi M, Tada T (1978) Studies on passive serum sickness. II. Factors determining the localization of antigen-antibody complexes in murine renal glomerulus. Lab Invest 38:253–262

24. Germuth FG Jr, Rodriguez E (1973) Immunopathology of the renal glomerulus. Immune complex deposit and anti-basement membrane disease. Little, Brown, Boston

25. Germuth FG Jr, Rodriguez E, Lorelle CA, Trump ER, Milano LL, Wise O (1979) Passive immune complex glomerulonephritis in mice: Models for various lesions found in human disease: II. Low avidity complexes and diffuse proliferative glomerulonephritis with subepithelial deposits. Lab Invest 41:366–371

26. Koyama A, Inage H, Kobayashi M, Ohta Y, Narita M, Tojo S, Cameron JS (1986) Role of antigenic charge and antibody avidity on the glomerular immune complex localization in serum sickness of mice. Clin Exp Immunol 64:606–614

27. Barnes JL, Radnik RA, Gilchrist EP, Venkatachalam MA (1984) Size and charge selective permeability defects induced in glomerular basement membrane by a polycation. Kidney Int 25:11–19

28. Barnes JL, Ventakachalam MA (1984) Enhancement of glomerular immune complex deposition by a circulating polycation. J Exp Med 160:286–293

29. Schmiedeke TMJ, Stöckl FW, Weber R, Sugisaki Y, Batsford S, Vogt A (1989) Histones have high affinity for the glomerular basement membrane: relevance for immune complex formation in Lupus nephritis. J Exp Med 169:1879–1894

30. Schmiedeke T, Stoeckl F, Muller S, Mertz A, Vogt A (1990) Detection of histone H3 and H2A in glomerular deposits of Lupus mice (abstract). Kidney Int 37:430

31. Gioud M, Ait Kaci M, Montier JC (1982) Histone antibodies in systemic Lupus erythematosus. Arthritis Rheum 25:407–413

32. Vogt A, Batsford S, Rodriguez-Iturbe B, Garcia R (1983) Cationic antigens in poststreptococcal glomerulonephritis. Clin Nephrol 20:271–279

33. Liu TY, Elliot SD (1971) Streptococcal proteinase. In: Buyer (ed) The enzymes, vol 3, 3rd edn. Academic, pp 609–647

34. Johnston KH, Zabriskie JB (1986) Purification and partial characterization of the nephritis strain-associated protein from streptococcus pyogenes, group A. J Exp Med 163:697–712

35. Lange K, Seligson G, Cronin W (1983) Evidence for the in situ origin of poststreptococcal glomerulonephritis: glomerular localization of endostreptosin and the clinical significance of the subsequent antibody response. Clin Nephrol 19:3–16

36. Mertz A, Batsford S, Stoeckl F, Vogt A (1990) Yersinia enterocolitica induced acute GN: Possible role of nucleic acid-binding proteins in immune complex formation (abstract). Kidney Int 37:423

37. Yousif Y, Mertz A, Batsford S, Vogt A (to be published) Cationic staphylococcal antigens have affinity for renal basement membrane: possible pathogenetic role in glomerulonephritis. Proceedings of the VIth international symposium on staphylococci and staphylococcal infections, September 4–8 1989 Warsaw, Poland. Jeljaszewicz J (ed) Gustav Fischer, Stuttgart

Pathogenesis of IgA Immune Complex-Mediated Glomerulonephritis

ABDALLA RIFAI[1]

SUMMARY. In a period of less than ten years, complementary experimental and clinical observations have contributed greatly to our understanding of various aspects of IgA immune complexes and their pathogenetic potential in IgA nephropathy. The primary mechanism of glomerular IgA deposition has been discussed in the light of experimental data. These findings indicate that the molecular form of IgA is critical for the formation of large- and intermediate-sized complexes that result in glomerular deposition. Glomerular IgA deposits, however, appear to develop in a continuum of preformed polymeric IgA complexes and in situ formed monomeric IgA complexes. Removal of IgA immune complexes from the circulation is mediated by the liver, with no evidence of any removal dysfunction in IgA nephropathy patients. IgA macromolecules are unable to activate the complement pathway in vitro or as a glomerular deposit. Complement activation, however, is shown to be an antigen-mediated process. Participation of the complement system in induction of glomerular injury associated with IgA nephropathy needs further investigation. Experimental evidence supports the hypothesis that in IgA immune complex-mediated nephropathy, the repertoire of IgA immune complexes that induce mesangial proliferation and glomerular sclerosis consists of IgA-bound nephritogenic antigens which determine the extent and outcome of glomerular injury.

Introduction

Glomerular IgA deposits represent the diagnostic hallmark of primary IgA nephropathy. This feature is also a consistent finding in and characteristic of Schonlein-Henoch purpura-associated glomerulonephritis. A secondary form of IgA nephro-

---

[1]Departments of Pathology, Rhode Island Hospital and Brown University, Providence, RI 02903, USA

pathy with identical glomerular immunohistochemical features is occasionally associated with alcoholic liver disease, portal systemic shunt, celiac disease, dermatitis herpetiformis, ankylosing spondylitis, and a number of other diverse diseases [1–3].

Several abnormalities are implicated in the pathogenesis of primary and secondary IgA nephropathy. Some of these abnormalities include: bacterial infections, viral infections, decreased T cell suppressor function, increased T cell helper function, increased polyclonal B cell activation, increased polymeric IgA synthesis, enhanced alpha chain switch region expression, IgM autoantibodies, IgG antibodies, IgA rheumatoid factors, collagen binding IgA, fibronectin-binding IgA, IgA anti-galactosyl reactivity, genetic predisposition, familial association, complement dysfunction, phagocytic dysfunction, anti-endothelial antibodies, anti-bovine serum albumin, anti-gluten, and anti-idiotypic antibodies. If at least 20 such abnormalities are to be accommodated in an experimental model, then the simple factorial rule (n!) would yield 2.4×10^{18} combinatorial models. Undoubtedly, no single experimental model aimed at elucidating the pathogenesis of IgA nephropathy can be developed to include all these abnormalities. IgA immune complexes, however, remain the most commonly reported and implicated immunopathologic abnormality. Accordingly, we have focused our studies on the mechanisms that lead to glomerular IgA immune deposit formation and, in particular, the potential role of the IgA, complement, and antigen in the development of glomerular injury.

IgA Immune Complexes

The first described experimental model for IgA nephropathy examined the ability of IgA immune complexes (IgA-IC) to induce glomerular injury [4]. This model took advantage of two important technical approaches. First, a well characterized monoclonal IgA (MOPC 315) anti-dinitrophenol was used as a source of purified antibody. Second, the hapten dinitrophenol (DNP) could be conjugated to a variety of carrier molecules, such as bovine serum albumin (DNP-BSA), or a chemically modified polysaccharide (DNP-Ficoll) to serve as an antigen. Thus, well characterized IgA-IC could be prepared in vitro and used for passive administration. Complexes of IgA-DNP-BSA prepared over a wide range of antigen/antibody ratio resulted in glomerular IgA immune deposits with the characteristic granular immunofluorescent patterns of IgA and complement component C3. The immunofluorescent pattern of bovine serum albumin in the deposits was identical with the IgA and confirmed the immune complex nature of the mesangial IgA.

Using two different experimental protocols, glomerular IgA immune deposits were also induced in vivo. In the first protocol, DNP-BSA administered to normal mice was followed by the injection of IgA. In the second protocol, DNP-BSA was administered to mice bearing the MOPC 315 myeloma, with predetermined levels of circulating IgA anti-DNP. Both protocols resulted in histopathological changes, representing primarily glomerular PAS positive material, that correlated well with the level of circulating IgA and administered antigen. Of importance in these findings were the mesangial IgA immune deposits which developed over a wide concentration range of IgA (antibody excess) and antigen (antigen excess) in the complexes.

There are seminal clinical observations that support the causal role of IgA-IC. First, the granular immunofluorescent pattern of the IgA and C3 deposits is usually indicative of an immune deposit. Second, electron dense deposits, a common feature of IgA nephropathy, were identified immunohistochemically to be IgA [5]. Third, extrarenal systemic vascular IgA deposits have also been reported in patients with IgA nephropathy. Fourth, a vast number of studies have reported the presence of circulating IgA-IC in primary and secondary forms of IgA nephropathy [6–9]. Most importantly, a correlation between serum level of circulating macromolecular IgA (IgA immune complexes) and hematuria has also been documented [10].

Mechanisms of Glomerular IgA Deposits Formation

The primary pathogenetic mechanism of immune complex-mediated glomerulonephritis is the formation or glomerular deposition of the IC. In IgA nephropathy, the role that the IgA molecular form (monomeric or polymeric) plays in the development of glomerular immune deposits is based largely on experimental observations. Large amounts of purified monomeric IgA anti-DNP mixed with DNP-BSA at different antigen-antibody ratios did not induce glomerular deposits. In contrast, smaller amounts of polymeric IgA were potent in inducing glomerular immune deposits [4]. In a comparative analytical study, in vitro preformed monomeric IgA and polymeric IgA immune complexes prepared with the same antigen (DNP-Ficoll) showed, by gradient polyacrylamide gel electrophoresis, that monomeric IgA formed only small-sized complexes. In contrast, polymeric IgA formed large- and intermediate-sized complexes. These results suggest that the size of the IgA immune complex plays a critical role in glomerular deposition [11].

To determine the relationship between immune complex formation, size, and glomerular deposition, analytical and kinetic double radioisotope studies were performed in vivo. In those studies, ^{131}I-antigen (DNP-Ficoll) was injected intravenously and ^{125}I-labelled monomeric or polymeric IgA anti-DNP were administered intraperitoneally [12]. At timed intervals, plasma samples were obtained and analyzed by gradient gel electrophoresis. Two important findings were revealed by these studies. First, large- and intermediate-sized IgA-IC composed only of polymeric IgA emerged in the circulation prior to glomerular deposition. Thus, glomerular IgA deposits were detectable only in mice that received polymeric IgA and DNP-Ficoll. A second important finding was that although monomeric IgA failed to bind or complex with polymeric IgA-IC in the circulation it did bind to the polymeric IgA immune deposits in the glomerulus. These findings indicate that glomerular IgA immune deposits evolve through a continuum process, initiated by the localization of preformed circulating polymeric IgA complexes and perpetuated by an in situ monomeric IgA-mediated complex formation.

Several clinical studies, utilizing immunohistochemical techniques, demonstrated that polymeric IgA is present in the glomerular immune deposits in patients with IgA nephropathy. The presence of J chain, the binding of secretory component to IgA immune deposits, and size analysis of renal eluates all confirmed the presence or predominance of polymeric IgA [13,14]. The participation or contribution of monomeric IgA to immune deposit formation, however, awaits further clinical investigation.

Removal of IgA Immune Complexes from Circulation

The presence of circulating and glomerular deposits of IgA-IC in IgA nephropathy patients propelled a series of experimental investigations to determine the kinetics, tissue distribution, and fate of IgA immune complexes. Because the antigen usually affects the clearance of immune complexes [15], we used model IgA immune complexes, prepared by covalent cross-linking of purified IgA anti-DNP with a specific affinity labeling antigen (Bis-dinitrophenyl pimelic acid ester). Removal of model IgA-IC from circulation was according to size. Large-sized IgA macromolecules were removed rapidly ($t_{1/2} < 2$ min), whereas small-sized polymers persisted in the circulation. Through the use of these covalently cross-linked IgA oligomers, we were able to determine the minimal composition of four dimeric IgA which was required for rapid elimination [16]. Tissue distribution results showed the liver as the major organ for removal of macromolecular IgA. Immunofluorescence microscopy and electron microscopy autoradiography showed macromolecular IgA to be associated with Kupffer cells [17]. With increasing doses of injected macromolecular IgA the clearance velocity approached a maximum, thus prolonging the circulation of macromolecular IgA. Further kinetic, morphologic, and binding specificity studies demonstrated in vivo the presence of specific receptors on Kupffer cells that bind and remove macromolecular IgA from circulation.

An impairment in the reticulophagocytic function of patients with IgA nephropathy has been postulated as the potential cause for the persistence of IgA immune complexes in the circulation that consequently lead to their glomerular deposition [18,19]. Since the fate and removal mechanisms of circulating macromolecular IgA are unknown in humans, equipped by our experience from animal studies, we examined the blood clearance and organ uptake of purified human IgA macromolecules and polymers in patients with IgA nephropathy and in normal controls [20]. The IgA macromolecules, serving as a probe of IgA-IC, were prepared by covalent cross-linking of purified human polymeric IgA with a heterobifunctional reagent, N-Succinimidyl 3-(2-pyridyldithio) propriante. After intravenous injection, large-sized IgA macromolecules were removed from the circulation of patients ($t_{1/2} = 3.8 \pm 1.0$ min) and normal controls ($t_{1/2} = 4.9 \pm 1.5$ min). Dynamic gamma camera scintigraphy revealed the liver as the major organ that mediates the removal of the macromolecular IgA, with no significant difference in the rate of hepatic uptake for patients ($t_{1/2} = 3.4 \pm 0.6$ min) and controls ($t_{1/2} = 3.3 \pm 0.9$ min). No significant amount of radioactivity could be detected in the lungs, kidneys, and spleen. These findings have general significance in showing the liver as a major organ for removal of macromolecular IgA. In addition, the results have specific importance in showing that patients with IgA nephropathy do not suffer from an IgA-removal dysfunction. Collectively, the similarity of these clinical and experimental results emphasizes the value of the experimental model.

IgA Immune Complexes and Complement

Although the central component (C3) of the classical and alternative pathways is found in mesangial deposits in many cases of IgA nephropathy, clinical studies have failed to detect systemic activation of the complement system [21]. Detection of other components of the alternative pathway and the membrane attack complex [22] have focused attention on the potential role of the complement system as mediator of glomerular injury.

The ability of aggregated human IgA to activate the complement system has been a subject of several conflicting reports. To address this issue in a manner relevant to IgA nephropathy, we examined in vitro the interaction of covalently cross-linked IgA macromolecules or naturally occurring IgA immune complexes with fresh normal human serum [23]. We demonstrated the lack of activation of C3 or factor B. Similar studies by Waldo and Cochrane [24] confirmed our findings. Administration of human IgA immune complexes or IgA macromolecules to mice resulted in glomerular deposition. Despite the presence of intense glomerular IgA deposits no C3 was detected. Collectively, these findings suggest that neither soluble nor renal localized human IgA deposits activate the complement system.

Although the above studies demonstrate the inability of human IgA to activate the complement system, the cause of the presence of complement in the glomerular deposits remains unknown. We entertained the possibility that the antigen might cause complement activation. A series of experiments were performed in order to determine how IgA immune complex activates complement and generates the mesangial complement deposits [25]. The first experiment was designed to determine whether the presence of an antigen within a glomerular IgA deposit is required for complement activation. In these experiments, covalently cross-linked model IgA macromolecules of anti-DNP with free antigen-binding sites were administered into two groups of mice. Following disappearance of the majority of macromolecules from circulation, either DNP-conjugated antigen or buffer was injected. After six hours both groups were killed. As expected, both groups showed glomerular IgA deposits. Yet only the group that received the DNP-conjugate, a known activator of the alternative pathway, showed C3 deposits. In the second series, a paired comparison of IgA immune complexes prepared with the same monoclonal IgA anti-phosphorylcholine and antigen-carrier, but differing only in a single antigenic feature (DNP), also demonstrated that glomerular C3 deposits developed with a DNP-conjugated antigen. The third series of experiments also showed, using immunoassay analysis, negligible or no conversion of normal serum C3 to inactive C3b (iC3b) upon treatment with soluble or insoluble large-sized IgA aggregates. In contrast, the antigen alone was able to induce maximal conversion of C3 to iC3b. Collectively, these findings indicate that the nature of the antigen in a glomerular IgA immune deposit is the major mediator of complement activation.

Although complement activation can be induced by the antigen in glomerular IgA deposits it is unknown whether such activation causes glomerular injury. Experimentally, we could not detect any histologic features that differentiated between glomeruli with or without C3 deposits within the same renal biopsy. Also, comparative experiments of induced glomerular IgA immune complexes in C3-depleted mice and normal mice showed no histopathologic difference. A number of studies have reported intense C3 deposits with no or minimal glomerular changes in IgA nephropathy. Although there is an agreement between clinical and preliminary experimental observations that the complement system does not appear to mediate glomerular injury, complement activation may be of importance in induction of hematuria, as shown experimentally by Emancipator et al. [26].

Influence of Antigen on Glomerular Injury

One of the most poorly defined areas relative to the role of immune complexes in IgA nephropathy is precise identification of the antigen involved. The close temporal relationship between upper respiratory tract or gastrointestinal infection and episodes of gross hematuria has been described as a frequent feature of IgA nephropathy [27]. The fact that this has also been associated with circulating IgA immune complexes [28] strongly implicates infectious agents as the source of antigen.

In most passive and active experimental models of immune complex-mediated glomerulonephritis, the antigen used is usually a heterologous serum protein consigned to aggregating the antibody without itself being detrimental. In IgG immune complex-mediated glomerulonephritis, the effector function of IgG, as in complement activation, is considered to be the main cause of glomerular injury. As described above, however, IgA has very little or lacks the ability to activate the complement system. As also emphasized, despite intense C3 deposits there is little or no evidence of glomerular injury in several cases of IgA nephropathy. The antigen may then be the major variable that may account for the spectrum of histopathologic patterns observed in IgA nephropathy.

In order to test the pathogenetic potential of the antigen in IgA-IC-mediated glomerulonephritis, we compared the effect of immune complexes formed in vivo with the same IgA anti-phosphorylcholine, and two different antigens, pneumococcal C-polysaccharide and phosphorylcholine-conjugated Ficoll (PC-Ficoll) that share phosphorylcholine (PC) as a common antigenic determinant [29]. Only the C-polysaccharide-containing IgA immune complexes resulted in renal injury. Recently we developed an animal model whereby glomerular IgA immune deposits, composed exclusively of IgA or IgA/IgA-IC, can capture circulating antigens in situ [30]. In this model, glomerular IgA deposits (IgA/IgA-IC) were induced by administration of a constant amount of IgA anti-DNP (antibody) and DNP-conjugated IgA anti-PC as antigen. The latter also served as antibody to capture, in situ, circulating PC-containing antigens. Mice that received only IgA/IgA-IC developed glomerular IgA and C3 deposits and a focal increase in mesangial cells and matrix, but no evidence of renal damage. Diffuse increase in mesangial cells and matrix developed in mice treated with IgA/IgA-IC and either PC-Ficoll or PC-conjugated bovine serum albumin. No significant alterations were noted in these groups. In contrast, mice that received IgA/IgA-IC and pneumococcal C-polysaccharide developed severe diffuse mesangial hypercellularity with segmental necrosis and thrombosis. These mice also developed proteinuria and hematuria. These studies demonstrate that the antigen plays a critical role in the development of glomerulonephritis associated with IgA immune complexes.

Conclusion

The experimental model of IgA immune complex-mediated glomerulonephritis has come of age. Conceptual and technical approaches have begun to provide accurate information regarding the factors and mediators that are involved in pathogenesis. In composing this review I have focused on an experimental system with emphasis on its relevance to human IgA nephropathy. I realize that this course is accompanied by obvious risks of misinterpretation. I hope that the benefits of intellectual challenge outweigh the pitfalls of misconception, and trust my composition provides adequate distinction between fact and fantasy. Finally, I predict that many of the observations made in this model, that appear now to be intriguing, will serve as a lead in the investigation of the pathogenesis of IgA nephropathy, once they are demystified by acquisition of thorough, substantiated information.

Acknowledgments. The presented experimental work was supported by NIH grant 32379. I am indebted to my collaborators whose contributions made this work possible. To the many investigators who have not been cited due to publisher restrictions, but who have contributed to the development of the knowledge presented in this review, my apologies and thanks. The secretarial assistance of Laura Gantt is highly appreciated.

References

1. Clarkson AR, Woodroffe AJ, Aarons I, Hiki Y, Hale G (1987) IgA nephropathy. Annu Rev Med 38:157-68
2. D'Amico G (1987) The commonest glomerulonephritis in the world: IgA nephropathy. Q J Med 245:709-27
3. Emancipator SN, Lamm ME (1989) IgA nephropathy: pathogenesis of the most common form of glomerulonephritis. Lab Invest 60:168-83
4. Rifai A, Small PA, Teague PO, Ayoub EM (1979) Experimental IgA nephropathy. J Exp Med 150:1161-73
5. Kanatsu K, Doi T, Sekita K, Yoshida H, Nagai H, Hamashima Y (1983) A comparative immunologic study of IgA nephropathy. Am J Kidney Dis 2:618-25
6. Woodroffe AJ, Gormly AA, McKenzie PE, Wootton AM, Thompson AJ, Seymour AE, Clarkson AR (1980) Immunologic studies in IgA nephropathy. Kidney Int 18:366-74
7. Hall RP, Stachura I, Cason J, Whiteside TL, Lawely TJ (1983) IgA-containing circulating immune complexes in patients with IgA nephropathy. Am J Med 74:56-63
8. Coppo R, Basolo B, Piccoli G, Mazzucco G, Roccatello D (1984) IgA1 and IgA2 immune complexes in primary IgA nephropathy and Henoch-Schonlein nephritis. Clin Exp Immunol 57:583-90
9. Egido J Sancho J, Rivera F, Hernando L (1984) The role of IgA and IgG immune complexes in IgA nephropathy. Nephron 36:52-9
10. Valentijn RM, Kauffmann RH, de la Riviere GB, Daha MR, van Es LA (1983) Presence of circulating macromolecular IgA in patients with hematuria due to primary IgA nephropathy. Am J Med 74:375-81
11. Rifai A, Millard K (1985) Glomerular deposition of immune complexes prepared with monomeric or polymeric IgA. Clin Exp Immunol 60:363-68
12. Chen A, Wong SS, Rifai A (1988) Glomerular immune deposits in experimental IgA nephropathy: A continuum of circulating and in situ formed immune complexes. Am J Pathol 130:216-22
13. Bene MC, Faure G, Duheille J (1982) IgA nephropathy: characterization of the polymeric nature of mesangial deposits by in vitro binding of secretory component. Clin Exp Immunol 47:527-34
14. Monteiro RC, Halbwachs-Mecarelli L, Roque-Barreira, Noel LH, Berger J, Lesavre P (1985) Charge and size of mesangial IgA in IgA nephropathy. Kidney Int 28:666-71

15. Finbloom DS, Magilavy DB, Harford JB, Rifai A, Plotz PH (1981) The influence of antigen on immune complex behavior in mice. J Clin Invest 68:214–24
16. Rifai A, Mannik M (1983) Clearance kinetics and fate of mouse IgA immune complexes prepared with monomeric or dimeric IgA. J Immunol 130:1826–32
17. Rifai A, Mannik M (1984) Clearance of circulating IgA immune complexes is mediated by a specific receptor on Kupffer cells in mice. J Exp Med 160:125–37
18. Lawrence S, Pussel BA, Charlesworth JA (1983) Mesangial IgA nephropathy: Detection of defective reticulophagocytic function in vivo. Clin Nephrol 16:280–83
19. Nicholls K, Kincaid-Smith P (1984) Defective in vivo Fc- and C3b-receptor function in IgA nephropathy. AM J Kidney Dis 4:128–34
20. Rifai A, Schena FP, Montinaro V, Mele M, D'Addabbo A, Nitti L, Pezzullo JC (1989) Clearance kinetics and fate of macromolecular IgA in patients with IgA nephropathy. Lab Invest 61:381–388
21. Miyazaka R, Kuroda M, Akiyama T, Tofuku Y, Takeda R (1984) Glomerular deposition and serum levels of complement control proteins in patients with IgA nephropathy. Clin Nephrol 21:335–40
22. Rauterberg EW, Lieberknecht HM, Wingen AM, Ritz E (1987) Complement membrane attack (MAC) in idiopathic IgA-glomerulonephritis. Kidney Int 31:820–29
23. Imai H, Chen A, Wyatt RJ, Rifai A (1988) Lack of complement activation by human IgA immune complexes. Clin Exp Immunol 73:479–83
24. Waldo FB, Cochran AM (1989) Mixed IgA-IgG aggregates as a model of immune complexes in IgA nephropathy. J Immunol 142:3841–3846
25. Rifai A, Chen A, Imai H (1987) Complement activation in experimental IgA nephropathy: an antigen-mediated process. Kidney Int 32:838–44
26. Emancipator SN, Ovary Z, Lamm ME (1987) The role of mesangial complement in the hematuria of experimental IgA nephropathy. Lab Invest 57:269–76
27. Indraprasit S, Boonpucknavig V, Boonpucknavig S (1985) IgA nephropathy associated with enteric fever. Nephron 40:219–22
28. Davin JC, Malaise M, Foidart J, Mahieu P (1987) Anti-alpha-galactosyl antibodies and immune complexes in children with Henoch-Schonlein purpura or IgA nephropathy. Kidney Int 31:1132–9
29. Imai H, Chen A, Endoh M, Rifai A (1987) Influence of the antigen on experimental IgA nephropathy. Semin Nephrol 7:283–285
30. Montinaro et al. (to be published)

Anti-Thymocyte Antibody Induced Mesangiolytic Nephritis

Nobuaki Yamanaka and Masamichi Ishizaki[1]

Summary. Recently, an experimental model of mesangiolytic nephritis, induced by the anti-thy 1 antibody, was established. The thy 1 antigen is known as the cell surface antigen of the mouse thymocyte and is found to be expressed also on the rat mesangial cell membrane, as thy 1.1 antigen. A single intravenous administration of anti-thymocyte serum (ATS) immediately induces complement-mediated mesangiolytic destruction of the glomerulus, followed by proliferative changes of mesangial cells. Reconstruction of the glomerular structure results from the mesangial proliferation associated with revascularization. Between day 30 and day 45 after administration of ATS, most of the glomeruli had reverted to almost their original structure, with occasional focal and segmental defective changes. This model is characterized by acute mesangial proliferation and the rapid repair process of a drastically deformed glomerular structure, demonstrating the self-repair function of the glomerulus.

Overloading some conditions on this model, such as repeated injection of ATS or renal lymphatic ligation after ATS administration, for example, modifies the natural course of this self-limited proliferative change and is useful for analyzing the glomerular lesions.

This experimental model will make a contribution as a good tool for use in elucidating not only the mechanisms of proliferative glomerulonephritis, but also for elucidating the various functions of mesangial cells.

Introduction

Following the significant influence contributions made toward elucidating glomerular injuries by studies based on Masugi's experimental animal models of nephrotoxic nephritis, there have been recent similar attempts to adapt normal glomerular com-

---

[1]Department of Pathology, Nippon Medical School, 1-1-5, Sendagi. Bunkyo-ku, Tokyo, 113 Japan

ponents other than glomerular basement membrane (GBM), as antigen sources in aiming toward the establishment of a new experimental model. Such components as the epithelial cell [1], endothelial cell [2], mesangial cell, [3] and mesangial matrix, have been selected [4,5]. Selective injuries of mesangial cells induced by the immune mechanism will contribute to the analysis of many aspects of proliferative changes in the glomerulus. However, the appropriate experimental model whose target antigen is in the mesangium has not been successful, although some trials have been reported [3–5]. Recently, an experimental model of mesangiolytic nephritis which is induced by the anti-thymocyte antibody in the rat has been in the spotlight, because the antibody reacts with the mesangial cell itself with a high incidence of successive proliferative changes.

Thy 1 Antigen and Mesangial Cells

In 1980, Ishizaki found that the thy 1 antigen, which is known as the cell surface marker antigen of the mouse thymocyte, is also expressed on the cell surface of the rat mesangial cell [6]. In the same year, Morris et al., based on their immunofluorescent study of thy 1 cell surface differentiation antigen in connective tissue, briefly described the fact that this antigen is expressed in the rat mesangial cell [7]. Following this description, the studies of Harada et al. [8], Paul et al. [9], Bagchus et al. [10], and Yamamoto et al. [11], established the fact that this antigen is present on the cell surface of the rat mesangial cell.

The presence of thy 1 antigen is recognized in other tissue cells in mouse as well as in rat thymocytes [12]. It is known that there are two sorts of thy 1 antigen, thy 1.1 and thy 1.2 antigens [13]. Only thy 1.1 antigen was found on the surface of the rat mesangial cell. In our laboratory, it was found that the thy 1.1 antigen is also expressed on the surface of mesangial cells of the Mongolian gerbil [14]. This animal, which lives in the desert, is commonly called the sand rat. So far, no other species have been found to express thy 1 antigen in mesangial cells. Interestingly, neither thy 1.1 nor thy 1.2 antigen are present in the mouse mesangial cell.

Immunofluorescent microscopy, using mouse monoclonal antibody against thy 1.1 antigen, shows that the antigen has limited distribution, exclusively in the mesangial area, and in some regions it appears to exist circumferentially. Immunoelectron microscopy, using mouse monoclonal antibody, reveals that thy 1.1 antigen localizes on the surface of mesangial cells of the rat.

Anti-Thymocyte Antibody Induced Mesangial Lesions

In 1980, in his paper (in Japanese), Ishizaki briefly described this phenomenon: an intravenous administration of anti-rat thymocyte rabbit serum in the rat induced destruction of the mesangium, which was followed by segmental proliferation of mesangial cells [15]. We have continued to study the details of this phenomenon, and we have published our analysis of the results, in English this time [16]. In the same year Bagchus et al., using mouse monoclonal antibody against the rat thymocytes, had almost the same results [17,18]. Yamamoto et al., using polyclonal anti-thymocyte serum, also demonstrated an extensive analysis of similar glomerular lesions [11,19,20]. The methods and results of these three different groups are some-what different in details; however, the main evolution of the disease is basically the same. That is to say, the heterologous antibody binds to the mesangial cell in the short term, subsequent autologous complement activation is induced, and as a result, cytolysis of the mesangial cell occurs, followed by mesangial proliferation.

According to our data [16], in immunofluorescent microscopy, rabbit IgG localizes in the region of the rat mesangium from at least 5 minutes after the intravenous administration of anti-thymocyte serum (ATS) and completely fixes within 15 minutes. The localization of rat C3 in the rat glomerulus is observed within 30 minutes of the administration of ATS. It demonstrates almost the same positive pat-tern as the distribution of rabbit IgG.

The electron micrograph reveals that 30 minutes after the administration of ATS, the mesangial cell severely degenerates, with shrinkage and dark appearance of the cytoplasm, suggesting an ongoing necrotic process. Two hours after the administra-tion of ATS, a majority of mesangial cells lyse and disappear from the mesangial area, while GBM is always well preserved. Endothelial cells are also preserved in spite of the significant destruction of the mesangium. In the lysed mesangial areas, there is an accumulation of blood components, including blood plasma and blood cells. Yamamoto et al. [19] and Bagchus et al. [18] demonstrated that the C5b–C9 complement components are also positive in almost the same pattern as mesangial C3 deposition, thus establishing the involvement of the membrane attack complex in this cytolytic process. Yamamoto et al. performed studies on the depletion of com-plement activation by using cobra venom and proved the complement-dependency of the lytic phenomenon in the mesangium in this model [19]. Bagchus et al. demon-strated that IgG 1, which is a subclass of IgG and is unable to activate rat comple-ment, is able to bind to the antigen on the mesangial cell, but is not able to induce subsequent cytolytic changes. On the other hand, IgG 2, which is able to activate rat complement, can cause cytolysis [17].

Aneurysmal cystic lesion of the glomerular capillary is observed 24 hours after administration of ATS, with margination of leukocytes and an accumulation of plate-lets and fibrin. The lesion highly resembles the glomerular lesion induced by snake venom and is regarded as an extremely severe state of mesangiolysis [21]. The GBM is usually preserved and the evidence of rupture is rare.

Figure 1 shows chronological glomerular changes followed by mesangiolysis dem-onstrated by methenamine silver staining. At 24 hours after ATS administration, the glomerulus exhibits a cystic mesangiolytic lesion containing accumulated cells with neutrophils (Fig. 1a). The glomerulus shows leukocytic infiltration with a predomi-nance of monocytes, and the initiation of mesangial cell proliferation from day 2 to day 4 after ATS administration (Fig. 1b). The matrix component is rarely present in this region. The glomerulus in Fig. 1c exhibits the changes on day 8. It shows the sig-nificant proliferation of mesangial cells in a segmental fashion, with a decreased number of leukocytes, which is equivalent to the state of proliferative glomerulo-nephritis. The silver-positive matrix components among the proliferated mesangial cells are recognized, as well as the regression of the diseased segment, together with irregular increase of capillary lumens. On day 18, there is a decrease of cell prolifera-tion, with evident reconstruction of capillary structure, decrease of matrix compo-nents, and disappearance of leukocytes in the segmental lesion (Fig. 1d). These findings appear to be the expression of rapid repair of the drastic cystic lesion of

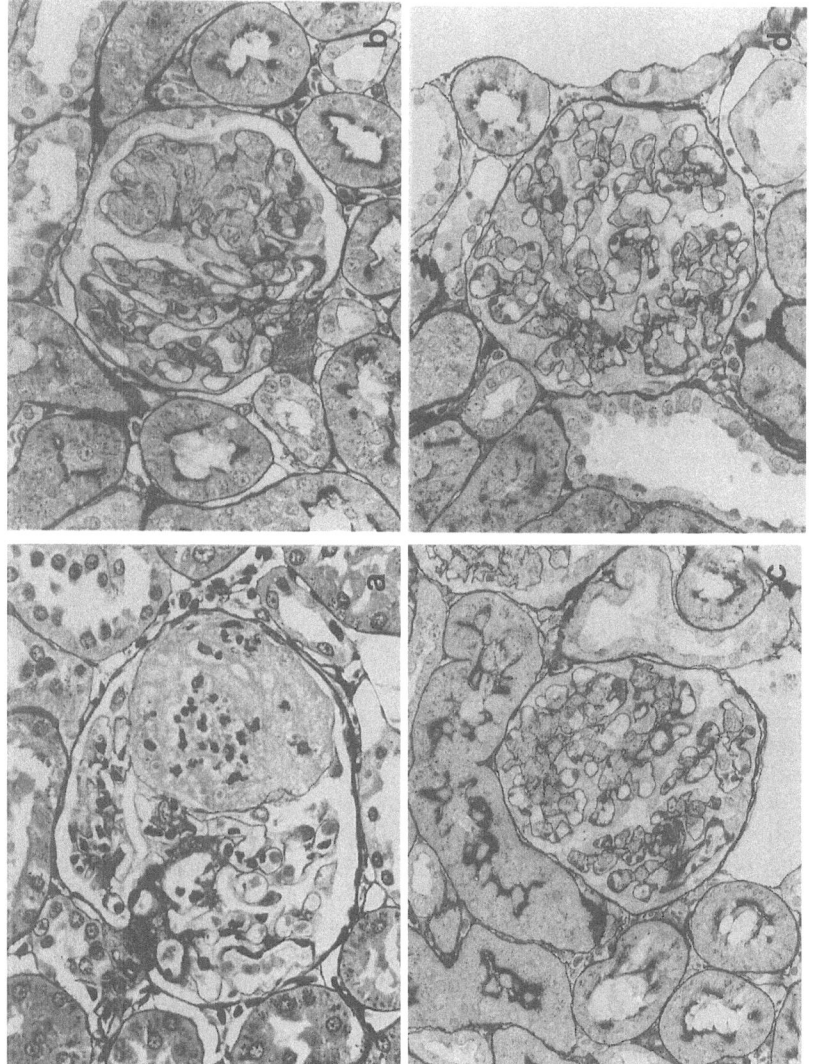

Fig. 1a–d. Chronological glomerular changes after administration of ATS (PAM stain). **a** 24 hours: cystic mesangiolytic lesion with accumulated neutrophils, **b** 2–4 days: initiation of mesangial proliferation with monocyte infiltration, **c** 8 days: proliferation of mesangial cells with a decreased number of leukocytes and increased matrix components, **d** 18 days: decrease of cell proliferation and matrix components with reconstruction of capillary structure

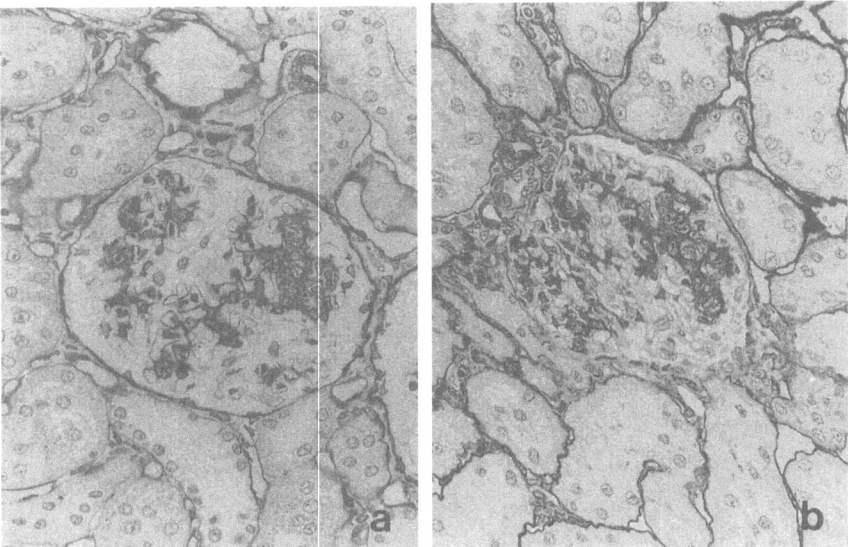

Fig. 2a,b. Immunostaining of increased matrix components in the injured glomerulus 12 days after ATS administration, demonstrated by immunoperoxidase (*PAP*) method. **a** type IV collagen, **b** laminin

mesangiolysis. The electron micrograph from around day 6 exhibits prominent mesangial proliferation with evident increase of the matrix, which occupies the site of the preforming cystic mesangiolytic change. Proliferation of endothelial cells and reconstruction of the glomerular vasculature are also demonstrated.

The process of protein excretion shows massive transient proteinuria with the peak around day 4 and gradual decrease to a normal level until around day 21. This movement of proteinuria is well correlated with the morphological changes of rapid reconstruction of the glomerular structure.

From day 30 to day 45 after the administration of ATS, most of the glomeruli had virtually reverted to their original structure, with focal and segmental sclerosis, partial appearance of collagen fibers or focal remnants of proliferative change, and occasional deformation. No proteinuria was detected at this stage. This model shows the characteristics of the rapid repair process of a drastically deformed glomerulus with mesangiolysis in the case of a one-shot charge of antibody. This model indicates that the glomerulus has a self-repair function which can reconstruct the breaking of its structure, and the proliferation of the mesangial cells in such situations may be the expression of the repair reaction of the living body.

Another characteristic of the model is that, in the rat, there is only heterologous reaction and no autologous antibody formation. It is probable that this defect of the autologous phase is the cause of the rapid recovery of the glomerular lesions.

Detection of changes in the matrix components in these diseased processes by the immunohistological method, reveal an overt increase of type IV collagen associated with mesangial cell proliferation. The distribution of laminin shows almost the same

Table 1. Evolution of anti-thymocyte antibody-induced glomerular injury

Antigen-antibody binding followed by activation of complement
Complement-mediated cytolysis of mesangial cell
Various degrees of mesangiolysis
Mesangial hypercellularity with leukocytic infiltration
 1 Polymormphonuclear neutrophils (PMN) → monocyte-macrophage, aggregation of platelets
 2 monocyte-macrophage + mesangial cell proliferation
Mesangial cell proliferation and increase of matrix components
Mesangial cell proliferation with revascularization
Remodelling of the glomerular structure
Defect healing with occasional focal segmental sclerosis

pattern as that of type IV collagen (Fig. 2). Proliferated mesangial cells and increased matrix components are reorganized in the stalk regions in accordance with the reconstitution of the glomerulus due to revascularization; gradually these components distribute in an almost normal fashion. These processes resemble mesangial development during glomerular embryogenesis [22].

The process of glomerular injury caused by anti-thymocyte antibody will progress in the manner proposed in Table I. The characteristics of this experimental model are as follows: 100% of the glomerular lesions will be induced by the administration of heterologous antibody; these lesions will be followed by complement-dependent drastic mesangiolysis. In the initial stage, there are inflammatory changes characterized by leukocyte infiltration and aggregation of platelets, followed by a prominent proliferation of mesangial cells. The increase of matrix components occurs among the proliferated mesangial cells, as does revascularization, which will contribute to the reconstruction of glomerular structure. In the case of a one-shot charge of antibody, most of the glomeruli repair morphologically within a short period of from 30 to 45 days.

Our studies on this model reveal that the degree of mesangiolysis induced by ATS administration is varied, and that mild mesangiolysis is a more common finding than aneurysmal cystic lesions. The proliferative response to mild mesangiolysis is rapid and mild mesangial cell proliferation tends to occur in the early period. Judging from these processes, the mesangial proliferation in this model may be the expression of the mesangial repair mechanism.

Bagchus et al. demonstrated these mesangiolytic glomerular changes by using only a small amount of monoclonal antibody [17,18]. Their results are very important because they show that these continuous histological changes of glomerular proliferation can be induced by administration of monoclonal antibody.

Thy 1 Antigen in Newborn Rat Kidney

Using mouse monoclonal antibody, the distribution of thy 1.1 antigen in the newborn rat kidney is found to reveal positive immunofluorescence in the cleft of the S-shaped body, which is the most immature glomerulus. Positive findings increase in accordance with the maturity of the primitive glomeruli. The most mature glomerulus in the newborn rat shows overt positive fluorescence encircling each mesangial cell in

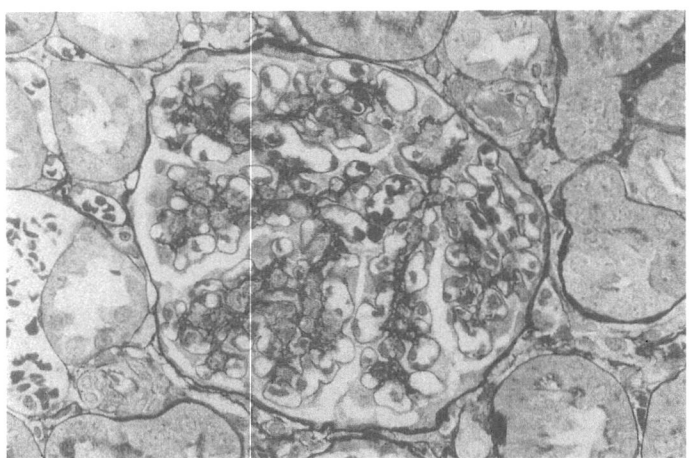

Fig. 3. Prolonged mesangial cell proliferation with increased matrix components due to repeated charges of ATS (PAM stain)

the simplified glomerular structure. These findings suggest the possibility of the induction of a mesangial lesion even in such primitive glomeruli.

Repeated Charges of ATS

According to our ongoing studies with repeated charges of polyclonal anti-thymocyte serum in the rat, the repair process of the damaged glomerulus is markedly retarded, demonstrating significant widening of the mesangial area due to diffuse increase of the cellular components and matrix (Fig. 3). These findings resemble the histological findings of chronic proliferative glomerulonephritis in human material. Appropriate applications of this experimental model will contribute to the analysis of the mechanism of human glomerulonephritis.

Influences of Lymphatic Ligation

In our laboratory, we have observed retardation of mesangial pathway flow by carrying out complete ligation of the renal lymph vessels at the renal hilus in the rat. In the ligated groups, the mesangiolytic changes of the glomerulus are mild, compared to those in the non-ligated groups, and no cystic lesions of mesangiolysis were observed (Fig. 4). These observations are interpreted as hindrance of antigen-antibody binding on the mesangial cell surface caused by retardation of flow through the mesangial pathway. In our observation of the glomerular changes which occurred after one-shot administration of ATS, the repair process progressed through a relatively short period in the nonligated group; however, this repair process was markedly hindered in the lymphatic ligated group during the mesangiolytic stage,

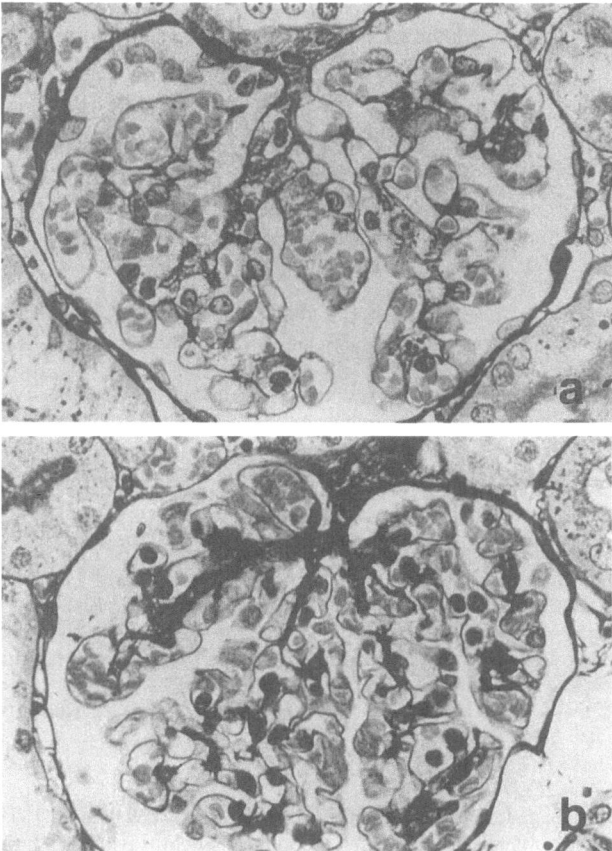

Fig. 4a,b. Influence of lymphatic ligation at renal hilus before ATS administration (PAM stain). **a** overt mesangiolytic change with no lymphatic ligation, **b** mild mesangiolytic change with lymphatic ligation

due to retardation of the mesangial pathway flow. As shown in these examples, by overloading some conditions on this self-limited proliferative model, the creation of an experimental setting for continuous mesangial change will be possible.

Conclusions

We will be able to analyze various factors in mesangial proliferation by using this model. Johnson et al., for example, reported on platelet mediation in glomerular cell proliferation by using this anti-thymocyte antibody model [23]. Sophisticated utilization of this experimental condition will contribute not only to analyzing the mechanism of glomerulonephritis, but also to elucidating the various functions of the mesangial cell. We now have great expectations for the use of this simple and clear model as a good tool in the elucidation of various problems in nephrology, other than the problem of mesangial proliferation.

References

1. Kerjaschki D, Farquhar MG (1983) Immunocytochemical localization of the Heymann nephritis antigen (gp330) in glomerular epithelial cells of normal Lewis rats. J Exp Med 157:667–686
2. Matsuo S, Fukatsu A, Taub ML, Caldwell PRB, Brentjens JR, Andres G (1987) Glomerulonephritis induced in the rabbit by antiendothelial antibodies. J Clin Invest 79:1798–1811
3. Seelig HP, Seelig R, Roth E (1975) Antibodies reacting with the glomerular mesangium: isolation and immunopathology. Virchows Arch [A] 336:313–330
4. Mendrick DL, Rennke HG (1986) Immune deposits formed in situ by a monoclonal antibody recognizing a new intrinsic rat mesangial matrix antigen. J Immunol 137:1517–1526
5. Batsford SR, Rohrback R, Takamiya H, Kluthr R, Vogt A (1979) Autoantibody specific for the glomerular mesangium and Bowman's capsule in man. Clin Nephrol 12:163–167
6. Ishizaki M, Sato S, Sano J, Fukuda Y, Sugisaki Y, Masugi Y (1980) The presence of Thy-1.1 antigen in rat glomerular mesangial cells. Biomed Res 1:438–442
7. Morris RJ, Ritter MA (1980) Association of Thy-1 cell surface differentiation antigen with certain connective tissues in vivo. Cell Tissue Res 206:459–475
8. Harada K, Yamamoto T, Hara M, Kihara I (1982) Antigenic association between kidney and thymocyte. Acta Pathol Jpn 32:483–489
9. Paul LC, Rennke HG, Milford EL, Carpenter CB (1984) Thy-1.1 in glomeruli of rat kidneys. Kidney Int 25:771–777
10. Bagchus WM, Donga J, Ronzing J, Hoedemaeker PhJ, Bakker WW (1984) The specificity of nephritogenic antibodies. IV. Binding of monoclonal anti-thymocyte antibodies to rat kidney. Transplantation 41:739–745
11. Yamamoto T, Yamamoto K, Kawasaki K, Yaoita E, Shimizu F, Kihara I (1986) Immunoelectron microscopic demonstration of Thy-1 antigen on the surface of mesangial cells in the rat glomerulus. Nephron 43:293–298
12. Douglas TC (1972) Occurrence of a theta-like antigen in rats. J Exp Med 136:1054–1062
13. Reif AE, Allen JM (1966) Mouse thymic iso-antigens. Nature 209:521–523
14. Ishizaki M, Shimizu M, Shichinoe K, Masuda Y, Sugisaki Y, Yamanaka N, Masugi Y (1989) The presence of Thy-1.1 antigen in Mongolian gerbils. Biomed Res 10:413–416
15. Ishizaki M (1980) The presence of Thy 1.1 antigen in rat glomerular mesangial cells (in Japanese, with abstract in English). Allergy 29:816–826
16. Ishizaki M, Masuda Y, Fukuda Y, Sugisaki Y, Yamanaka N, Masugi Y (1986) Experimental mesangioproliferative glomerulonephritis in rats induced by intravenous administration of anti-thymocyte serum. Acta Pathol Jpn 36:1191–1203
17. Bagchus WM, Hoedemaeker PJ, Rozing J, Bakker WW (1986) Acute glomerulonephritis after intravenous injection of monoclonal antithymocyte antibodies in the rat. Immunol Lett 12:109–113
18. Bagchus WM, Hoedemaeker PJ, Rozing J, Bakker WW (1986) Glomerulonephritis induced by monoclonal anti-Thy 1.1 antibodies. A sequential histological and ultrastructural study in the rat. Lab Invest 55:680–687

19. Yamamoto T, Wilson CB (1987) Complement dependence of antibody induced mesangial injury in the rat. J Immunol 138:3758–3765
20. Yamamoto T, Wilson CB (1987) Quantitative and qualitative studies of antibody-induced mesangial cell damage in the rat. Kidney Int 32:514–525
21. Morita T, Churg J (1983) Mesangiolysis. Kidney Int 24:1–9
22. Yamanaka N (1988) Development of the glomerular mesangium. Pediatr Nephrol 2:85–91
23. Johnson R, Garcia RI, Pitzl P, Alpers CE (1990) Platelets mediate glomerular cell proliferation in immune complex nephritis induced by anti-mesangial cell antibodies in the rat. Am J Pathol 136:369–374

Experimental Nephritis—Other Models and Future Directions

CURTIS B. WILSON[1]

SUMMARY. Almost all of the advances in understanding the nephritogenic process responsible for human immune, glomerular, and tubulointerstitial renal injury have their basis in animal models. A large number of model systems are now available, with recent interest focused on producing selective glomerular cell injury. Antimesangial cell and anti-epithelial cell surface antigens participate in these processes. An almost parallel set of models are available for understanding the immune processes responsible for tubulointerstitial nephritis. These processes, which include immune deposit formation through antibody reactions with structural and cellular antigens, immune complex formation, and cellular immune reactions, are reviewed. Possible future directions for model use are described. A search for models of disease produced by antigens present only in activated or stimulated cells is suggested and should lead to a better understanding of the immunopathogenesis of vasculitis. Extensions of current model systems to better define the contribution of cytokine and growth factor cascades responsible for glomerular and renal cell contributions to injury are discussed, including the use of the isolated perfused kidney. A number of other possible extensions are mentioned, including selective immunotherapies using antibodies to the T cell receptor Vbeta gene, utilization of SCID mice for development of models of human autoimmunity, the possible role of transgenic mice, and, finally, the utilization of models of selective renal cell injury to further the understanding of renal pathophysiology.

Studies of model systems have produced great strides in understanding the immunologic basis of glomerular disease since the early work of Lindemann, Masugi, Kay, and von Pirquet (Table 1). These studies have been the subject of review [1,2]. The classical Masugi nephritis employs heterogenous anti-glomerular basement membrane (GBM) antibodies (Abs), reactive with a variety of GBM components, to cause acute glomerular capillary wall damage and glomerulonephritis

---

[1]Department of Immunology, Research Institute of Scripps Clinic, La Jolla, CA 92037, USA

1014

Table 1. Immune models of glomerular injury

Ab reactions with glomerular Ags to form immune deposits
  Basement membrane and extracellular matrix Ags
  Trapped or planted Ags
  Immune complex formation/dynamic interchange
  Glomerular cell surface Ags
?? Ab reactions without immune deposits
Cellular immune mechanisms
?? Activation of immune mediator pathways

(GN) in a dose-dependent fashion, largely through the recruitment of systemic mediator systems. This model, combined with the models inducing autoimmune anti-GBM reactions in sheep introduced by Stebley and co-workers, laid the groundwork for recognition of the role of anti-GBM Ab-related injury in humans. The heterologous anti-GBM Ab bound to the GBM in the Masugi model, in turn, served as a trapped antigen (Ag) during the autologous phase of injury, when the host's own Ab response to it caused a second wave of inflammation. The trapped Ag concept now encompasses a wide variety of Ags capable of binding to the glomerular capillary for a number of physicochemical reasons, including lectin binding and charge interactions.

The concept of selective glomerular localization or trapping of a potentially nephritogenic Ag in the glomerular capillary wall for subsequent Ab reaction, and the concept of Ag/Ab reactions in the circulation which form immune complexes (ICs) that can subsequently accumulate in the glomerular capillary, provide a complicated interface between planted Ag mechanisms and IC-based immunopathogenic processes. Except for instances in which Ag can be trapped before the appearance of Ab, as in the Masugi nephritis model, Ag and Ab are typically present together, making quantitative separate or trapping with in situ Ab reaction from IC formation and accumulation difficult. No matter what the major factor is in initiating the glomerular and vascular accumulation of IC, the subsequent dynamic interaction of Ag and Ab in the deposit causes considerable reshaping of the deposit relative to the concentrations of Ag and Ab in the immediate environment; the interchange is modified by physicochemical factors that retain Ag or Ab at the site. Secondary immune reactions, such as anti-idiotypic Abs or rheumatoid factor production, also alter this interchange, depending on the degree of cross-linking produced.

The concept of Ab reactions with the glomerular capillary wall of the Masugi nephritis model has recently been expanded by the recognition of specific reactions with glomerular cell surface Ags, leading to selective injury or modulation of individual glomerular cell types. The mesangial cell lesions, associated with an Ab reactive with a Thy-1-like Ag on the mesangial cell surface, caused complement-mediated cell death and subsequent proliferation of residual mesangial cells, which resolved with focal mesangial matrix increase [3,4]. As with the Masugi nephritis model, quantitative features of anti-Thy-1 Ab binding can be related to the extent of cell injury, degree of proliferation, or to re-injury by additional Ab. The ability to selectively damage one glomerular cell type allows the study of the cell's function and pathophysiology.

Necrotizing and crescentic GN, associated with vasculitis, can occur in patients without evidence of immune deposits, suggesting that other mechanisms of immune injury remain to be defined (see ahead). Cellular immune mechanisms are not pre-

Table 2. Ab reactions with glomerular cell Ags leading to immune deposit formation and/or cell injury

Fx1A-associated Ags (gp330, dipeptidyl peptidase IV, etc), Thy-1, ACE, other Ags recognized by monoclonal Abs, ? infectious agents, phagocytosed materials, ?MHC Ags, ? trapped Ags, ? expressed Ags

ACE, angiotensin converting enzyme

dominant in most instances of GN; however, interesting models in chickens and a recent example in rats indicate the need for additional study [5,6]. Activation of immune mediator systems may also participate, as in Type II membranoproliferative GN.

A topic which originally was planned to be the subject of a separate discussion during the symposium was that of the Ab reactions with a glomerular cell in the long-studied Heymann's nephritis model. Initially, this model was considered to be an example of an autologous IC mechanism involving a proximal tubular brush border Ag. More recently, evidence has accumulated that a selective reaction of Ab with Ags, in particular gp330, shared between the glomerular epithelial cell podocytes and the brush border of the proximal renal tubule, is responsible [7,8]. The molecule has cysteine-rich 40-amino acid repeats, which are also a feature of the human low-density lipoprotein (LDL) receptor; similarity with some regions of epidermal growth factor precursor is also present [9]. A 76 kDa serum protein is reported that may be a ligand for gp330; the 76 kDa material also binds with nephritogenic autoAb eluted from glomerular deposits [10]. Additional Ags may be involved in the full blown Heymann's nephritis lesion. The membrane attack complex of complement (MAC) pays a major role in mediation of this non-inflammatory glomerular lesion [11,12].

In Heymann's nephritis, the mechanism of injury is related to Ab-induced cross-linking of the epithelial cell surface Ag, with shedding of the complex as an immune deposit at the subepithelial aspect of the GBM, where the podocytes abut the GBM [13,14]. Other epithelial Ags, including dipeptidyl peptidase IV, lead to more transient Ab binding [15–17] (see Table 2). It remains difficult to completely exclude ICs, due to the complexity of different crude Ags used for induction and the possibility of anti-idiotypic contributions. The relationship of the Heymann's nephritis model to human membranous glomerulopathy remains unclear, although there are occasional reports of possible anti-gp330 reactions and reports that some anti-glomerular epithelial cell antibodies can react with human or monkey glomeruli with redistribution of surface Ag [18,19]. A spontaneous GN, with subepithelial deposits in rabbits, may represent a similar type of immune mechanism with a glomerular Ag that is also prominent in human glomeruli [20].

We have learned a lot from these models regarding the effects of antibody binding; in terms of quantity and tempo, the site of binding, the accessibility of the reactive antigen which governs these parameters, and the ever increasing complexity of the mediator systems, both systemic and intrinsic, within the glomerular cells themselves, that can produce the injury signaled by the specific interaction of antibody molecules.

It is now apparent that virtually all the immune mechanisms defined in the study of glomerular injury models have counterparts in tubulointerstitial nephritis (TIN) as well (Table 3) (reviewed in [21]). In some of these models, cellular immune mechanisms play major roles. The tubular basement membranes (TBMs) are prominent Ags

Table 3. Immune tubulointerstitial nephritis (TIN)

Ab reactions with tubular Ags to form immune deposits
  Basement membrane and extracellular matrix Ags
    TBM, TBM/GBM, ? TBM/Drug conjugates
  ?? Trapped or planted Ags
    Drugs, microbial Ags, DNA, etc.
  Immune complex formation/dynamic interchange
    Serum proteins, drugs, products of infectious agents, tissue components, idiotypic Ags, etc.
  Tubular cell surface Ags
    Brush border Ags, Tamm Horsfall protein

Cellular immune mechanisms
  Ags associated with delayed type hypersensitivity
    Aggregated proteins, cell surface Ags, TBM Ags, ? drugs
  Ags in cellular forms of TIN
    Isologous kidney, homologous renal basement membrane, heterologous TBM, tubular Ag/TBM Ag in
      kdkd mice, ?non-native materials (drugs, infectious agents, etc.)
?? Activation of immune mediator pathways

which, when used as immunogens in adjuvants, can elicit predominantly humoral (guinea pigs, rats) or cellular (mice) immune mononuclear leukocyte-dominated reactions, surrounding the tubules with linear Ig deposits in the TBM. The circulating and eluted anti-TBM Abs react with Ags confined to the proximal TBM; the Ags are genetically variable in rats and in humans [22]. The allotypic differences can induce anti-TBM Ab in association with renal transplantation. TBM/drug conjugates have been suggested to induce anti-TBM antibody reactions in humans [23]. Sodium aurothiomalate and mercuric chloride can also induce Ab reactive with TBM [24,25]. A different set of immune reactions in rats is directed toward Ags shared with GBM/TBM, as seen in human anti-GBM Ab disease and Goodpasture's syndrome.

The anti-TBM Ab disease of the guinea pig or rat is transferable with immune serum. In the rat, the kinetics of binding have been studied, and reveal a gradual increase in fixation over 5–6 days, suggesting that the Ag is relatively sequestered [26]. The molecule carrying the reactive Ag may vary somewhat in size depending on extraction methods. It has been termed 3M-1 and is about 30 kDa in mice, 42–45 or 48 kDa in rats, and 48 kDa in rabbits and humans (reviewed in [27]). cDNA defines the 3M-1 as a complex, novel structure containing five distinct amino acid termini, all sharing a common framework domain [28]. Comparisons of the anti-TBM Ab binding sequence suggest a 37% non-repetitive structural similarity with some intermediate filament-associated proteins (E.G. Neilson personal communication). A peptide fragment synthesized from the sequence encoding this common framework domain was able to bind to a monoclonal 3M-1 reactive anti-TBM Ab and stimulate the growth of 3M-1-reactive helper T cells, as well as induce nephritogenic effector T cells capable of producing TIN (E.G. Neilson personal communication). These findings indicate that a small and unique, immunodominant region of the 3M-1 Ag, evolutionarily related to the family of intermediate filament-associated proteins, provides a sufficient recognition structure for the model of TIN.

Reactions with renal tubular cell Ags also occur in models that parallel, to some extent, those reactive with glomerular cell Ags. Active or passive immunization to Fx1A type Ags leads to immune deposits in and around the proximal tubular cell;

striking damage to the brush border is found when the Ab gains access to the tubular urine [29]. The reaction is thought to represent another example of Ab-induced cross-linking of Ag [30]. Numerous Ags would be candidates for this type of reaction and anti-tubular brush border Abs are sometimes identified in humans with tubular damage (reviewed in [27]). Another tubular protein that has been studied in a similar type of reaction is the Tamm-Horsfall protein [31] and angiotensin converting enzyme which may react with the basolateral compartment of the proximal tubular cell [32]. A wide variety of monoclonal Abs reactive with tubular cell Ags have a similar potential. The concept of molecular mimicry, in which short segments of amino acid homology are shared between molecules, can also lead to cross-reactions with renal tubular Ags. For example, we have found that a number of monoclonal anti-viral Abs also react with renal tubular (or glomerular) structures.

As they do in immune glomerular injury, ICs can accumulate in the tubulointerstitial tissues in serum sickness, and in murine and human examples of systemic lupus erythematosus (SLE) or presumed IC disease. Regarding circulating versus in situ formed ICs, the same factors as those in the glomeruli must be taken into consideration, as well as the dynamic interchange of Ag and Ab (see above). The possibility of trapping of Ag within the tubulointerstitial tissue for subsequent Ab reaction is another possibility, although good models are lacking as yet.

In TIN, cellular immune reactions play a more striking role than in GN, and a variety of models of delayed type hypersensitivity reactions are described (reviewed in [27]). The TIN of SJL mice induced by immunization with heterologous TBM, as noted above, is largely cellular in nature, with the development of a MHC class I restricted, Lyt-2+ effector cell which can adaptively transfer the disease [33-36]. The proximal tubular epithelial cell line producing the 3M-1 Ag expresses MHC class II Ags and can support the proliferation of MHC class II restricted helper T cell lines in culture [37]. Anti-3M-1 Abs down regulate MHC class II expression of the 3M-1 synthesizing cells in vitro [38]. Proximal tubular enhancement of MHC class II expression is also found in the MRL/1pr lupus mice [39]. The SJL model is being used very successfully to explore therapeutic approaches, including the evaluation of suppressor cell networks capable of inhibiting the disease, via injection of spleen cells coupled with TBM Ag [40]. At least two suppressor subsets are defined and soluble factors from spleen cells of mice treated to induce suppressor cells are able to inhibit development of interstitial lesions in an Ag-specific, genetically restricted manner [41,42]. These models hold considerable promise for better understanding of treatment (see ahead).

Lewis rats (lacking reactive TBM Ag), when immunized with Brown Norway rat TBM, develop a severe nodular granulomatous form of TIN [43]. The lesion is easily transferred with immune cells and there is little evidence for an Ab role in the model. The kdkd mouse, a congenic subline of the CBA/Ca strain, also appears to have a cell-mediated form of TIN [44]. As considered in glomerular disease, immune mediation activation, particularly that of complement, may occur in the tubulointerstitial tissue, associated with ammonia increases during compromised renal function.

The models of GN and TIN are responsible for our current understanding of the immunopathogenesis of renal disease. The growth of knowledge in the past few years, based on molecular biologic techniques and glomerular cell culture, has been outstanding, but much of it is yet to be transferred to the intact kidney models or the human counterparts. The models can be expected to play a more prominent role as the basic information is translated in vivo. The request by the program organizers to look into the next century is difficult and it is a bit presumptuous to predict how the current or new models will be used; however, some suggestions will be made.

A new mechanism of injury, such as that recently defined by the glomerular cell surface reactions, may emerge in the broad field of Ag accessibility and induced Ag expression. In the former case, evidence is accumulating that alveolar basement membrane Ags are not readily available for anti-GBM Ab reaction unless the integrity of the alveolar wall is first altered, as determined in model studies [45]. If this is also true for human anti-GBM Abs, it could explain episodes of pulmonary hemorrhage in Goodpasture's syndrome. In the case of Ag expression, the renal syndromes associated with vasculitis serve as a starting point. In these conditions, glomerular disease may be severe, without the usual evidence of immune deposits. This suggests a new immunopathogenic mechanism. In Kawasaki's syndrome, for example, the Abs present are capable of lysis of activated, but not normal, cultured human endothelial cells [46,47]. In one type, IgG and IgM Abs lyse interleukin-1 (IL-1) and tumor necrosis factor (TNF)-treated endothelial cells. In the other type, IgM Abs lyse INF gamma treated endothelial cells via different Ags. Complement-fixing IgG and IgM Abs are reported in acute hemolytic uremic syndrome, which can lyse umbilical vein endothelial cells, but not after INF treatment [48]. A number of less well defined anti-endothelial cell Abs have been reported in Wegener's granulomatosis, other vasculitis, and IgA nephropathy. The cytokine effects on endothelium have been reviewed [49] and, in addition to modulating a number of coagulation related proteins, including tissue factor, thrombomodulin, and PAI, they also increase surface adhesion of leukocytes. The latter is via expression of endothelial leukocyte adhesion molecule (ELAM-1) and intracellular adhesion molecule (ICAM-1, CD54)J. ICAM-1 is a ligand for LFA-1 (CD11a/CD18) of the leukocyte adhesion CD11/18 complex, which also includes Mac-1 and p150,95, all having common beta chains and unique alpha chains (reviewed in [50]).

In addition to changes in the endothelium with the expression of Ags, one must also consider a similar observation in the neutrophil, the target of anti-neutrophil (and macrophage) cytoplasmic Ab (ANCA), subsets of which are seen in various forms of vasculitis and in idiopathic necrotizing and crescentic GN [51,52]. Of great interest is the recent observation that neutrophils may need to be "activated" with cytokines to be able to express the reactive Ag on their surface [53]. These Ag expression observations should serve as a base for a new use of model systems in advancing understanding of the immunopathogenesis of the poorly understood class of vasculitis-associated renal injury that occurs without the usual immune deposit formation.

The models of glomerular injury have been widely used to study systemic mediator pathways of immune GN, and, to a lesser extent, TIN, injury (Table 4). Almost all that we know was derived first from observation of possible reactants and subsequent mediator depletion in models. These studies have been coupled, in many instances, with identification of similar factors in humans. It is to be expected that the models will continue to be used for these purposes. In addition, there has been an explosion of information derived from glomerular cell culture and application of molecular biologic techniques. This incorporation points to the potential large contribution of factors from the glomerular cells themselves to the inflammatory process and to the sclerosis that often follows (Table 5). It is in this area that the models, particularly the models in which selective glomerular cell damage can be produced, will have a great deal of play

Table 4. Models and isolated kidney for the study of systemic mediators of inflammation

Ab effects and the MAC
? Integrins, glomerular cell products
Neutrophils and macrophages
  Oxidants, proteinases, cationic proteins, eicosanoids, cytokines, growth factors, coagulation factors
Platelets
  Neutrophil interaction, PAF, platelet factor 4, eicosanoids
Lymphocytes

MAC, membrane attack complex; PAF, platelet activating factor

in the next few years. The determination of cytokine/growth factor cascades in glomerular inflammation will employ molecular biology techniques, bioassays, and cytochemical staining in models employing selective systemic mediator depletion. It is also expected that the isolated perfused kidney will find great usefulness in the study of immune injury in the absence of systemic mediators. The perfused kidney can also be used to study the direct glomerular effects of initial factors in the cascades, to confirm their roles. It is anticipated that the isolated perfused kidney will be used to manipulate pivotal factors, using Ab, peptide, or molecular techniques, so that the most suitable approaches for therapy in the intact models and, subsequently, in human glomerular disease can be determined. Interference with receptor binding, with peptide blocking such as the RGD (arg-gly-asp) sequence [54], or with gene expression, through the administration of anti-sense RNA, [55] has potential usefulness that can be tested in the isolated perfused kidney and in the models.

The T cell-mediated models will be used to advantage to study the effects of immunologically specific therapy, such as that utilizing T cell receptor Vbeta-specific antibodies, as in experimental allergic encephalomyelitis [56,57]. In experimental allergic encephalomyelitis, only two T cell receptor Vbeta gene segments, Vbeta8.2 and Vbeta13, and two distinct Valpha gene segments, Valpha2.3 and Valpha4.3, are identified in the myelin basic protein-specific T helper cells. This limited use of the T cell receptor V region genes, in response to myelin basic protein, allowed the specific treatment of the disease, including reversal of paralysis, with a combination of monoclonal Vbeta8.2 and Vbeta13 specific antibodies [58].

The recent identification of the SCID mice, which have sufficient immunodeficiency to allow implantation and growth of human immune cells, allows the construction of models of laboratory animal based human disease. In mice given peripheral blood leukocytes from patients with systemic lupus erythematosus, antinuclear antibodies develop and glomerular immune deposits resembling lupus nephritis are found [59]. The model expands the potential for directly evaluating the

Table 5. Potential contribution of glomerular cells to inflammation

Interleukin — 1(IL-1alpha, beta), Tumor necrosis factor (TNF), interleukin-6 (IL-6), insulin-like growth
  factor (IFG-I), tissue plasminogen activator (t-PA), plasminogen activator inhibitor (PAI), platelet
  activating factor (PAF), platelet derived growth factor (PDGF), tissue factor (TF), oxidative products,
  neutral proteinase and its inhibitor, thrombospondin, renin, eicosanoids, endothelial cell adhesion
  molecules
Growth factors; epidermal growth factor (EGF), receptors for transforming growth factor beta
  (TGFbeta), beta1-integrin, fibronectin production

influence of cellular and humoral functions in the progression of the disease and expands the potential for evaluating various possible therapies in several mice from the same donor. We have been successful in establishing anti-GBM Ab production in SCID mice, with transfer of peripheral blood leukocytes from patients with active disease, so that the study of numerous autoimmune diseases with renal features appears to be possible.

The development of mesangial proliferative GN has been noted in IL-6 transgenic mice [60], and mesangial proliferation and progressive glomerulosclerosis has been observed in mice expressing growth hormone and growth hormone releasing factor [61,62]. The heavy metal-inducible promoter of the mouse metallothione in I gene, among others, can be used to express genes in the kidneys of transgenic mice. It is much easier, currently, to express a gene than to delete the function of one. As currently employed, the technique of homologous recombination used for the latter is demanding [63]. It is to be expected that systems will be available, however, which will use transgenic animals to alter gene expression for a variety of purposes in the study of immune renal injury. Extensions of the studies evaluating the role of cytokines and growth factors should be possible, as noted above. Alteration in Ag expression and manipulation of Ab production or T cell receptor functions should also be of interest.

Another use of the models, either of those now available or of those that could be developed, would be in the examination of the pathophysiologic effects of selective glomerular or tubular cell injury. We have used the anti-mesangial cell injury model to look at the effect of acute mesangial cell lysis at 24 hours after antibody administration; we found a reduction in glomerular ultrafiltration coefficient as plasma was shunted into the lytic mesangial space away from the filtering surface [64]. During the proliferative phase of injury, 3–5 days later, the ultrafiltration coefficient remained low during the increase in mesangial volume and decreased capillary luminal volume and surface area.

Acknowledgments. This work was supported in part by USPHS Grants Nos. AI-07007, DK20043, DK32353, DK40251, AG04342, and Biomedical Research Support Grant RR0-5514.

References

1. Wilson CB (to be published) The renal response to immunological injury. In: Brenner BM, Rector FC Jr (eds) The kidney, 4th edn. Saunders, Philadelphia
2. Wilson CB (1988) Antibody reactions with native or planted glomerular antigens producing nephritogenic immune deposits or selective glomerular cell injury. IN: Wilson CB (guest ed) Contemporary issues in nephrology, vol 18. Churchill-Livingstone, New York, pp 1–34
3. Yamamoto T, Wilson CB (1987) Complement dependence of antibody-induced mesangial cell injury in the rat. J Immunol 138:3758–3765
4. Yamamoto T, Wilson CB (187) Quantitative and qualitative studies of antibody-induced mesangial cell damage in the rat. Kidney Int 32:514–525
5. Bolton WK, Tucker FL, Sturgill BC (1984) New avian model of experimental glomerulonephritis consistent with mediation by cellular immunity. Nonhumorally mediated glomerulonephritis in chickens. J Clin Invest 73:1263–1276

6. Rennke HG, Klein PS, Mendrick DL (1990) Cell-mediated immunity (CMI) in hapten-induced interstitial nephritis and glomerular crescent formation in the rat (abstract). Kidney Int 37:428
7. Kerjaschki D, Farquhar MG (1982) Identification of membrane glycoprotein from kidney brush border as the pathogenic antigen of Heymann's nephritis. Proc Natl Acad Sci USA 79:5557–5561
8. Ronco P, Neale TJ, Wilson CB, Galceran M, Verroust P (1986) An immunopathologic study of a 330-kD protein defined by monoclonal antibodies and reactive with anti-RTE-alpha-5 antibodies and kidney eluates from active Heymann nephritis. J Immunol 136:125–130
9. Raychowdhury R. Niles JL, McCluskey RT, Smith JA (1989) Autoimmune target in Heymann nephritis is a glycoprotein with homology to the LDL receptor. Science 244:1163–1165
10. Kanalas JJ, Makker SP (1988) A possible ligand of serum origin for the kidney autoantigen of Heymann nephritis. J Immunol 141:4152–4157
11. Salant DJ, Belok S, Madaio MP, Couser WG (1980) A new role for complement in experimental membranous nephropathy in rats. J Clin Invest 66:1339–1350
12. Cybulsky AV, Rennke HG, Feintzeig ID, Salant DJ (1986) Complement-induced glomerular epithelial cell injury. Role of the membrane attack complex in rat membranous nephropathy. J Clin Invest 77:1096–1107
13. Andres G, Brentjens JR, Caldwell PRB, Camussi G, Matsuo S (1986) Formation of immune deposits and disease. Lab Invest 55:510–520
14. Kerjaschki D, Miettnen A, Farquhar MG (1987) Initial events in the formation of immune deposits in passive Heymann nephritis. J Exp Med 166:109–128
15. Mendrick DL, Rennke HG (1988) Epitope specific induction of proteinuria by monoclonal antibodies. Kidney Int 33:831–842
16. Quigg RJ, Abrahamson DR, Cybulsky AV, Badalamenti J, Minto AWM, Salant DJ (1989) Studies with antibodies to cultured rat glomerular epithelial cells. Subepithelial immune deposit formation after in vivo injection. Am J Pathol 134:1125–1133
17. Verroust PF (1989) Kinetics of immune deposits in membranous nephropathy. Kidney Int 35:1418–1428
18. Fukatsu A, Yuzawa Y, Olson L, Miller J, Milgrom M, Zamlauski-Tucker, Van Liew JB, Campagnari A, Niesen N, Patel J, Doi T, Striker L, Striker G, Milgrom F, Brentjens J, Andres G (1989) Interaction of antibodies with human glomerular epithelial cells. Lab Invest 61:389–403
19. Makker SP, Kanalas JJ (1989) Autoantibodies to human gp330 in sera of patients with idiopathic membranous nephropathy. Kidney Int 35:211
20. Neale TJ, Woodroffe AJ, Wilson CB (1984) Spontaneous glomerulonephritis in rabbits: Role of a glomerular capillary antigen. Kidney Int 26:701–711
21. Wilson CB (1989) Study of the immunopathogenesis of tubulointerstitial nephritis using model systems. Kidney Int 35:938–953
22. Wilson CB, Lehman DH, McCoy RC, Gunnells JC Jr, Stickel DL (1974) Antitubular basement membrane antibodies after renal transplantation. Transplantation 18:447–452
23. Border WA, Lehman DH, Egan JD, Sass HJ, Glode JE, Wilson CB (1974) Antitubular basement-membrane antibodies in methicillin-associated interstitial nephritis. N Engl J Med 291:381–384
24. Ueda S, Wakashin M, Wakashin Y, Yoshida H, Iesato K, Mori T, Mori Y, Akikusa B, Okuda K (1986) Experimental gold nephropathy in guinea pigs: Detection of autoantibodies to renal tubular antigens. Kidney Int 29:539–548
25. Guery C-J, Hedrich HJ, Mercier P, Reetz IC, Mandet C, Mahieu P, Neilson EG, Druet P (1989) Mapping of a gene for the M_r 48000 tubular basement membrane antigen in the rat. Immunogenetics 29:350–354

26. Bannister KM, Wilson, CB (1985) Transfer of tubulointerstitial nephritis in the Brown Norway rat with anti-tubular basement membrane antibody: Quantitation and kinetics of binding and effect of decomplementation. J Immunol 135:3911–3917
27. Wilson CB (to be published) Nephritogenic tubulointerstitial antigens. Kidney Int
28. Neilson EG, Sun MJ, Emergy J, Kelly CJ, Haverty T, Clayman M, Cooke NE (1989) Molecular cloning of the 3M-1 nephritogenic antigen (abstract). Kidney Int 35:358
29. Noble B, Mendrick DL, Brentjens Jr, Andres GA (1981) Antibody-mediated injury to proximal tubules in the rat kidney induced by passive transfer of homologous anti-brush border serum. Clin Immunol Immunopathol 19:289–301
30. Brodkin M, Noble B (1988) Antibody-mediated proliferation of proximal tubule cells requires cross-linking of antigenic determinants. Clin Exp Immunol 72:315–320
31. Ishidate T, Hoyer JR, Seiler MW (1983) Influence of altered glomerular permeability on renal tubular immune complex formation and clearance. Lab Invest 49:582–588
32. Fukatsu A, Yuzawa Y, Niesen N, Matsuo S, Caldwell PRB, Brentjens JR, Andres G (1988) Local formation of immune deposits in rabbit renal proximal tubules. Kidney Int 34:611–619
33. Neilson EG, Phillips SM (1982) Murine interstitial nephritis. I. Analysis of disease susceptibility and its relationship to pleiomorphic gene products defining both immune-response genes and a restrictive requirement for cytotoxic T cells at H-2K. J Exp Med 155: 1075–1085
34. Zakheim B, McCafferty E, Phillips SM, Clayman M, Neilson EG (1984) Murine interstitial nephritis II. The adoptive transfer of disease with immune T lymphocytes produces a phenotypically complex interstitial lesion. J Immunol 133:234–239
35. Mann R, Kelly CJ, Hines WH, Clayman MD, Blanchard N, Sun MJ, Neilson EG (1987) Effector T cell differentiation in experimental interstitial nephritis. I. The development and modulation of effector lymphocyte maturation by I-J⁺ regulatory T cells. J Immunol 138:4200–4208
36. Kelly CJ, MoK H, Neilson EG (1988) The selection of effector T cell phenotype by contrasuppression modulates susceptibility to autoimmune injury. J Immunol 141:3022–3028
37. Haverty TP, Kelly CJ, Hines WH, Amenta PS, Wattanabe M, Harper RA, Kefalides NA, Neilson, EG (1988) Characterization of a renal tubular epithelial cell line which secretes the autologous target antigen of autoimmune experimental interstitial nephritis. J Cell Biol 107:1359–1368
38. Haverty TP, Wattanabe M, Neilson EG, Kelly CJ (1989) Protective modulation of class II MHC gene expression in tubular epithelium by target antigen-specific antibodies. Cell-surface directed down-regulation of transcription can influence susceptibility to murine tubulointerstitial nephritis. J Immunol 143:1133–1141
39. Wuthrich RP, Yui MA, Mazoujian G, Nabavi N, Glimcher LH, Kelley VE (1989) Enhanced MHC class II expression in renal proximal tubules precedes loss of renal function in MRL/1pr mice with lupus nephritis. Am J Pathol 134:45–51
40. Neilson EG, McCafferty E, Mann R, Michaud L, Clayman M (1985) Tubular antigen-derivatized cells induce a disease-protective, antigen-specific, and idiotype-specific suppressor T cell network restricted by I-J and Igh-V in mice with experimental interstitial nephritis. J Exp Med 162:215–230
41. Mann R, Neilson EG (1986) Murine interstitial nephritis. V. The auto-induction of antigen-specific Lyt2⁺ suppressor T cells diminishes the expression of interstitial nephritis in mice with antitubular basement membrane disease. J Immunol 136:908–912
42. Neilson EG, Kelly CJ, Clayman MD, Hines WH, Haverty T, Sun MJ, Blanchard N (1987) Murine interstitial nephritis. VII. Suppression of renal injury after treatment with soluble suppressor factor TsF↓. J Immunol 139:1518–1524
43. Bannister KM, Ulich TR, Wilson CB (1987) Induction, characterization, and cell transfer of autoimmune tubulointerstitial nephritis in the Lewis rat. Kidney Int 32:642–651

44. Kelly CJ, Neilson EG (1987) Contrasuppression in autoimmunity. Abnormal contrasuppression facilitates expression of nephritogenic effector T cells and interstitial nephritis in kdkd mice. J Exp Med 165:107–123

45. Queluz TH, Pawlowski I, Brunda MJ, Brentjens JR, Vladutiu AO, Andres G (1990) Pathogenesis of an experimental model of Goodpasture's hemorrhagic pneumonitis. J Clin Invest 85:1507–1515

46. Leung DYM, Geha RS, Newburger JW, et al. (1986) Two monokines, interleukin 1 and tumor necrosis factor, render cultured vascular endothelial cells susceptible to lysis by antibodies circulating during Kawasaki syndrome. J Exp Med 164:1958–1972

47. Leung Dym, Collins T, Lapierre LA, et al. (1986) Immunoglobulin M antibodies present in the acute phase of Kawasaki syndrome lyse cultured vascular endothelial cells stimulated by gamma interferon. J Clin Invest 77:1428–1435

48. Leung DYM, Moake JL, Havens PL, et al. (1988) Lytic anti-endothelial cell antibodies in haemolytic-uraemic syndrome. Lancet II:183–186

49. Cotran RS, Pober JS (1989) Effects of cytokines on vascular endothelium: Their role in vascular and immune injury. Kidney Int 35:969–975

50. Arnaout MA (1990) Structure and function of the leukocyte adhesion molecules CD11/CD18. Blood 75:1037–1050

51. Falk RJ, Jennette JC (1988) Anti-neutrophil cytoplasmic autoantibodies with specificity for myeloperoxidase in patients with systemic vasculitis and idiopathic necrotizing and crescentic glomerulonephritis. N Engl J Med 318:1651–1657

52. Cohen Tervaert JW, Goldschmeding R, Elema JD, et al. (1990) Autoantibodies against myeloid lysosomal enzymes in crescentic glomerulonephritis. Kidney Int 37:799–806

53. Falk RJ, Terrell RS, Charles LA, Jennette JC (1990) Anti-neutrophil cytoplasmic autoantibodies induce neutrophils to degranulate and produce oxygen radicals in vitro. Proc Natl Acad Sci USA 87:4115–4119

54. Hynes RO (1986) Fibronectins. Sci Am 254:42–51

55. Stein CA, Cohen JS (1988) Oligodeoxynucleotides as inhibitors of gene expression: a review. Cancer Res 48:2659–2668

56. Urban JL, Kumar VK, Kono DH, Gomez C, Horvath SJ, Clayton J, Ando DG, Sercarz EE, Hood L (1988) Restricted use of T cell receptor V genes in murine autoimmune encephalomyelitis raises possibility of antibody therapy. Cell 54:577–592

57. Acha-Orbea H, Mitchell DJ, Timmermann L, Wraith DC, Tausch GS, Waldor MK, Zamvil SS, McDevitt HO, Steinman L (1988) Limited heterogeneity of T cell receptors from lymphocytes mediating autoimmune encephalomyelitis allows specific immune intervention. Cell 54:263–273

58. Zaller DM, Osman G, Kanagawa O, Hood L (1990) Prevention and treatment of murine experimental allergic encephalomyelitis with T cell receptor Vbeta-specific antibodies. J Exp Med 1943–1955

59. Duchosal MA, McConahey PJ, Robinson CA, Dixon RJ (to be published) Transfer of human systemic lupus erythematosus in SCID mice. J Exp Med

60. Suematsu S, Matsuda T, Aozasa K, Akira S, Nakano N, Ohno S, Miyazaki J, Yamamura K, Hirano T, Kishimoto T (1989) IgG1 plasmacytosis in interleukin 6 transgenic mice. Proc Natl Acad Sci USA 86:7547–7551

61. Doi T, Striker LJ, Quaife C, Conti FG, Palmiter R, Behringer R, Brinster R, Striker GE (1988) Progressive glomerulosclerosis develops in transgenic mice chronically expressing growth hormone and growth hormone releasing factor but not in those expressing insulin-like growth factor-1. Am J Pathol 131:398–403

62. Quaife CJ, Mathews LS, Pinkert CA, Hammer RE, Brinster RL, Palmiter RD (1989) Histopathology associated with elevated levels of growth hormone and insulin-like growth factor I in transgenic mice. Endocrinology 124:40–48

63. Zijlstra M, Li E, Sajjadi F, Subramani S, Jaenisch R (1989) Germ-line transmission of a disrupted beta$_2$-microglobulin gene produced by homologous recombination in embryonic stem cells. Nature 342:435–438
64. Yamamoto T, Mundy C, Wilson CB, Blantz RC (1988) Antibody induced mesangial cell (MC) lysis and proliferation: Glomerular hemodynamic consequences (abstract). Kidney Int 33:327

Nephrolithiasis: New Ideas in Pathophysiology, New Facts in Therapy

Chair: Philippe Jaeger (Switzerland)
Kenkichi Koiso (Japan)

Idiopathic Hypercalciuria: Proposal for a New Cascade

Pierre Bataille, Albert Fournier, Bernard Boudailliez, Pierre François Westeel, Najeh El Esper, Jean Michel Achard[1], Catherine Bergot[2], and Roger Bouillon[3]

SUMMARY. Idiopathic hypercalciuria (IH) is defined by a 24 hour urinary excretion of calcium greater than 4 mg or 0.1 mmol/kg of body weight on a calcium diet of 1 g and greater than 3 mg or 0.07 mmol/kg on a Ca diet of 400 mg, while there is no excess of sodium (120–180 mmol) nor of protein (1–1.3 g/kg per day). IH with fasting hypercalciuria but without secondary hyperparathyroidism represents in our experiece the most prevalent subtype of IH. Since bone mineral density has been shown to be decreased in this undetermined subtype (Pak's classification), as in patients with absorptive hypercalciuria type I or with renal hypercalciuria, the clinical relevance of this classification is questioned. A primary bone hyperresorption seems to be the main explanation of IH, since in this group as a whole, fasting hypercalciuria is correlated positively with fasting hydroxyprolinuria which is higher than in controls. This bone resorption may be favored by protein intake of non-dairy origin due to a higher meat intake and hypersensitivity of bone resorption to meat intake, as evidenced by a higher daily urinary excretion of urea on a diet without dairy products and a steeper slope of the regression of fasting calciuria versus 24 hour urea excretion. Furthermore, calcitriol synthesis is increased, probably because of a hypersensitivity of 25 OH vitamin D 1α hydroxylase to phosphate, as evidenced by the fact that plasma calcitriol correlates negatively with plasma phosphate which, however, remains in the normal range. High plasma calcitriol is not responsible for the bone hyperresorption, since it correlates negatively with fasting hypercalciuria and positively with bone density and postprandial calciuria (an index of calcium absorption).

Since Pacifici has recently shown that Ca stone formers with fasting hypercalciuria have an increased synthesis of interleukin I by their peripheral monocytes, and that interleukin I may stimulate prostaglandin E2, which can be responsible for both bone resorption and increased activity of the 25 OH vitamin D 1α hydroxylase, a new cascade of pathophysiological events originating from a monocyte disease has been

[1] Hôpital Sud, Service de Néphrologie du CHRU d'Amiens, 80054 Amiens Cédex, France
[2] Service de Radiologie de l'Hôpital St. Louis, Paris, France
[3] Laboratoire d'Endocrinologie, Université de Leuven, Leuven, Belgium

presented. The therapeutic consequences of these new pathophysiological insights are: 1/ dietary restriction in protein of non dairy origin, so that the calcium intake remains around 1000 mg to prevent worsening of bone loss; 2/ thiazide therapy which decreases calciuria not only by a direct tubular effect, but also by a decrease of prostaglandin E2 synthesis.

Introduction

Hypercalciuria is found in about one-half of patients with idiopathic calcium lithiasis, i.e., Ca lithiasis not explained by a well individualized disease which is responsible either for secondary hypercalciuria, such as primary hyperparathyroidism, sarcoidosis, distal tubular acidosis, neoplasia, hyperthyroidism, Cushing's syndrome, vitamin D intoxication and milk alkali syndrome, or for frank hyperoxaluria (primary or enteric hyperoxaluria). Hypercalciuria is therefore the most frequent risk factor of idiopathic Ca lithiasis. Despite recent advances in the knowledge of its pathogenesis, hypercalciuria is still a controversial subject for many reasons: 1/ the statistical difficulty of assigning an upper limit of calcium excretion in a normal population; 2/ the role of dietary factors other than calcium intake; and 3/ the interrelation of many metabolic abnormalities.

In this paper, we shall consider successively the definition of hypercalciuria, the dietary factors influencing calcium excretion, the classical types and subtypes of idiopathic hypercalciuria as proposed by Pak, the evidence for disordered calcitriol synthesis, the evidence for bone involvement, and data suggesting a primary monocyte disorder which could be an overall explanation for the spectrum of this so called idiopathic hypercalciuria.

Definition of Hypercalciuria and its Relation with Dietary Factors Influencing Calcium Excretion

Because of an upward skew of calciuria values in a normal population on a free diet, it is preferable to take as the upper limit of normal not the sum of the mean plus 2 standard deviations, but the limit below which is found the calciuria of 90% of the population [1]. There is a considerable overlap between calciuria histograms of controls and stone-formers, the latter being shifted upwards by 75 mg/day [2,3].

Calciuria is an extremely variable parameter, which depends on a constitutional parameter such as weight and dietary parameters: intakes not only of calcium, but also of protein, phosphate, sodium, and carbohydrate.

The expression of calciuria adjusted to the creatinine excretion or, as is more usually done, to the body weight, makes unnecessary the use of the term *"constitutional hypercalciuria"* proposed by Broadus [4] to describe high values of calciuria in relation only to larger patient size, and not to specific metabolic abnormalities.

Increasing calcium intake from 400 mg/day to 1000 mg/day induces an increase of calciuria both in normal controls and in Ca stone formers, but this increase is much greater in the latter (120 mg/24h) than in the normals (40 mg/24h) [5]. In evaluating calciuria, it is thus necessary to have data for calciuria measured in controls who are on the same known dietary intake of calcium as the Ca stone formers.

Dietary protein intake is likewise an important determinant of urinary calcium. In a normal subject, calcium excretion doubles as daily protein intake increases from 0.5 g/kg of body weight to 2g/kg. As a matter of fact, daily urea excretion, which is an index of protein intake, is positively correlated with calciuria [6]. The mechanism of the dependency of calcium excretion upon protein intake is not clear. Initially it was thought to be linked to an increased fixed acid production producing mild metabolic acidosis, which would increase calcium excretion by inhibition of tubular calcium reabsorption and by stimulation of bone resorption related to skeletal buffering of retained acids [5]. Actually the decreased tubular calcium reabsorption seems rather to be linked to the increase of urinary sulfate concentration observed after protein loads rich in methionine. Sulfate is a poorly reabsorbed anion which is available for complexing urinary calcium; this thus limits its tubular reabsorption [7]. Indeed, this explains the fact that prevention of metabolic acidosis does not correct the protein-induced hypercalciuria [7]. Whatever the actual mechanism of protein-induced hypercalciuria, high dietary protein intake induces a negative calcium balance which favors bone loss [8,9].

Dietary phosphate intake variation in the usual range, from 600 to 1500 mg/day, does not significantly influence calciuria. However, extreme phosphate restriction (< 300 mg of phosphate/day) is accompanied by hypercalciuria which is responsible for a negative calcium balance, in spite of a fall in parathyroid hormone (PTH) secretion [7].

Infusion of sodium chloride or increasing dietary sodium intake increases urinary calcium. In controls, urinary calcium increases by about 25 mg per 100 mEq of additional dietary sodium chloride and a strong relationship is observed between daily urinary sodium and urinary calcium excretions [10,11]. The sodium load depresses both proximal and distal tubular calcium reabsorption. After 28 days, sodium-induced hypercalciuria is, however, no longer observed in normal subjects [12]. In calcium stone formers the dependence of calcium excretion upon sodium intake exists on a short term basis (1 week) [13] and persists after 2 months [14]. The influence of sodium intake on calciuria is so strong in Ca stone formers that it influences even fasting calciuria, so that high Na intake may be responsible for factitious renal hypercalciuria (see Pak's classification) [13].

Refined carbohydrates increase calcium excretion by inducing hyperinsulinism, which enhances tubular sodium reabsorption and decreases tubular calcium reabsorption [15,16]. Alcohol also seems to favor hypercalciuria probably by way of an identical mechanism. The clinical importance of alcohol and carbohydrate excess remains unclear for the moment.

The importance of dietary factors is all the more great in that *the hypercalciuric effect of protein and sodium is more pronounced in Ca stone-formers than in normal subjects.* The slopes of the relationship between calcium and sodium or urea excretion are, respectively, 3 times [13] and 5 times [6,17] greater in stone-formers.

Thus, in order to appropriately evaluate calcium excretion, results must be weight or creatinine adjusted and interpreted in relation to calcium, sodium, protein, and, possibly, carbohydrate intakes. According to our own data [17] and those in the literature, *we propose the following values as upper limits of normal for calciuria according to diet:*

1) 4 mg or 0.1 mmol/kg per day on a diet providing 1 g calcium, 130 mmol of sodium, and 1–1.3 g/kg of protein daily;

2) 3 mg or 0.07 mmol/kg per day after 4 days of low calcium intake (excluding all dairy products ≈ 400 mg calcium daily) and 115 mmol of sodium and 1–1.3 g/kg of protein daily.

In clinical practice it is, however, important to first evaluate the patient, as an outpatient, on his or her usual diet, i.e., the diet followed spontaneously before any dietary advice, for at least 2 days (because of the variability of calciuria). Then, to properly classify the calciuria, it is important to measure it again, in 24 hour urine, for at least 4 days while the patient is on a known calcium intake. We recommend evaluating the patients on both 1000 mg and 400 mg calcium diets. As a matter of fact, a 1000 mg calcium diet is now the diet recommended for calcium stone formers in order to prevent bone loss (see below) and marginal hyperoxaluria induced by calcium restriction [17]; a 400 mg calcium diet is the diet recommended so that fasting calciuria according to Pak [18] can be appropriately evaluated.

Calciuria exceeding the upper limit of normal on 400 and 1000 mg Ca diets while sodium, protein, and carbohydrate intakes are concomitantly controlled defines true idiopathic hypercalciuria, once well defined diseases responsible for secondary hypercalciuria have been eliminated (see introduction). It must be pointed out that in most previous reports in the literature, authors have classified patients as having idiopathic hypercalciuria, without taking into account sodium, protein, and carbohydrate intakes. Thus, dietary hypercalciuria, an expression which was formerly used to designate only hypercalciuria related to gluttony for calcium-rich food, may now also be applied to hypercalciuria related to gluttony for salt-, protein-, and carbohydrate-rich food, although these types of hypercalciuria were formerly classified as idiopathic hypercalciuria.

Classification of Idiopathic Hypercalciuria (IH) According to Pak

Some years ago, Pak proposed to classify IH into two main types, namely absorptive hypercalciuria (AH), and renal hypercalciuria (RH) [18].

In AH, he further distinguished 3 subtypes (Table I): *type II*, actually a dietary hypercalciuria related to an excess calcium intake; *type I*, due to a primary selective jejunal hyperabsorption of calcium, since the calcitriol levels are normal or low [19]; and *type III*, in which the hyperabsorption of calcium is linked to an increased synthesis of calcitriol, secondary to a hypophosphoremia induced by a primary tubular leak of phosphate. This phosphate leak hypothesis is supported by several pieces of evidence: (*1*) the high prevalence of hypophosphatemia and decreased Tm P/GFR in patients with IH [2,4,7]; (*2*) the increased levels of circulating calcitriol in response to hypophosphatemia observed in normal subjects [20] and the partial reversal of the syndrome in patients after treatment with oral phosphate [21,22]; (*3*) the inverse relationship between plasma calcitriol level and phosphate concentration [23,24]; and (*4*) the recently described syndrome of IH with renal phosphate leak and increased plasma calcitriol occurring in a Bedouin tribe, some of whose members presented with hereditary hypophosphatemic rickets along with hypercalciuria [25].

Renal hypercalciuria (RH) is differentiated from AH mainly on the basis of fasting hypercalciuria (fasting UCa/UCr > 0.12 mg/mg or > 0.33 mmol/mmol) and of secondary hyperparathyroidism. As a matter of fact it is thought to be due to a primary renal leak of calcium which would promote negative calcium balance which would

Table 1. Possible primary mechanisms of hypercalciuria and their pathophysiological consequences

Primary mechanism	Primary hyperparathyroidism	Excessive dietary intake of				Primary intestinal Ca hyperabsorption	Hypersecretion of calcitriol			Primary bone resorption	Monocyte disease[e]
		Ca	Na	Protein	Sugar alcohol		Renal PO4 leak	Renal Ca leak	Primary		
Pak's classification[a]	–	AH II	–	–	–	AH I	AH III	RH	–	–	–
24 hour calciuria on fixed Ca intake[b]	↗	N	↗	↗	↗	↗	↗	↗	↗	↗	↗
Fasting calciuria[c]	↗	N	↗	↗	N	N	N	↗	↗	↗	↗
Δ UCa after 1 g of oral Ca[d]	↗	N	?	?	?	↗	↗	↗	↗	N	↗
Fractional intestinal absorption of Ca	↗	N	?	?	?	↗	↗	↗	↗	N	↗
Plasma calcium	↗	N	N	N	N	N	N	N	N	N	N
Plasma phosphate	↘·N	N	N	N	N	N	↘	N	N	N	N
PTH or nephrogenic cAMP — fasting	↗	N·↘	?	?	?	N·↘	N·↗	↗	N·↘	N·↘	N·↘
PTH or nephrogenic cAMP — after Ca load	↗	↘	?	?	?	↘	N·↗	N	N·↘	N·↘	N·↘
Fasting plasma calcitriol	↗	↘·N	?	↗	?	N	↗	↗	↗	N·↘	↗
Hydroxyprolinuria	↗	N	?	↗	?	N	?	↗	?	↗	↘
Bone density	↘	N	?	↘	?	N·↘?	?	↘	?	↘	↘

[a] According to Pak: AHI - II - III, absorptive hypercalciuria type I - II - III; RH, renal calciuria
[b] Upper limit of normal per kg BW/day is 4 mg or 0.1 mmol on 1000 mg of Ca, and 3 mg or 0.07 mmol on 400 mg of Ca
[c] Upper limit of normal of fasting hypercalciuria is <0.12 mg/mg creatinine or 0.33 mmol/mmol creatinine
[d] The upper limit of normal increase of calciuria after 1 g of oral calcium is <0.17 mg/mg creatinine or 0.50 mmol/mmol
[e] Monocyte disease responsible for hypersecretion of interleukin I, hypersecretion of calcitriol and bone resorption
N, normal; ↗, increased; ↘, decreased; ?, uncertain or unknown; PTH, parathyroid hormone

therefore stimulate, primarily PTH secretion and secondarily, calcitriol synthesis and increase intestinal absorption of calcium. This secondary hyperparathyroidism is, however, suppressed by an oral calcium load [24], as shown by the normalization of plasma PTH or nephrogenic cAMP in the urine.

However, this clear-cut classification has been challenged for various reasons:

1) the classification does not take into account the dependence of IH on dietary factors other than calcium intake [6];
2) the overprevalence of AH I in Pak's experience (60%) is in blatant contradiction with the calcium balance data which show a negative balance in two-thirds of patients [2,26] (the average calcium balance for the hypercalciuric stone former is -1.0 ± 2.7 mmol/day, whereas it is $+0.7\pm2.4$ mmol/day in healthy controls [2]);
3) primary disorders of intestinal calcium absorption and tubular reabsorption of calcium or phosphate appear to be variously associated in the same patients, making their classification within distinct pathogenetic subtypes not always possible [4,26,27];
4) Pak's classification is not able to classify all patients, namely those with fasting hypercalciuria not related to a high sodium diet: most of these patients, in fact, do not have high plasma concentrations of PTH, but on the contrary, have normal or low PTH levels, excluding the hypothesis of renal hypercalciuria [24,28]. In patients with fasting hypercalciuria not associated with secondary hyperparathyroidism a subtle renal leak of calcium may, however, be suspected. In patients with fasting hypercalciuria, a proximal tubular defect has been demonstrated by successive acute administration of diuretics [27]. These subtle renal disorders could explain the hypersensitivity to sodium, acidosis, or high protein diet in IH patients, discussed previously (Fig. 1).

Increased Calcitriol Production

Plasma calcitriol concentration is extremely sensitive to variations in calcium intake in normal controls as well as in patients with IH. Most of the studies which have taken calcium diet into account have shown increased levels of plasma calcitriol in calcium stone-formers with IH and normal PTH levels [7]. Direct evidence for a disordered control of calcitriol production has been clearly demonstrated by Broadus in patients with AH. In these patients, when a high normal calcium diet is continued for several weeks, calcitriol plasma levels initially decrease, but after 2 weeks an escape phenomenon with a rebound increase in circulating calcitriol level and a pronounced fall in T mP/GFR [29] is observed.

The mechanism accounting for this increased calcitriol synthesis remains controversial. As discussed above, several pieces of evidence favor a tubular phosphate leak. However, the frequency of hypophosphatemia in IH is controversial, probably because of a lack of data regarding diurnal variations in serum phosphate; this impedes detection of subtle hypophosphatemia. For instance, in normal man, a decrease of dietary phosphorus which induces a 35% decrease of afternoon serum phosphate, induces a 58% increase in fasting serum levels of calcitriol, while no change is observed in the morning fasting levels of phosphorus [30]. In patients with IH, we observed a negative correlation between plasma calcitriol and plasma phos-

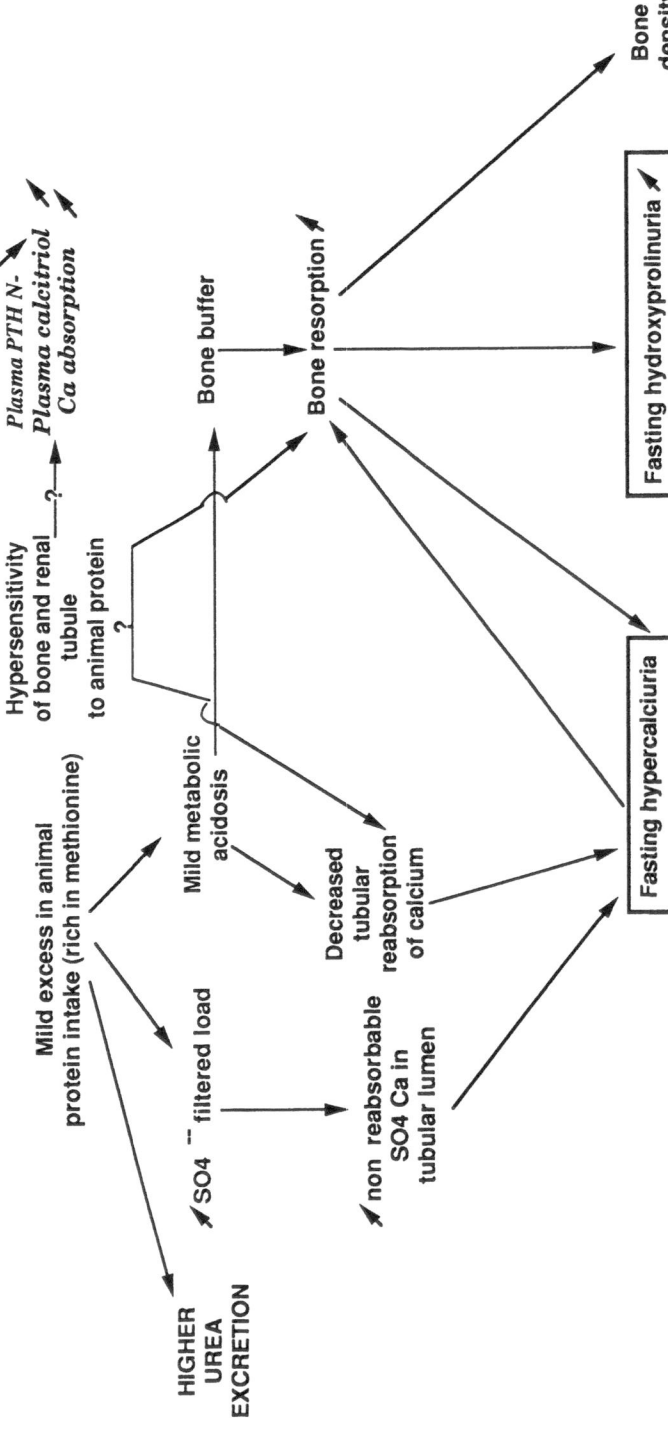

Fig. 1. This figure is an attempt to put into perspective the pathophysiological events derived from the exaggerated protein-induced hypercalciuria observed in calcium stone formers with idiopathic hypercalciuria (*IH*). Mild excess in meat intake and hypersensitivity of the renal tubule and skeleton to mild acidosis secondary to the protein-induced production of acids (especially H_2SO_4, derived from methionine) may explain the fasting hypercalciuria. The fasting hyperhydroxyprolinuria is an index of increased bone resorption, which may be secondary to the primary renal calcium leak because of sulfate overproduction and mild acidosis and the consumption of bone buffer because of the mild acidosis. This scheme does not account for the fact that in IH, parathyroid hormone (*PTH*) levels are normal or low while plasma calcitriol levels and intestinal absorption of calcium are increased. ☐ Parameter correlating positively with 24 hour UREA EXCRETION on Ca restricted diet

phate which, however, remained in the normal range [17]. On the basis of this negative correlation, we suggest that the increased synthesis of calcitriol in IH may be due to a hypersensitivity of 25 OH vitamin D 1α hydroxylase to phosphate.

An alternative hypothesis which would explain this disordered control of calcitriol and the tendency to hypophosphatemia would be hypersensitivity of 25 OH vitamin D 1α hydroxylase to PTH. This possibility remains dubious because no correlation exists between PTH and calcitriol and because PTH levels are normal or low in most patients with fasting hypercalciuria.

Finally, as will be discussed below, another explanation for increased calcitriol synthesis could be a monocyte disease.

Bone Involvement in Idiopathic Hypercalciuria

While overt bone disease with pain and fractures is extremely rare in hypercalciuric patients, the frequently observed mild negative calcium balance suggests that bone may be the primary source of the extra calcium appearing in the urine. This possibility is supported by the positive relationships observed between fasting calcium and hydroxyprolinuria [17,31,32] or fasting calciuria and alkaline phosphatases [31], and by radiocalcium kinetic data showing increased bone turnover [33].

Indeed, loss of bone mass has been detected by various techniques in calcium stone formers with hypercalciuria: photonabsorptiometry of the distal radius [34] or the lumbar spine [35], radiological density of the proximal radial shaft [36], in vivo neutron activation of the trunk and upper thighs [37], and single energy computerized tomography (CT) densitometry of the vertebrae [17,38].

In most of these studies the type of hypercalciuria was not clearly defined. In Lawoyin's study [39] this was done and decreased bone mineral content of the radius was observed only in renal hypercalciuria patients, but not in absorptive hypercalciuria patients. In the study of Pacifici et al. [38] vertebral mineral density was decreased in all calcium stone formers, whether with normocalciuria, absorptive hypercalciuria, or fasting hypercalciuria with normal PTH, but the decrease was greater in the last-mentioned group. In our experience [17] vertebral mineral density was decreased comparably in fasting hypercalciuria with normal PTH, in one case of renal hypercalciuria, and in absorptive calciuria type I, but not in absorptive calciuria type II.

Moreover, scarce histomorphometric evaluations have shown bone abnormalities, such as increased bone resorption with normal bone formation [40] and normal bone resorption with decreased bone formation and mineralization rate [41]. The recent study of 33 patients with recurrent stone formation and idiopathic hypercalciuria with hypophosphatemia and normal PTH carried out by Steiniche et al. [42] confirms the existence of a moderate mineralization defect (reduced adjusted appositional rate, prolonged mineralization lag time), with increased eroded surfaces but without decrease of the trabecular bone volume.

What is the origin of this increased bone loss? In most of these patients mild hyperparathyroidism is excluded by normal or low values of plasma PTH. A bone resorbing effect of calcitriol has been suspected according to the following observations: (1) in normal subjects put on a low calcium diet fasting calciuria is increased by oral calcitriol elevating serum 1,25 (OH)2 D3 concentration [43]; (2) in organ cultures of bone, 1,25 (OH)2 D3 has a bone resorbing effect [44]. Therefore, in IH patients put on a low calcium diet, a high level of calcitriol could lead to bone loss in spite of a normal PTH level. However, this is probably not the case, at least in our experience: after 4 days of low calcium diet, plasma calcitriol was, on the contrary, negatively correlated with fasting calciuria and was positively correlated with vertebral mineral density and with calcium absorption (as assessed by calciuria increase after oral calcium load). These data suggest that a high level of calcitriol has a protective effect which is mediated by increased intestinal calcium absorption [17].

Nutritional factors also have to be considered. A dietary restriction of calcium, as treatment for hypercalciuric patients, may worsen the bone problem. Sequential measurements of bone density have shown that patients chronically submitted to a low calcium diet increase their bone loss [36,45].

A high protein intake has also been shown to favor osteoporosis [46]. Urea excretion on a low calcium diet was significantly higher in our IH patients than in the controls, suggesting that their protein intake of non dairy origin (i.e., meat) was greater than that of the controls. Furthermore, plasma bicarbonates were lower than in controls and the correlation between fasting calciuria and 24 hour urea excretion of the previous day was much steeper in this group of patients than in controls. The urea excretion of the IH patients was also correlated with fasting hydroxyprolinuria [17]. These data support the hypothesis that in our patients with IH, higher protein intake could favor bone loss by inducing mild acidosis (Fig. 1). In Ca stone formers, Fellström [47] has demonstrated that a short term animal protein intake simultaneously increases calciuria and hydroxyprolinuria.

Thus, such nutritional factors as low calcium diet and high meat intake may favor bone loss in IH. However, they do not account for all the observed metabolic abnormalities, especially the high plasma calcitriol levels along with normal-low PTH levels and increased calcium absorption. This leads to a search for a broader disorder which could encompass all these various data. Such a disorder could be an immunological disorder involving the monocyte. This could be proposed as a global explanation depending on a new cascade of mechanisms which we now wish to discuss.

Idiopathic Hypercalciuria as a Monocyte Disease

Some recent data favor an immunological involvement in bone resorption. Pacifici et al. [38] have recently described an increased production of interleukin I. The interleukin I is produced by peripheral blood monocytes in association with increased hydroxyproline excretion and decreased vertebral mineral density. Interleukin I activity was related positively to hydroxyprolinuria and negatively to vertebral mineral density, suggesting that interleukin I may induce bone resorption. This bone resorbing effect might either be direct or be mediated by prostaglandins, well known bone resorbing agents, which have been shown to be stimulated by interleukin I [48]. In patients with fasting hypercalciuria, the administration of a powerful prostaglandin synthesis inhibitor, with (diclofenac) or without (sulindac) effect on the renal cyclooxygenase system, decreases calcium excretion with a rise in PTH levels [48]. These results suggest that in fasting IH, the hypercalciuria is secondary to a prostaglandin mediated bone resorption which suppresses PTH secretion. This interpretation of the results excludes the alternative explanation for the association of increased interleukin I production by monocyte and increased bone resorption,

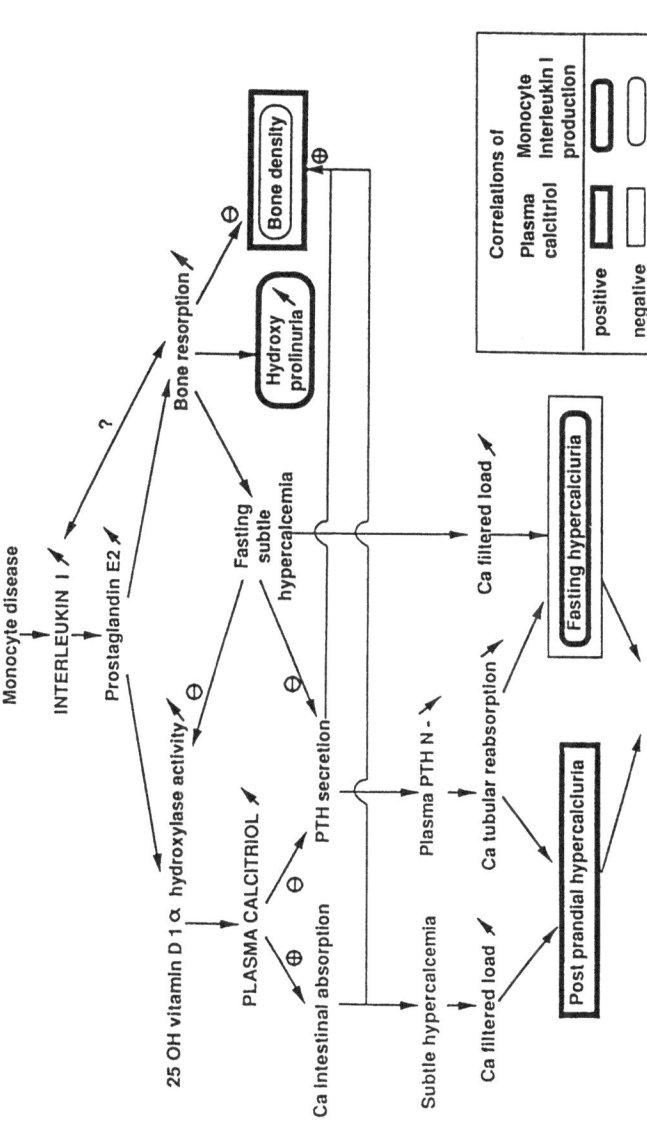

Fig. 2. A monocyte disease leading to increased production of interleukin I favors bone resorption directly or by stimulating prostaglandin E2 synthesis. Increased bone resorption explains fasting calciuria, fasting hyperhydroxyprolinuria, and decreased bone density. Therefore there are positive correlations of interleukin I production with fasting calciuria and hydroxyprolinuria, and a negative correlation between interleukin I production and bone density. The activity of 25 OH vitamin D 1α hydroxylase is increased because of increased production of prostaglandin E2. Resulting high plasma calcitriol levels explain calcium intestinal hyperabsorption and parathyroid hormone (*PTH*) suppression (together with the calcium coming from bone): these factors favor post prandial hypercalciuria (hence the positive correlation between plasma calcitriol and post prandial hypercalciuria).

The effect of calcitriol on calcium absorption and PTH secretion has a beneficial effect on bone density, thus explaining the positive correlation of plasma calcitriol and bone density namely, that products such as TGFβ, coming from resorbing bones, stimulate the production of Interleukin I.

The disordered control of calcitriol synthesis found in IH may also be explained by the same immunological cascade (Fig. 2). In idiopathic hypercalciuria with normal vitamin D nutritional status, the disordered control of calcitriol synthesis is characterized by its dependence upon plasma 25 OH D, as is the case in vitamin D depleted patients [49]. In IH, an increase of plasma calcitriol induced by ultraviolet radiation is associated with increased plasma levels of calcitriol [50], whereas such a phenomenon is not observed in normal men [51] and plasma calcitriol is positively correlated to plasma calcidiol [17]. The nature and the site of this disturbed metabolism is unknown. A disordered monocyte, mimicking, for instance, what is observed in granulomatous disease such as sarcoidosis would be a possible explanation. As a matter of fact, a very high and positive correlation between plasma calcidiol and plasma calcitriol is observed in patients with hypercalcemic-sarcoidosis [52]. An abnormal monocyte,, producing interleukin I in excess, could induce increased calcitriol synthesis mediated by prostaglandins [53]. In IH, urinary prostaglandins have been shown to be increased [54,55].

Therefore an abnormality of the monocyte in calcium stone-formers provides a seductive explanation for an apparent primary bone disease and a disturbed 1,25 dihydroxyvitamin D metabolism. The cascade of events (Table I and Fig. 2) could be: increased interleukin I production by abnormal monocyte stimulates the synthesis of prostaglandins E2, which have been proven to stimulate the synthesis of prostaglandins E2, which have been proven to stimulate both bone resorption and calcitriol synthesis. Thus, the two apparently contradictory phenomena that we have found in our patients with IH, namely, increased bone resorption leading to reduction of bone density and the protective effect of high plasma calcitriol levels [17], could be explained by a monocyte disease recently discovered by Pacifici et al.

Therapeutic Implications

The observation of decreased bone mineral content in patients with idiopathic hypercalciuria and the two new cascades that we propose for explaining hypercalciuria, namely the protein cascade, and the monocyte cascade, suggest the following therapeutic conclusions:

1) Protein intake of non-dairy origin should be restricted, so that the total daily intake is of the order of 1 g/kg per day.
2) Dairy products should, however, not be restricted so that calcium intake will be 800–1000 mg/day in order to prevent bone loss worsening and to prevent the marginal hyperoxaluria of the Ca stone former. This hyperoxaluria increases when dietary calcium is decreased, leading to a lack of improvement in the probability index of stone formation in idiopathic hypercalciuria [56].
3) Thiazides appear to be an appropriate therapy for all types of idiopathic hypercalciuria, since we have found decreased vertebral mineral density in all subtypes [17]. As a matter of fact, thiazides have a hypocalciuric effect explained not only by a direct tubular effect, but also by the inhibition of prostaglandin E synthesis, this latter accounting for a decrease of 25 OH vitamin D 1α hydroxylase activity [57] and a decrease of prostaglandin mediated bone resorption [58].

Because thiazides have already been proven both to decrease the recurrence of Ca stones [2] and to decrease the risk of femoral neck fracture [59], they should be considered as the treatment of reference. Pending the results of ongoing trials, prostaglandin synthetase inhibitors which can reduce hypercalciuria and bone resorption cannot presently be recommended, especially considering their possible long term hazards on renal function.

References

1. Hodgkinson A, Pyrah LN (1958) The urinary excretion of calcium and inorganic phosphate in 344 patients with calcium stone of renal origin. Br J Surg 46:10–11
2. Lemann J (1980) Idiopathic hypercalciuria. In: Coe FL, Brenner BM, Stein IH (eds) Nephrolithiasis. Churchill Livingstone, New York, pp 86–115
3. Robertson WG, Peacock M, Marshall BW, et al. (1978) Risk factors in calcium stone disease of the urinary tract. Br J Urol 50:449–454
4. Broadus AE, Burdis WJ, Oren DA (1987) Concerning the pathogenesis of idiopathic hypercalciuria. In: Linari F, Marangella M (eds) The pathogenesis and treatment of nephrolithiasis. Contrib Nephrol 36:127–136
5. Lemann J, Adams NC, Gray BW (1979) Urinary calcium excretion in human beings. N Engl J Med 301:535–541
6. Goldfard S (1988) Dietary factors in the pathogenesis and prophylaxis of nephrolithiasis. Kidney Int 34:544–555
7. Lemann J, Worcester ER (1989) Nephrolithiasis. In: Massry S, Glassock R (eds) Textbook of nephrology. Williams and Wilkins, Baltimore, pp 920–941
8. Walker RM, Linkswiler HM (1972) Calcium retention in the adult human male as affected by protein intake. J Nutr 102:1297–1302
9. Aller LH, Oddoye EA, Margen S (1979) Protein induced hypercalciuria a longer term study. Am J Clin Nutr 32:741–749
10. Kleeman CR, Bohannan J, Bernstein D, Living S, Maxwell MH (1964) Effect of variations in sodium intake on calcium excretion in normal humans. Soc Exp Biol Med 115:29–32
11. McCarron DA, Rankin LI, Bennet WM (1981) Urinary calcium excretion at extremes of sodium intake in normal man. Am J Nephrol 1:84–90
12. Kirkendall WM, Connar WE, Abbou DF, Rastogi SP, Anderson TA, Fry M (1976) The effect of dietary sodium chloride on blood pressure, body fluids, electrolytes, renal function of normotensive man. J Lab Clin Med 87:418–434
13. Muldowney FP, Freaney B, Moloney MF (1982) Importance of dietary sodium in the hypercalciuric syndrome. Kidney Int 22:292–296
14. Bataille P, Fournier A, Locquet P, Idrissi A, Renaud H, Finet M, Leflon P, Rogez JC, Plaquet R (1987) Hydrochlorothiazide-amiloride association in calcium stone formers: increase of oxalate tolerance and critical role of calcium and sodium intake on their hypocalciuric effect. In: Puschett JB, Greenberg A (eds) Diuretic II: chemistry, pharmacology and clinical applications. Elsevier Science, pp 438–444
15. Lemann J (1985) Urinary calcium excretion and net acid excretion: effects of dietary protein, carbohydrate and calories. In: Schwille PO, Smith LH, Robertson WG, Finlayson B (eds) Urolithiasis and Related Clinical Research. Plenum, New York, pp 53–60
16. Ulmann A, Aubert J, Bourdeau A (1982) Effects of weight and glucose ingestion on urinary calcium and phosphate excretion: implications for urolithiasis. J Clin Endocrinol Metab 54:1063–1068
17. Bataille P, Fournier A, Bouillon R (to be published) Vertebral mineral density in hypercalciuric Ca stone formers. Its relation to calcium and protein intake and vitamin D

metabolism. Evidence for primary bone resorption in dietary calcium independent hypercalciuria favored by high protein intake of non dairy origin and suppressed by high plasma concentration of calcitriol. Kidney Int (submitted)

18. Pak CYC, Galosy RA (1979) Fasting urinary calcium and cyclic adenosine 3', 5' monophosphate: a discriminant analysis for the identification of renal absorptive hypercalciuria. J Clin Endocrinol Metab 48:260–265

19. Pak CYC, Britton F, Petterson R (1980) Ambulatory evaluation of nephrolithiasis. Am J Med 69:19–30

20. Gray BW, Wilz DR, Caldas AE (1977) The importance of phosphate in regulating plasma 1,25 (OH)2 vitamin D levels in humans: studies in healthy subjects, in calcium stone-formers and in patients with primary hyperparathyroidism. J Clin Endocrinol Metab 45:299–306

21. Van Den Berg CY, Kumar B, Wilson DM, Heath H, Smith LH (1980) Orthophosphate therapy decreases urinary calcium excretion and serum 1,25 dihydroxyvitamin D concentrations in idiopathic hypercalciuria. J Clin Endocrinol Metab 51:998–1001

22. Barilla DE, Zerwekh JE, Pak CYC (1979) A critical evaluation of the role of phosphate in the pathogenesis of absorptive hypercalciuria. Min Electrol Metab 2:301–309

23. Shen FH, Baylink DJ, Nielsen RL (1977) Increased serum 1,25 (OH)2 D3 in patients with idiopathic hypercalciuria. J Lab Clin Med 90:955–961

24. Bataille P, Bouillon R, Fournier A (1986) Increased plasma concentrations of total and free 1,25 (OH)2 D3 in calcium stone formers with idiopathic hypercalciuria. In: Linari F, Marengella M (eds) Pathogenesis and treatment of nephrolithiasis. Contrib Nephrol 58: 50–53

25. Tieder M, Modai D, Samuel B (1987) "Idiopathic" hypercalciuria and hereditary hypophosphatemic rickets. N Engl J Med 316:125–129

26. Coe FL, Bushinsky DA (1984) Pathophysiology of hypercalciuria. Am J Physiol 247: F1–F13

27. Sutton R, Walker V (1980) Responses to hydrochlorothiazide and acetazolamide in patients with calcium stones. Evidence suggesting a defect in renal tubular function. N Engl J Med 302:709–715

28. Burckhardt P, Jaeger P (1981) Secondary hyperparathyroidism in idiopathic renal hypercalciuria: fact or theory? J Clin Endocrinol Metab 53:550–551

29. Broadus AE, Insogna KL, Lang R (1984) Evidence for disordered control of 1,25 (OH)2 D production in absorptive hypercalciuria. N Engl J Med 311:73–80

30. Portale A, Halloran BP, Morris C (1989) Physiologic regulation of the serum concentration of 1,25 dihydroxyvitamin D by phosphorus in normal men. J Clin Invest 83:1494–1499

31. Messa P, Mioni G, Montanaro D (1987) About primitive osseous origin of the so-called idiopathic hypercalciuria. In: Linari F, Marangella M (eds) Pathogenesis and treatment of nephrolithiasis. Contrib Nephrol 58:106–110

32. Sutton R, Walker V (1986) Bone resorption and hypercalciuria in calcium stone formers. Metabolism 6:485–486

33. Liberman V, Sperling O, Atsman A (1969) Metabolic and calcium kinetic studies in idiopathic hypercalciuria. J Clin Invest 47:2580–2590

34. Alhava EM, Juuti M, Karjalainen P (1976) Bone mineral density in patients with urolithiasis. Scand J Urol Nephrol 10:154–156

35. Malvasi L, Sartori L, Giannini S, Al Awady M, Musaio F, Varotto S, D'Angelo A (1988) Mineral metabolism and bone mineral content in calcium nephrolithiasis with and without hyperparathyroidism. Urological Res 16:190

36. Velentzas C, Oreopoulos DG, Meema S, Meema HE, Nutsuga T, Alison E, Katirtzoglou A, Crassweller P (1981) Dietary calcium restriction may be good for patients' stones but not for their bones. In: Smith LH, Robertson WG, Finlayson B (eds) Urolithiasis clinical and basic research. Plenum, New York, pp 847–854

37. Barkin J, Wilson DR, Manuel MA, Bayley A, Murray T, Harrison J (1985) Bone mineral content in idiopathic calcium nephrolithiasis. Min Electrol Metab 11:19-24
38. Pacifici R, Rothstein M, Rifas L, Lau KHW, Baylink DG, Avioli LV, Hruska K (1990) Increased monocyte interleukin-I activity and decreased vertebral bone density in patients with fasting hypercalciuria. J Clin Endocrinol Metab
39. Lawoyin S, Sismilich S, Browne B, Pak CYC (1979) Bone mineral content in patients with calcium orolithiasis. Metabolism 28:1250-1254
40. Bordier P, Ryckwaert A, Gueris J (1977) On the pathogenesis of the so-called idiopathic hypercalciuria. Am J Med 63:398-402
41. Malluche HH, Tschoepe W, Ritz E (1980) Abnormal bone histology in idiopathic hypercalciuria. J Clin Endocrinol Metab 50:654-658
42. Steiniche T, Mosekilde L, Christensen MS, Melsen F (1989) A histomorphometric determination of iliac bone remodeling in patients with recurrent renal stone formation and idiopathic hypercalciuria. A.P.M.I.S. 4:309-316
43. Maierhofer W, Lemann JJ, Gray R (1984) Dietary calcium and serum 1,25 (OH)2 D concentrations as determinants of calcium balance in healthy men. Kidney Int 26:752-759
44. Raisz DG, Trummel CL, Holick MF, De Luca MF (1972) 1,25 dihydroxycholecalciferol: a potent stimulator of bone resorption in tissue culture. Science 175:768-769
45. Fuss M, Pepersack T, Van Geel J, Corvilain J, Vandewall JC, Bergman P, Simon P (1990) Involvement of low-calcium diet in the reduced bone mineral content of idiopathic renal stone formers. Calcif Tissue Int 46:9-13
46. Wachman A, Bernstein DS (1968) Diet Osteoporosis. Lancet I:958-959
47. Fellström B, Danielson BG, Karlström B (1986) Effect of high intake of dietary animal protein on mineral metabolism and urinary supersaturation of calcium oxalate in renal stone formers. Brit J Urol 56:263-269
48. Filipponi P, Mannarelli C, Pacifici R, Grossi E, Moretti I, Tini S, Carloni C, Blass A, Morucci P, Hruska KA, Avioli LV (1988) Evidence for a prostaglandin-mediated bone resorptive mechanism in subjects with fasting hypercalciuria. Calcif Tissue Int 43:61-66
49. Bouillon R, Auwery JH, Lissens WD, Pelemans W (1987) Vitamin D status in the elderly: seasonal substrate deficiency causes 1,25 dihydroxycholecalciferol deficiency. Am J Clin Nutr 45:755-763
50. Varghese M, Godman JS, William CG (1989) The effect of ultraviolet B radiation treatment on calcium excretion and vitamin D metabolites in kidney stone formers. Clin Nephrol 31:225-231
51. Bell NH, Greene V, Sharry J, Shaw J (1986) Evidence that 25-hydroxyvitamin D has a role in the regulation of calcium metabolism in man (abstract). J Bone Mineral Res 1:380
52. Sandler LM, Winearls CG, Fraher LJ, Clemens TL, Smith R, O'Riordan JLH (1984) Studies on the hypercalcemia of sarcoidosis: effect of steroids and exogenous vitamin D3 on the circulating concentrations of 1,25 dihydroxyvitamin D3. Q J Med New Series 53:165-180
53. Yamade M, Matrumoto T, Takahashi N, Suda T, Ogada E (1983) Stimulatory effect of prostaglandin E2 on 1α 25 dihydroxyvitamin D3 synthesis in rats. Biochem J 216:237-240
54. Roche CH, Rodriguez-Iturbe B, Henera J, Parra G (1988) Increased urinary excretion of prostaglandin E in patients with idiopathic hypercalciuria. Clin Sci 75:581-587
55. Houser M, Zimmerman B, Davidson M, Smith C, Smaiko A, Fish A (1984) Idiopathic hypercalciuria associated with hyperreninemia and high urinary prostaglandin E. Kidney Int 26:176-182
56. Bataille P, Charransol G, Grégoire I, Daigre JC, Fournier A (1983) Effect of calcium restriction on renal excretion of oxalate and the probability of stones in the various pathophysiological groups with calcium stones. J Urol 130:218-223
57. Calo L, Cantaro S, Marchini F, Giannini S, Castrignano B, Gambaro G, Antonello A, Baggio B, D'Angelo A, Williams H, Borsatti A (1990) Is hydrochlorothiazide-induced hypocalciuria due to inhibition of prostaglandin E2 synthesis? Clin Sci 78:321-325

58. Lemann J, Gray RW, Maïerhofer WJ, Cheung HS (1985) Hydrochlorothiazide inhibits bone resorptions in men despite experimentally elevated serum 1,25 dihydroxy vitamin D concentrations. Kidney Int 28:951–958

59. Lacroix AZ, Wienpahl J, White LR, Wallace RB, Scherr PA, George LK, Cornoni-Huntley J, Ustfeld AM (1990) Thiazide diuretic agents and the incidence of hip fracture. N Engl J Med 322:286–290

Extracorporeal Shock Wave Lithotripsy (ESWL): Past, Present, and Future

CHRISTIAN G. CHAUSSY[1] and GERHARD J. FUCHS[2]

SUMMARY. Extracorporeal shock wave lithotripsy (ESWL) has now been in clinical use for 10 years and has replaced other treatment techniques for the majority of surgical calculi located in the upper urinary tract. For the first time it provides a completely noninvasive method for the treatment of renal and ureteral stones. The current range of its indications includes approximately 70% of nonselected urinary stone patients. An additional 25% of patients with more complex stones in the upper urinary tract can receive treatment with the lithotripter (E.S.W.L. (R)) when combining the method with endourological procedures (see Table 1).

Introduction

The first experimental efforts at using extracorporeally induced shock waves to disintegrate human kidney stones were made in Munich (West Germany) in 1972. After extensive in vitro testing had proven the disintegration of stones of various chemical composition by focussed shock wave energy to be feasible, an animal stone model was finally used to demonstrate that shock waves generated outside the body could noninvasively disintegrate kidney stones to a size allowing their spontaneous passage [1–5].

In February 1980, extracorporeal shock wave lithotripsy (ESWL) was introduced clinically at the Department of Urology, University of Munich, as the first noninvasive method to treat patients suffering from upper urinary tract stones [3,4]. It only took a short time to prove the efficacy, safety, and reliability of the method, dramatically changing the management of upper urinary stones.

[1]Department of Urology, Staedtisches Krankenhaus, München-Harlaching, Federal Republic of Germany

[2]UCLA Stone Center, Division of Urology, Los Angeles, CA 90024, USA

1043

Table 1. Historical development of ESWL

1972–1980	Development of extracorporeal shock wave lithotripsy (ESWL)	
ä	Ludwig Maximillian Universität, Departments of Surgical Research and Urology, München,	
ü	Germany Dornier Medical Systems, Friedrichshafen, Germany	
2/80–5/82	Human model no 1 (HM-1)	Indications
ü	-First clinical application of ESWL (München, Germany) 200 patients	renal pelvic stones + caliceal stones <1 cm. (approx. 20%)*
5/82–10/83	Human model no 2 (HM-2)	
ü	(München, Germany) 800 patients	+ selected ureteral stones + infected stones + stones up to 2.5 cm. + partial staghorn stones (approx. 60–70%)*
10/83	Human model no 3 (HM-3)	
	-Beginning of series production and distribution of the lithotripter	+ staghorn stones + combination with percutaneous surgery (approx. 95%)
12/1984	Food and Drug Administration (U.S.A.) -PMA Approval for Dornier HM-3 lithotripter	
1984-Present	-More than 2.000.000 treatments Distribution to 700 centers in 32 countries worldwide Clinical trials with new second generation lithotripters (Table 2)	

*percentage of unselected stone patients eligible for ESWL(R)

Physical Principles

The underlying physical principles of shock wave treatment of calculi in the human urinary tract are 1) generation of shock waves outside the body, 2) focusing of the shock wave onto an area distant from the generation area, 3) coupling of the shock wave into the body and, 4) localization and positioning of the respective treatment target into the treatment focus. The selective utilization of the destructive potential of shock waves for the disintegration of brittle stone material without damage to surrounding tissues constitutes a major breakthrough of modern medical technology [1–5].

Lithotripter Hardware Features

In the recent past, clinical trials involving new lithotripters have been performed at a number of centers in Europe, Japan, and the United States. The basic features of these devices are described in Table 2 [6,7]. Preliminary clinical data and product information furnished by the various manufacturers indicate that changes of the

Table 2. Comparison of technology of various shock wave lithotripters

Lithotripter	Energy source	Focusing device	Coupling medium	Localization	Anesthesia
Dornier HM-3	Spark gap	Ellipsoid	Bath	X-ray	regional, SDA
modified Dornier HM-4	Spark gap	Ellipsoid	Membrane	X-ray	SDA
Dornier MPL 9000	Spark gap	Ellipsoid	Membrane	Ultrasound	No, SDA
Dornier MFL 5000	Spark gap	Ellipsoid	Membrane	X-ray	No, SDA
Technomed	Modified spark gap	Ellipsoid	Limited bath	Ultrasound, X-ray	No, SDA
Yashiyoda	Microexplosive	Ellipsoid	Bath	X-ray	SDA
Siemens	Electromagnetic	Lens	Membrane	X-ray	SDA
Wolf	Piezoelectric	Bowl	Limited bath	Ultrasound	No
EDAP	Piezoelectric	Bowl	Membrane	Ultrasound	No, (SDA)
Medstone	Spark gap	Ellipsoid	Membrane	X-ray	SDA
Direx	Spark gap	Ellipsoid	Membrane	X-ray	SDA
Nitech	Spark gap	Ellipsoid	Membrane	Ultrasound	SDA

SDA, Sedoanalgesia

major lithotripter components (energy source, focusing device, coupling medium, stone localization system) result in distinctly different treatment parameters.

Preliminary results with the new lithotripters indicate that the various energy sources are all effective in fragmenting kidney stones [7]. Compared to the original device, however, a lower percentage of stone fragmentation is noted for most of the new devices, resulting in a higher number of repeat treatments [7].

In particular, the non spark gap devices, the PESE and EMSE energy sources currently used, fall short in this regard. Focusing of the shock wave onto a distant focal area utilizes different principles, as depicted in Table 2.

Depending on the characteristic features of the focusing devices (ellipsoid, acoustical lens, self-focusing), areas of high energy density ranging from 0.3 cm times 0.6 cm to 4.5 cm times 6.0 cm are measured. Energy density at the skin level and the maximum energy applied determines the need for anesthesia. Since the introduction of ESWL several anesthesia techniques have been employed.

Most groups working with the original device utilize regional anesthesia (epidural catheter anesthesia); only about 25% of users routinely employ general anesthesia. Several centers use local infiltration anesthesia of the skin entry area in an effort to reduce the amount of anesthetic required. Some of the newer devices require much less anesthesia (IV sedation and IM analgesics) due to changed physical parameters of shock wave generator energy and focusing devices [7]. Other devices even offer the prospect of anesthesia free shock wave treatment, owing to the different characteristics of the shock wave at the skin entry site and lower overall energy density [6,7]. This mainly applies to the piezoelectric devices, to machines using larger ellipsoids in conjunction with lower generator energy levels, and to the EMSE system. Clinical trials have shown this concept to be applicable at the expense of a significantly higher number of repeat treatments.

Ultrasound as a means of stone localization is utilized with several of the newer devices (Table 2). With the use of sophisticated ultrasound equipment this may offer reduced X-ray exposure and cost savings. Preliminary results of groups using ultrasound localizing devices, who have extensive experience with conventional shock wave lithotripsy, are encouraging. The problem areas are the technical limitations of

Table 3. Exclusion criteria for ESWL

Medical	-uncorrected bleeding disorder
	-uncorrected hypertension
	-pregnancy (stone treatment rarely necessary, placement of internal stent or percutaneous nephrostomy)
	-aortic or renal artery aneurysm (calcifications of aorta and renal artery are relative contraindications)
	-pacemakers (standby–cardiologist recommended)
Technical	-depending on type of lithotripter
	-general problems: stone location relative to energy source and patient positioning system (determinants: patient size, patient obesity, skeletal anomalies and ectopic kidneys, radioopacity of stone)
Urological	-severe anatomical or functional alterations precluding proper elimination of debris
	-stenosis distal to the stone (calyceal neck, ureteropelvic junction, ureter, hypertrophy of prostate requiring surgical correction, urethral stricture)
	-stone bearing calyx grossly distended (especially dependent calyces)
	-functional impairment of ureteral mobility (neurogenic, immobile patient)

current ultrasound equipment, the unfamiliarity of many lithotripter operators with proper ultrasound interpretation, and the time needed for proper ultrasound localization [7]. Owing to the difficulty of detecting ureteral stones with ultrasound, the range of indications for these stones is limited.

Current State of the Clinical Use of Extracorporeally Induced Shock Waves

Contraindications

Less than 5% of all stone patients are excluded from ESWL routine treatment as they present with one of the still existing contraindications (Table 3). High risk patients, i.e., patients with bleeding disorders, hypertension or a heart condition have been treated with extracorporeal shock wave lithotripsy (ESWL) [5,7–9].

Indications

The range of indications, initially established in Munich, was soon confirmed by other centers [6, 8–10]. Owing to the high success rate of extracorporeal shock wave lithotripsy, the low rate of periprocedural complications, and the absence of long term adverse effects, the range of indications has been expanded over the years to include most of the urinary stones (Tables 4 and 5). Approximately 70% of non-selected stone patients are eligible for extracorporeal shock wave lithotripsy monotherapy [5–7,9,11–14]. This group includes single and multiple stones of an added stone mass of up to 2.5 cm in the kidney, selected ureteral stones above the iliac crest and below the pelvic brim (pelvic window), and staghorn stones which fill a non-dilated collecting system (in the absence of intrarenal stenosis or dilatation). The aforementioned stones are found in approximately 70%–80% of patients that are referred to a urinary stone center, depending on certain referral biases. The

Table 4. Selection criteria for extracorporeal shockwave lithotripsy of renal stones

---

Variables determining treatment approach
  -stone burden (period of stone passage and rate of auxiliary procedures increase proportionally with stone size)
  -intrarenal stone distribution (pelvis vs. calyces)
  -presence of intrarenal stenosis
  -isolated dilatation of calyces
  -stone composition (calcium-oxalate monohydrate and cystine stones respond poorly to ESWL)
  -patient compliance (prolonged period of time before treatment is completed, depending on stone size)

---

remainder of patients present with more complex stone disease, or with stones which need auxiliary procedures to maximize the advantage of extracorporeal shock wave lithotripsy. Into the latter group fall radiolucent and small semiopaque stones which need to be made visible by use of contrast medium, as they cannot be primarily identified on the X-ray screen (with the exception of ultrasound based localization lithotripters).

Controversy still exists over the treatment of staghorn stones and ureteral stones. For these two subgroups, different treatment strategies have evolved (monotherapy with extracorporeal shock wave lithotripsy vs the combined treatment of endourological procedures and subsequent extracorporeal shock wave lithotripsy) [5-11,15]. Success with extracorporeal shock wave lithotripsy of kidney stones is dependent upon (1) the overall stone burden in the kidney, (2) the shape of the renal collecting system, (3) the architecture of the dependent calyces, and (4) stone composition [5,6,8-11,13,15,16]. Based on these criteria the following guidelines for the treatment of staghorn stones have been established at our institution. In partial and complete staghorn stones, monotherapy with extracorporeal shock wave lithotripsy (in conjunction with the use of indwelling ureteral catheters) is preferable to other treatment modalities only in cases where the stone fills a nondilated collecting system [5-7,9]. A planned staged extracorporeal shock wave lithotripsy procedure is usually performed in staghorn stones which fill a slightly dilated collecting system [7,9]. It has to be pointed out, however, that with increasing stone burden the rates for second sessions and follow up complications are considerably higher than those encountered with smaller stones.

Also, the period of stone passage is significantly prolonged compared to percutaneous stone surgery or the combination therapy. The liberal use of indwelling ureteral catheters has not had any proven effect on these parameters; however, it reduces perioperative morbidity and the need for auxiliary procedures to relieve ureteral obstruction. Auxiliary procedures, namely percutaneous nephrostomy tube placement and

Table 5. Selection criteria for extracorporeal shock wave lithotripsy of ureteral stones

---

Variables determining treatment approach
  -approach individualized according to expansion space and stone location
  -no standard treatment protocol for all ureteral stones available
  -depending on lithotripter used (X-ray or ultrasound stone localization)
  -depending on endourological experience

---

ureteroscopic ureteral manipulations are required in approximately 60% of patients after ESWL treatment of large branched stones [5-7,9,13].

Thus, in staghorn stones with (1) a large stone mass, filling a dilated renal collecting system, and (2) with intrarenal anatomical alterations, a percutaneous procedure is performed first for debulking the stone. In a second session, extracorporeal shock wave lithotripsy is employed for the disintegration of the remaining caliceal stone parts and under the same anesthesia the patient undergoes a second percutaneous procedure for removal of the stone gravel [5-7,9]. Although inherently more invasive than monotherapy with extracorporeal shock wave lithotripsy, this approach is of great benefit for the patient with regard to stone free rates, hospitalizations, and time lost from work.

Although 80% of all stones which become symptomatic are ureteral stones, only 10%-15% of those stones require interventional treatment; the remainder pass spontaneously. Ureteral stones have been primarily amenable to extracorporeal shock wave lithotripsy only if located above the bony pelvis in the mid or upper third of the ureter [5,7,9,10,12,14-16]. Only recently, stones in the terminal ureter below the pelvic brim have been treated successfully with ESWL through the pelvic window [7,14,17]. The prone position has been advocated for stones overlying the bony pelvis.

When ultrasound stone localization systems are used, treatment of ureteral stones becomes more difficult, especially for stones below the level of the lower pole of the kidney [7]. Experience has shown that even with a stone in a favorable position, the success rate of stone disintegration is dependent on particle expansion, which is low or nonexistent in the ureter surrounding an impacted stone [5-7,9,14]. To obviate this unfavorable condition, two modalities are available – namely, repositioning the stone(s) into the renal pelvis, and/or passing a ureteral catheter about the calculus. With both procedures the expansion chamber is increased, thereby resulting in a high rate of stone disintegration (>97%) [5-7,9,14]. Ureteral stones overlying the bony pelvis below the iliac crest and above the pelvic brim become amenable to extracorporeal shock wave lithotripsy only when repositioned into the upper ureter or ideally into the renal pelvis in a retrograde or antegrade fashion. Otherwise the shock wave energy would be absorbed by the bony structures and would therefore not suffice to fragment the stone. Prone positioning is a time-consuming alternative with less than optimal success rates. Stones which cannot be manipulated, or ESWL treatment failures are best managed ureteroscopically [5-7,9,14].

Although nephrolithiasis is a relatively rare incident in the pediatric age group, the advent of a noninvasive treatment modality for children was especially appreciated. Treatment by ESWL is particularly advantageous in this patient population, as it can be repeated without adverse effect.

Concerns have been raised with regard to the effect of high energy shock waves on immature bony tissue, growing renal tissue, long-term renal function, or the induction of hypertension [7,18]. The available clinical results indicate that extracorporeal shock wave lithotripsy does not lead to deterioration of long-term renal function or affect renal development; no juvenile hypertension has been noted after extracorporeal shock wave lithotripsy. Recently conducted research on the effects of high energy shock waves on immature bony tissue and renal growth confirms the safety of this treatment modality. Cautious use of the energy, however, is advocated [7].

Table 6. Results with extracorporeal shock wave lithotripsy (München, Dornier HM-1,2,3)

Extracorporeal shock wave lithotripsy Results of the Munich group (1980–1983)	
Stone free	90%
Spontaneously passable	9.3%
Surgery	0.7%
Renal function unchanged ($n = 50$, 1980–1984)	

Results with Extracorporeal Shock Wave Lithotripsy

The initial results of the Munich group for the first three years, when extracorporeal shock wave lithotripsy was used in Munich alone, revealed a success rate of 99%. Ninety percent of patients became completely stone free within a three month period. Only small and spontaneously passable fragments remained in 9.3% of patients. In 0.7% of cases an open surgical or endourological procedure was indicated to relieve a persisting ureteral obstruction (Table 6) [4,15,16].

Evaluation of pre and post-lithotripsy renal function showed no evidence of any adverse effects of extracorporeal shock wave lithotripsy on renal function. Over a four year period, it was found that the renal function of those patients treated with extracorporeal shock wave lithotripsy actually improved with time, which is attributable to those cases where obstructing stones had been successfully treated (Table 6). Comparison of these results with the results from other institutions using the same lithotripter, and with those results achieved with different machines is difficult, since there is no commonly accepted nomenclature or stratification system. It would therefore seem reasonable to agree on a nomenclature encompassing stone size, location, anatomy of the urinary tract, and stone composition. The reported annual stone recurrent rates of 4%–8% are reassuringly low and compare favorably to those of other treatment modalities. Approximately 25% of residual stones increase in size over a 2 year followup period. Long-term observation of the clinical fate of these patients is necessary to decide whether or not the regrowth rate and the associated need for auxiliary procedures are acceptable.

Complications of Extracorporeal Shock Wave Lithotripsy

Transient macroscopic hematuria is reported to occur in most patients, regardless of the energy source used. However, clinically significant bleeding with the development of perirenal hematoma is a rare exception (0.1%–0.66%) [7,9,18]. Recent discussion has focused on the relevance of short-term shockwave induced alterations on renal morphology, long-term function, and the possibility of so far unappreciated long-term adverse effects. With the advent of more sensitive imaging technology immediate changes in renal morphology, such as subcapsular bleeding, perirenal fluid collections and loss of corticomedullary differentiation, have been described in as many a 63% of patients following shockwave treatment for renal stones. Animal studies have revealed renal injury secondary to shock wave energy, including disruption of renal vessels, damage to tubular epithelium, and eventual formation of focal and segmental interstitial fibrosis when higher than clinically recommended levels of energy were employed. These studies identified the amount of energy used as a common denominator of damage. Unless exceedingly high levels of energy were used, however, the shock wave induced morphological changes were found to be transient. Clinically, no long-term adverse effects have been reported until recently, when various retrospective studies suggested an incidence of new onset hypertension of up to 8% within a 2 year period following extracorporeal lithotripsy treatment [7,18].

These figures, however, were obtained from retrospective observations and have not been reproduced so far in prospective studies, reflecting the difficulties of reliable assessment of small changes in blood pressure within a relatively short period. Urological post-lithotripsy complications are secondary to either insufficient stone disintegration or to ureteral obstruction with stone debris. Discomfort or pain is found in between 5% and 25% of all cases. Auxiliary procedures after extracorporeal shock wave lithotripsy are indicated when obstructive pyelonephritis (2%–6%) has to be relieved to prevent urosepsis. In our service we use percutaneous nephrostomy tube drainage liberally. This, together with appropriate antibiotic treatment, quickly relieves the acute symptoms (pain and/or infection). When ureteral Steinstrasse (accumulation of disintegrated stone debris in the ureter) is present without signs of infection, obstruction persistent for 4 weeks prompts us to use percutaneous nephrostomy drainage. In many cases fragments are then spontaneously discharged within a reasonable period, thus reducing the necessity for more invasive auxiliary procedures.

Conclusion

Undoubtedly, extracorporeal shock wave lithotripsy has become a most valuable asset to the urologist and greatly benefits urological stone patients. During the short time since the advent of extracorporeal shock wave lithotripsy the management of urinary stone disease has completely changed. Extracorporeal shock wave lithotripsy has almost completely supplanted open surgical and, to a lesser extent, endourological approaches.

Experience has shown that approximately 70% of patients can benefit from extracorporeal shock wave lithotripsy as monotherapy. More complex stones require auxiliary procedures, namely endourological procedures or, at times, open surgery. Those 25%–30% of cases which require combined endourological or open surgical techniques are technically demanding and should be reserved for the stone centers, where extensive experience with all alternative techniques of urinary stone treatment exists.

We certainly have not yet reached the endpoint of the development of this method and its clinical applications in urology and other medical fields. At this point it is certain that the progress of ESWL represents a dramatic change in the management of urinary stones, by which invasive approaches have been superseded by a noninvasive procedure. We, the urologists, and of course over and above all, the patient himself who gets rid of his stones, avoiding open surgery, have learned to appreciate the outstanding achievements of the recent past. From now on all other methods employed for the treatment of urinary stones will have to be judged against the results of this new methodology.

References

1. Chaussy C, Eisenberger F, Wanner K, Forssmann B, Hepp W (1976) The use of shock waves for the destruction of renal calculi without direct contact. Urol Res 4:175
2. Chaussy C, Schmiedt E, Forssmann B, Brendel W (1979) Contact free renal stone destruction by means of shock waves. Eur Surg Res 11:36
3. Chaussy C, Brendel W, Schmiedt E (1980) Extracorporeally induced destruction of kidney stones by shock waves. Lancet 12.3:1265
4. Chaussy C, Schmiedt E, Jocham D, Brendel W, Forssmann B, Walther W (1981) First clinical experience with extracorporeally induced destruction of kidney stones by shock waves. J Urol 125:417–420
5. Chaussy C, Schmiedt E, Jocham D, Fuchs G, Brendel W (1986) Extracorporeal shock wave lithotripsy, 2nd ed. In: Chaussy CG (ed) Karger, Munich
6. Fuchs G, Chaussy C (1987) Worldwide experience with, and future concepts of ESWL, In: Riehle R, Newman D (eds) Principles of extracorporeal shock wave lithotripsy. Livingstone, New York
7. Chaussy C, Fuchs G (1989) Current state and future development of noninvasive treatment of human stones with extracorporeal shockwave lithotripsy. J Urol 141:790
8. Drach G, Dretler S, Fair W, Finlayson B, Gillenwater J, Griffith D, Lingeman J, Newman D (1986) Report of the United States cooperative study of extracorporeal shock wave lithotripsy. J Urol 135:1127
9. Chaussy C, Fuchs G (1986) Extracorporeal shock wave lithotripsy (ESWL) for the treatment of urinary stones. In: Gillenwater J (ed) Textbook on adult and pediatric urology. Year Book Publishers, Chicago
10. Fuchs G, Miller K, Rassweiler J, Eisenberger F (1985) Extracorporeal shock wave lithotripsy: One-year experience with the Dornier Lithotripter. Eur Urol 11:145
11. Eisenberger, F, Fuchs G, Miller K, Rassweiler J (1985) Extracorporeal shock wave lithotripsy and endourology—an ideal combination for the treatment of kidney stones. World J Urol 3:41–47
12. Miller K, Fuchs G, Rassweiler J, Eisenberger F (1985) Treatment of ureteral stone disease: the role of ESWL and endourology. World J Urol 3:445
13. Winfield H, Clayman R, Chaussy C, Weyman P, Fuchs G, Lupu A (1988) Monotherapy of staghorn calculi: Comparative study between percutaneous nephrolithotomy and extracorporeal shock wave lithotripsy. J Urol 139:895
14. Fuchs G, Chaussy C, Riehle R (1987) The Use of ESWL for ureteral stones. In: Riehle R, Newman D (eds) Principles of extracorporeal shock wave lithotripsy. Livingstone, New York
15. Schmiedt E, Chaussy C (1984) Extracorporeal shock wave lithotripsy of kidney and ureteric stones. Urol Int 39:193–198
16. Chaussy C, Schmiedt E (1983) Shock wave treatment for stones in the upper urinary tract. N Amer Clin Urol vol 10, No 4:743–750
17. Chaussy C, Fuchs G (1987) Extracorporeal shock wave lithotripsy of distal ureteral calculi: Is it worthwhile? J Endourol 1:1
18. Lingeman J, Evan A (1987) Bioeffects of ESWL. J Endourol 1:89
19. Jocham D, Liedl B, Chaussy C, Schmiedt E (1987) Preliminary clinical experience with the HM-4 bath-free Dornier lithotriptor. World J Urol 5:4, 208

Extracorporeal Shock Wave Lithotripsy (ESWL): Late Consequences

JOHN C. PETERSON[1]

SUMMARY. Since its introduction, ESWL has had a great impact on the treatment of renal stone disease. This treatment is 90% successful for upper urinary tract stones less than 2 centimeters in diameter. The initial reports created tremendous enthisiasm and related few complications. Subsequent studies have raised concerns about stone recurrence rates and renal dysfunction, as well as hypertension, following lithotripsy. Studies on stone recurrence rates have yielded reassuringly low rates; however, the duration of follow-up in these studies is only 2 years and certainly more data concerning the 10%–30% of patients with remnant stone fragments are needed. Initial reports of tissue damage, consisting of subcapsular hematomas immediately following treatment and localized areas of interstitial fibrosis in more chronic animal models, provide a possible explanation for the reports of decreased renal blood flow correlated with hypertension in human subjects studied up to 4 years after lithotripsy. These studies contain small numbers of patients and corroborative studies are needed to document the risks of such complications.

Introduction

Renal stone disease accounts for approximately 1% of all hospital admissions in the United States and has an annual incidence of 7–21 cases per 10000 persons. Its peak incidence is between ages 20 and 30 years, thus it affects individuals during the height of career development [1]. Realizing the economic impact of this disease and the extraordinary technologic developments in its treatment over the past decade, the Office of Medical Applications of Research of the National Institute of Health (NIH) convened a Consensus Development Conference on the Prevention and Treatment of

[1]Division of Nephrology, Hypertension and Transplantation, University of Florida College of Medicine, Gainesville, FL 32610-0224, USA

Kidney stones in March of 1988. One of the topics discussed was the role of lithotripsy in treatment of renal stone disease. Their summary statement included the following comment: "Since ESWL is relatively new, the long-term effects of this therapy are unknown. Concerns relative to the effects of kidney function, ... increased new stone growth, and subsequent diseases, such as hypertension will require long term evaluation [1]."

Extracorporeal shock wave lithotripsy (ESWL) was first used by Chaussy in 1980 [2], was introduced to the United States in 1984 and, almost immediately, became the treatment of choice for the majority of cases of symptomatic upper urinary tract nephrolithiasis [3-5]. Initial reports suggested that ESWL had very few deleterious effects [6-7]. Early in our experience (late 1984) with ESWL, one patient developed flank pain and abrupt onset of hypertension within hours of treatment, and was found to have a markedly reduced effective renal plasma flow (by radionuclide renography) with a perirenal hematoma (by magnetic resonance imaging). This experience prompted a prospective study showing acute effects of ESWL on morphology and renal function [8], and a retrospective review of our first 79 patients suggested an increase in diastolic blood pressure several months following ESWL [9]. Subsequently, other reports have corroborated these findings [10-12] and reports concerning tissue effects—both acute and chronic—have suggested that ESWL does have a measurable effect on renal and on other tissues [13-16].

This paper will review the reported experience of long-term consequences of ESWL as enumerated by the NIH-convened consensus report, i.e., increased stone growth, effects on kidney function, and hypertension [1].

Increased or Recurrent Stone Growth

There is no debate concerning the efficacy of ESWL in removing stones which previously would have required surgery. Several large series have reported success rates of approximately 90% when pre-treatment stone diameter is less than 2 centimeters [17,18]. These success rates generally include 10%–30% of patients who are left with small (0.3–0.4 centimeters) stone fragments at the time of discharge, which subsequently pass, leaving the patient "stone-free" or with a remarkably reduced stone burden at 3 months as evaluated by plain film radiography. Whether these remnant stone fragments serve as a nidus for further stone formation was not addressed by these initial studies. Since the natural history of nephrolithiasis suggests that 40% of patients will have a recurrent stone (15% will recur in the first year) within five years after the first episode [19], the presence of stone fragments in 10%–30% of patients after 3 months is bothersome. Two recent reports show reassuringly low rates of new stone formation, approximating 6% [20,21]; however, these evaluations were at 19–26 months after ESWL and thus the long-term effects on stone recurrence must await further studies at longer time periods after ESWL. Additionally, the issue of regrowth of residual fragments will also require further study, since the values in different reports are not consistent. Since the clinical effectiveness of ESWL seems to be greater than its stone-removal (or stone-free) efficacy, future reports will need to include clinical correlation and to contain follow-up for periods longer than the current two-year studies.

Kidney Function and Hypertension

The second and third concerns enumerated by the NIH Consensus Report involve kidney function and hypertension, as well as the tissue effects of ESWL [1]. I shall attempt a collated discussion of these subjects, since it seems rational to suppose that long-term decrements in renal function are attributable to tissue damage incurred during ESWL, and recent evidence indicates a significant correlation between decrement in estimated renal plasma flow (ERPF) and increment in systolic and diastolic blood pressure [22].

As related above, our initial experience with hypertension, reduced renal plasma flow, and a perirenal hematoma in a single patient led us to do a retrospective study in which we found an increased diastolic blood pressure in 4% (3 out of 79) of patients up to several months after ESWL. Because all 3 cases had perirenal or subcapsular hematomas which subsequently resolved while the blood pressure remained elevated, we suggested the pathophysiology might involve a phenomenon known as the Page kidney [9]. In the same symposium, Kaude and co-workers, using magnetic resonance imaging, documented loss of corticomedullary demarcation and subcapsular hemorrhage in 24% of patients [23]. Studies in dog kidneys demonstrated pathologic changes in the kidney, which were dose-dependent on the number of shocks delivered [24], and demonstrated that fibrosis was a predictable event in the resolution of intraparenchymal hemorrhage following ESWL [14,15].

In the interim, in 1987 Lingeman and Kulb [10] reported a retrospective evaluation of 900 patients treated with ESWL; of follow-up patients examined, 8.2% (24 out of 295) had become hypertensive. Bomanji and co-workers then reported a significant decrement in glomerular filtration rate immediately after ESWL [25].

In 1988, Williams and co-workers reported an overall prevalence of hypertension, at 18 months after treatment, of 8% (7 out of 91). In a subgroup of 21 patients with decreased blood flow, 5 were hypertensive [12]. Sixteen of these patients were restudied 4 years after treatment and showed a further decline in blood flow to the treated kidney, with hypertension severe enough to require treatment present in 4 of 16 patients (25%). Interestingly, the decreased blood flow to the treated kidney correlated significantly with the increments in both systolic and diastolic blood pressure [22]. Lingeman and co-workers have recently reported results of follow-up blood pressure measurements in 731 patients at least 1 year after ESWL. They found no difference in annualized incidence of diastolic hypertension compared to a control group of patients who received urethroscopy or passed stones spontaneously (171 patients); however, the group as a whole had a significant rise in diastolic blood pressure after ESWL. Unfortunately their definition of hypertension included only diastolic values and no systolic values were reported [11]. A recent report from the same center documented findings in 8 patients with solitary kidneys who received ESWL five years ago. They showed a significant rise in serum creatinine, new onset of hypertension in 2 of 8 patients, and a decrement in renal blood flow that did not reach statistical significance (pre-327 ml/min and post-294 ml/min) [26].

In summary, although the numbers of patients studied are small and uncontrolled, the data to date suggest that hypertension and reduced renal function occur after ESWL and are maintained for at least 4 years. Even if further studies corroborate these findings, ESWL will continue to have a massive impact on the treatment of kidney stones. The stage has been set for the development of a multi-center, prospective evaluation of the long-term consequences of ESWL. This is currently underway and the results will be eagerly awaited.

References

1. Consensus development summaries (1988) Prevention and treatment of kidney stones. National Institutes of Health. Conn Med 52(7):415–420
2. Chaussy CG, Brendel W, Schmiedt E (1980) Extracorporeally induced destruction of kidney stones by shock waves. Lancet II:1265–1268
3. Fuchs G, Miller K, Rassweiler J, Eisenberger F (1985) Extracorporeal shock wave lithotripsy. Eur Urol 11:145–149
4. Lingeman JE, Newman DM, Mertz JHO, Mosbaugh PG, Steele RE, Kahnoski RJ, Coury TA, Woods JR (1986) Extracorporeal shock wave lithotripsy. J Urol 135:1134–1137
5. Drach G, Dretler SP, Fair W, Finlayson B, Gillenwater J, Griffith D, Lingeman J, Newman D (1986) Report of the United States cooperative study of extracorporeal shock wave lithotripsy. J Urol 135:1127–1133
6. Chaussy CG, Schmiedt E, Jocham D, Brendel W, Forssman B, Walther V (1982) First clinical experience with extracorporeally induced destruction of kidney stones by shock waves. J Urol 127:417–420
7. Chaussy CG, Schmiedt E (1983) Shock wave treatment for stones in the upper urinary tract. Urol Clin North Am 10:743–750
8. Kaude JV, Williams MC, Millner MR, Scott KN, Finlayson B (1985) Renal morphology and function immediately after extracorporeal shock wave lithotripsy. AJR 145:305–313
9. Peterson JC, Finlayson B (1986) Effects of ESWL on blood pressure. In: Gravenstein JS, Peter K (eds) Extracorporeal shock wave lithotripsy for renal stone disease. Butterworth, Stoneham, pp 145–150
10. Lingeman JE, Kulb TB (1987) Hypertension following extracorporeal shock wave lithotripsy. J Urol 137:142A
11. Lingeman JE, Woods JR, Toth PD (1990) Blood pressure changes following extracorporeal shock wave lithotripsy and other forms of treatment of nephrolithiasis. JAMA 263(13):1789–1794
12. Williams CM, Kaude JV, Newman RC, Peterson JC, Thomas WC (1988) ESWL: Long-term complications. AJR 150:311–315
13. Lingeman JE, McAteer JA, Kempson SA, Evan AP (1988) Bioeffects of extracorporeal shock wave lithotripsy. Urol Clin North Am 15:507–514
14. Newman R, Hackett R, Senior D, Feldman J, Sosnowski J, Finlayson B (1987) ESWL: pathologic effects on canine renal tissues. Urology 29:194–200
15. Jaeger P, Redha G, Uhlschmid G, Hauri D (1988) Morphological changes in canine kidneys following extracorporeal shock wave treatment. Urol Res 16:161–166
16. Haupt G, Haupt A, Donovan JM, Drach GW, Chaussy C (1989) Short-term changes of laboratory values after extracorporeal shock wave lithotripsy. J Urol 142:259–262
17. Roth RA, Beckmann CF (1988) Complications of extracorporeal shock wave lithotripsy and percutaneous nephrolithotomy. Urol Clin North Am 15(2):155–166
18. Schmiedt E, Chaussy C (1984) Extracorporeal shock wave lithotripsy of kidney and ureteric stones. Urol Int 39:193–198
19. Williams RE (1969) The natural history of renal lithiasis. In: Hodgkinson A, Nordin BEC (eds) Renal stone research symposium, Leeds (1968). Churchill, London, pp 65–70
20. Miles SG, Kaude JV, Newman RC, Thomas WC, Williams CM (1988) Extracorporeal shock wave lithotripsy: prevalence of renal stones 3 to 21 months after treatment. AJR 150:307–309

21. Graff J, Diederichs W, Schulze H (1987) Long-term follow-up in 1003 extracorporeal shock wave lithotripsy patients. J Urol 140:479–483
22. Williams CM, Thomas WC (1989) Permanently decreased renal blood flow and hypertension after lithotripsy. N Engl J Med 321:1269–1270
23. Kaude JV, Williams CM, Millner M, Finlayson B (1986) Magnetic resonance imaging of the kidney after ESWL. In: Extracorporeal shock wave lithotripsy for renal stone disease: technical and clinical aspects. Butterworth, Stoneham, pp 125–129
24. Delius M, Enders G, Xuan Z, Liebisch HG, Brendel W (1988) Biological effects of shock waves. Ultrasound Med Biol 14:117–122
25. Bomanji J, Boddy SAM, Britton KE, Nimmon CC, Whitfield HN (1987) Radionuclide evaluation pre- and post-extracorporeal shock wave lithotripsy for renal calculi. J Nucl Med 28:1284–1289
26. Brito CG, Lingeman JE, Newman DM, Kight JL, Heck LL (1990) Long term follow-up of renal function in ESWL-treated patients with solitary kidney. J Urol 143(4):299A

Nephrolithiasis—Extracorporeal Shock Wave Lithotripsy (ESWL): Current Status in Japan

Hiroshi Tazaki[1]

Introduction of ESWL to Japan

In December 1983, a survey team was sent to Munich and Stuttgart, Federal Republic of Germany, to study new lithotripters. Drs. Tazaki and Higashihara were there; they reported that the machine was effective for disintegrating kidney stones and that the side effects were minor. In 1984, four machines were installed in four institutions in Japan and treatments were initiated. The spark gap system ESWL was found to be so useful that the number of machines had increased to ten by the end of 1986. Membrane type and piezo type ESWL were introduced in 1987 and 1988. In November, 1989 at the seventh world congress of endourology and ESWL in Kyoto, all kinds of lithotripters were displayed at the exhibit and discussed. Multipurpose types of ESWL became more popular; since 1989 the Piezo type ESWL with ultrasound focusing has tended to be the preferred type.

As of the end of June, 1990, 244 ESWL machines are being operated in this country; the regional distribution and types of ESWL are shown in Figs. 1 and 2. Regional populations and patient ratio to machine are shown in Table 1. Wide differences in each region become more apparent when comparisons are made between prefectures. More ESWL machines are found on the Pacific coast; there are no machines in two prefectures along the sea of Japan; however, the incidence of stone disease is apparently higher on the Pacific side of Japan.

Clinical Investigation of ESWL

Results of clinical studies on urinary stone disintegration, using various types of ESWL, have been published. The results are almost the same as the reports from

[1]Department of Urology, School of Medicine, Keio University, 35, Shinanomachi, Shinjuku-ku, Tokyo, 160 Japan

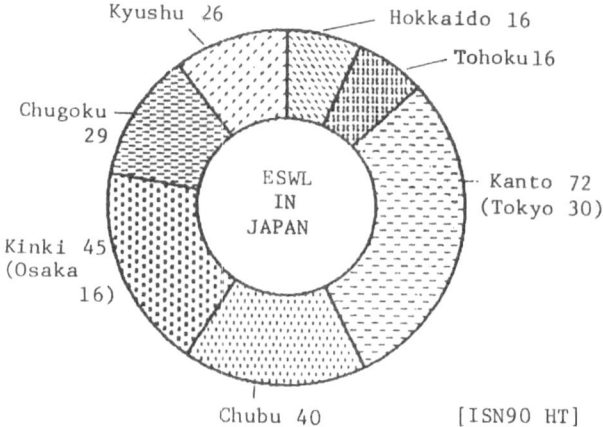

Fig. 1. Regional distribution of ESWL (June 1990)

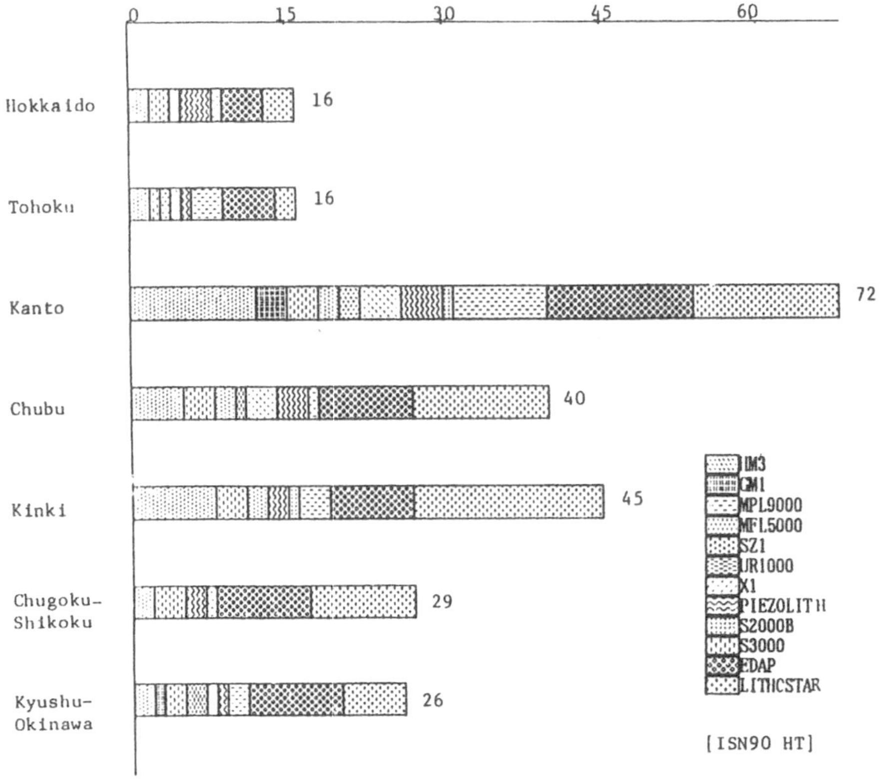

Fig. 2. Regional distribution of ESWL in Japan (June 1990)

Table 1. ESWL distribution and regional population

	Number of ESWL	Population (million)	Ratio (1: $\times 10^3$)
Hokkaido	16	5.6	350
Tohoku	16	9.8	610
Kanto	72	35.6	490
(Tokyo)	(30)	(11.5)	(380)
Chubu	40	20.3	510
Kinki	45	21.4	480
(Osaka)	(16)	(8.4)	(520)
Chugoku-Shikoku	29	12.0	410
Kyushu-Okinawa	26	14.3	550
	244	120.0	350–610

other countries, and so far on simple single stones in the renal pelvis the success rate has been shown to be nearly 90%. Some of these reports are summarized as follows:

HM3

The most significant report on the results of clinical investigation using HM3 was published by Higashihara et al. in the *Journal of Endourology and ESWL* in 1988 [1]. The study summarized 3702 cases treated with HM3 at 11 hospitals in Japan. Of these, 93% were treated by ESWL monotherapy; 7% of the cases required additional therapies such as percutaneous nephrolithotripsy (PNL), percutaneous nephrostomy (PCN), and transurethral ureterolithotripsy (TUL); the incidence of these therapies was 50%, 21% and 29%, respectively (Fig. 3). At 6 month follow-up in the same study residual fragments of 4mm or less were seen in 17% of cases; fragments over 4mm in size were seen in 4% of cases; however, 79% of cases were free of residual

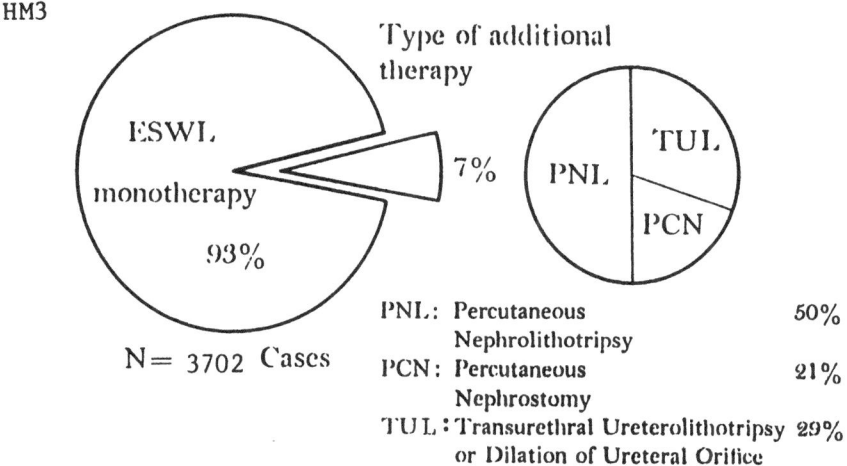

Fig. 3. Type of additional therapy. (From [1])

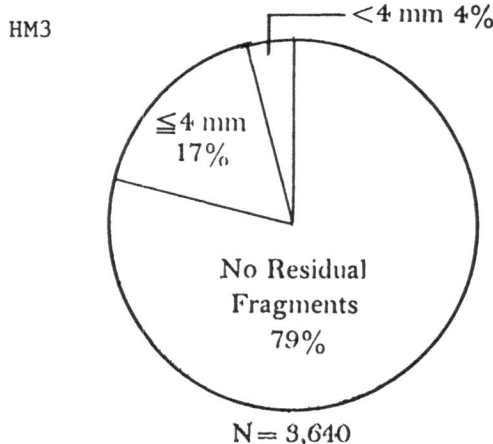

Fig. 4. Residual fragments at 6-month follow-up. (From [1])

fragments (Fig. 4). More reports on staghorn stones and complicated cases have been seen in 1989–1990, which have fairly good results using combinations of various endourological techniques.

Lithostar

Konishi et al. [2] reported their experience of 323 cases treated with the electromagnetic lithotripter, Lithostar, in 1988 and 1989. The study included 123 cases (35.1%) of upper ureteral stones (Table 2); good results were achieved. Many other reports have described the advantages to be gained with this ESWL machine.

Piezolith

Our experience with 183 cases, [3] using the piezoelectric type lithotripter, Piezolith 2200, at Keio University Hospital are shown in Tables 3 and 4. A great advantage of using this ESWL machine that it is anesthesia free; none of these 183 patients

Table 2. Lithostar

Number of cases	323 cases
Male:female	227:96
Age	13 ~ 89 (mean 49.6)
Stone location	
Kidney	111 (31.6%)
Upper ureter	123 (35.1%)
Middle ureter	39 (11.1%)
Lower ureter	70 (19.9%)
Bladder	8 (2.3%)

(From [2])

Table 3. Keio University Hospital, Tokyo Piezolith 117 cases in 1989

Location	No. of stones evaluated	Largest diameter (mm)
Pelvis and calyx	39	15.5±6.5
Calyx	103	8.4±5.4
UPJ	11	11.2±4.1
Upper ureter	7	9.0±3.2
Ureter:Pelvis (flush up)	23	7.8±2.3
Total	183	9.3±5.8

(From [3])

required even pretreatment sedation. Ultrasonographic imaging for focusing is good, but in cases with small stones focusing is difficult, especially in the ureter.

Other Studies and Complications

Experience with EDAP LT01, Sonolith 2000B, and other machines has been reported. Yachiyoda SZ1 is a Japanese made ESWL, using microexplosives for its energy source of shock waves; its characteristics are shown in Table 5. The results of the study described by Honda et al. in 1988 [4] indicate that, because of its lower residual stone rates, this ESWL machine has greater power to disintegrate stones with microexplosives.

Complications have been reported. Subcapsular hematomas, endotoxin shock and possibilities of hypertension have been reported following the therapy. From our experience with Piezolith, temporary elevation of plasma renin activity has been described by Baba et al. [3]; however, this may not indicate persistent hypertension so much as late complications; also, it is not specific to the piezoelectric system.

Socioeconomic Background of ESWL

In the early stages of the introduction of ESWL to Japan nobody could have predicted that this new therapeutic modality would take over from traditional treatments within 5 years. Apparently the government was so interested in new trends that reconsidera-

Table 4. Keio University Hospital, Tokyo Piezolith 117 cases in 1989

	Stone Size 3 Months after Tx.		
Stone free	<3mm	3~5mm	>5mm
66.7%	11.1%	7.4%	14.8%
67.0%	13.9%	2.6%	5.2%
81.8%	9.1%	9.1%	0%
85.7%	0%	14.3%	0%
95.7%	4.3%	0%	0%
73.8%	12.8%	3.7%	7.5%

(From [3])

Table 5. Characteristics of microexplosive ESWL

	Characteristics
• Energy source	Microexplosion (10 mg silver azide)
• Focus	X-rays
• Target	Moving the chair by computer control
• Coupling	Water bath
• Patient's position	Sitting
• Anesthesia	Not required
• Clinical results	Satisfactory (almost equivalent to conventional ESWL)
• Complications	Not severe (almost comparable with conventional ESWL)
• Cost of construction	Not expensive

(From [4])

tion of the socialized medical care system resulted in the formation of a new system called "High Technology Medicare" in 1985. However, ESWL and endourology were excluded from the system and the government set the treatment cost at the lowest level of 20000 points per treatment. This resulted in the installation of low running cost machines becoming preferable.

On the other hand, private insurance for stone disease can cover most expenses. As the aged population increases, those patients are not covered for a 100% increase and they must go to a local doctor for conventional therapy. The distribution of ESWL machines is greater in large cities and is still inadequate. Endourology is established in this country, but people wish to have totally non-invasive therapy, as they do in other countries. Other problems occurring coincidentally such as gall bladder stones can be treated. Most surgeons still like open surgery, but patients like less invasiveness. Organization in society is needed to promote ESWL and exclude endourology in the near future. As the machines become more sophisticated the cost per treatment becomes higher; new types of ESWL will replace old models.

Conclusion and the Remarks on the Future

Introducing ESWL to Japan was a culture shock. The shock continued for the next 5 years. At present the status of this therapy is in an early stage of recovery. The recovery must be complete with no scar remaining. The coming era will see the replacement of the 1st and 2nd generation machines by Japanese-made machines. It will be done serenely and peacefully.

References

1. Higashihara E (1988) Jpn J Endourol ESWL 1:24–25
2. Konishi T et al. (1989) Jpn J Endourol ESWL 2:105–109
3. Baba S et al. (1989) Jpn J Endourol ESWL 2:114–120
4. Honda M et al. (1988) Jpn J Endourol ESWL 1:28–29

New Drugs to Prevent Recurrence of Renal Stone Disease

Bo G. Danielson, B. Fellström, M. Lindsjö, S. Ljunghall, and B. Wikström[1]

SUMMARY. Many patients who are stone formers have recurrent stone formation, for which detailed clinical and biochemical work-up is necessary. Even if conventional treatments with thiazides, orthophosphate, or magnesium or potassium citrate are effective in many stone formers, their use may be limited by their way of acting or by their side effects. This is particularly the case in patients with increased urinary oxalate excretion.

Therefore, during recent years, two new approaches have been tried. Since it is known that glycosaminoglycans are potent inhibitors of calcium oxalate crystal growth, aggregation, and possibly also crystal adherence to the walls of the urinary tract, a pentosan polysulfate (PPS), has been tried as a prophylactic treatment in stone formers. Of the patients on PPS treatment 75% were free of recurrences, despite severe stone disease with previous frequent recurrences. Another 10% of the patients experienced considerable reduction in the frequency of the stone episodes.

In patients with enteric hyperoxaluria and severe stone disease, treatment with an organic marine hydrocolloid (OMH)—trade name Ox−absorb—was used to reduce gastrointestinal oxalate absorption. The OMH was shown to bind oxalate in vitro, and to reduce urinary oxalate by oxalate binding in the gut. It was very well tolerated, improved bowel function, showed promising effects on stone episode rate, and had very few side effects.

Introduction

During recent years less interest has been focused on basic mechanisms of stone formation and prophylactic treatment than on extracorporeal shock wave lithotripsy (ESWL) treatment and its consequences.

[1]Department of Internal Medicine, University Hospital, S-751 85 Uppsala, Sweden

However, there are many patients with severe stone disease, with frequent recurrences where repeated shock-wave treatment is less suitable and where prophylactic medical treatment is more advisable. Even if ESWL may be the easiest way to treat the stone former when he or she presents with a stone, the strategy for long-term treatment has to be considered. Therefore a clinical and metabolic work up of the recurrent stone former is essential.

Renal stone formation is basically a consequence of an imbalance between supersaturation of the urine and the inhibition of crystal formation, growth and aggregation [1]. Urine contains many substances which are claimed to modify the rate of crystallization of calcium oxalate and calcium phosphate.

Increased renal excretion of calcium, oxalate, and phosphate contributes to an increased risk of stone formation. The risk can be influenced by the presence of various promoters of nucleation, growth, and aggregation which could contribute to matrix formation and also to epitaxial growth.

However, the urine also contains many substances which inhibit crystal formation through one or two possible mechanisms. Firstly, they may act by complexing either calcium or oxalate ions, thereby reducing the level of calcium oxalate and calcium phosphate supersaturation in the crystallizing solution. Of the urinary inhibitors, citrate and magnesium fall into this group. The other group of inhibitors acts at relatively low concentrations by adsorbing to the surface of the crystals, thereby retarding the rate of crystal growth and agglomeration. Among this group could be mentioned pyrophosphate, heparinoids or glycosaminoglycans (GAGs) like chondroitin sulfate, heparin, heparan sulfate, dermatane sulfate, nephrocalcin, and Tamm-Horsefall mucopolysaccharide. Glycosaminoglycans including chondroitin sulfate, heparin sulfate, keratan sulfate and dermatane sulfate are naturally occurring in human urine. Heparin, however, is not excreted in human urine. It has been shown previously in experimental work that the inhibitor potential of GAGs is dependent on the degree of sulfation and that the inhibitor effect takes place because of reversible binding of the GAGs to the crystal surface, whereby further crystal growth and aggregation become blocked. Experimental studies have also included a pentosan polysulfate (PPS), which has been used for clinical trials in the treatment of urolithiasis.

In Vitro Study of PPS

The inhibition of calcium oxalate crystal growth was investigated by seeded crystal procedure, whereby seeded crystals of calcium oxalate were added to metastable calcium oxalate solution together with the inhibitor to be studied. The inhibition of calcium oxalate crystal growth by polyanionic GAGs, Tamm-Horsefall glycoprotein, and pyrophosphate was compared [2]. Using the same system, PPS was also added in order to compare the inhibitory effect. On a concentration basis pyrophosphate was found to be the most inefficient inhibitor tested. Among the polyanions, heparin was the most effective inhibitor, whereas chondroitin sulfate exerted about 40% of the inhibitory activity of heparin. The inhibitory effect of PPS was about 80% of the inhibitory activity found for heparin. The inhibition was directly proportional to the logarithm of the concentration of the polyanions.

In order to investigate the mechanism of inhibition, experiments were performed with radioactive-labeled heparin, chondroitin sulfate, and pentosan polysulfate, binding to calcium oxalate crystals; subsequent displacements were induced by increasing the amounts of non-radioactive ligands or by increasing ionic strength. It was then found that ligands with a high charge density bound more readily and with a seemingly higher affinity than ligands with a low charge density, but the former were also more suspectible to displacement when the ionic strength was increased [3]. It could be concluded that the higher affinity of the crystals may be the reason why highly charged glycosaminoglycans are more efficient inhibitors of calcium oxalate crystal growth.

Pharmacokinetic Studies of PPS

Following intravenous injection of PPS the plasma curve could be described by an exponential decline, indicating a two-compartment distribution [4]. The distribution half-life was 25 min for the first compartment and the plasma half-life, i.e., elimination phase, was 24 h. Renal clearance was about 4 ml/min and the renal excretion of unchanged PPS was 8%–10%.

When tritium-labeled PPS was given orally to healthy volunteers, about 3% of the given dose appeared unchanged in the urine, which is significantly more than the amount found using unlabeled PPS.

The distribution of PPS has also been studied using autoradiographic techniques, where it was found that PPS could be observed in the urinary tract, urinary bladder, the pelvis of the kidney, and in the urethra.

Clinical Results with PPS as Prophylactic Treatment

With these experimental and pharmacokinetic data as background, a clinical trial was started where PPS was evaluated as a prophylactic agent in renal calcium stone disease [5]. One hundred patients with recurrent renal calcium stones were the subjects; PPS treatment was given at a dose of 400 mg/day. The drug was given in the form of capsules two hours after meals. When the results were evaluated, patients who had been on the treatment for more than 12 months were included. The average follow-up time was nearly 3 years (12–56 months). The patients were 66 males and 34 females with a mean age of 47 years. The duration of the stone disease was 15 ± 10 years with the range between 1 and 43 years. Six patients had experienced more than 50 stones each and, when these were excluded, the average number of total stone episodes was 11 ± 9 stones, or 1.3 stones/year. About half of the patients had had surgical intervention because of stones. Each of the patients had had an average of 1.8 operations.

Of the 100 patients, 76 patients were free of recurrences. Of the 96 patients who were evaluated, 20 formed new stones during the main treatment time of 22 months. Four of these 20 patients had enteric disorders, one patient had celiac disease, and three had regional enteritis. One patient acquired a urinary tract infection caused by *Proteus*. Eight of the other 15 patients had fewer and smaller stones than before treatment.

Of the 100 patients initially included in the study, 16 patients were withdrawn because of side effects or other concomitant events. Nine of the patients had nausea, diarrhea, and other related gastrointestinal problems, their susceptibility perhaps related in part to a history of previous ulcers or gastritis found in many of them. Two patients were withdrawn because of pregnancy, one had a myocardial infarction, one died of intercurrent disease, one had eczema (probably not related to PPS), and two patients with regional enteritis and severe stone disease which continued were withdrawn.

The excretion of urinary electrolytes such as calcium, oxalate, magnesium, urate and citrate was not altered in response to treatment.

It could be concluded that the experimental and clinical results favoured the concept of PPS as a potent inhibitor of calcium oxalate crystal growth. The clinical results showed that about 75% of the patients who had been on treatment for more than 12 months had been free of recurrences of stone production and another 10% of the patients were improved.

However, gastrointestinal side effects may occur, particularly in patients with a history of enteric disease. Special attention has therefore to be focussed on how the drug is administered, in order to reduce the gastrointestinal side effects. A lower effective dose and administration of the drug together with meals could help to reduce adverse reactions. However, in patients with inflammatory or intestinal bowel disease the risk that the uptake of the drug may be reduced has to be considered. From the clinical results it seems that pentosan polysulfate inhibits calcium oxalate growth and may also inhibit stone formation by preventing microcrystal adherence to the wall of the urinary tract.

Treatment of Patients with Enteric Hyperoxaluria and Renal Stones

Calcium oxalate is the main constituent of most renal stones. Urinary oxalate is of great significance for stone formation, since even a small increase of urinary oxalate concentration exerts a great influence on the degree of urinary saturation. A group with often severe kidney stone disease are those patients with enteric hyperoxaluria due to gastrointestinal disorders, i.e., inflammatory bowel disease. (For a review, see [6]).

Oxalate is basically a non-essential metabolic end product in man. Under normal circumstances about 90% of urinary oxalate is derived from endogenous oxalate and only 10% from exogenous oxalate in the diet. Ascorbate and glyoxalate are the main precursors of oxalate, each contributing 30%–50% to urinary oxalate. The gastrointestinal absorption of oxalate is mainly a passive diffusion process, which takes place in the entire intestine. More than half of the dietary oxalate in man is decomposed by bacteria in the large intestine.

The intestinal absorption of oxalate in healthy subjects is in the range of 5%–14%, dependent on the amounts given and whether the subjects were fasting or not. A substantial decrease in urinary oxalate excretion occurs during a low oxalate diet, not only in patients with enteric hyperoxaluria, but also in healthy individuals. The uptake of oxalate is also known to be influenced by various dietary components, such as calcium, but magnesium, iron, trace metals, fatty acids, bile salts, and perhaps fibers can also influence the absorption. Binding of oxalate to calcium in the gut lowers the concentration of free oxalate and reduces the oxalate uptake. Conversely oxalate absorption increases when calcium is restricted. Intraluminal fatty acids bind calcium, which will reduce the amount of calcium available for binding of oxalate. Bile salts may increase the absorption of oxalate in the colon by altering mucosa permeability. It has also been suggested that fibers and fatty acids might affect oxalate absorption, mainly by binding to calcium, leaving more oxalate available for absorption.

In contrast to healthy subjects, where the fractional gastrointestinal oxalate absorption is in the range of 5%–10%, idiopathic stone formers may have moderately increased oxalate absorption of up to 15%, but patients with enteric hyperoxaluria caused by, e.g., regional enteritis, celiac disease, or intestinal bypass operations could have significantly increased absorption of oxalate – up to 60% of the ingested oxalate.

Urinary oxalate intake in the ordinary western diet is less than 500 μmol/24 h. In various groups of idiopathic stone formers a moderately increased urinary oxalate excretion could be found, up in the range of 400–600 μmol/24 h.

A diagnosis called mild metabolic hyperoxaluria has been suggested, where typical findings for oxalate excretion are in the range of 500–800 μmol/24 h, in combination with renal calcium stone formation and a raised urinary glycolate concentration, indicating a metabolic and not absorptive cause of hyperoxaluria. Some of these patients have been reported to have responded to pyridoxine treatment.

In patients with enteric hyperoxaluria increased urinary oxalate, in the range of 600–1200 μmol/24 h, is found. This disease is often complicated with severe renal stone disease and is due to gastrointestinal disorders, i.e., inflammatory bowel disease, celiac disease, and pancreatic insufficiency. In some patients the increased oxalate excretion is due to previous surgical intervention, e.g., small bowel resection or jejunoileal bypass operations, done for example, because of obesity. The origin of the increased urinary oxalate in patients with enteric hyperoxaluria is the diet.

This group of patients also has fat malabsorption; a strong correlation between urinary oxalate and degree of steatorrhea has been found. Non-absorbed fatty acids form soaps with interluminal calcium, which leaves unbound oxalate available for absorption. In addition, non-absorbed fatty acids and bile acids in the colon are supposed to increase colonic permeability to oxalate. In healthy subjects oxalate absorption takes place along the entire gastrointestinal tract, but in patients with enteric hyperoxaluria, increased oxalate absorption is due to increased absorption in the colon. In patients with ileostomy no hyperoxaluria has been observed.

A particular group of patients are those who have undergone jejunoileal bypass operations because of obesity. They have an increased risk of renal stone formation and also an increased risk of interstitial nephritis with renal failure, probably due to renal tubular dysfunction and renal tubular acidosis. They often have low excretion of citrate and magnesium, but high oxalate excretion.

Treatment of Hyperoxaluria

The contribution of the diet to hyperoxaluria may be reduced by dietary measures. A logical approach to treatment of enteric hyperoxaluria is to avoid oxalate-rich foodstuffs. A low fat diet has been shown to further reduce urinary oxalate. Binding of the oxalate in the gut seems logical; aluminum or cholestyramin have been used for this purpose, but have not always been successful. Cholestyramin may also bind bile salts and fatty acids and could then reduce the effect of the increased colonic permeability for calcium.

Calcium supplementation has been reported to reduce urinary oxalate by binding oxalate in the gut. However, there is a risk of increased calcium absorption and increase of urinary calcium, which may counteract the binding of the oxalate in the gut. Magnesium therapy can result in an increase of both urinary magnesium and citrate, which may be beneficial, but it may cause further deterioration of bowel function. Potassium citrate, by complexing calcium, has also been reported to have favourable clinical effects on patients with low citrate excretion, but may be of disadvantage in patients with hyperoxaluria. Orthophosphate has also been used in stone patients with primary hyperoxaluria and has been shown to have a beneficial effect on the stone recurrence rate in patients with primary and mild metabolic hyperoxaluria. Pyridoxine deficiency may occasionally be a cause of hyperoxaluria; pyridoxine treatment could be of value in patients with primary hyperoxaluria, but is probably not of any value in patients with enteric hyperoxaluria.

Reduction of Gastrointestinal Oxalate Absorption with OMH

In patients with enteric hyperoxaluria a markedly increased gastrointestinal absorption of oxalate leads to high urinary oxalate excretion. One approach to therapy might therefore be to reduce the gastrointestinal uptake of oxalate by binding dietary oxalate in the gut. In the present study an organic marine hydrocolloid (OMH) used in the treatment of enteric hyperoxaluria was investigated [7]. This group of substances consist of polymers of high molecular weight, derived from alginates and carrageenans extracted from plants and seaweeds. The OMH (Ox-Absorb, Vitaline, Ashland, Oregon, USA) used for this purpose was specially processed and charged with calcium and zinc. It can be formulated as tablets or capsules. In this case each 1 g tablet contained 100 mg calcium and 1.2 mg of zinc. The OxAbsorb was given 3 tabl t.i.d. with meals. This group of substances have no toxic properties and are also licensed as food additives. They also have the capacity to increase water binding, which might be of beneficial effect to soften and enlarge patients' stools. This hydrocolloid was investigated with respect to its capacity to bind oxalate, its effect on oxalate excretion, and also its effect on crystal inhibition in recurrent stone formers with hyperoxaluria.

In Vitro Binding Experiments with OMH

Binding of oxalate to OMH was studied in vitro by incubation of the substance with sodium oxalate at different pH. For measurements of the oxalate binding ^{14}C-oxalate was used. The results showed that a maximum binding of 3.4 mmol of oxalate/g OMH was achieved.

Patient Studies with OMH

Patients with recurrent renal stone formation and hyperoxaluria due to jejunoileal bypass or MbCrohn with ileal resection were included in two studies, namely a *short-*

term (two-week pilot study where 5 females and 4 males, mean age 46 years, as well as one patient with ulcerative colitis and ileostomy with normal urinary oxalate excretion were included) and a *long-term study* (six months, where 18 females and 2 males, mean age 41 years, range 22–63 years, were included). The main purpose of these two studies was to measure the urinary oxalate excretion during short- and long-term treatment, respectively. In the two-week pilot study there was a significant reduction of the 24-hour urinary oxalate excretion with a mean reduction of 133 ± 92 $\mu mol/24$ h. There was no difference in the excretion of electrolytes such as calcium, magnesium, phosphate, or urate. During the long-term study urinary oxalate excretion was also significantly reduced.

A simple estimate of the ionic product for calcium oxalate (AP_{CaOx}) was calculated on each 24 h collection of the patients who participated in the long-term study. The activity product index decreased significantly despite a moderate increase of urinary calcium excreted on treatment. The activity product index decreased in 8 of the 10 patients included in the study. Even if the studies were too short to evaluate the stone episode rate, it was found, in addition to biochemical effects, that 7 of the 10 patients with diarrhea reported considerable improvement in bowel function. Although OMH is capable of binding water and swelling, the marked clinical improvement may also have been due to the binding of free fatty acids in the bowel. The patient studies referred to here do not permit any evaluation with respect to the effects of treatment on the long-term risk of stone formation. However, in a few patients who have been on treatment for up to 5 years, there has been a prompt reduction of stone formation, which encourages further clinical trials with this group of substances.

Conclusions

It can therefore be concluded that patients with enteric hyperoxaluria often have severe kidney stone disease. It has been shown that OMH (Ox-Absorb) binds oxalate in vitro. Treatment with this marine hydrocolloid, in patients with enteric hyperoxaluria, resulted in reduced gastrointestinal absorption and urinary excretion of oxalate, often with drastic improvement of diarrheas. In the few patients treated so far on a long-term basis, substantial reduction in stone formation was achieved.

References

1. Robertson WG, Hughes H, Barkworth SA, Walker VR (1988) Competition between the known inhibitors and promoters of calcium oxalate crystallization in urine. In: Martelli A, Buli P, Marchesini B (eds) Inhibitors of Crystallization in Renal Lithiasis and their Clinical Application. Acta Medica, Bologna, pp 193–195
2. Fellström B, Danielson BG, Ljunghall S, Wikström B (1986) Crystal inhibition: the effects of polyanions on calcium oxalate crystal growth. Clin Chim Acta 158:229–235
3. Fellström B, Lindsjö M, Danielson BG, Karlsson FA, Ljunghall S (1989) Binding of glycosaminoglycan inhibitors to calcium oxalate crystals in relation to ionic strength. Clin Chim Acta 3:213–220
4. Fellström B, Björklund U, Danielson BG, Eriksson H, Odlind B, Tengblad A (1986) Pentosan polysulphate (Elmiron): pharmacokinetics and effects on the urinary inhibition of crystal growth. Fortschr Urol Nephrol 25:340–344

5. Danielson BG, Fellström B, Wikström B (1989) Glycosamino-glycans as inhibitors of renal stone formation. In: Walker VR, Sutton RAL, Cameron ECB, Pak CYC, Robertson WG (eds) Urolithiasis. Plenum, New York, pp 101–104
 6. Lindsjö M (1989) Oxalate metabolism in renal stone disease. Scand J Urol Nephrol [Suppl] 119:1–54
 7. Lindsjö M, Fellström B, Ljunghall S, Wikström B, Danielson BG (1989) Treatment of enteric hyperoxaluria with a calcium containing organic marine hydrocolloid. Lancet II:701–704

Molecular Action of Diuretics

Chair: Neil A. Kurtzman (USA)
Yoshimasa Orita (Japan)

The Mode of Action of Diuretics

E. Lohrmann[1], R.B. Nitschke[1], R. Nitschke[1], I. Burhoff[1],
B. Masereel[2], B. Pirotte[2], E. Schlatter[1], J. Delarge[2], H.J. Lang[3],
H.C. Englert[3], M. Salomonsson[4], A.E.G. Persson[4], O. Eidelman[5],
Z.I. Cabantchik[5], and R. Greger[1]

SUMMARY. This review will address several recent findings regarding the interaction of so called loop diuretics of the furosemide type with the $Na^+2Cl^-K^+$ cotransporter in the thick ascending limb of the loop of Henle (TAL): (i) The organ selectivity of these transport inhibitors is caused by their secretion by the proximal tubule leading to an increase in their luminal concentration. We have examined whether probenecid, a selective inhibitor of proximal organic anion secretion, reduces the diuretic effect of known loop diuretics. We show that all compounds tested: furosemide (FUR), piretanide (PIR), bumetanide (BUM), and azosemide (AZO) lose part of their diuretic effect when administered in the presence of probenecid. (ii) Previously, we have shown that all loop diuretics of the furosemide type require an acidic group for binding to the $Na^+2Cl^-K^+$ cotransporter. This is a carboxylate group in the case of FUR, PIR, and BUM; a tetrazolic acid group in the case of AZO; and a sulfonylurea group in the case of torasemide (TOR). Now we show that TOR-derivates with an even less acidic sulfonylurea group ($pK_a > 8$) are still very potent inhibitors of the $Na^+2Cl^-K^+$ cotransporter. Experiments at various pH values indicate that, even for these substances, it is only the anionic form which inhibits the $Na^+2Cl^-K^+$ cotransporter. (iii) Most of the loop diuretics, with the exception of TOR, are rather hydrophilic (FUR, PIR, BUM, AZO). Now we have examined whether one can design compounds which sustain their inhibitory effect on the $Na^+2Cl^-K^+$ cotransporter, although they are highly lipophilic. We found that cyclo-alkyl substitutions at the tolyl- and sulfonylurea-moieties of TOR led to highly lipophilic compounds with very high affinity for the $Na^+2Cl^-K^+$ cotransporter. (iv) Previous data suggested that loop diuretics bind to the $Na^+2Cl^-K^+$ cotransporter at the extracellular side of the

[1]Albert-Ludwigs-Universität, Freiburg, Federal Republic of Germany
[2]Institut de Pharmacie, Université de Liège, Belgium
[3]Hoechst Pharma, Frankfurt/Main, Federal Republic of Germany
[4]Department of Physiology and Biophysics, University of Lund, Sweden
[5]Department of Biological Chemistry, Hebrew University, Jerusalem, Israel

luminal membrane. Now we have designed impermeable macromolecular derivatives of PIR and we show that these macromolecular probes inhibit the Na⁺2Cl⁻K⁺ cotransporter as well as PIR. (v) Previous data indicated that loop diuretics interrupt the macula densa feedback mechanism, and circumstantial evidence suggested that the uptake of Cl⁻ and/or Na⁺ by macula densa cells may occur via the Na⁺2Cl⁻K⁺ cotransporter. Now we show that macula densa cells sense the luminal NaCl concentration via FUR sensitive Na⁺2Cl⁻K⁺ cotransport.

The Mode of Action of Loop Diuretics

Loop diuretics bind to the Na⁺2Cl⁻K⁺ cotransporter of the thick ascending limb (TAL) of the loop of Henle [1,2] and inhibit the coupled uptake of all participating ions. This effect is instantaneous and easily reversible. The inhibition of Na⁺ influx reduces the requirement to remove Na⁺ from the cell via (Na⁺+K⁺)-ATPase, and thus reduces the ATP [3,4] and O_2 consumption of TAL cells [5]. Hence this nephron segment is protected against hypoxic or ischemic damage [6]. From studies with a large number of derivatives [7–10] we have some understanding of the molecular requirements for interaction of a compound with the Na⁺2Cl⁻K⁺ cotransporter. Figure 1 shows several loop diuretics: furosemide (FUR), piretanide (PIR), bumetanide (BUM), azosemide (AZO), and torasemide (TOR), and gives the concentrations for the half maximal inhibition (IC_{50}) of active NaCl reabsorption in the rabbit cortical thick ascending limb of the loop of Henle (cTAL). It is important to note that all these molecules have several properties in common: (1) All substances are more or less acidic. The pK_u-values of the -COOH group (FUR, PIR, BUM) are around 4, the value for the tetrazolic group (AZO) is around 5, and that for the sulfonylurea (TOR) is around 7. (2) All substances except TOR possess a sulfonamide group. In the case of TOR, the nitrogen of the pyrimidine ring, probably serves the same function [11]. (3) All substances possess a secondary or tertiary amine, and (4) all have apolar residue. Still, most of these substances, except for TOR, are rather hydrophilic.

  In the following paper we will address, on the basis of recent findings from our laboratories, a few loosely related questions regarding (1) the secretion of loop diuretics by the proximal tubule and the inhibition of this secretion by probenecid, (2) the relevance of the acidic moiety of loop diuretics, (3) the lipophilicity of loop diuretics, (4) the site of interaction of loop diuretics with the TAL, and (5) the effect of FUR on macula densa cells.

Secretion by the Proximal Tubule, a Prerequisite for the Inhibitory Effect of Loop Diuretics

It has recently been shown [12] that loop diuretics are secreted by the proximal tubule via basolateral uptake through the so-called PAH-system. This prompted us to ask whether the secretion of all used loop diuretics is equally sensitive towards an inhibitor of basolateral anion uptake, namely, probenecid [13]. This question could be clinically relevant because it cannot be anticipated that proximal secretion of all loop diuretics would be equally affected by other organic acids such as probenecid.

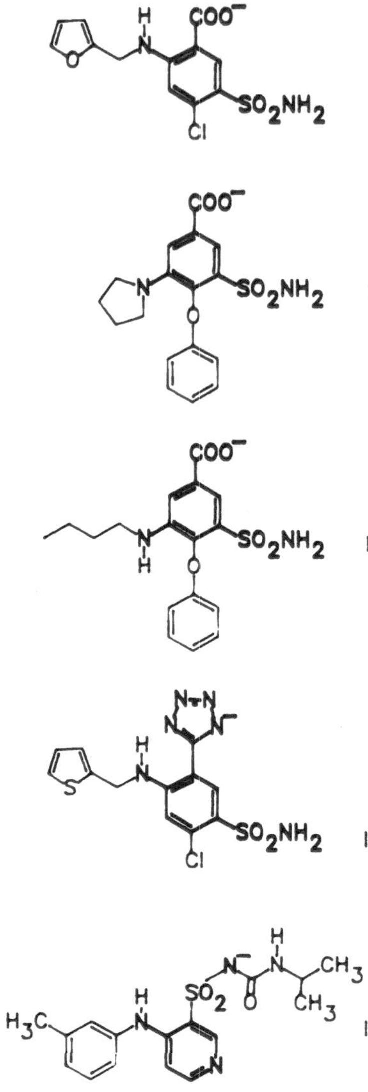

Furosemide
IC_{50}: $3 \cdot 10^{-6}$ mol/l

Piretanide
IC_{50}: $1 \cdot 10^{-6}$ mol/l

Bumetanide
IC_{50}: $2 \cdot 10^{-7}$ mol/l

Azosemide
IC_{50}: $6 \cdot 10^{-6}$ mol/l

Torasemide
IC_{50}: $3 \cdot 10^{-7}$ mol/l

Fig. 1. Chemical structures of diuretics and the concentrations required for half maximal inhibition of equivalent short circuit current (IC_{50} values) in isolated in vitro perfused rabbit thick ascending limbs of Henle's loop

Figure 2 summarizes the results from rat clearance experiments for PIR, BUM, FUR, and AZO. It is evident that comparable diuretic responses to any of these diuretics were almost equally attenuated by increasing doses of probenecid. These findings indicate: (1) The secretion of all these loop diuretics is highly relevant for their effect in the TAL segment. The increase in luminal concentration by secretion

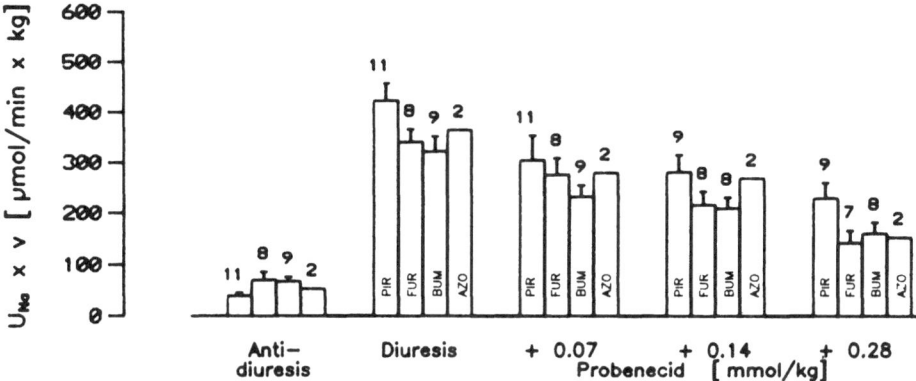

Fig. 2. Rat clearance experiments. Urinary Na^+ (U_{Na}) excretion is given for the control period, after the respective diuretic, and after additional application of probenecid. Note that probenecid attenuates the natriuretic response equally well for all diuretics used. Attenuation of the diuretic response to FUR, furosemide, 90 μmol/kg prime and same dose over one hour; PIR, piretanide, 17 μmol/kg and same dose over one hour; BUM, bumetanide, 27 μmol/kg and same dose over one hour; and AZO, azosemide, 90 μmol/kg and same dose over one hour, by increasing doses of probenecid (0.07–0.28 mmol/kg)

and by water reabsorption is the only cause for the organ selectivity of these drugs. In fact, the $Na^+2Cl^-K^+$ cotransporter is present in many cells of the body, and its sensitivity towards loop diuretics appears to be similar in all these cells [2,14]. (2) None of the diuretics tested has any detectable advantage over the others, i.e., a comparable diuretic effect is attenuated in a comparable way by probenecid, irrespective of the diuretic used. This finding is surprising, since the doses of the diuretics used were quite different: 17 μmol/kg of PIR, 27 μmol/kg of BUM, 90 μmol/kg of FUR and AZO. The finding may be explained by the presence of affinity sequences for the basolateral membrane organic anion transporter comparable to those on the $Na^+2Cl^-K^+$ cotransporter.

All Loop Diuretics Inhibit in Their Anionic Form

Previous data has suggested that all loop diuretics act in their anionic form [7]. For example, the pK_a of 3.6 for FUR predicts that some 99.9% of the total luminal concentration of FUR will be in the anionic form. On the other hand, we have found that TOR and its derivatives are also strong inhibitors of the $Na^+2Cl^-K^+$ cotransporter [8,15], but the pK_a values of these compounds are much less acidic. Recently, we examined even less acidic derivatives [16] with pK_a values as high as 9.0, and found that these substances were still strong inhibitors of the $Na^+2Cl^-K^+$ cotransporter in the rabbit cTAL segment. In the case of the compound BM 10 (cf Fig. 4), pK_a value 9.0, only 2.5% would be anionic at pH 7.4, at which pH we carried out the experiments. Rabbit cTAL segments were perfused with solutions containing 0.5 μmol/l

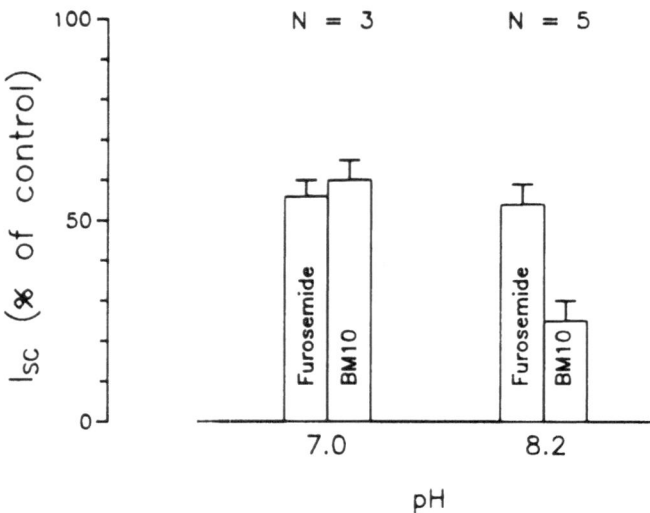

Fig. 3. pH dependence of the inhibitory effect of a sulfonylurea diuretic (BM 10, structural formula c.f. Fig. 4) in isolated perfused rabbit cTAL segments. The remaining equivalent short circuit current (I_{SC}) (in percent of control) is shown for different luminal pH values. The total concentration of BM 10 was 0.5 µmol/l at both pH values. The anionic form was 0.005 and the protonated form 0.495 µmol/l at pH 7.0, and 0.07 and 0.43 µmol/l, respectively, at pH 8.2. Note that the anionic form determines the inhibitory effect

BM 10 at various pH-values. The results are shown in Fig. 3. It is evident that the inhibitory effect is enhanced with alkaline pH. This indicates that only the anionic moiety of this compound interacts with the $Na^+2Cl^-K^+$ cotransporter. By extension, this finding implies that the IC_{50}-value for this compound, which was determined at pH 7.4, would be almost two decades lower if expressed as the concentration of the anionic moiety of this compound (IC_{50} = 12 nmol/l instead of 0.5 µmol/l).

Inhibitors of the $Na^+2Cl^-K^+$ Cotransporter can be Designed as Highly Lipophilic Compounds

Most loop diuretics are rather hydrophilic (FUR, PIR, BUM, AZO). Only TOR shows an octanol/water partition of around 3. It was tempting to examine whether one could design even more lipophilic compounds related to TOR, which would still be inhibitors of the $Na^+2Cl^-K^+$ cotransporter [16]. This effort was triggered by the hypothesis that such compounds would dissolve into a larger volume of distribution and, hence, would be excreted more slowly. Furthermore, such compounds might be able to cross the blood brain barrier more easily and have direct effects on the volume of glial cells (BM and JD unpublished work). Figure 4 shows several derivates of TOR and summarizes the pK_a values, the octanol/water partition (as log P = [octanol]/[water]), and the IC_{50} value in rabbit cTAL segments. It is evident that the

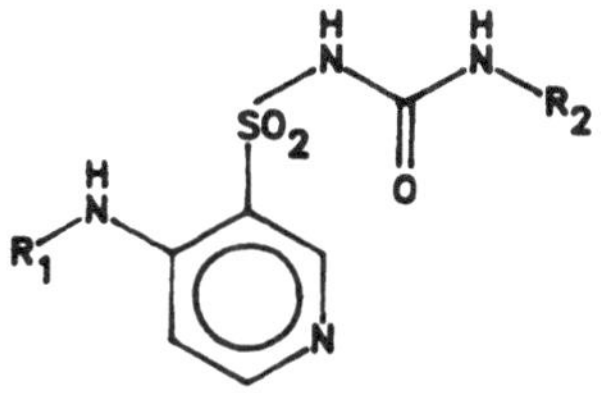

	R_1	R_2	pKa	log P	IC_{50}	IC_{50}^{cor}
					(umol/l)	
TOR	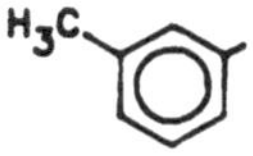 (3-methylphenyl)	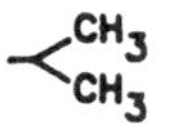 CH(CH$_3$)$_2$	6·82	0·449	0·30	0·24
BM2	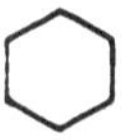 cyclohexyl	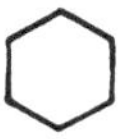 cyclohexyl	9·03	1·331	19	0·43
BM8	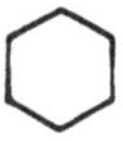 cyclohexyl	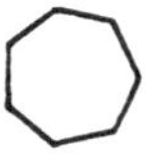 cycloheptyl	9·39	1·717	9·6	0·097
BM4	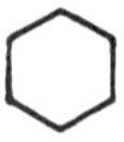 cyclohexyl	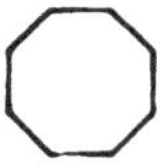 cyclooctyl	9·15	2·074	14	0·24
BM3	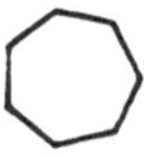 cycloheptyl	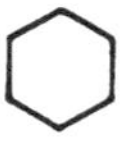 cyclohexyl	9·30	1·665	3·5	0·043
BM27	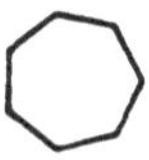 cycloheptyl	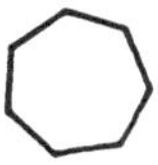 cycloheptyl	n·t·	2·062	2·8	n·t·
BM10	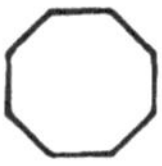 cyclooctyl	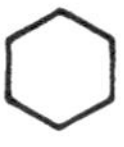 cyclohexyl	8·98	2·063	0·47	0·012
BM6	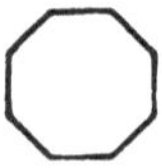 cyclooctyl	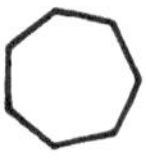 cycloheptyl	9·13	2·449	2·0	0·036
BM9	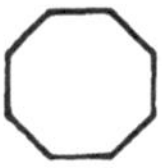 cyclooctyl	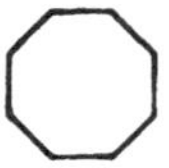 cyclooctyl	7·70	2·704	0·56	0·18

Fig. 4. Lipophilic sulfonylurea diuretic compounds. The chemical structure, the pK$_a$ value, the log of the octanol/water partition (log P), the total luminal concentration for half maximal inhibition of equivalent short circuit current in isolated perfused rabbit cTAL segments (IC_{50} in μmol/l), and the concentration of the anionic form (IC_{50}^{cor}) are given for the individual compounds. Note that the highly lipophilic compound BM 10 has a very strong inhibitory effect R_1, radical 1; R_2, radical 2

tolyl and isopropyl residues of TOR can be replaced by cyclo-alkyls. This leads to an increase in the octanol/water partition, an increase in pK_a value, and a reduction in the IC_{50} value, indicating that these compounds have a very high affinity for the $Na^+2Cl^-K^+$ cotransporter. An optimal structure is, e.g., the compound BM 10, with apparent IC_{50} values of 0.5 μmol/l. The IC_{50} values would be even smaller if one took into account the finding above that the inhibition was caused only by the anionic moiety (IC_{50}^{cor} values in Fig. 4). We conclude that it is possible to design highly lipophilic loop diuretics which may offer some therapeutical advantages.

The Interaction with the $Na^+2Cl^-K^+$ Cotransporter in the Luminal Membrane of the cTAL Segment Occurs at an Extracellular Binding Site

Several findings have suggested that drugs like FUR need not be incorporated into the cTAL cell to exert their effect. (i) We have noted that the effect of FUR [1] and of PIR [4] was instantaneous and rapidly reversible. Inhibition occurred as rapidly as we were able to change the lumen perfusate ($\ll 1$ s), and recovery after removal of the drugs was complete within a few seconds. These findings would not be expected for a compound entering the cell. (ii) We measured the cytosolic Cl^--activity with ion selective microelectrodes in cTAL cells [17]. The used ion exchanger was several hundreds of times more sensitive for FUR when compared to Cl^-. Still, we were able to show that the apparent cytosolic Cl^--activity signal fell rapidly after the addition of furosemide. Both arguments, even though strongly suggestive, do not prove that FUR interacts at the extracellular side. Therefore, we designed macromolecular probes of piretanide, with a molecular mass of 5300 daltons, and examined their effects in rabbit cTAL segments [18]. We found that dextran as well as polyethyleneglycol macromolecules inhibited the $Na^+2Cl^-K^+$ cotransporter with IC_{50} values very similar to those for PIR. Hence, we conclude that the binding site for loop diuretics of the $Na^+2Cl^-K^+$ cotransporter is easily accessible at the extracellular side of the luminal membrane. These and other macromolecular probes of PIR are currently used to design antibodies against the $Na^+2Cl^-K^+$ carrier. When given systematically these macromolecular PIR derivatives show only a very moderate diuresis. This indicates that these substances cannot be secreted by the proximal tubule (c.f. above).

Macula Densa Cells Sense Luminal NaCl Concentration via Furosemide Sensitive $Na^+2Cl^-K^+$ Cotransport

It has been known for some time that loop diuretics inhibit the so called feedback response between macula densa cells and single nephron filtration rate [19]. Furthermore, it has been shown that the feedback response is produced by luminal Na^+ [20] or Cl^- concentration [21]. This has prompted us to examine directly whether macula densa cells possess the $Na^+2Cl^-K^+$ cotransporter. We used an electrophysiological approach to examine this question. Rabbit cTAL segments with the glomerulus and

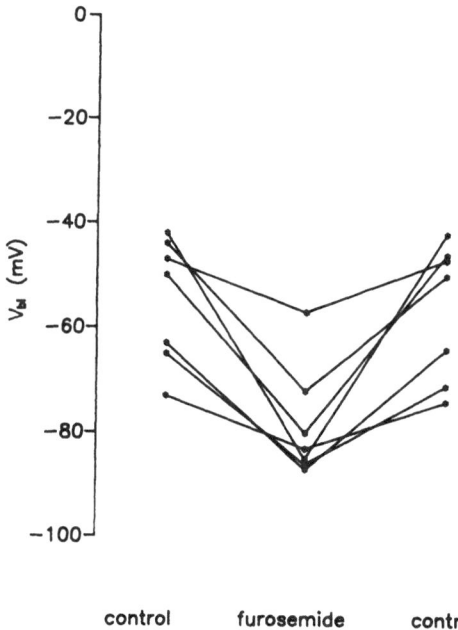

Fig. 5. Basolateral membrane voltage (V_{bl}) of macula densa cells of isolated in vitro perfused rabbit cTAL segments containing the macula densa region. Note that V_{bl} is hyperpolarized by luminal furosemide (10 μmol/l)

the macula densa segment attached were perfused in vitro and the transepithelial voltages, as well as the membrane voltage across the basolateral membrane, of macula densa cells was examined [22]. The key finding is shown in Fig. 5. The basolateral membrane voltage (V_{bl}) of macula densa cells hyperpolarized by some 14 mV when FUR was added to the luminal perfusate. Similarly, a hyperpolarization of V_{bl} was observed when the NaCl concentration in the lumen was reduced from 150 to 30 mmol/l. Examination of the conductance properties of these cells revealed that the luminal membrane was K^+-, and the basolateral membrane was Cl^--conductive [22]. All these findings are compatible with the view that the luminal membrane of macula densa cells is equipped with the $Na^+2Cl^-K^+$ cotransporter, and that the general cell model of the macula densa cells is identical to that described for the TAL segment [2,23]. It should be noted, however, that the transport rates across macula densa cells are much lower than those across the TAL segment [22]. Thus, it is likely that the $Na^+2Cl^-K^+$ carrier-mediated uptake in macula densa cells serves to sense the concentrations in the tubule lumen and to trigger a, thus far unknown, transducing mechanism which translates the cytosolic signal in macula densa cells into the response of renin producing cells.

Acknowledgments. Supported by Deutsche Forschungsgemeinschaft Gr 480/10 and by German Israeli Foundation GIF I-86-100.1/88.

References

1. Greger R, Schlatter E (1983) Cellular mechanism of the action of loop diuretics on the thick ascending limb of Henle's loop. Klin Wochenschr 61:1019–1027
2. Greger R (1985) Ion transport mechanisms in thick ascending limb of Henle's loop of mammalian nephron. Physiol Rev 65:760–797
3. Greger R (1985) Wirkung von Scheifendiuretika auf zellulärer Ebene. Nieren-Hochdruck-krankheiten 14(6):217–220
4. Greger R, Wangemann PH (1987) Loop diuretics. Renal Physiol 10:174–183
5. Eveloff J, Bayerdörffer E, Silva P, Kinne R (1981) Sodium-chloride transport in the thick ascending limb of Henle's loop. Oxygen consumption studies in isolated cells. Pflugers Arch 389:263–270
6. Brezis M, Rosen S, Silva P, Epstein FH (1984) Renal ischaemia: A new perspective. Kidney Int 26:375–383
7. Schlatter E, Greger R, Weidtke C (1983) Effect of "high ceiling" diuretics on active salt transport in the cortical thick ascending limb of Henle's loop of rabbit kidney. Correlation of chemical structure and inhibitory potency. Pflugers Arch 396:210–217
8. Wittner M, Di Stefano A, Wangemann P, Delarge J, Ligeois JF, Greger R (1987) Analogues of torasemide-structure function relationships. Experiments in the thick ascending limb of the loop of Henle of rabbit nephron. Pflugers Arch 408:54–62
9. Greger R, Lang HJ, Englert HC, Wangemann P (1987) Blockers of the Na$^+$2Cl$^-$K$^+$ carrier and of chloride channels in the thick ascending limb of the loop of Henle. In: Puschett JB (ed) Diuretics II. Elsevier, Amsterdam, pp 33–38
10. Greger R, Wangemann P, Wittner M, Di Stefano A, Lang HJ, Englert HC (1987) Blockers of active transport in the thick ascending limb of the loop of Henle. In: Andreucci VE, Dal Canton A (eds) Diuretics: Basic, pharmacological, and clinical aspects. Martinus Nijhoff, Boston, pp 33–38
11. Wangemann P, Wittner M, Di Stefano A, Englert HC, Lang HJ, Schlatter E, Greger R (1987) Cl$^-$-channel blockers in the thick ascending limb of the loop of Henle. Structure activity relationship. Pflugers Arch 407(Suppl 2):S128–S141
12. Ullrich KJ, Rumrich G, Klöss S (1989) Contraluminal organic anion and cation transport in the proximal renal tubule: V. Interaction with sulfamoyl- and phenoxy diuretics, and with β-lactam antibiotics. Kidney Int 36:78–88
13. Braitsch R, Lohrmann E, Greger R (1990) Effect of probenecid on loop diuretic induced saluresis and diuresis. In: Puschett J (ed) Diuretics III, chemistry, pharmacology, and clinical applications. Elsevier, New York, pp 137–139
14. Greger R (1986) Chlorid-transportierende Epithelien. In: Bromm B (ed) Physiologie Aktuell, Band 2. Gustav Fischer, Stuttgart, pp 47–58
15. Wittner M, Di Stefano A, Schlatter E, Delarge J, Greger R (1986) Torasemide inhibits NaCl reabsorption in the thick ascending limb of the loop of Henle. Pflugers Arch 407:611–614
16. Lohrmann E, Masereel B, Nitschke R, Pirotte B, Delarge J, Greger R (1990) Action of diuretics at the cellular level. In: Reyes AJ (ed) Diuretics. Gustav Fischer, Stuttgart, in press
17. Greger R, Oberleithner H, Schlatter E, Cassola AC, Weidtke C (1983) Chloride activity in cells of isolated perfused cortical thick ascending limbs of rabbit kidney. Pflugers Arch 399:29–34
18. Nitschke R, Schlatter E, Eidelman O, Lang HJ, Englert HC, Cabantchik ZI, Greger R (1989) Piretanide-dextran and piretanide-polyethylene glycol interact with high affinity with the Na$^+$ 2Cl$^-$ K$^+$ cotransporter in the thick ascending limb of the loop of Henle. Pflugers Arch 413:559–561

19. Wright FS, Schnermann J (1974) Interference with feedback control of glomerular filtration rate by furosemide, triflocin and cyanide. J Clin Invest 53:1695–1708
20. Thurau K, Schnermann J (1965) Die Natriumkonzentration an den Macula Densa Zellen als regulierender Faktor für das Glomerulumfiltrat (Mikropunktionsversuche). Klin Wochenschr 43:410–413
21. Schnermann J, Ploth DW, Hermle M (1976) Activation of tubuloglomerular feedback of chloride transport. Pflugers Arch 362:229–240
22. Schlatter E, Salomonsson M, Persson AEG, Greger R (1989) Macula densa cells sense luminal NaCl concentration via the furosemide sensitive Na-2Cl-K cotransporter. Pflugers Arch 414:286–290
23. Greger R, Schlatter E (1981) Presence of luminal K^+, a prerequisite for active NaCl transport in the thick ascending limb of Henle's loop of rabbit kidney. Pflugers Arch 392:92–94

Biochemical Action of Loop Diuretics

Yoshimasa Orita[1], Masaru Yamazaki[2], and Yoshifumi Fukuhara[3]

SUMMARY. We have investigated the quantum-chemical and physico-chemical properties of hydrochlorothiazide and its related molecules. Negative charge of the 7th carbon in the benzothiadiazine ring, hydrophobicity, and van der Walls volume, play important roles in contacting the sodium chloride channel of the renal tubule. Binding of hydrochlorothiazide to erythrocytes of human and rabbit was analyzed. Three different binding sites were demonstrated. This property could contribute to the high bioavailability and long duration of mild diuretic activity of hydrochlorothiazide. Ethacrynic acid acts as both an uncoupler and an inhibitor of the electron transport system of mitochondria. These biochemical properties of ethacrynic acid might be one of the causes of its inhibition of sodium chloride transport in the thick ascending limb of Henle's loop.

Introduction

The site of action of diuretics in the nephron has been extensively studied [1,2]. The physiological basis of the mode of action of diuretics also has been explored [3,4]. But few studies on the biochemical properties of diuretics have been reported. Since physiological function is supported by biochemical reaction or process, attention should be paid to the biochemical properties of diuretics. Recently, the molecular structure of transporter and channel was clarified by molecular biological techniques [5]. The interaction of these molecules and diuretics under physico-chemical forces might be expected. The physico-chemical properties of diuretics should be explored.

[1]College of Biomedical Technology Osaka University, 1-1, Machikaneyama-cho, Toyonaka, 560 Japan
[2]Faculty of Pharmaceutical Science Osaka University, 1-6, Yamadaoka, Suita, 565 Japan
[3]Department of Medicine, Osaka University Medical School, 1-1-50, Fukushima, Fukushima-ku, Osaka, 553 Japan

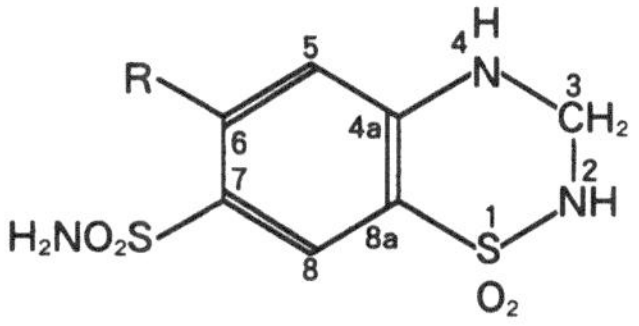

R	diuretic activity
Cl	+ + + +
NO₂	+ + +
OCH₃	+ +
CH₃	+
F	+
NH₂	−
H	−

Fig. 1. Diuretic activity of hydrochlorothiazide and its related molecules (deStevens)

Quantum-Chemical and Physico-Chemical Properties of Hydrochlorothiazide

The chemical structure of hydrochlorothiazide and its related molecules are shown in Fig. 1 [6]. The molecular geometry of hydrochlorothiazide is cited from an X-ray crystallographic study [7]. To examine the electronic effect of the sulfamoyl group on the benzothiadiazine ring, the electronic state of imaginary molecules with substituents in the 7th carbon of the benzothiadiazine ring were also calculated. The substituents were chloride, methyl, amino, fluorine, methoxy, hydrogen, and amino [8]. Molecular orbital calculation with CNDO/2 (complete neglect of differential overlap, all valenced electron approximation with $3d\pi$) was carried out.

The van der Waals volume of the substituents of the 7th carbon was calculated by Bondi's method. The hydrophobic parameter of Hansch was used. It was found that the negative charge of the 7th carbon in the benzothiadiazine ring seems to be essential to diuretic activity. Diuretic activity, van der Waals volume, and the hydrophobic parameter of the substituent of the 6th carbon in hydrochlorothiazide and its related molecules are shown in Table 1. The highest index of correlation was obtained by the regression equation

Table 1. Diuretic activity, van der Waals volume, and the hydrophobic parameter of hydrochlorothiazide and its related molecules

Substituent of the 6th position	Diuretic activity[a]	van der Waals volume[b]	Hydrophobic parameter[c]
Cl	4+	0.178	0.71
CH₃	1+	0.167	0.56
OCH₃	2+	0.248	−0.02
NO₂	3+	0.200	−0.28
H	−	0.013	0.00
NH₂	−	0.112	−1.23

[a] By deStevens in the dog
[b] By Bondi's method
[c] By C. Hansch

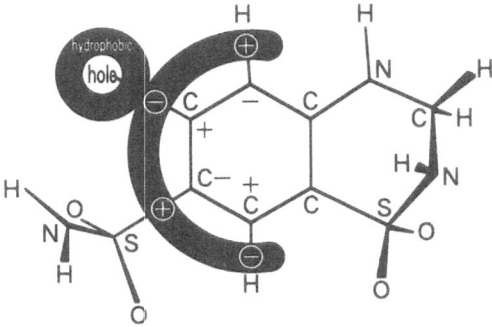

Fig. 2. A proposed model of the interaction site for thiazide diuretics in the apical membrane of the distal convoluted tubule. (From [8] with permission)

$$\ln y = 0.2695 \times 10^{-3}\, \pi + 7.62535\ \text{V.W.} + 15.7681\ \text{Fc}_7 + 0.98501$$

where $r = 0.980$ $(P < 0.01)$

π, hydrophobic parameter of the substituent of the 6th carbon;
V.W., van der Waals volume of the substituent of the 6th carbon;
Fc_7, the formal charge of the 7th carbon.

We proposed a model of the action site of hydrochlorothiazide in the tubular membrane, particularly the apical side of the distal convoluted tubule (Fig. 2). This site consisted of a rather larger hydrophobic (lipophilic) hole and an electrostatic reaction with a positive charge to the negative charge of the 7th carbon of the benzothiadiazine ring of hydrochlorothiazide. The result shown in Table 1 suggests that the van der Waals volume has a close relation to diuretic activity. The significance of the van der Waals volume in the biological membrane has been pointed out [9,10]. Considering the lipid rich biological membrane and an electrostatic interaction between diuretics and the sodium chloride channel consisting of polypeptide, the proposed site of action of hydrochlorothiazide in the sodium chloride channel in the distal convoluted tubule seems to be reasonable. Hydrochlorothiazide has been reported to be excreted in the urine in unchanged form [11,12]. Hydrochlorothiazide could act on the channel of the distal convoluted tubule before being excreted in the urine.

Binding of Hydrochlorothiazide to Erythrocyte

We have already reported that concentrations of hydrochlorothiazide in the erythrocytes of humans and animals were always about ten times higher than those in plasma [11]. We have attempted to clarify the kinetics of hydrochlorothiazide binding to erythrocyte [13]. Fresh blood was drawn from rabbits and immediately centrifuged to separate erythrocytes. The erythrocytes were suspended in phosphate buffered saline (PBS) containing varying amounts of hydrochlorothiazide (1, 10, 100 µg/ml). These samples were incubated at 37°C for up to 4 hours; after incubation, the samples were centrifuged and hemolyzed. Hydrochlorothiazide concentration in erythrocytes was determined using column chromatography on Sephadex G-75 [14].

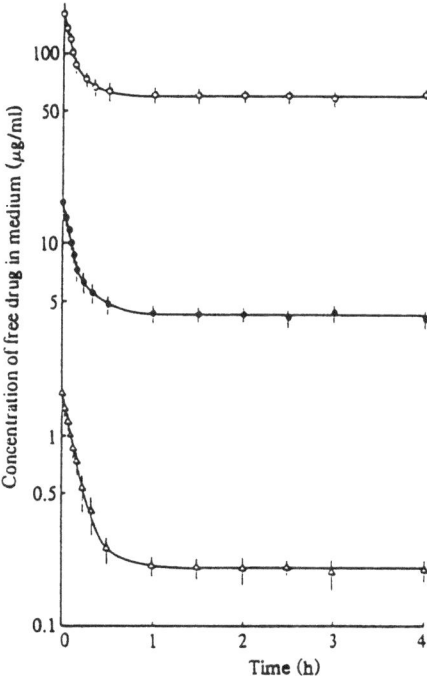

Fig. 3. Decrease of hydrochlorothiazide in the incubation medium by uptake by erythrocytes. Each point represents the mean ± S.D. of four data. Initial concentration in erythrocyte suspension: 100 μg/ml (○), 10 μg/ml (●), 1 μg/ml (△). (From [13] with permission)

Using a similar experimental method, the effect of HgCl$_2$ or acetazolamide on hydrochlorothiazide binding to erythrocytes was studied.

The disappearance kinetics of hydrochlorothiazide in PBS for up to 4 hours are shown in Fig. 3. The kinetics showed similar monoexponential curves. Percentage binding by erythrocytes was 65%, 75%, and 88% at 100, 10, and 1 μg/ml of the initial hydrochlorothiazide concentration respectively. Preincubation of erythrocytes with HgCl$_2$ had no affect on the uptake amount of hydrochlorothiazide (Table 2). On

Table 2. Effect of HgCl$_2$ and acetazolamide on the binding of hydrochlorothiazide to erythrocyte

Inhibitor	Concentration (μM)	Amount of hydrochlorothiazide in erythrocyte (%)
HgCl$_2$	0	100.0 ± 1.2
	5.00	102.2 ± 2.8
	10.00	97.6 ± 3.5
Acetazolamide	1.67	98.6 ± 2.9
	16.7	87.4 ± 2.3
	167.00	73.2 ± 5.3

Each value represents the mean ± S.D. of 5 experiments. The concentration of hydrochlorothiazide in suspension is 16.7 μM. (From [13] with permission)

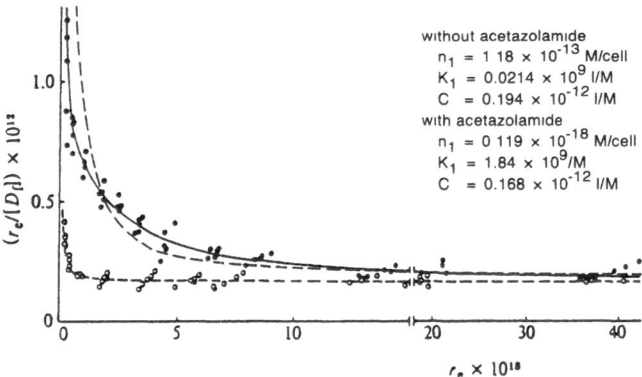

Fig. 4. Scatchard plot of the binding of hydrochlorothiazide with ($\bigcirc$) and without ($\bullet$) acetazolamide. The *broken lines* are the least-square regression line obtained from Eq. 3 as 3-parameter model. The *solid line* is obtained from Eq. 4 as 5-parameter model. (See text for equations). (From [13] with permission)

the other hand, acetazolamide, an inhibitor of carbonic anhydrase, dose-dependently significantly decreased the uptake of hydrochlorothiazide (Table 2). These data were converted to a Scatchard plot (Fig. 4); r_e is the number of moles of hydrochlorothiazide bound per erythrocyte and $[D_f]$ is the concentration of free hydrochlorothiazide. The curve for hydrochlorothiazide binding without acetazolamide has a curvature with nearly horizontal asymptote at higher r_e. The addition of acetazolamide discharged the majority of the first phase observed at lower r_e, but the phase characterized by extremely high affinity and low capacity still remained. Blanchard et al. [15] reported a model with three parameters to describe binding data involving multiple binding sites (equation 3).

$$r/[D_f] = n_1 K_1/(1 + K_1[D_f]) + C$$

$$r = [D_b]/[M_t]$$

where r is the number of moles of preservative bound per mole of macromolecule;
$[D_f]$ and $[D_b]$ are the concentrations of free and bound drug, respectively;
$[M_t]$ is the concentration of macromolecule;
K_1 is the association constant;
n_1 is the number of binding sites per macromolecule;
$C = n_2 K_2$

The parameters were calculated by the non-linear least-squares computer program MULTI [16]. The theoretical lines obtained are illustrated as broken lines in Fig. 4.

By analysis of the curve of hydrochlorothiazide binding with acetazolamide, the presence of binding sites showing an extremely high binding affinity was observed. The model with five parameters was used and the plots for hydrochlorothiazide binding without acetazolamide were fitted for the equation (equation 4) which is written as:

$$\frac{r_e}{[D_f]} = \frac{n_1 K_1}{1 + K_1[D_f]} + \frac{n_2 K_2}{1 + K_2[D_f]} + C$$

The parameters obtained were as follows: K_1, 1.84×10^9 l/M; K_2, 0.158×10^6 l/M; n_1, 0.119×10^{-18} M/cell; n_2, 3.21×10^{-18} M/cell; C, 0.170×10^{-12} l/M

    r_c: the number of moles of drug preservatively bound per mole of macromolecule

K_1,K_2: the association constant of the first binding site and the second binding site, respectively;

n_1,n_2: the number of the first binding sites per macromolecule and the second binding sites per maculomolecule respectively

The theoretical line obtained by this equation is shown as the solid line in Fig. 4. This line fitted well to the plots of hydrochlorothiazide binding without acetazolamide.

    The presence of a high capacity binding site in erythrocytes implies a high bioavailability of hydrochlorothiazide [17,18]. In a therapeutic range, the second sites (inhibited by acetazolamide) seem to play an important role, because serum hydrochlorothiazide concentration is about 1–10 μM. Long acting diuretic activity is explained by this binding ability of hydrochlorothiazide to erythrocytes.

Effect of Ethacrynic Acid on Mitochondrial Electron Transport System and Oxidative Phosphorylation

The physiological basis of the site of action of ethacrynic acid has been well defined [19,20]. However, some questions remain concerning the biochemical properties of ethacrynic acid. One perplexing problem is whether or not ethacrynic acid acts as an uncoupler [21–23]. We have attempted to determine whether ethacrynic acid is an uncoupler or not and whether it is an inhibitor of the electron transport system in mitochondria. The mitochondrial enzymes which are sensitive to ethacrynic acid

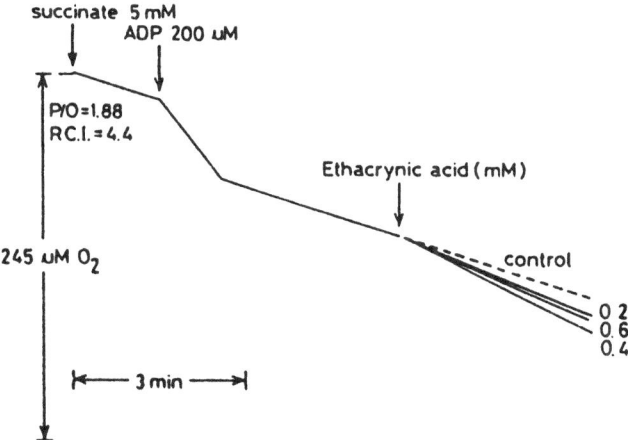

Fig. 5. The effect of ethacrynic acid on succinate oxidation in intact rat liver mitochondria (state 4). The final mitochondrial concentration was about 0.5 mg protein/ml. The cell volume of the oxygen electrode apparatus was 2.7 ml. (From [24] with permission)

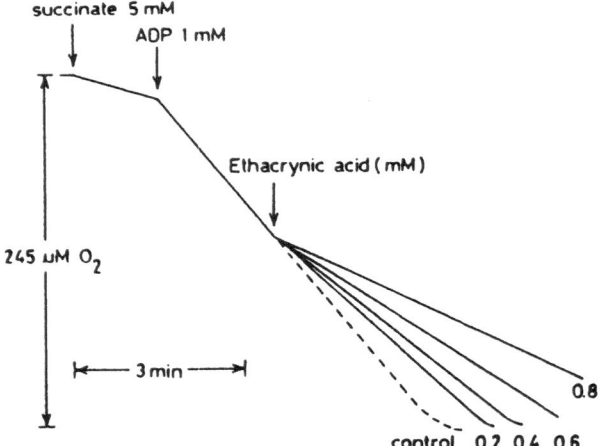

Fig. 6. The effect of ethacrynic acid on succinate oxidation in intact rat liver mitochondria (state 3). The final mitochondrial concentration was about 0.5 mg protein/ml. (From [24] with permission)

have not been identified. Another aim of this study was to identify the enzymes affected by ethacrynic acid.

Mitochondria were obtained from the liver, the renal cortex, and the renal medulla of the rat [24]. Further, mitochondria were obtained from the heart of freshly slaughtered cows [25].

Measurement of oxygen consumption was made with a galvanic electrode in each incubation medium [24]. Oxygen consumption of the mitochondria of rat liver, renal

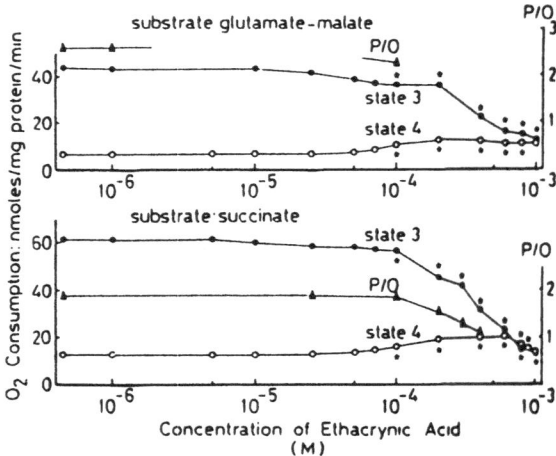

Fig. 7. The effect of ethacrynic acid on state 3 and state 4 respiration and P/O ratio of rat liver mitochondria. The final mitochondrial concentration was about 0.5 mg protein/ml. The results are the means of from two to eight experiments. *$P < 0.05$. (From [24] with permission)

cortex, and renal medulla was measured. Oxygen consumption of rat liver mitochondria treated with oligomycin was also measured. The P/O ratio was calculated by the method of Chance [26]. Using frozen bovine heart mitochondria, the enzyme activities of NADH (reduced form of nicotinamide adenine dinucleotide)-DCIP (2,6-dichloroindophenol) reductase, NADH-cytochrome c reductase, succinate dehydrogenase, and succinate-cytochrome c reductase were assayed [27].

As shown in Fig. 5, state 4 respiration of rat liver mitochondria in succinate oxidation was stimulated by ethacrynic acid.

Figure 6 shows that ethacrynic acid dose-dependently inhibited the respiration of phosphorylating mitochondria (state 3) in succinate oxidation. Ethacrynic acid stimulated state 4 respiration (substrate; glutamate-malate). On the other hand, ethacrynic acid inhibited state 3 respiration (substrate; glutamate-malate). Figure 7 shows the relationship between the concentration of ethacrynic acid and the respiration of mitochondria in rat liver. A slight, but significant, stimulation was observed at the concentration of 10^{-4} M/l. A significant inhibition of state 3 respiration was observed dose-dependently from the concentration of 10^{-4} M/l. The same effects of ethacrynic acid on mitochondria were observed in the mitochondria of renal cortex (Fig. 8). Ethacrynic acid at concentrations of 10^{-4} M/l, 5×10^{-4} M/l, and 10^{-3} M/l

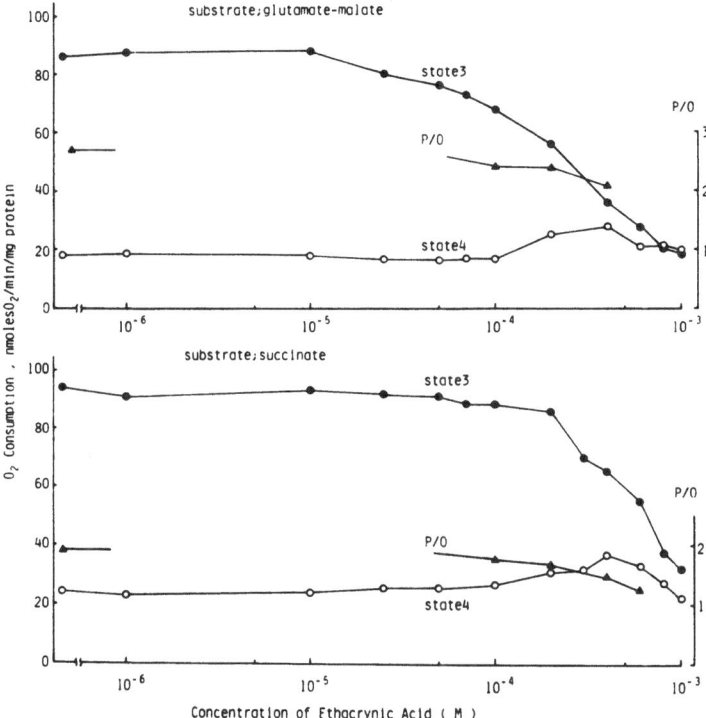

Fig. 8. The effect of ethacrynic acid on state 3 and state 4 respiration and P/O ratio in rat renal cortex mitochondria. Final mitochondrial concentrations used were about 0.5 mg protein/ml. The results are means of two to eight experiments. (From [24] with permission)

Table 3. The effects of ethacrynic acid on respiration inhibited by oligomycin

	Substrate: glutamate-malate	n	Substrate: succinate	n
Control	14.9 ± 0.6	4	15.1 ± 0.7	4
(ADP 500 μmol/l + oligomycin 1 μmol/l)				
Ethacrynic acid (mmol/l)				
0.1	16.3 ± 0.3*	4	16.8 ± 0.4*	4
0.5	21.4 ± 0.6***	4	20.0 ± 0.8**	4
1.0	17.9 ± 0.7*	4	14.1 ± 0.3	4
10.0	11.8 ± 0.6**	4	11.1 ± 0.4**	4

Rate of oxygen consumption expressed as nmol/mg protein per min
$*P < 0.01$, $**P < 0.005$, $***P < 0.001$
(From [24] with permission)

Table 4. The effects of ethacrynic acid (*EA*) on enzyme activities of bovine heart mitochondria

Enzyme	Control	n	EA 1 mmol/l	n	% inhibition
NADH-DCIP reductase[a]	150.0 ± 2.1	4	128.8 ± 2.5	4	14.2 $P < 0.001$
NADH-cytochrome c reductase[b]	440.7 ± 34.3	5	277.7 ± 12.3	5	37.0 $P < 0.005$
Succinate dehydrogenase[a]	106.7 ± 5.1	4	79.6 ± 2.2	4	25.4 $P < 0.005$
Succinate-cytochrome c reductase[b]	335.9 ± 7.7	4	255.9 ± 8.1	4	23.8 $P < 0.001$

[a]Expressed as nmol DCIP reduced/mg protein per min
[b]Expressed as nmol cytochrome c reduced/mg protein per min
(From [24] with permission)

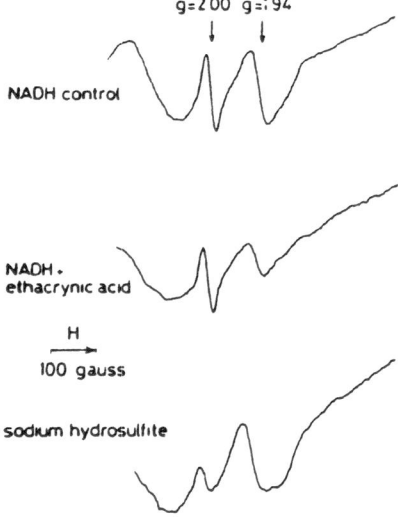

Fig. 9. The effect of ethacrynic acid on EPR absorption spectrum of bovine heart mitochondria. The EPR absorption spectrum is shown in the region between g = 3.0 and g = 1.0. Mitochondria were suspended at a concentration of about 30 mg protein/ml in 0.1 mol/l potassium phosphate buffer at pH 8.0 and 20 °C and were frozen in liquid nitrogen after 1 min incubation with 0.2 mmol/l NADH at 20 °C. All spectra were recorded at a sample temperature 100 °K. The EPR absorption spectrum of fully reduced mitochondria by the addition of hydrosulfite is shown in the *bottom* panel. EPR, electron paramagnetic resonance. (From [24] with permission)

stimulated the respiration of rat liver mitochondria inhibited by oligomycin, but a much higher concentration of ethacrynic acid (10^{-2}M/l) significantly inhibited this respiration when the substrate was glutamate-malate. When the substrate was succinate, ethacrynic acid at 10^{-4}M/l and 5×10^{-4}M/l stimulated the respiration of rat liver mitochondria inhibited by oligomycin. But a much higher concentration of ethacrynic acid (10^{-2}M/l) significantly inhibited this respiration (Table 3).

Ethacrynic acid at the concentration of 10^{-3}M/l significantly inhibited the activity of NADH-DCIP reductase and the activity of NADH-cytochrome c reductase in mitochondria of the frozen-thawed bovine heart (Table 4). The activity of succinate dehydrogenase and that of succinate-cytochrome c reductase were significantly inhibited by 10^{-3}M/l of ethacrynic acid.

Ethacrynic acid at the concentration of 10^{-3}M/l remarkably reduced the signal height in electron paramagnetic resonance (EPR) at electron value g = 1.94 of mitochondria of frozen-thawed bovine heart after 1 min incubation with 0.2 mM/l NADH (Fig 9). In contrast, when the substrate was succinate, reduction of signal height, g = 1.94 was not observed (Fig. 10).

The results obtained are summarized in Fig. 11. In general, uncouplers, such as dinitrophenol and pentachlorophenol, stimulate state 4 respiration at lower concentration and inhibit electron transport at higher concentration [28]. However, ethacrynic acid stimulates state 4 respiration and inhibits the electron transport system at the same concentration. To identify the site of electron transport inhibition,

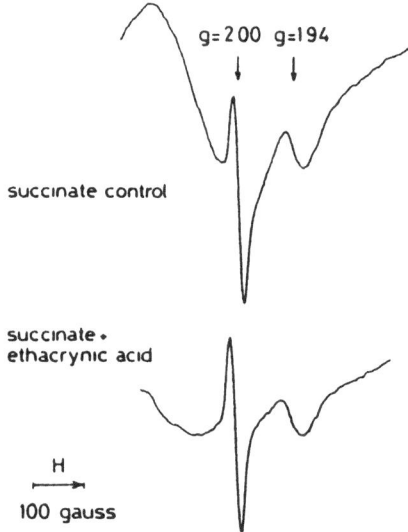

Fig. 10. The effect of ethacrynic acid on EPR absorption spectrum of bovine heart mitochondria. The EPR absorption spectrum is shown in the region between g = 3.0 and g = 1.0. Mitochondria were suspended at a concentration of about 30 mg protein/ml in 0.1 mol/l potassium phosphate buffer at pH 7.4 and 20°C and were frozen in liquid nitrogen after 1 min incubation with 10 mmol/l succinate at 20°C. All spectra were recorded at a sample temperature 100°K. EPR, electron paramagnetic resonance. (From [24] with permission)

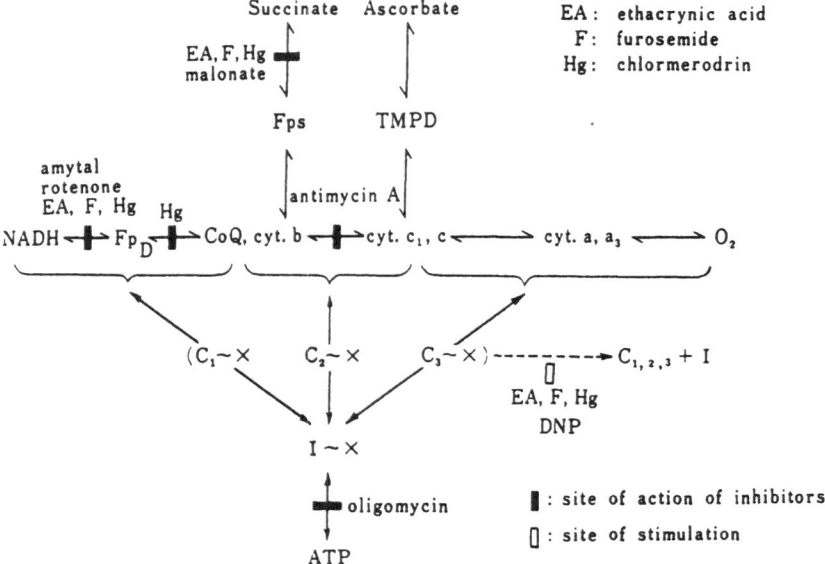

Fig. 11. A possible inhibitory site by some diuretics in the mitochondrial electron transport system. EA, ethacrynic acid; F, furosemide; Hg, chlormerodrin; TMPD, tetramethyl-*p*-phenyline-diamine; Fps, flavoproteins; DNP, 2,4-dinitrophenol

the effects of ethacrynic acid on the enzyme activities of the electron transport system were studied. The method of Hatefi [27] was used to purify the enzymes from bovine heart mitochondria. No differences have been observed between animal species and tissue types in the properties of electron transfer systems [29]. Our experimental results suggest that ethacrynic acid inhibits mitochondrial NADH dehydrogenase, since ethacrynic acid inhibited NADH-cytochrome c reductase more strongly than it inhibited NADH-DCIP reductase. Further, the results suggest that ethacrynic acid inhibits succinate dehydrogenase, but does not inhibit the electron transport system between succinate dehydrogenase and cytochrome c. In order to clarify the site of electron transport inhibition between NADH dehydrogenase and cytochrome c, the effects on ethacrynic acid of the reduction of nonhem iron were studied. The reduced form of nonhem iron has an EPR absorption at low temperature with a characteristic electron g value [29]. We have determined the reduction of non-hem iron by the signal height of the EPR spectrum at g = 1.94. Our results suggest that ethacrynic acid inhibits the electron transport system from flavin of NADH dehydrogenase to nonhem iron. Therefore, ethacrynic acid could inhibit the activity of NADH-cytochrome c reductase more strongly than it inhibits the activity of NADH-DCIP reductase, and could inhibit the activities of succinate dehydrogenase and succinate-cytochrome c reductase to a similar extent. We submit that ethacrynic acid inhibits the mitochondrial electron transport system at several sites: NADH dehydrogenase, succinate dehydrogenase, and the reduction of nonhem iron. Ethacrynic acid is considered to be one of the phenol derivatives [31]. The electron accepting nature of phenol derivatives was reported to be important for their uncoupling activity [32]. We have previously reported the electron accepting nature of ethacrynic acid [33]. These biochemical actions of ethacrynic acid were noted at concentrations above 10^{-4}M/l. This concentration is more than ten times that required to inhibit sodium transport of the isolated, perfused renal tubule [19]. However, in kidney slices ethacrynic acid was reported to accumulate in a concentration almost ten times that of the incubation medium [34]. This raises the possibility that ethacrynic acid inhibits sodium reabsorption by interfering with energy generation in the renal tubule.

References

1. Greger R, Frömter E (1980) Time course of oubain and furosemide effects on transepithelial potential difference in cortical thick ascending limbs of rabbit nephron. In: Kidney and body fluids. Pergamon, Budapest, p 375
2. Burg MB, Stoner L, Cardina J, Green N (1973) Furosemide effect on isolated perfused tubules. Am J Physiol 225:119-124
3. Malnic G, Klose RM, Giebisch G (1966) Micropuncture study of distal tubular potassium and sodium transport in rat nephron. Am J Physiol 211:529-547
4. Grantham JJ, Burg MB, Orloff J (1970) The nature of transtubular Na and K transport in isolated rabbit renal collecting duct. J Clin Invest 49:1815-1826
5. Hediger MA, Coady MJ, Ikeda TS, Wright EM (1987) Expression, cloning and cDNA sequencing of Na$^+$/glucose co-transporter. Nature 330:379-381
6. deStevens G (1963) Diuretics, chemistry and pharmacology. Academic, New York, p 99
7. Dupont L, Diedeberg O (1972) Structure cristalline et l'Hydrochlorothiazide. Acta Cryst B 28:2340-2347
8. Orita Y, Ando A, Yamabe S, Nakanishi T, Arakawa Y, Abe H (1983) Quantum-chemical and physico-chemical properties of hydrochlorothiazide. Arzneimittelforsch 33:688-691
9. Hansch C, Rockwell SD, Jow PY, Leo A, Stellar EE (1972) Substituent constants of correlation analysis. J Med Chem 20:304-308
10. Moriguchi I, Kanada Y (1977) Use of van der Waals volume in structure-activity studies. Chem Pharm Bull (Tokyo) 25:926-935
11. Orita Y, Nakanishi T, Nakahama H, Fukuhara Y, Ando A, Abe H, Yamazaki M, Itoh S, Itoh Y (1984) Diuretics I, Chemistry, Pharmacology, Clinical Applications. Elsevier, New York, pp 546-548
12. Patel RB, Patel UR, Rogge MC, Shah VP, Prasad VK, Selen A, Welling PG (1984) Bioavailability of hydrochlorothiazide from tablets and suspensions. J Pharm Sci 73:359-361
13. Yamazaki M, Itoh S, Okuda T, Tanabe K, Nakahama H, Fukuhara Y, Orita Y (1989) Binding of hydrochlorothiazide to erythrocytes. J Pharmacobiodyn 12:423-428
14. Dieterle W, Wangere J, Faigle J (1976) Binding of chlorthalidone to blood components in man. Eur J Clin Pharmacol 10:37-42
15. Blanchard J, Fink W, Duffy J (1977) Effect of sorbitol on interaction of phenolic preservatives with polysorbate. J Pharm Sci 66:1470-1473
16. Yamaoka K, Tanigawara Y, Nakagawa T, Uno T (1981) A pharmacokinetic analysis program (MULTI) for microcomputer. J Pharmacobiodyn 4:879-885
17. Yamazaki M, Itoh T, Yaginuma H, Itoh S, Kamada A, Orita Y, Nakama H, Nakanishi T, Ando A (1984) High-performance liquid chromatographic method of determination of hydrochlorothiazide in plasma, urine, blood cells and bile. Chem Pharm Bull (Tokyo) 32:2387-2394

18. Welling PG (1986) Pharmacokinetics of the thiazide diuretics. Biopharm Drug Dispos 7:501–535
19. Burg MB, Green N (1973) Effect of ethacrynic acid on the thick ascending limb of Henle's loop. Kidney Int 4:301–308
20. Greger R (1985) Ion transport mechanisms in thick ascending limb of Henle's loop of mammalian nephron. Physiol Rev 65:760–797
21. Sawa H, Weinman EJ, Hyde SE, Ekynoyan G (1976) Renal and hepatic mitochondrial effect of diuretics in the rat. Biochem Pharmacol 25:2649–2655
22. Mannuel MA, Weiner MW (1976) Effects of ethacrynic acid and furosemide on isolated rat kidney mitochondria. J Pharmacol Exp Ther 198:209–221
23. Landon EJ, Fritzpartick DF (1972) Ethacrynic acid and kidney cell metabolism. Biochem Pharmacol 21:1561–1568
24. Yanase M, Orita Y, Fukuhara Y, Okada N, Ando A, Abe H (1983) Effect of ethacrynic acid on mitochondrial electron transport system and oxidative phosphorylation. Arzneimittelforsch 33:120–124
25. Azzone GF, Colonna R, Zieche B (1979) Preparation of bovine heart mitochondria in high yield. Methods Enzymol 55:46–50
26. Chance B, Williams GR (1956) The respiratory chain and oxidative phosphorylations. Adv Enzymol 17:65–134
27. Hatefi Y, Haavik AG, Jurtshuk P (1961) Studies on the electron transport system, DPNH-cytochrome reductase. Biochim Biophys Acta 52:106–118
28. Heytler PG (1979) Uncouplers of oxidative phosphorylation. Methods Enzymol 55:462–472
29. Singer TP (1979) Mitochondrial electron-transport inhibitors. Methods Enzymol 55:454–462
30. Lehninger AL (1975) Biochemistry. Worth, New York, pp 477–508
31. Schultz EM, Cragoe EJ Jr, Bricking JB, Bolhofer WA, Sprague JM (1962) α, β-unsaturated ketone derivatives of aryloxyacetic acid acids, A new class of diuretics. J Med Pharmacol Chem 5:660–662
32. Kean EA (1968) An ihibitor of mitochondrial oxidations. Arch Biochem Biophys 127:528–533
33. Orita Y, Ando A, Takamitsu Y, Shirai D, Urakabe S, Furukawa T, Abe H (1968) A quantum biological analysis of thiazide diuretics and ethacrynic acid. Jpn Circ J 32:547–554
34. Charnock JS, Almeida AF (1972) Ethacrynic acid accumulation by renal tissue. Biochem Pharmacol 21:647–655

Molecular Properties of the Na-K-Cl-Cotransporter

Rolf K.H. Kinne[1]

SUMMARY. Since 1980, when the transporter was first characterized in Ehrlich Ascites tumor cells [1], the Na-K-Cl cotransport system has been found to play a major role in volume regulation in cells in general, and in transepithelial active chloride transport in epithelia in particular [2]. This contribution first summarizes our still very limited knowledge on the molecular properties, in the strictest sense, of the transport system and then deals with some peculiarities of the transporter which set it apart from other "simple" sodium cotransport systems: i.e., the polyfunctionality and variability of the transport activity. Finally the question of the intrarenal distribution of the transporter is addressed.

Molecular Properties

During recent years various laboratories have aimed to define the molecular weight of the cotransport system and to isolate it in an active form. A summary of these attempts is given in Table 1 [3–7]. In most instances the protein was identified by, or purified via, its interaction with loop diuretics. This interaction is dependent on the presence of sodium and potassium and requires in addition a small amount of chloride, higher chloride concentrations being inhibitory. These results indicate that the loop diuretics interact with the Na-K-Cl cotransport system at one of its anion binding sites [8]. Thus far the molecular weights proposed for the transporter vary, however, quite substantially. This might be due to a lack of specificity of labeling or might reflect an oligomeric structure of the protein—similar to that of the sodium-D-glucose cotransport system [9,10].

With regard to the specificity and affinity of the transporter for anions and cations the transport system has been relatively well characterized, as summarized in Table 2 [11–15]. The points worth mentioning are the very high affinity of the sodium and

---

[1]Max-Planck-Institut für Systemphysiologie, Rheinlanddamm 201, 4600 Dortmund, Federal Republic of Germany

Table 1. Tentative molecular mass of the Na-K-Cl cotransporter

Author	Method of identification	Material	Molecular mass	Comments
Haas & Forbush [4]	Photolabeling with [³H]-BSTBA, high affinity, potassium, sodium, and chloride dependence	Dog kidney membranes	~150 kDa	Nonreducing SDS-PAGE
Haas & Forbush [5]	Photolabeling with [³H]-bumetanide, high affinity	Dog kidney membranes	~150 kDa	
Feit et al. [6]	Affinity chromatography on bumetanide column	Ehrlich ascites cell plasma membranes	~135 kDa	Cholate gel
Kinne et al. (unpublished work)	Radiation inactivation	Rabbit kidney outer medulla microsomes	~76 kDa ~83 kDa	Reducing SDS-PAGE
Deutscher et al. (unpublished work)	Photolabeling with [³H]-bumetanide, chloride dependence	Shark rectal gland plasma membranes	~42 kDa	Reducing SDS-PAGE
	Affinity chromatography on piretanide column, chloride-dependent labeling of isolated protein with [³H]-bumetanide	Shark rectal gland plasma membranes	~42 kDa	Reducing SDS-PAGE
Haas & Forbush [4]	Photolabeling with [³H]-BSTBA, low affinity, sodium dependence of labeling	Dog kidney membranes	~50 kDa	Nonreducing SDS-PAGE
Jørgensen et al. [7]	Photolabeling with [³H]-bumetanide, competition with cold bumetanide	Rabbit kidney membranes	~34 kDa	Reducing SDS-PAGE

BSTBA, 4-benzoyl-5-sulfamoyl-3-(3-phenyloxy) benzoic acid; SDS-PAGE, sodium dodecylsulfate polyacrylamide gel electrophoresis

Table 2. Properties of the Na-K-Cl cotransporter in various renal cells

	Rabbit TALH [2,11–13]	LLC-PK$_1$ [14]	MDCK Cells [15]
Sodium binding site			
Affinity	1.8-3.5 mM	0.5 mM	9 mM
Specificity	Na > Li > > NH$_4$	ND	Na > Li
Potassium binding site			
Affinity	0.3 mM	ND	9 mM
Specificity	K = Rb > NH$_4$ > Cs	ND	K = Rb > NH$_4$ > Cs
Chloride binding site 1			
Affinity	~1.0 mM	~5.1 mM	ND
Specificity	Br = Cl > > J = NO$_3$ = SCN	ND	Br = Cl
Chloride binding site 2			
Affinity	~15 mM	~55.2 mM	~48 mM
Specificity	Br > Cl > J = NO$_3$ = SCN	ND	ND
Interaction with loop diuretics			
Affinity (bumetanide)	~10^{-6} M	~10^{-6} M	ND
Specificity	bumetanide > piretanide > furosemide		

TALH, thick ascending limb of Henle's loop; ND, not done

the potassium site of the transporter and the presence of two different anion binding sites. One site has a high affinity and selectivity for chloride (and bromide) and a second which, when the first binding site is occupied by chloride, shows a broad substrate specificity and is probably one site of interaction of the loop diuretics with the carrier. As depicted in Fig. 1 one diuretic with a very high affinity for the transporter is a molecule which carries a SO$_3$ at C$_1$ (Hoe 758) instead of a COO$^-$ as does furosemide. The SO$_3$ group probably interacts with the second anion binding site of the transporter as demonstrated recently by Shetlar et al. in Xenopus oocytes (R. Shetlar et al., unpublished work). However, substitutions at other positions of the diuretic also change the apparent affinity of the diuretic to the transporter. This holds, as demonstrated in Fig. 2, for positions at the aromatic ring, as well as for the deletion of the sulfamoyl group [16,17]. These results suggest a very complex and very flexible (cooperative) interaction of the transporter with its substrates as well as with its inhibitors.

With regard to the amino acid residues essential for these interactions, the study of George and Turner [18] is worth mentioning. In isolated basal-lateral plasma membrane vesicles of salivary glands it was demonstrated that N-ethylmaleimide — which interacts mainly with SH-groups — inhibits KCl-dependent ^{22}Na uptake. Substrate protection studies suggest that this SH-group is closely associated with the anion binding site to which loop diuretics also bind.

Further studies are needed to unravel the molecular basis of the Na-K-Cl cotransporter — a challenge endowed with a higher probability of success after the cloning of the Na-glucose cotransporter has been achieved [19].

Polyfunctionality of the Transporter

As is evident from the data presented in Table 2 on the substrate specificity of the Na-K-Cl cotransporter, NH$_4$ can very effectively and with a high affinity replace potassium at its binding site [20]. It can also substitute for potassium as a cotransported

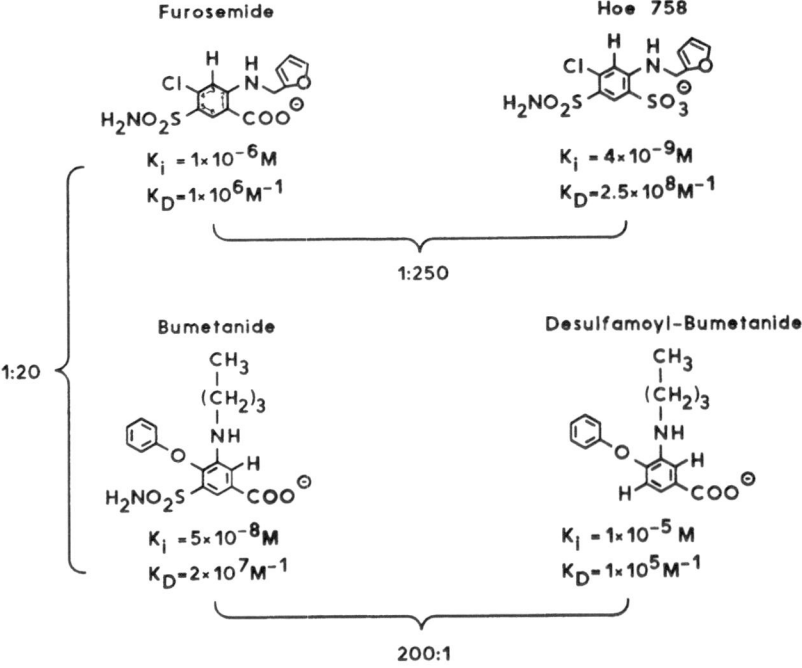

Fig. 1. Effect of side group modifications on the affinity of loop diuretics. K_i = concentration of the diuretic which led to 50% inhibition of transport activity in chloride-containing modified Ringer's solution. The numbers given in the figure compare relative affinities based on the ratios of the dissociation constants K_D. K_D values represent the reciprocals of the K_i values. (Data from [16] and [17])

ion. This results in a Na-NH$_4$-Cl cotransport which, together with a rather low permeability of the luminal thick ascending limb of Henle (TALH) membrane for NH$_3$, forms the basis for active ammonium reabsorption in this segment [21]. Thus, application of loop diuretics also interferes with the way in which ammonium is handled by the kidney. The same holds for anions other than chloride; as physiologically relevant iodide, which is also accepted by the anion binding site of the cotransporter, might be mentioned [13].

Variability of Cotransport Activity

Due to its high stoichiometry for chloride translocation and the coupling of sodium and chloride movement to an uptake of potassium into the cell, this transport system is exquisitely sensitive to alterations in transmembrane driving forces. Such an example is shown in Table 3, where the driving forces for the transporter at the beginning and at the end of the TALH have been estimated [22]. Assuming that the intracellular ion composition is identical, the decrease in intratubular sodium and chloride

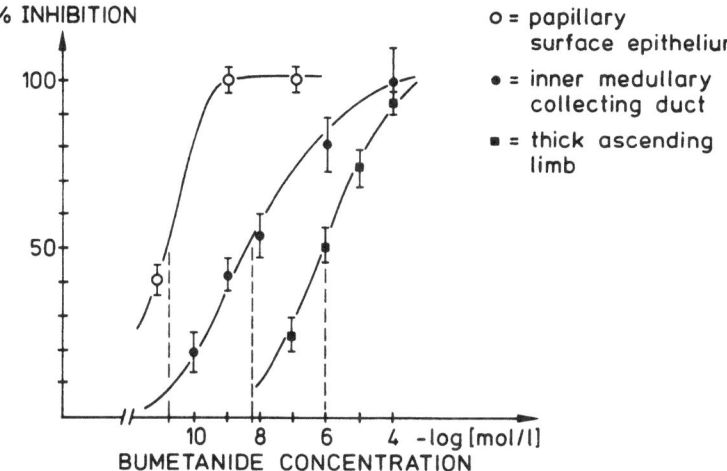

Fig. 2. Effect of bumetanide on Na-K-Cl cotransport in various renal epithelia. Data for the papillary surface epithelia are from [23]; data for the inner medullary collecting duct are from [24]. (After [3] with permission)

suffices to reduce the driving forces, and thereby active chloride transport, to zero. The same can be achieved by lowering the extracellular potassium content. Experiments in low potassium medium suggest that in such instances the transporter acts as a major potassium leak for the cell [15]. Similarly, changes in intracellular ion composition markedly affect the rate of Na-K-Cl cotransport. Thus, a decrease in intracellular chloride by stimulation of an independent chloride channel increases the rate of transport, as does an activation of the Na-K-ATPase [11]. Therefore, sometimes the responsiveness of the transporter to inhibitors such as the loop diuretics, as well as to endogenous regulators such as cAMP, cGMP, and antidiuretic hormone (ADH) might vary, depending on the experimental conditions employed. This different *set-point* of the transporter can explain the sometimes contradictory results [23].

Table 3. Driving forces for the Na-K-Cl cotransporter

	Luminal sodium	Luminal chloride	Luminal potassium	Driving force
Initial TALH	137 mM	150 mM	2.5 mM	
	$E_{Na} = 66$ mV	$E_{Cl} = 96$ mV	$E_K = -100$ mV	+62 mV
End of TALH	25–40 mM	25–40 mM	6.0 mM	
	$E_{Na} = 23$–34 mV	$E_{Cl} = 6.4$–30 mV	$E_K = -79$ mV	-49 / -15 mV
Intracellular ions	Na 10 mM			
	K 140 mM			
	Cl 22 mM			

Intrarenal Distribution of the Na-K-Cl Cotransport System

The renal Na-K-Cl cotransport system was first demonstrated in the thick ascending limb of Henle's loop (TALH) of mammals and in the diluting segment of amphibia and was considered to represent a transport system specific for this renal segment [11]. Accordingly, it was assumed that loop diuretics acted exclusively on this part of the nephron. In recent years, however, Na-K-Cl cotransport activity has been detected in the papillary surface epithelium of the rabbit [24], covering the surface of the renal papilla, and in isolated inner medullary collecting duct cells of rat kidney [25]. The sensitivity of these three renal Na-K-Cl cotransporters to inhibition by bumetanide is compared in Fig. 2. It is evident that within the rabbit kidney the transport system in the papillary surface epithelium is much more sensitive to the loop diuretic than the transport system in the TALH. The consequences of this additional action of loop diuretics have not been investigated thus far. It is interesting to note that the papillary surface epithelium has been postulated to participate in the exchange of water and solutes between pelvic urine and medullary tissue [26] and to facilitate the function of pelvic refluxes in aiding the diluting processes of the urine.

The transport activity found in rat inner medulla also seems to have a high sensitivity to loop diuretics. This transport system, as in other cells [27], is activated by cell shrinkage and mediates regulatory volume increase [28]; an inhibition of this system by diuretics might impair the capability of the collecting duct cells to regulate volume.

Conclusion

The renal Na-K-Cl cotransport system is thus far only poorly characterized with regard to its biochemical molecular properties; the biophysical events which ultimately lead to the translocation of the four ions are essentially unknown. Similarly, the detailed interactions of diuretics with the transporter remain to be elucidated. Phenomenologically and thermodynamically, the transporter is well characterized and some peculiarities such as high cooperativity, polyfunctionality, and variability of transport activity can be explained based on these phenomenological parameters. In considering the renal site of action of loop diuretics, recent evidence suggests that the transport system is not only present in the thick ascending limb of Henle's loop, but is also present distally in the inner medullary collecting duct and in the papillary surface epithelium. The extent to which the latter locations contribute to the action of diuretics or the extent to which they may lead to unexpected side effects remains to be determined.

Acknowledgment. The travel support by Hoechst Japan and Hoechst Germany is gratefully acknowledged. The skillful secretarial work of Mrs. D. Mägdefessel is also greatly appreciated.

References

1. Geck P, Heinz E (1986) The Na-K-2Cl cotransport system. J Membr Biol 91:97–105
2. Kinne R, Hannafin JA, König B (1985) Role of NaCl-KCl cotransport system in active chloride absorption and secretion. Ann NY Acad Sci 456:198–206

3. Kinne RKH (1989) The Na-K-Cl cotransporter in the kidney. Ann NY Acad Sci 574:63–74
4. Haas M, Forbush III B (1987) Photolabeling of a 150-kDa (Na + K + Cl) cotransport protein from dog kidney with a bumetanide analogue. Am J Physiol 253:C243–C250
5. Haas M, Forbush III B (1987) Na,K,Cl-cotransport system: characterization by bumetanide binding and photolabelling. Kidney Int 32:S134–S140
6. Feit PW, Hoffmann EK, Schiødt M, Kristensen P, Jessen F, Dunham PB (1988) Purification of proteins of the Na/Cl cotransporter from membranes of Ehrlich ascites cells using a bumetanide-sepharose affinity column. J Membr Biol 103:135–147
7. Jørgensen PL, Petersen J, Rees WD (1984) Identification of a Na⁺, K⁺, Cl⁻-cotransporter protein of M_r 34000 from kidney by photolabeling with [³H]bumetanide. The protein is associated with cytoskeleton components. Biochim Biophys Acta 775:105–110
8. Haas M, McManus TJ (1983) Bumetanide inhibits (Na + K + Cl) cotransport at a chloride site. Am J Physiol 245:C235–C240
9. Lin J-T, Szwarc K, Kinne R, Jung CY (1984) Structural state of the Na⁺/D-glucose cotransporter in calf kidney brush-border membranes. Target size analysis of Na⁺-dependent phlorizin binding and Na⁺-dependent D-glucose transport. Biochim Biophys Acta 777:201–208
10. Jung CY (1987) Radiation target size measurement of glucose transport function in animal cells. In: Venter JC, Jung CY (eds) Target-Size Analysis of Membrane Proteins. Alan R. Liss, New York, pp 137–151
11. Greger R (1985) Ion transport mechanisms in thick ascending limb of Henle's loop of mammalian nephron. Physiol Rev 65:760–797
12. Kinne RKH (1988) Sodium cotransport systems in epithelial secretion. Comp Biochem Physiol [A] 90:721–726
13. Kinne R, Kinne-Saffran E, Schölermann B, Schütz H (1986) The anion specificity of the sodium-potassium-chloride cotransporter in rabbit kidney outer medulla: Studies on medullary plasma membranes. Pflügers Arch 407:S168–C173
14. Brown CDA, Murer H (1985) Characterization of a Na:K:2Cl cotransport system in the apical membrane of a renal epithelial cell line (LLC-PK₁). J Membr Biol 87:131–139
15. Saier Jr MH, Boyden DA (1984) Mechanism, regulation and physiological significance of the loop diuretic-sensitive NaCl/KCl symport system in animal cells. Mol Cell Biochem 59:11–32
16. Schlatter E, Greger R, Weidtke C (1983) Effect of "high ceiling" diuretics on active salt transport in the cortical thick ascending limb of Henle's loop of rabbit kidney. Correlation of chemical structure and inhibitory potency. Pflügers Arch 396:210–217
17. Amsler K, Kinne R (1986) Specific irreversible inhibition of Na⁺-K⁺-Cl⁻ cotransport activity by exposure to bumetanide and near UV light. In: Alvarado F, van Os CH (eds) Ion-Gradient-Coupled Transport. INSERM Symposium No. 26. Elsevier, Amsterdam, pp 295–298
18. George JN, Turner RJ (1989) Inactivation of the rabbit parotid Na/K/Cl cotransporter by N-ethylmaleimide. J Membr Biol 112:51–58
19. Hediger MA, Turk E, Pajor AM, Wright EM (1989) Molecular genetics of the human Na⁺/glucose cotransporter. Klin Wochenschr 67:843–846
20. Kinne R, Kinne-Saffran E, Schütz H, Schölermann B (1986) Ammonium transport in medullary thick ascending limb of rabbit kidney. Involvement of the Na⁺,K⁺,Cl⁻-cotransporter. J Membr Biol 94:279–284
21. Garvin JL, Burg MB, Knepper MA (1988) Active NH_4^+ absorption by the thick ascending limb. Am J Physiol 255:F57–F65
22. Kinne R (to be published) Selectivity and direction: Plasma membranes in renal transport. Am J Physiol
23. Haas M (1989) Properties and diversity of (Na-K-Cl) cotransporters. Annu Rev Physiol 51:443–457

24. Sands JM, Knepper MA, Spring KR (1986) Na-K-Cl cotransport in apical membrane of rabbit renal papillary surface epithelium. Am J Physiol 251:F475–F484
25. Grupp C, Pavenstädt-Grupp I, Grunewald RW, Stokes III JB, Kinne RKH (1989) A Na-K-Cl cotransporter in isolated rat papillary collecting duct cells. Kidney Int 36:201–209
26. Schmidt-Nielsen B (1990) Function of the pelvis. Comp Physiol 2:103–140
27. Geck P (1990) Volume regulation in Ehrlich Cells. Comp Physiol 4:26–58
28. Grunewald JM, Grunewald RW, Kinne RKH (1990) Osmoregulation in isolated rat renal inner medullary collecting duct (IMCD) cells. FASEB J 4:A563

The Cellular Receptor for Thiazide-Type Diuretics

DARRELL D. FANESTIL, ZUOFANG CHEN, JOHAN M. TRAN, DUKE A. VAUGHN, and KEVIN BEAUMONT[1]

SUMMARY. ^{3}H-metolazone has been developed by our laboratory as a marker for the density of the thiazide diuretic receptor. The identity of the high affinity binding site for ^{3}H-metolazone with the receptor for thiazide-type diuretics is supported by three lines of investigation: (i) pharmacological specificity, (ii) autoradiographic localization in distal nephron, and (iii) the influence of the presumed transported ions, sodium and chloride, on the affinity. This development is beginning to impact upon our understanding of the renal regulation of excretion of sodium and chloride. Heretofore, there has been a lack of attention to the potential role of physiological and pathophysiological regulation of the thiazide-sensitive segment of the nephron in the homeostatic control of sodium, chloride, calcium, and acid-base homeostasis. The published and unpublished studies reviewed in this paper point out that the thiazide-sensitive transporter can be rapidly (within minutes) regulated, is influenced by both sex and adrenal steroid hormones, and is altered in two types of pathophysiological condition – experimental genetic hypertension and experimental genetic hypercalciuria. We predict with confidence that future work will provide additional appreciation for the role of the thiazide-sensitive Na-Cl transporter in renal physiology and pathophysiology.

Introduction

Thiazide diuretics (benzothiadiazides) have been utilized since the 1950s for the treatment of edema and hypertension [1]. Relatively little is known about the molecular and cellular mechanisms of action of thiazides, despite this long history of clinical utility in edema and hypertension. Moreover, the mode of their antihypertensive action is not firmly established [2]. However, thiazide-type diuretics are known to

---

[1]Division of Nephrology, Department of Medicine, University of California San Diego, La Jolla, CA 92093-0623, USA

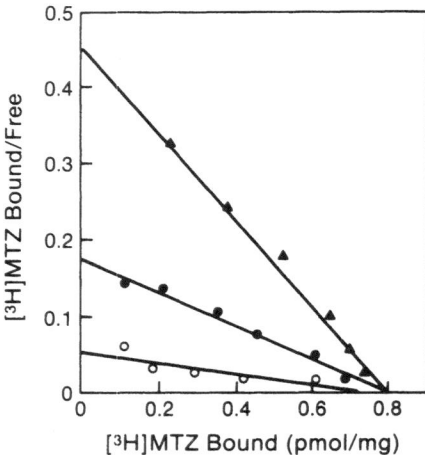

Fig. 1. Effect of sodium and of chloride on the binding of ³H-metolazone by rat kidney membranes. Membranes were incubated with various concentrations of ³H-metolazone in the presence of no added salt (*solid circles*), 25 mM Na$_2$SO$_4$ (*triangles*), or 50 mM NaCl (*open circles*). Results are plotted according to Scatchard, in which the intercept with the abscissa defines the maximal binding capacity and the slope of the line reflects the affinity. The maximal binding of ³H-metolazone was not affected by the ions. In contrast, the apparent affinity of the binding of ³H-metolazone, expressed as the equilibrium dissociation constant, was 3.56 nM in the absence of salt ($n=10$), 1.32 nM in the presence of 50 mM sodium ($n=5$), and 9.27 nM ($n=10$) in the presence of 50 mM sodium chloride. (From [9] with permission of The American Physiological Society)

inhibit reabsorption of NaCl and increase reabsorption of calcium from the renal tubule [3,4], probably by inhibition of a Na-Cl electroneutral symporter in the distal nephron [5,6,7].

Identification and Model of the Thiazide Receptor

The deficit in knowledge about the cellular and molecular mechanism of action of this important class of diuretics is undergoing rapid rectification. Our laboratory has recently developed and utilized ³H-metolazone to identify the putative pharmacological receptor for thiazide-type diuretics by ligand-binding technology [8,9]. Two classes of binding sites for ³H-metolazone, distinguished by differing affinities, were identified. The binding of ³H-metolazone to the class of sites with lower affinity could be inhibited by a variety of drugs with calcium channel-blocking activity (at micromolar concentration). In contrast, the high affinity binding site for ³H-metolazone exhibited characteristics expected of the pharmacological receptor for thiazide diuretics. Indeed, the identity of the high-affinity specific binding site for ³H-metolazone with the thiazide receptor is indicated by three major sets of data. *First*, the pharmacological specificy of the binding of ³H-metolazone to rat kidney membranes is as expected for the receptor for thiazide-type diuretics [8]. The biological potency of 12 thiazide-type diuretics correlated ($r=0.75$, $P<0.01$) with their

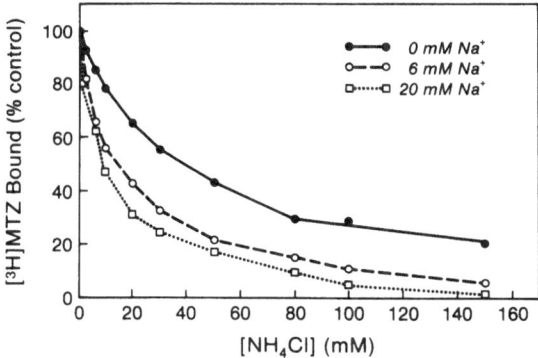

Fig. 2. Effect of Sodium on the ability of chloride to inhibit binding of ^{3}H-metolazone. Renal membranes were incubated with 1 nM ^{3}H-metolazone in the absence or presence of the indicated concentrations of sodium (as the SO_4 salt) and in the presence of the indicated concentrations of chloride (as the ammonium salt). (From [9] with permission of The American Physiological Society)

affinity for the putative receptor [8]. *Second*, the high affinity site for ^{3}H-metolazone has been localized by autoradiography to short and sparsely distributed segments of renal cortical tubules [10], a pattern consistent with a localization to the distal convoluted tubule (DCT). *Third*, the affinity of the binding of ^{3}H-metolazone is altered by the presumed transported ions [9]. The affinity of the thiazide receptor for ^{3}H-metolazone is increased by sodium ions and is decreased by chloride ions, as shown in Fig. 1. Moreover, the ability of chloride to inhibit binding of ^{3}H-metolazone to the thiazide receptor is modulated by the presence of cations. The concentration of chloride needed to produce 50% inhibition of binding (IC_{50}) of ^{3}H-metolazone in the presence of no added cation was 47 ± 3 mM. However, the IC_{50} decreased in the presence of 6 and 20 mM Na^+ to 19 ± 3 and 10 ± 2 mM chloride, respectively (Fig. 2). An additional important observation was that the Hill slopes characterizing the stimulation of binding by sodium and the inhibition of binding by chloride were not significantly different from unity. Therefore, there is no need to implicate more than one class of binding sites for either cation or anion. These findings enabled Tran et al. [9] to propose a conservative model for the transport of sodium/chloride by the transporter (see Fig. 3). The model predicts (a) that the transporter contains two binding sites, one for sodium and one that recognizes chloride and metolazone in a mutually exclusive/competitive fashion and (b) that occupancy of the sodium site increases the affinity of the second site for chloride/metolazone. Normally, the carrier is loaded with sodium from the tubular fluid (Step II, Fig. 3), resulting in an increase in the affinity for chloride, which is loaded in turn (Step III). The lower concentration of sodium in the tubular cell (from the action of Na-K-ATPase) provides a tubular fluid to intracellular concentration gradient for sodium that enables a favorable conformational change in the loaded Na-Cl carrier, such that sodium dissociates into the cell. This decreases the affinity of the carrier for the Cl and, consequently, results in the dissociation of Cl from the carrier into the cell (Step IV). Metolazone and other thiazide-type diuretics exert their action by binding to the transporter from the

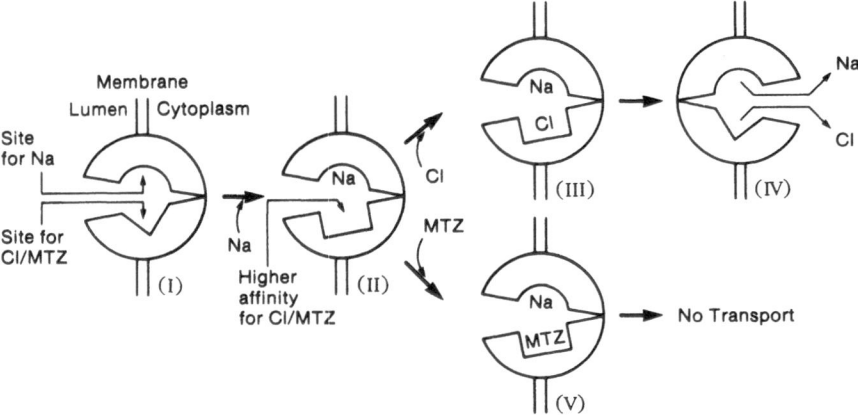

Fig. 3. Model for the mechanism of NaCl cotransport by the thiazide receptor. (From [9] with permission of The American Physiological Society)

tubular side, where their binding affinity is increased as a result of the loading of the carrier with sodium. However, the Na-thiazide carrier complex prevents the loading of chloride, and hence its transport, by the carrier (Step V).

Role of Thiazide-Sensitive Transport in Sodium Homeostasis

Regulation of the reabsorption of sodium by the renal tubule has been under long-term and extensive investigation by numerous laboratories. These studies have led to the following (admittedly overly simplified) appreciation of the complexity of the renal regulation of excretion of sodium. (i) In the proximal tubule, current evidence indicates that sodium transport regulators include angiotensin, the sympathetic nervous system, and dopamine. (ii) In the thick ascending limb of Henle, sodium transport regulators include antidiuretic hormone (in some species), PGE_2, and parathyroid hormone. (iii) In the collecting tubule and ducts, sodium transport regulators include aldosterone, antidiuretic hormone, atrial natriuretic peptide and others. In contrast, there is a paucity of information about regulation of transport of sodium by the DCT.

The lack of information about regulation of the handling of sodium and chloride by the DCT is now in the process of change. Kaissling and Stanton [11,12] and Ellison et al. [13] have recently shown that the DCT responds to increased sodium delivery by changing morphology, including an increase in the basolateral surface area of DCT cells, and an increase in the rate at which sodium is reabsorbed by the DCT.

Our development of ^3H-metolazone as a new method for quantitating specific binding sites for thiazide-type diuretics provides the opportunity to determine for the first time if the density of the thiazide receptor is regulated by physiological or pathophysiological conditions. We have learned the following about the regulation of the density of the thiazide receptor in vivo.

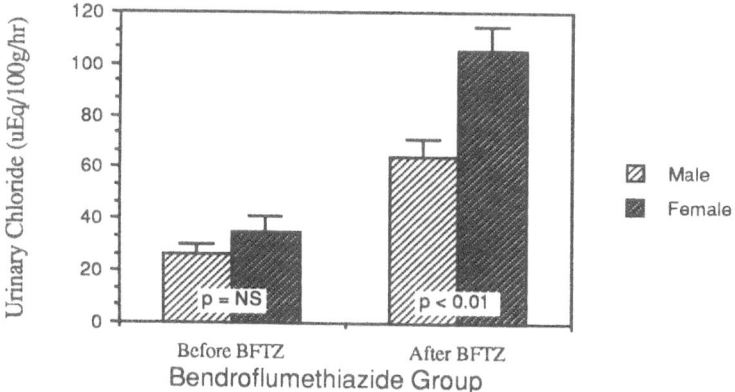

Fig. 4. Effect of treatment with bendroflumethiazide (BFTZ) on urinary excretion of chloride in males and females. The figure shows the hourly rate of excretion of chloride during six hours after treatment with vehicle (before BFTZ) or drug (after BFTZ) in 12 animals of each gender. (Data from [14])

The Thiazide Receptor is Regulated by Gender/Sex Hormone Status

Chen and co-workers [14] have found the following regarding the thiazide receptor in Sprague-Dawley rats: (a) a greater density in 12-week-old female (0.770 ± 0.048 pmol/mg protein) than in age-matched male animals (0.433 ± 0.040 pmol/mg protein); (b) a decrease in density after ovariectomy (0.529 ± 0.051 pmol/mg protein); and (c) an increase in density after orchiectomy (0.793 ± 0.076 pmol/mg protein). Importantly, in unpublished studies, the gender-related difference in binding of ^{3}H-metolazone was accompanied by a demonstrable difference in the renal response to administration of bendroflumethiazide (BFTZ). (Bendroflumethiazide was selected because of its low carbonic anhydrase inhibitory activity.) Urinary excretion of sodium, potassium, and chloride was quantitated during six hours after intraperitoneal administration of diluent or BFTZ. Bendroflumethiazide increased the excretion of sodium in both sexes and the magnitude of the increase was not different between the sexes. In contrast, the excretion of chloride after BFTZ rose to a greater extent in females than in males (Fig. 4). The rate of excretion of chloride was not significantly different between the sexes before BFTZ, but was greater ($P < 0.01$) in females than in males after BFTZ. Since urine pH was less than 6.0 in all animals after BFTZ, the drug did not appreciably inhibit carbonic anhydrase. This greater chloriuresis in females than in males is a finding consistent with the greater density of the thiazide receptor in females than in males.

The Thiazide Receptor is Altered by Adrenocortical Status

Our preliminary studies indicate that the thiazide receptor: (a) decreased in density 5 days post adrenalectomy ($0.248 \pm .027$ pmol/mg protein) vs that in sham operated, age matched control males (0.597 ± 0.048); (b) in another experiment, increased in density after 7 days from 0.117 ± 0.012 pmol/mg in adrenalectomized animals receiving diluent via minipump to 0.383 ± 0.010 pmol/mg in adrenalectomized animals receiving aldosterone (5 μg/100 g per day for 7 days by osmotic minipump), and to 0.445 ± 0.24 pmol/mg in adrenalectomized animals receiving dexamethasone (30 μg/100 g per day for 7 days). This level of replacement of aldosterone was chosen in order to produce a plasma level of aldosterone that was intermediate between that found in animals on a normal vs a low salt diet [15]. This level of administration of dexamethasone was selected in order to produce a maximal glucocorticoid effect, as judged by the ability to decrease the weight of the thymus [16].

The Thiazide Receptor is Increased by Adrenomedullectomy

In unpublished studies (M. Ziegler), adrenal medullectomy resulted in a 50% increase in density from $0.431 \pm .036$ pmol/mg in control animals to 0.652 ± 0.025 pmol/mg 4 days post adrenomedullectomy. The adequacy of the medullectomy was confirmed by measurement of adrenal epinephrine content.

The Thiazide Receptor is Altered by Prior Administration of Chloriuretic Diuretics [17]

The density of the binding of ³H-metolazone was increased 47% by acute (60 min) administration of hydrochlorothiazide and 39% by acute administration of furosemide (Fig. 5). In contrast, acute acetazolamide produced no change in binding (Fig. 5), though eliciting a dramatic diuresis, natriuresis, and kaliuresis. Acetazolamide did not produce chloriuresis. Chronic hydrochlorothiazide (5 days) and chronic furosemide (7 days) increased binding of ³H-metolazone by 46% and 101%, respectively. In contrast, variation in dietary sodium intake over a range that allowed normal growth of the animal and that produced urinary excretion of sodium varying from 0.28–2.62 mEq/100gm per day failed to alter the density of the binding of ³H-metolazone. These results do not support the postulate that the receptor is "upregulated" by increased sodium at the lumen of the distal convoluted tubule, since the acetazolamide-treated animals undoubtedly had increased delivery of sodium to the distal convoluted tubule [18,19]. However, we cannot eliminate either of two other postulates regarding the potential signal or mechanism whereby these changes in the density of the thiazide receptor are elicited: The increase in density of the thiazide receptor might be regulated (i) by increased delivery or concentration of chloride in distal convoluted tubular fluid or (ii) by occupancy of the thiazide receptor by either chloride or diuretic.

The Thiazide Receptor is Decreased by Anoxia/Ischemia

Ten minutes of in situ ischemia (produced by cross-clamping the renal pedicle) decreased the density of binding by 90%. Subsequent reperfusion (produced by releasing the cross-clamp) for 10 minutes restored binding ⅔ of the way to normal [20]. In pursuing the in vivo effects of ischemia in vitro, we determined that small segments of rat kidney incubated in physiological salt solution also responded to anoxia or to inhibitors of oxidative phosphorylation with a decrease in density of the thiazide receptor. The in vitro effect of anoxia was reversible upon restoration of oxy-

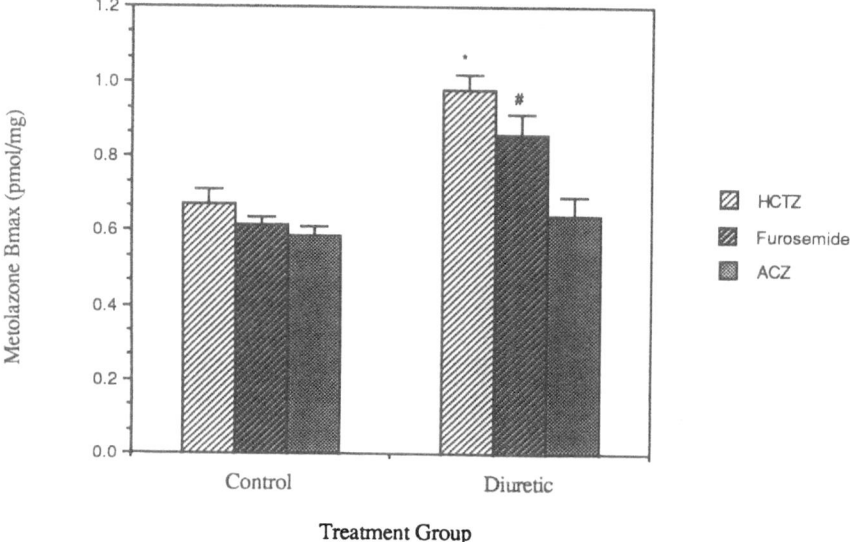

Fig. 5. Acute effect of diuretics on binding of ³H-metolazone. Animals were treated with hydrochlorothiazide (*HCTZ*), furosemide or acetazolamide (*ACZ*) 60 min prior to removal of the kidneys for determination of the density of the thiazide receptor. * and # indicate significantly different from the respective, simultaneously analyzed control groups at $P \leq 0.01$. (Data from [17])

gen (just as in vivo ischemia had been), even after 30 minutes of incubation under a 100% nitrogen environment [20].

The Thiazide Receptor is Increased in Genetic Hypercalciuria

Dr. David Bushinsky has selectively bred rats for hypercalciuria [21]. He presented convincing evidence that the primary defect is gastrointestinal hyperabsorption of calcium, since the animals are in positive calcium balance. We have collaborated in a preliminary study on the thiazide receptor in these animals. The rationale was: if the thiazide-sensitive transporter were so intimately related to control of urinary excretion of calcium as is suggested by the pharmacological actions of thiazide-type diuretics on the DCT, an appropriate homeostatic response to hyperabsorption of calcium would be secondary hyperactivity of the thiazide-sensitive system, in order to facilitate excretion of the increased body burden of calcium. Dr. Bushinsky harvested and rapidly froze kidneys from hypercalciuric animals and their normocalciuric controls. The daily rate of excretion of calcium by the hypercalciuric animals was increased about 5-fold above the control. The kidney weights from the two groups of animals did not differ. However, the density of the thiazide receptor, measured by saturation binding studies with ³H-metolazone, was increased from $0.872 \pm .045$ pmol/mg to $1.102 \pm .057$, P=.005.

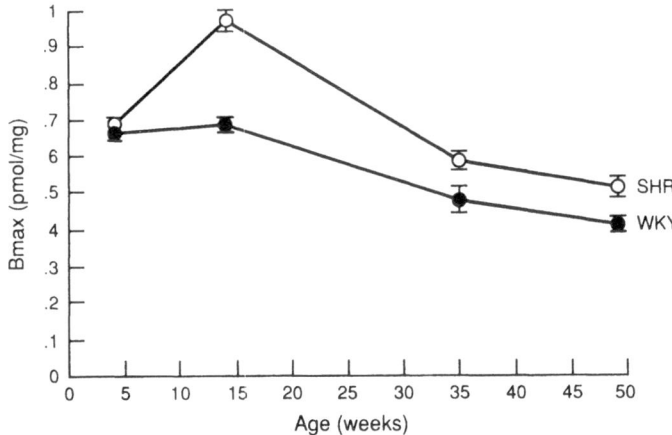

Fig. 6. Alteration of the density of the thiazide diuretic receptor in kidneys from female spontaneously hypertensive (*SHR*) and Wistar Kyoto control (*WKY*) rats. Values are means ± sem for 6–9 animals in each group. SHR and WKY differ significantly at all except 4 weeks of age. (From [22] by courtesy of Marcel Dekker, Inc.)

The Thiazide Receptor is Increased in the Spontaneously Hypertensive Rat (SHR)

Fig. 6 shows a comparison of the density of the receptor in SHR females at several ages, compared with the normotensive Wistar-Kyoto control (WKY) [22]. There was increased receptor density at 14, 35, and 49 weeks of age in female animals and at 35 weeks of age in male animals (the only age tested in males – data not shown). The density was not different in SHR females at 4 weeks of age. Since GFR is low in 5-week-old SHR but normal in older SHR [23,24,25], the density of the thiazide receptor per unit of GFR is likely greater in SHR than in WKY at all ages tested. Thus, the thiazide receptor could mediate increased reabsorption of sodium/chloride per unit GFR in SHR at all ages! An intuitive interpretation of these findings would be that the increase in thiazide receptor in SHR would lead to retention of sodium/chloride and cause or contribute to the generation of hypertension. It is important to note that the increase in thiazide receptor density in hypertensive SHR was not a non-specific effect of elevated renal perfusion pressure, since the receptor density was not different in the clipped vs. unclipped kidney in 2 Kidney-1 Clip animals whose systemic systolic blood pressure was at a level similar to that of the SHR [22]. The relationship between the genes that cause hypertension in SHR and the development of the increased density of the thiazide receptor are fruitful areas for future investigation. Moreover, this finding raises the possibility that the alteration in calcium homeostasis known to occur in SHR [26,27] might be secondary, in SHR, to alteration in calcium reabsorption in the thiazide-sensitive segment of the renal tubule.

The Thiazide Receptor is Dependent Upon Age

The density of the receptor decreases in spontaneously hypertensive (SHR) and Wistar Kyoto control (WKY) females after 15 weeks of age (Fig. 6). This observation has been confirmed in Sprague-Dawley animals in our laboratory (unpublished data).

Conclusions

Development of ^{3}H-metolazone as a marker for the density of the thiazide diuretic receptor is beginning to impact upon our understanding of the renal regulation of excretion of sodium and chloride. Heretofore, there has been a lack of attention to the potential role of physiological and pathophysiological regulation of the thiazide-sensitive segment of the nephron in the homeostatic control of sodium, chloride, calcium, and acid-base homeostasis. The published and unpublished studies reviewed in this paper point out that the thiazide-sensitive transporter can be rapidly (within minutes) regulated, is influenced by both sex and adrenal steroid hormones, and is altered in two types of pathophysiological conditions – experimental genetic hypertension and experimental genetic hypercalciuria. We predict with confidence that future work will provide additional appreciation for the role of the thiazide-sensitive Na-Cl transporter in renal physiology and pathophysiology.

References

1. Wilkins RW, Hollander W, Chobanian AV (1959) Chlorothiazide in hypertension: studies on its mode of action. Ann NY Acad Sci 71:465–472
2. O'Connor DT, Preston RA, Mitas JA, Frigon RP, Stone RA (1981) Urinary kallikrein activity and renal vascular resistance in the antihypertensive response to thiazide diuretics. Hypertension 3:139–147
3. Costanzo LS, Windhager EE (1978) Calcium and sodium transport by the distal convoluted tubule of the rat. Am J Physiol 246:F492–F506
4. Costanzo LS (1985) Localization of diuretic action in microperfused rat distal tubules: Ca and Na transport. Am J Physiol 248:F527–F535
5. Velazquez H, Good DW, Wright FS (1984) Mutual dependence of sodium and chloride absorption by renal distal tubule. Am J Physiol 247:F904–F911
6. Ellison DH, Velazquez H, Wright FS (1987) Thiazide-sensitive sodium chloride cotransport in the early distal tubule. Am J Physiol 253:F546–F554
7. Kunau RT, Weller DR, Webb HL (1975) Clarification of the site of action of chlorothiazide in the rat nephron. J Clin Invest 56:401–407
8. Beaumont K, Vaughn DA, Fanestil DD (1988) Thiazide diuretic receptors in rat kidney: identification with [3-H]metolazone. Proc Natl Acad Sci USA 85:2311–2314
9. Tran JM, Farrell MA, Fanestil DD (1990) Effect of ions on the binding of the thiazide-type diuretic metolazone to kidney membranes. Am J Physiol 258:F908–F915
10. Beaumont K, Vaughn DA, Healy DP (1989) Thiazide diuretic receptors: Autoradiographic localization in rat kidney with [3H]-metolazone. J Pharmacol Exp Ther 250:414–419
11. Kaissling B, Stanton BA (1988) Adaptation of distal tubule and collecting duct to increased sodium delivery. I. Ultrastructure. Am J Physiol 255:F1256–F1268

12. Stanton BA, Kaissling B (1988) Adaptation of distal tubule and collecting duct to increased Na delivery. II. Na⁺ and K⁺ transport. Am J Physiol 255:F1269–F1275

13. Ellison DH, Velazquez H, Wright FS (1989) Adaptation of the distal convoluted tubule of the rat. Structural and functional effects of dietary salt intake and chronic diuretic infusion. J Clin Invest 83:113–126

14. Chen Z, Vaughn DA, Cochoit J, Fanestil DD (to be published) Influence of gender, sex hormone status and pregnancy on binding of 3H-metolazone in kidney.

15. Martin RS, Jones WJ, Hayslett JP (1983) Animal model to study the effect of adrenal hormones on epithelial function. Kidney Int 24:386–391

16. Khalid BAK, Lim AT, Funder JW (1982) Steroid effects on protein synthesis: Mineralocorticoids and glucocorticoids, thymus and pituitary. Excerpta Medica 598:289–294

17. Chen Z, Vaughn DA, Beaumont K, Fanestil DD (1990) Effects of diuretic treatment and of dietary sodium on renal binding of 3H-metolazone. J Am Soc Nephrology 1:91–98

18. Cogan MG, Maddox DA, Warnock DG, Lin ET, Rector JFC (1979) Effect of acetazolamide on bicarbonate reabsorption in the proximal tubule of the rat. Am J Physiol 237:F447–F454

19. Kunau RT (1972) The influence of the carbonic anhydrase inhibitor benzolamide (Al-11,366) on the reabsorption of chloride, sodium and bicarbonate in the proximal tubule of the rat. J Clin Invest 51:294–306

20. Beaumont K, Vaughn DA, Maciejewski AR, Fanestil DD (1989) Reversible downregulation of thiazide diuretic receptors by acute renal ischemia. Am J Physiol 256:F329–F334

21. Bushinsky DA, Favus MJ (1988) Mechanism of hypercalciuria in genetic hypercalciuric rats. J Clin Invest 82:1585–1591

22. Beaumont K, Vaughn DA, Casto RL, Printz MP, Fanestil DD (1990) Thiazide diuretic receptors in spontaneously hypertensive rats and 2-kidney 1-clip hypertensive rats. Clin Exp Hypertens [A]12:215–226

23. Arendshorst WJ, Beierwaltes WH (1979) Renal tubular reabsorption in spontaneously hypertensive rats. Am J Physiol 237:F38–F47

24. Arendshorst WJ, Beierwaltes WH (1979) Renal and nephron hemodynamics in spontaneously hypertensive rats. Am J Physiol 237:F246–F251

25. Beierwaltes WH, Arendshorst WJ, Klemmer PJ (1982) Electrolyte and water balance in young spontaneously hypertensive rats. Hypertension 4:908–915

26. Hsu CH, Chen P-S, Smith DE, Yang C-S (1986) Pathogenesis of hypercalciuria in spontaneously hypertensive rats. Min Electrol Metab 12:130–141

27. McCarron DA (1989) Calcium metabolism and hypertension. Kidney Int 35:717–736

Application of the Amiloride Series in the Study of Ion Transport

Thomas R. Kleyman[1]

SUMMARY. Amiloride and amiloride analogs have been extensively used as inhibitors of Na^+-selective transport proteins. The interaction of amiloride analogs with the epithelial Na^+ channel, Na^+/H^+ exchanger, and Na^+/Ca^{2+} exchanger is summarized. The potential use of amiloride analogs as biochemical probes for amiloride-sensitive transport proteins, and as immunologic tools for development of antibodies directed against these proteins is discussed, as are some of the limitations and problems encountered using amiloride analogs as "specific" inhibitors of defined transport proteins.

Introduction

The search for diuretics with antikaliuretic properties lead to the generation of the amiloride series [1,2]. Both the natriuresis and antikaliuresis following oral adminis-tration of amiloride occur as a result of inhibition of the epithelial Na^+ channel present in the distal nephron [3]. The concentration of amiloride required to inhibit the epithelial Na^+ channel by 50% (IC_{50}) is less than 1 µM. Higher concentrations inhibit other transport proteins (see Table 1) including Na^+/H^+ exchanger, Na^+/Ca^{2+} exchanger, Na^+,K^+-ATPase, Na^+-d-glucose cotransporter, Na^+-1-alanine cotran-sporter, Na^+-PO_4^{3-} cotransporter, voltage-gated Na^+ channel, voltage-gated Ca^{2+} chan-nel, delayed rectifier K^+ channel, and the nicotinic acetylcholine receptor (for review, see [4]).

Amiloride inhibits most Na^+-selective transport proteins, and kinetic studies of amiloride's interaction with the Na^+/H^+ exchanger [5], Na^+/Ca^{2+} exchanger [6], and Na^+-hexose cotransporter [7] suggest that amiloride binds to a Na^+ recognition or binding site on these transporters. Studies of the interaction of amiloride with the epithelial Na^+ channel in several model systems have also suggested that amiloride

[1]Renal and Electrolyte Section – 700 CRB, University of Pennsylvania, Philadelphia, PA 19104-6144, USA

Table 1. Amiloride-sensitive transport proteins

Epithelial Na$^+$ channel
Na$^+$/H$^+$ exchanger
Na$^+$/Ca^{2+} exchanger
Na$^+$,K$^+$-ATPase
Na$^+$-d-glucose cotransporter
Na$^+$-l-alanine cotransporter
Na$^+$-PO$_4^{3-}$ cotransporter
Voltage-gated Na$^+$ channel
Voltage-gated Ca^{2+} channel
Delayed rectifier K$^+$ channel
Nicotinic acetylcholine receptor

and Na$^+$ share a common binding or recognition site, which is presumably in or near the pore of the channel [8,9,10]. However, examination of the site of interaction of amiloride with the Na$^+$ channel is complicated by the voltage-dependent interaction of amiloride (a monovalent cation) with the channel [11,12], as the varied Na$^+$ concentrations used in these studies could change the electric potential across the plasma membrane and, as a secondary effect, alter the binding of amiloride.

Inhibition of Transport Proteins

Amiloride is a substituted pyrazinoylguanidine. Its structure is illustrated in Fig. 1. In addition, two major classes of amiloride analogs have been used as ion transport inhibitors. These include analogs with hydrophobic groups on the terminal nitrogen of the guanidino moiety of amiloride, such as benzamil (Fig. 1), and analogs with hydrophobic groups on the 5-amino moiety of the pyrazine ring, such as EIPA

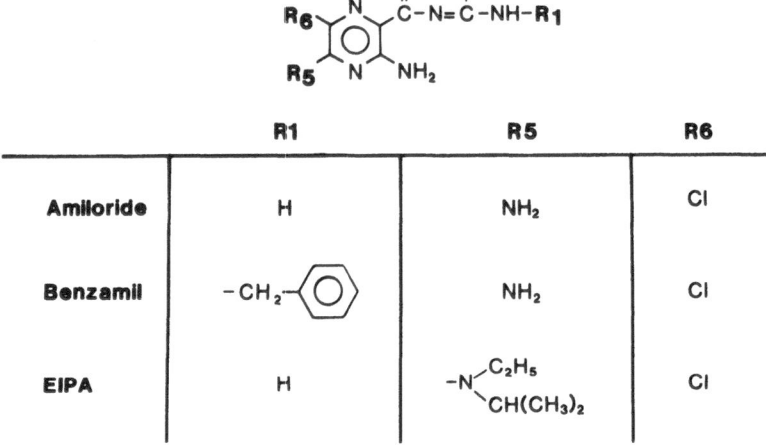

Fig. 1. Structures of amiloride and the amiloride analogs benzamil and EPIA

Table 2. IC_{50} (μM) of amiloride or amiloride analogs

	Na$^+$ channel	Na$^+$/H$^+$ exchange	Na$^+$/Ca^{2+} exchange
Amiloride	0.35	84	1,100
Benzamil	0.04	> 1,000	100
EIPA	> 10	0.38	140

The concentrations of amiloride, benzamil, and EIPA required to achieve half maximal inhibition (IC_{50}) of the A6 cell epithelial Na$^+$ [4] channel, neutrophil Na$^+$/H$^+$ exchanger [15], and GH$_3$ cell Na$^+$/Ca^{2+} [6] exchanger are listed

(Fig. 1). Amiloride is a reversible inhibitor of ion transport and it is the protonated form of amiloride which is required to block transport [6,13,14]. The interaction of amiloride or amiloride analogs with ion transporters has been most extensively characterized in three systems: the epithelial Na$^+$ channel, Na$^+$/H$^+$ exchange, and Na$^+$/Ca^{2+} exchange. A summary of the IC_{50}s of amiloride, benzamil, and EIPA for the apical epithelial Na$^+$ channel [4], Na$^+$/H$^+$ exchanger (in neutrophils) [15], and Na$^+$/Ca^{2+} exchanger [6] is listed in Table 2.

Epithelial Na$^+$ Channel

The epithelial Na$^+$ channel is expressed on the apical plasma membrane of high-resistance, Na$^+$-transporting epithelia, such as renal collecting tubule, distal colon, urinary bladder, and trachea (for review, see [16]). Amiloride inhibits the Na$^+$ channel at a site which is accessible from extracellular fluid. The IC_{50} for amiloride is in the range of 0.1–0.5 μM, when measured in the presence of a physiologic concentration of Na$^+$ [4]. Lowering the extracellular Na$^+$ concentration will decrease the IC_{50} by up to ~ 10 fold [4,17]. As discussed above, the kinetics of amiloride binding to the Na$^+$ channel in the presence of a varying apical plasma membrane potential suggest that amiloride senses between 10%–45% of the membrane electric field [11,12]. This observation, together with studies in voltage-clamped cells demonstrating that amiloride binding kinetics are altered by Na$^+$ or Li$^+$ loading cells in order to generate an outward current through the channel [18,19], support the notion that the amiloride-binding site is likely within the pore of the channel, possibly at a Na$^+$ binding or recognition site.

Amiloride analogs with hydrophobic groups on the guanidino moiety tend to lower the IC_{50} and increase the specificity for the Na$^+$ channel [4,20]. Analogs with hydrophobic groups on the 5-amino moiety of the pyrazine ring both raise the IC_{50} and decrease the specificity for the channel [4,20].

Na$^+$ channels with a low affinity for amiloride (IC_{50}s in the range of 1–20 μM) have recently been described [21,22]. The interaction of these channels with amiloride analogs differs from that observed with the high affinity Na$^+$ channels described above, in that the IC_{50}s for amiloride analogs with hydrophobic groups on the guanidino moiety or on the 5-amino moiety of the pyrazine ring are similar to the IC_{50} for amiloride. These channels were described in membrane vesicles isolated from urinary bladder and colon. A Na$^+$ conductive pathway, with an IC_{50} for amiloride of 13 μM, was recently observed in the basolateral plasma membrane of toad urinary bladder [23], suggesting that these channels are expressed on the basolateral plasma membrane of high-resistance, Na^+-transporting epithelia.

Na^+/H^+ Exchange

The Na^+/H^+ exchanger is a 110 kDa glycoprotein [24] which is constitutively expressed in most mammalian cells and participates in regulation of intracellular pH [25]. This transporter is also expressed at the apical plasma membrane of low-resistance epithelia and facilitates vectorial transport of Na^+ and HCO_3^- (or H^+) [25]. Amiloride inhibits the Na^+/H^+ exchanger with an IC_{50} in the range of 3–30 μM, when measured in the presence of a low Na^+ concentration [5,14,26,27]. The IC_{50} is dependent on the extracellular Na^+ concentration, in that lowering the extracellular Na^+ concentration will decrease the IC_{50}. Certain amiloride analogs with hydrophobic groups on the 5-amino moiety of the pyrazine ring have a lower IC_{50}, relative to amiloride, for the exchanger and at low concentrations are specific inhibitors of the exchanger [4,14,15,26,27]. In contrast, analogs with hydrophobic groups on the guanidino moiety inhibit the Na^+/H^+ exchanger with IC_{50}s greater than amiloride.

In epithelia, basolateral and apical transporters differ in their apparent affinity for amiloride. The apical transporter has a higher IC_{50} for both amiloride and the analog EIPA, relative to the basolateral transporter. The IC_{50} of EIPA for the basolateral transporter is ~ 300-fold lower than that for the apical transporter [28].

Na^+/Ca^{2+} Exchange

The Na^+/Ca^{2+} exchanger is expressed at the plasma membrane of a variety of cell types and participates in intracellular Ca^{2+} regulation. Amiloride's IC_{50} is ~ 1 mM [6]. The IC_{50} for amiloride is dependent on the extracellular Na^+ concentration, in that lowering the extracellular Na^+ concentration will decrease the IC_{50}. Analogs with hydrophobic groups on either the 5-amino moiety of the pyrazine ring and/or on the guanidino moiety lower the IC_{50} for the exchanger [4,6]. Certain amiloride analogs which inhibit Na^+/Ca^{2+} exchange may inhibit Ca^{2+} channels with equal or lower IC_{50}s [29].

Amiloride Analogs as Probes for Na^+-Selective Transport Proteins

Aside from the use of amiloride analogs as inhibitors of ion transporters, amiloride analogs have been successfully used as probes for biochemical characterization of transport proteins. Radioactive amiloride derivatives have been used to examine binding of amiloride analogs to the Na^+ channel and Na^+/H^+ exchanger [30–33]. Two groups have recently used the binding of a radiolabeled amiloride analog as a marker to purify the epithelial Na^+ channel [32,34].

Photoactive amiloride analogs have also been used to identify the amiloride-binding subunit of the epithelial Na^+ channel. Two classes of photoactive amiloride

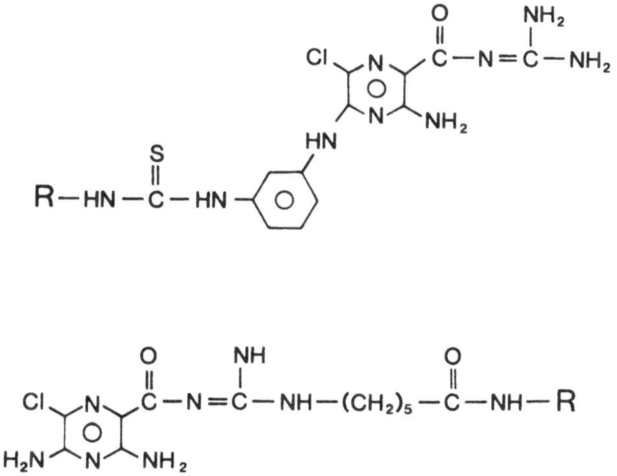

Fig. 2. Structures of amiloride analogs coupled to carrier protein (R). Amiloride was coupled to albumin either through the 5-amino group on the pyrazine ring or through the guanidino group

analogs with different reactive groups were used to affinity label the amiloride-binding subunit of the Na$^+$ channel [30,34,35]. The first class of compounds, which include bromobenzamil and bromomethylamiloride, utilize the halide (bromo) on the 6-position of the pyrazine ring on the amiloride molecule as the photoreactive moiety. A second class of photoactive amiloride analogs was developed with an aromatic ether attached to amiloride through its guanidino moiety. One member of this group, 2-methoxy-5-nitrobenzylamiloride, was used to label the amiloride-binding subunit of the Na$^+$ channel [35]. The 2-methoxy-5-nitrobenzyl group undergoes photoactivation and incorporates into proteins through a mechanism of aromatic nucleophilic photosubstitution [36]. This type of photochemical reaction has several major advantages. First, it is a high efficiency reaction, as labeling of more than 30% of amiloride-binding sites was noted [35]. Second, only one reactive intermediate is formed, with a half-life of less than 10^{-7} s [36], which markedly reduces nonspecific photolabeling. The Na$^+$ channel is an oligomeric protein [34]. The amiloride-binding subunit of the channel identified in photoaffinity labeling studies is a polypeptide subunit with an apparent molecular weight in the range of 130–180 kDa [30,34,35].

Amiloride analogs with spacer arms have been synthesized with terminal carboxyl or amino groups to allow for coupling to immobilized resins or to carrier protein (see Fig. 2) [37,38]. Since amiloride analogs with hydrophobic groups on the guanidino moiety of amiloride are specific high affinity inhibitors of the Na$^+$ channel, amiloride coupled through its guanidino group to albumin was used as an immunogen to raise anti-amiloride antibodies. These antibodies bind amiloride analogs in a manner similar to that of the Na$^+$ channel [39]. In contrast, antibodies raised against amiloride conjugated to albumin through its 5-amino group bound amiloride analogs in a manner similar to that of the Na$^+$/H$^+$ exchanger [39]. These antibodies raised against the different amiloride-albumin conjugates recognize distinct epitopes on amiloride.

The anti-amiloride antibodies have proven to be useful in detecting a photoactive amiloride analog covalently bound to the Na^+ channel [35], and as tools for raising anti-idiotypic antibodies which recognize the Na^+ channel. This approach for raising anti-Na^+ channel antibodies is based on the apparent structural mimicry of the amiloride-binding domain on the anti-amiloride antibody and on the Na^+ channel. The anti-idiotypic antibody can mimic the effect of amiloride by inhibiting Na^+ transport across a Na^+-transporting epithelium (A6 cells) (Kleyman TR, Kraehenbuhl JP, and Ernst SA, J. Biol. Chem. in press).

Problems Encountered Using Amiloride Analogs as Ion Transport Probes

Amiloride analogs are often added to extracellular fluid in order to inhibit ion transport proteins expressed on the plasma membrane. Unfortunately, amiloride analogs do not remain in the extracellular space and will accumulate within cells. The cellular uptake of amiloride occurs by simple diffusion [40,41], although transport across the plasma membrane has been observed in hepatocytes [42]. The intracellular concentration may reach levels greater than the extracellular concentration, assuming that measured "cellular" amiloride was free in solution and not bound to lipid, nor compartmentalized. In neutrophils 75% of the intracellular amiloride was considered to be in the lysozomal compartment [40]. In other cell types, the extent to which intracellular amiloride is compartmentalized is uncertain. Amiloride diffuses across red blood cell and neutrophil plasma membranes with a permeability coefficient of approximately 10^{-7} cm•sec^{-1} [40,41]. As amiloride is a permeable weak base, cellular accumulation of amiloride could alter intracellular pH.

Amiloride and amiloride analogs have gained widespread use as inhibitors of ion transport proteins. However, the specificity of these drugs may be limited by inhibition of cellular processes other than ion transport. Amiloride binds to or inhibits a number of enzymes, which are listed in Table 3 (for review, see [4]). The inhibition of protein kinase activity is competitive with respect to ATP, suggesting that amiloride interacts with, or binds to an ATP binding site on protein kinases [43]. As inhibition of a particular enzyme might have a direct (or indirect) influence on a specific

Table 3. Amiloride-sensitive enzymes

Acetylcholinesterase
Adenylate cyclase
DNA Topoisomerase II
Monoamine oxidase
Na^+,K^+-ATPase
Renal kallikrein
Urokinase type plasminogen activator
Type I cAMP dependent protein kinase
Type II cAMP dependent protein kinase
Epidermal growth factor receptor protein kinase
Platelet derived growth factor receptor protein kinase
Insulin receptor protein kinase
Protein kinase C

ion transporter protein, it is of value to be cognizant of the effects of amiloride analogs on these enzymes when using amiloride analogs as "selective" inhibitors of ion transport.

Amiloride analogs have been observed to effect other cellular processes as well. These include inhibition of oxidative phosphorylation and depletion of cellular ATP levels, and inhibition of DNA, RNA, and protein synthesis [14,26,42,44] (for review, see [4]). The extent of inhibition may vary with the cell type studied. These effects may be both direct, as well as indirect, as a result of inhibition of ion transport [14].

Amiloride is a fluorescent aromatic compound with excitation maxima at 286 and 360 nm and emission maxima at 410–414 nm [4,43]. The major absorption peaks of amiloride are at 360–370 nm, 265–290 nm, and 215–235 nm [4]. The fluorescence and absorption properties of amiloride may interfere with techniques which utilize fluorescent probes to measure intracellular pH and intracellular Ca^{2+}.

Protonation of the guanidino group is required for amiloride to inhibit ion transport. The pK_a of the guanidino group is 8.8, and at a pH of 7.4, more than 95% of amiloride will be protonated [4]. However, the pK_a is significantly lowered in certain amiloride analogs with substituents on the guanidino group, which can considerably alter the concentration of the amiloride analog which is in its active, or protonated form.

Review

The amiloride series was initially developed with the goal of identifying new diuretics with antikaliuretic properties. These compounds subsequently found widespread use as inhibitors of Na^+-selective transport proteins. Amiloride or amiloride analogs are often used as specific inhibitors of ion transporters; however, the use of these compounds as selective inhibitors should be tempered by knowledge of their effects on enzymes and other cellular processes which could indirectly alter ion transport. Despite these limitations, amiloride analogs have provided valuable probes for the isolation and biochemical characterization of the epithelial Na^+ channel, and for the generation of antibodies directed against this channel. As amiloride and its analogs bind to a Na^+ recognition or binding site on several of the Na^+-selective transport proteins, these compounds may provide useful tools to define structural features on these proteins which participate in Na^+ binding.

Acknowledgments. This work was supported by grants from the Cystic Fibrosis Foundation and the Department of Veterans Affairs.

References

1. Cragoe EJ Jr, Woltersdorf OW Jr, Bicking JB, Kwong SF, Jones JH (1967) Pyrazine diuretics. II. N-amidino-3-amino-5-substituted 6-halopyrazine-carboxamides. J Med Chem 10:66–75
2. Cragoe EJ Jr (1983) Pyrazine diuretics. In: Cragoe EJ Jr (ed) Diuretics: chemistry, pharmacology, and medicine. John Wiley and Sons, New York, pp 303–343

3. Kleyman TR, Cragoe EJ Jr (1988) Mechanism of action of amiloride. Semin Nephrol 8:242–248

4. Kleyman TR, Cragoe EJ Jr (1988) Amiloride and its analogs as tools in the study of ion transport. J Membr Biol 105:1–21

5. Kinsella JL, Aronson PS (1981) Amiloride inhibition of the Na^+/H^+ exchanger in renal microvillus membrane vesicles. Am J Physiol 241:F374–F379

6. Kaczorowski GJ, Barros F, Dethmers JK, Trumble MJ (1985) Inhibition of Na^+/Ca^{2+} exchange in pituitary plasma membrane vesicles by analogues of amiloride. Biochemistry 24:1394–1403

7. Cook JS, Shaffer C, Cragoe EJ Jr (1987) Inhibition by amiloride analogues of Na^+-dependent hexose uptake in LLC-PK_1/CL_4 cells. Am J Physiol 253:C199–C204

8. Li JH-Y, Lindemann B (1983) Competitive blocking of epithelial sodium channels by organic cations: the relationship between macroscopic and microscopic inhibition constants. J Membr Biol 76:235–251

9. Cuthbert A (1981) Sodium entry step in transporting epithelia – results of ligand-binding studies. In: Schultz S (ed) Ion transport by epithelia. Raven, New York, pp 181–196

10. Gottlieb GP, Turnheim K, Frizzell RA, Schultz SG (1978) p-Chloromercuribenzene sulfonate blocks and reverses the effect of amiloride on sodium transport across rabbit colon in vitro. Biophys J 22:125–129

11. Palmer LG (1984) Voltage-dependent block by amiloride and other monovalent cations of apical sodium channels in the toad urinary bladder. J Membr Biol 80:153–165

12. Hamilton K, Eaton D (1985) Single-channel recordings from amiloride-sensitive epithelial sodium channel. Am J Physiol 249:C200–C207

13. Benos DJ, Simon SA, Mandel LJ, Cala PM (1976) Effect of amiloride and some of its analogues on cation transport in isolated frog skin and thin lipid membranes. J Gen Physiol 68:43–63

14. L'Allemain G, Franchi A, Cragoe EJ Jr, Pouyssegur J (1984) Blockade of the Na^+/H^+ antiport abolishes growth factor-induced DNA synthesis in fibroblasts. Structure-activity relationships in the amiloride series. J Biol Chem 259:4313–4319

15. Simchowitz L, Cragoe EJ Jr (1986) Inhibition of chemotactic-factor activated Na^+/H^+ exchange in human neutrophils by analogues of amiloride: structure-activity relationships in the amiloride series. Mol Pharmacol 30:112–120

16. Sariban-Sohraby S, Benos DJ (1986) The amiloride-sensitive sodium channel. Am J Physiol 250:C175–C190

17. Cuthbert AW, Shum WK (1974) Amiloride and the sodium channel. Naunyn Schmiedebergs Arch Pharmacol 281:261–269

18. Li JH-Y, Lindemann B (1982) Movement of Na and Li across the apical membrane of frog skin. In: Emrich HM, Aldenhoff JB, Lux DH (eds) Basic mechanisms in the action of lithium. Excerpta Medica, Amsterdam, pp 28–35

19. Van Driessche W, Erlij P (1983) Noise analysis of inward and outward Na^+ currents across the apical border of ouabain-treated frog skin. Pflugers Arch 398:179–188

20. Cuthbert AW, Fanelli GM (1978) Effects of some pyrazinecarboxamides on sodium transport in frog skin. Br J Pharmacol 63:139–149

21. Asher C, Cragoe EJ Jr, Garty H (1987) Effects of amiloride analogues on Na^+ transport in toad bladder membrane vesicles. J Biol Chem 262:8566–8573

22. Bridges RJ, Cragoe EJ Jr, Frizzell RA, Benos DJ (1989) Inhibition of colonic Na^+ transport by amiloride analogues. Am J Physiol 256:C67–C74

23. Garty H, Warncke J, Lindemann B (1987) An amiloride-sensitive Na^+ conductance in the basolateral membrane of toad urinary bladder. J Membr Biol 95:91–103

24. Sardet C, Counillon L, Franchi A, Pouyssegur J (1990) Growth factors induce phosphorylation of the Na/H antiporter, a glycoprotein of 110 kD. Science 247:723–726

25. Seifter JL, Aronson PS (1986) Properties and physiologic roles of the plasma membrane sodium-hydrogen exchanger. J Clin Invest 78:859–864

26. Zhuang Y, Cragoe EJ Jr, Shaikewitz T, Glaser L, Cassel D (1984) Characterization of potent Na/H exchange inhibitors from the amiloride series in A431 cells. Biochemistry 23:4481–4488

27. Vigne P, Frelin C, Cragoe EJ Jr, Lazdunski M (1984) Structure-activity relationships of amiloride and certain of its analogues in relation to the blockade of the Na^+/H^+ exchange system. Mol Pharmacol 25:131–136

28. Haggerty JG, Agarwal N, Reilly RF, Adelberg EA, Slayman CW (1988) Pharmacologically different Na/H antiporters on the apical and basolateral surfaces of cultured porcine kidney cells (LLC-PK_1). Proc Natl Acad Sci USA 85:6797–6801

29. Garcia ML, King VF, Shevell JL, Slaughter RS, Suarez-Kurtz G, Winquist RJ, Kaczorowski GJ (1990) Amiloride analogs inhibit L-type calcium channels and display calcium entry blocker activity. J Biol Chem 265:3763–3771

30. Kleyman TR, Yulo T, Ashbaugh C, Landry D, Cragoe EJ Jr., Karlin A, Al-Awqati Q (1986) Photoaffinity labeling of the epithelial sodium channel. J Biol Chem 261:2839–2943

31. Sariban-Sohraby S, Benos DJ (1986) Detergent solubilization, functional reconstitution, and partial purification of epithelial amiloride binding protein. Biochemistry 25:4639–4646

32. Barbry P, Chassande O, Vigne P, Frelin C, Ellory C, Cragoe EJ Jr, and Lazdunski M (1987) Purification and subunit structure of the [^{3}H]phenamil receptor associated with the renal apical Na^+ channel Proc Natl Acad Sci USA 84:4836–4840

33. Vigne P, Frelin C, Audinot M, Borsotto M, Cragoe EJ Jr, Lazdunski M (1984) [^{3}H]ethyl-propylamiloride, a radio-labelled diuretic for the analysis of the Na^+/H^+ exchange system. EMBO J 3:2647–2651

34. Benos DJ, Saccomani G, Sariban-Sohraby S (1987) The epithelial sodium channel. Subunit number and localization of the amiloride binding site. J Biol Chem 262:10613–10618

35. Kleyman TR, Cragoe EJ Jr, Kraehenbuhl JP (1989) The cellular pool of Na^+ channels in the amphibian cell line A6 is not altered by mineralocorticoids. Analysis using a new photoactive amiloride analog in combination with anti-amiloride antibodies. J Biol Chem 264:11995–12000

36. Cornelisse J, Havinga E (1975) Photosubstitution reactions of aromatic compounds. Chem Rev 75:353–388

37. Kleyman TR, Rajagopalan R, Cragoe EJ Jr, Erlanger BF, Al-Awqati Q (1986) New amiloride analogue as hapten to raise anti-amiloride antibodies. Am J Physiol 250:C165–C170

38. Cassel D, Rotman M, Cragoe EJ Jr, Igarashi P (1988) Preparation of 6-^{125}I-labeled amiloride derivatives. Anal Biochem 170:63–67

39. Kleyman TR, Kraehenbuhl JP, Rossier BC, Cragoe EJ Jr, Warnock DG (1989) Distinct epitopes on amiloride. Am J Physiol 257:C1135–C1141

40. Simchowitz L, Woltersdorf OW Jr, Cragoe EJ Jr (1987) Intracellular accumulation of potent amiloride analogues by human neutrophils. J Biol Chem 262:15875–15975

41. Benos DJ, Reyes J, Shoemaker DG (1983) Amiloride fluxes across erythrocyte membranes. Biochim Biophys Acta 734:99–104

42. Leffert HL, Koch KS, Fehlmann M, Heiser W, Lad PJ, Skelly H (1982) Amiloride blocks cell-free protein synthesis at levels attained inside cultured rat hepatocytes. Biochem Biophys Res Commun 108:738–745

43. Davis RJ, Czech MP (1985) Amiloride directly inhibits growth factor receptor tyrosine kinase activity. J Biol Chem 260:2543–2551

44. Koch KS, Leffert HL (1979) Increased sodium ion influx is necessary to initiate rat hepatocyte proliferation. Cell 18:153–163

Target Cell Metabolism of Corticosteroids Mediating Antisteroid Effects

Klaus Hierholzer, Helmut Bühler, and Frank H. Perschel[1]

Introduction

Anticorticosteroid hormones have attracted attention, since they not only provide useful tools for evaluating mechanisms of corticosteroid (CS) action but also since they constitute powerful therapeutic agents. Thus, antimineralocorticosteroids are applied in treating hypertension, antiglucocorticosteroids are useful in counteracting glucocorticosteroid (GCS) excess syndromes, and antiprogestins are widely used in interrupting the luteal phase, in counteracting early pregnancy, and may be useful in inhibiting mammary tumor growth.

In Principle, Antisteroid Effects Can Be Induced

1) By interfering with CS production either at the level of the adrenals or by reducing the availability of releasing and/or trophic hormones,
2) by interfering with CS effects in target cells, i.e., by anti-CS action in the classical sense which (competitively) binds to target cell receptors and inhibits the function of endogenous agonists; or
3) by interfering with steps subsequent to hormone-receptor interaction at the transcriptional level, or even further downstream.

Recent developments in the field have been covered in several excellent publications [1–22].

---

[1]Institut für Klinische Physiologie, Klinikum Steglitz, Freie Universität Berlin, Hindenburgdamm 30, 1000 Berlin 45, Federal Republic of Germany

A fourth principle of modulating physiological CS effects is inhibition (or stimulation) of CS-metabolizing enzymes. This aspect has recently attracted attention. It can be documented that many target organs are equipped with CS transforming enzymes that share the potency to convert CS to metabolites with biological properties which may differ quantitatively, as well as qualitatively, from the respective mother hormones. It is this fourth aspect which shall be addressed in the present paper. This is pertinent for the present discussion, since the 11-hydroxysteroid dehydrogenase (11-HSD) system constitutes a diuretic principle and, in turn, inhibition of 11-HSD results in Na^+ and fluid retention.

Materials and Methods

Experiments were performed with male Sprague Dawley rats (250–400 g). Renal tissue slices, microsomes and solubilized 11-HSD were incubated in vitro with ^{3}H-labelled corticosterone (B) or 11-dehydro B. Metabolites were identified by reversed phase high pressure liquid chromatography (RP-HPLC). The techniques used are described in detail elsewhere [23–26].

Sources of steroids and chemicals were: 1] ^{3}H-B from New England Nuclear, Dreieich, FRG, 2] ^{3}H-11 dehydro B prepared in our laboratory from 1, 3] β-glycyrrhetinic acid from Sigma, Deisenhofen, FRG, 4] detergents: CHAPS series from Calbiochem, Frankfurt/Main, FRG, Triton X-100 from Boehringer Mannheim, FRG, 5] bile acids from Calbiochem and Sigma, and 6] ginseng root extract and ginsenosides from Tsumura Co., Japan.

CS Metabolism in Peripheral Target Organs

Figure 1 indicates the sites of the steroid skeleton where metabolic transformations occur, as shown, in different tissues such as kidney, liver, intestinal tract, salivary glands, gonads, placenta, toad bladder, and fish gills (for references see [24,25]).

In our studies we initially concentrated on the rat kidney. Isolated perfused organs, tissue slices, and subcellular fractions such as microsomes, nuclei, mitochondria and cytoplasm were incubated with the respective endogenous ^{3}H-CS; the metabolites formed were identified by HPLC and mass spectrometry [23,27]. It can be shown that mammalian renal tissue converts aldosterone into reduced di- and tetrahydro metabolites. B is converted at C_{11} and C_{20} and is subsequently reduced to pregnane. From a quantitative point of view the enzyme 11-HSD seems to be most important. Thus, we concentrated on this enzyme (system).

Some of the relevant properties of the enzyme are listed in Table 1. Of particular interest seem to be results obtained in microbiochemical studies with microdissected single tubules, which demonstrated highest activities of 11-HSD in the proximal pars recta [28]. Furthermore, a peculiar distribution pattern of immunoreactive enzyme in cortex and papilla was obtained in immunohistochemical studies using a specific mouse anti-11-HSD monoclonal antibody. The latter studies identified intra-epithelial localization of 11-HSD in cortex and interstitial cell staining in renal

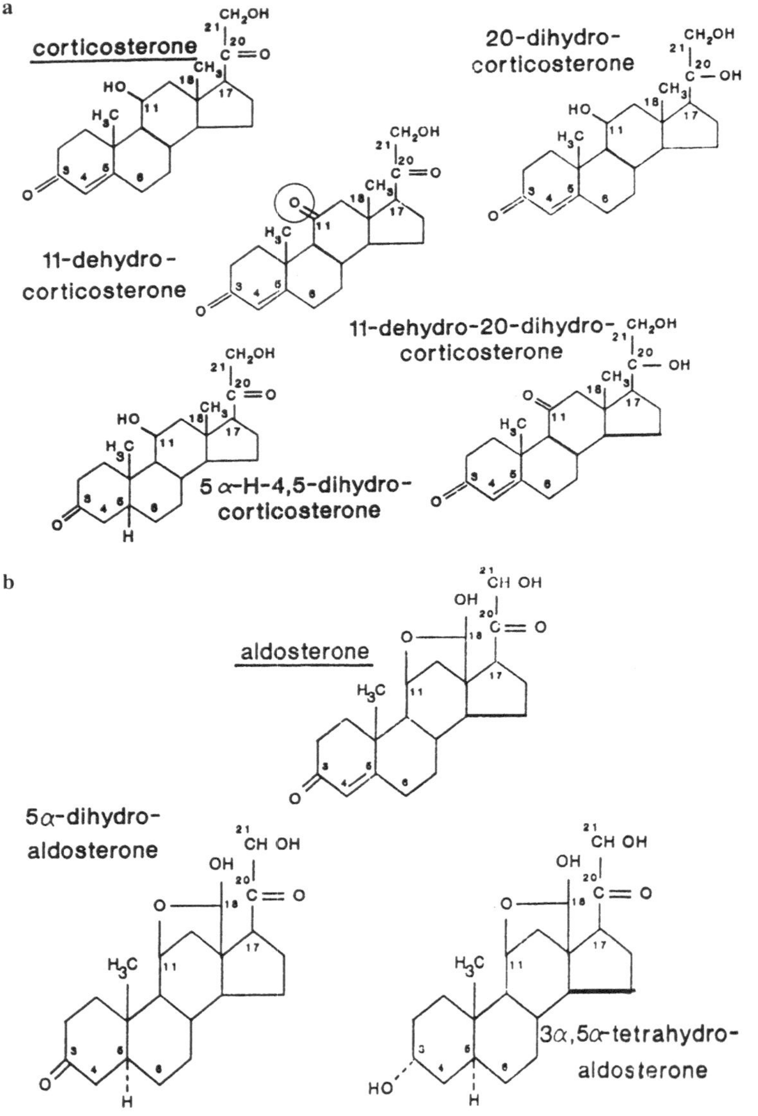

a

corticosterone

20-dihydro-
corticosterone

11-dehydro-
corticosterone

11-dehydro-20-dihydro-
corticosterone

5 α-H-4,5-dihydro-
corticosterone

b

aldosterone

5α-dihydro-
aldosterone

3α,5α-tetrahydro-
aldosterone

Fig. 1a,b. Structure of corticosterone with possible sites of renal metabolism **a.** corticosterone **b.** aldosterone

Table 1. 11-Hydroxysteroid-dehydrogenase (rat kidney)

(E.C. 1.1.1.146)
- Membrane bound (micros., nuclear)
- Identified in a) liver, gonads b) transporting epithelia (kidney, GIT, lung, placenta, toad bladder)
- Bidirectional? (oxidoreductase?) $11-OH-CS \longleftrightarrow 11=O-CS$
- Properties:
  a) molecular weight 34 kDa
  b) $K_m \sim 10^{-7}$ M
  c) $P_I \sim 5.9$ (ox. and red)
  d) pH $opt_{ox} \sim 9$, pH $opt_{red} \sim 6-7$
- Biological significance:
  CGS (in)activation
  Control of apparent MCS specificity

medulla [29]. The potential biological relevance of this differing distribution pattern has recently been discussed [30,31].

Inhibitors of 11-HSD (and other CS Transforming Enzymes)

The evaluation of the potential biological significance of the 11-HSD enzyme system has recently benefitted from experiments with specific enzyme inhibitors [30–36].

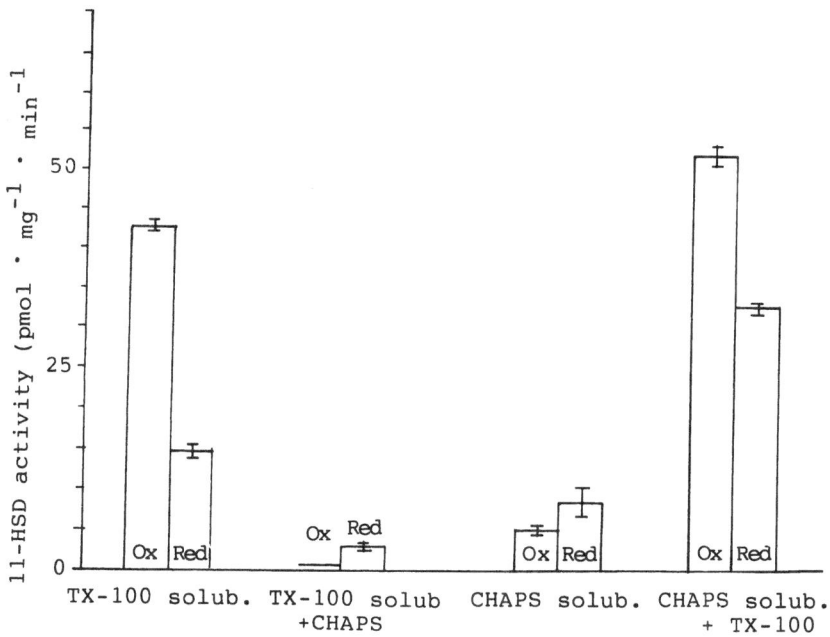

Fig. 2. Interference of different detergents with 11-HSD. Triton X (*TX*)-100 solubilized 11-HSD was incubated with 0.1% CHAPS; CHAPS solubilized 11-HSD was incubated with 0.1% Triton X-100. Ox, Oxidase; Red, Reductase. (X±SEM) (From [25])

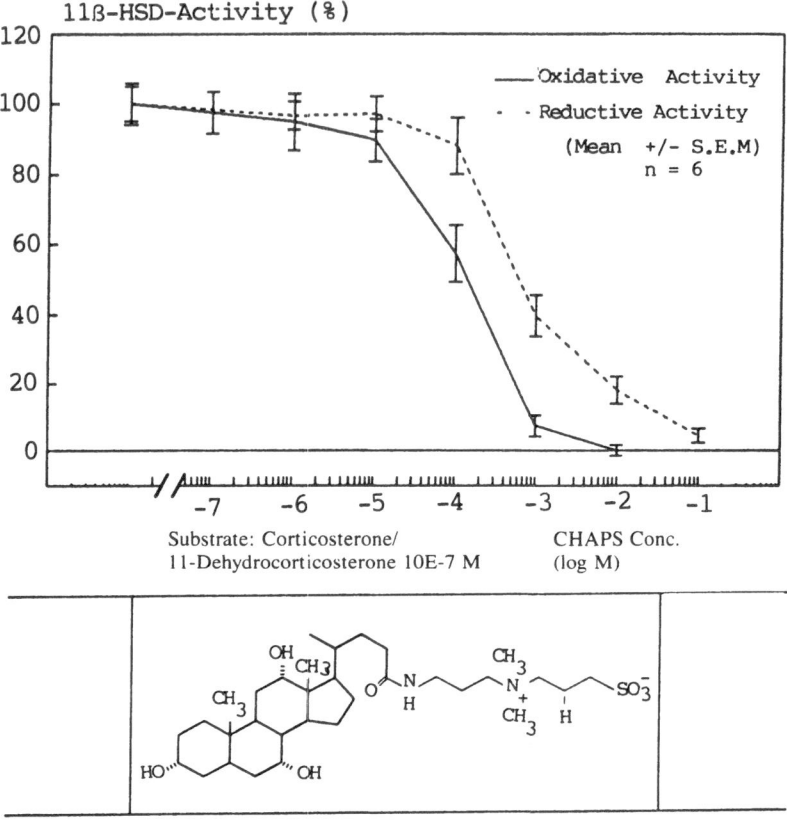

Fig. 3. Inhibition of 11-HSD by CHAPS. Aliquots of rat renal microsomes (adjusted to 20 μg protein/ml HEPES buffer) were incubated (pH 8. 37°C, 30 min). Corticosterone (*B*) + ^{3}H-B or 11-dehydro B + ^{3}H-11-dehydro B (10^{-7} M) and cosubstrates (NADP$^+$ or NADPH, 10^{-3} M) were added; metabolites were measured using RP-HPLC. (Adapted from [31])

Exogenous Inhibitors of 11-HSD

A first group of inhibitors was detected when we tried to solubilize 11-HSD from rat renal microsomes with different detergents, such as TX-100, Zwittergent, N-octylglucoside, and the CHAPS series. In contrast to all mentioned nonsteroidal detergents, CHAPS seemed to be rather ineffective in solubilizing oxidative activity [25]. Since the oxidative activity of the solubilized fraction could be reconstituted in vitro simply by dilution of the CHAPS concentration to less than 0.01% (Fig. 2) [25] we tested whether or not CHAPS, a steroidal detergent, might inhibit 11-HSD. The results shown in Fig. 3 document that both oxidative, and to a lesser degree, reductive activities are inhibited by concentrations ranging from 10^{-5} to 10^{-1} M. Comparable results were obtained with Big CHAP and Deoxy Big CHAP, which differ from CHAPS only in the hydrophilic head segment.

Table 2. Effects of licorice (L.) and/or glycyrrhetinic acid (Gl.Ac.)

− L. exerts DOC-like activity	Moluysen et al.	(1950). [37]
− L. causes hypertension, hypokalemia, ↓ plasma renin-activity (PRA), ↑ aldosterone	Epstein et al.	(1977), [38]
− Gl.Ac. binds to CS-receptors	Ulmann et al.	(1975), [39]
∼ Addision patients and adx. rats do not respond to L.	Borse et al.	(1953), [40]
	Card et al.,	(1953), [44]
− L. causes high urinary cortisol (at normal plasma cortisol)	Epstein et al.	(1978), [41]
∼ L. effect inhibited by spironolactone	Salassa et al.	(1982), [42]
− L. effect inhibited by dexamethasone	Hoefnagels et al.	(1983), [43]
− Gl.Ac. inhibits 11-HSD	Stewart et al.	(1987), [32]

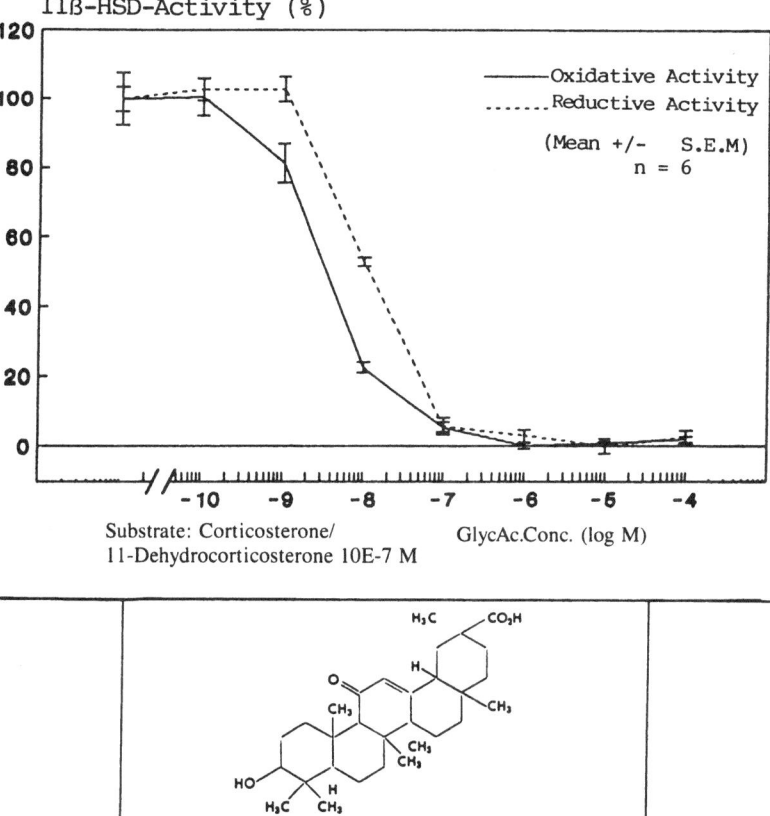

Substrate: Corticosterone/
11-Dehydrocorticosterone 10E-7 M

GlycAc.Conc. (log M)

Fig. 4. Inhibition of 11-HSD by β-glyc. acid; experiments and presentation as in Fig. 3 glyc., glycyrrhetinic acid (Adapted from [31])

A second group of inhibitors of 11-HSD consists of licorice and its active principles, glycyrrhitic acid, glycyrrhetinic acid, and the succinate ester carbenoxolone
[30–36]. As shown in Table 2 this group gained attention when clinical studies
pointed to a desoxycorticosterone (DOC)-like effect of licorice which could not be
explained on the basis of the weak binding properties of the active principle to miner-
alocorticosteroid (MCS)-receptors, but could apparently be explained by its effect on
cortisol metabolism [32,37–44].

Stewart et al. [32] were the first who demonstrated that glycyrrhetinic (glyc.) acid
was a potent inhibitor of 11β-HSD; they proposed the concept that the inhibitor plays
an important role in controlling the access of GCS such as B and cortisol (F) to the
MCS-receptor. Relevant data from our laboratory are shown in Fig. 4. It was demonstrated that glyc. acid inhibited 11-HSD in vitro in a dose-dependent manner; effective concentrations ranged from 10^{-9} to 10^{-6} M.

Similar results have been obtained with a mixture of glycyrrhitic acid, cysteine,
and glycine (REMEFA S kindly provided by Dr. Falk, Pharma GmbH, Freiburg, Federal Republic of Germany, distributed in Japan as "Stronger Neo-Minophagen C").

The biologic function of glyc. acid as an 11-HSD inhibitor has been tested in in-
vitro preparations. Thus, Dr. Fromm in our laboratory was able to show that addition
of the inhibitor (10^{-6} M) to totally stripped rat rectal colon unmasked an apparent
MCS effect of B (10^{-8} M) on amiloride inhibitable short circuit current. The apparent
MCS effect was indistinguishable from the maximal aldosterone effect [31]. Comparable effects have been observed in isolated toad bladders by Gaeggeler et al. [45]
and by Brem et al. [46].

A third class of inhibitors stems from Japanese traditional medicine. We have come
across the fact that ginseng root contains steroid-like compounds which might exhibit

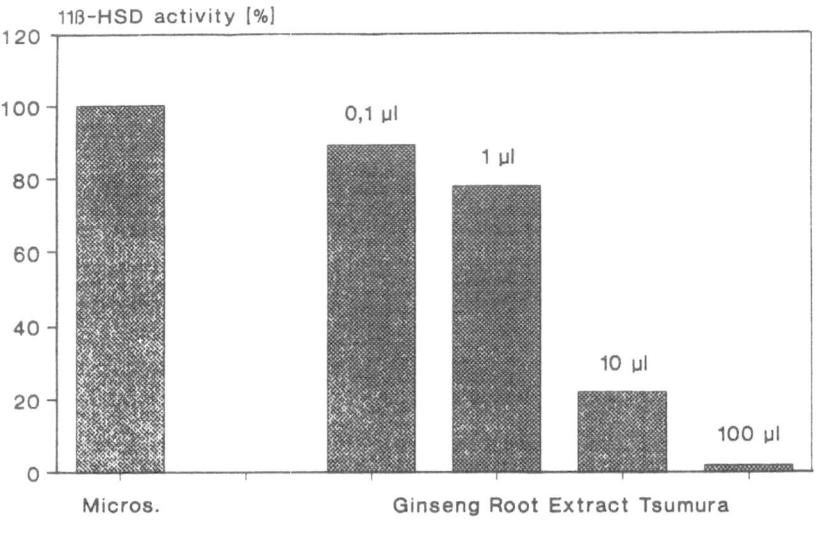

Fig. 5. Effect of ginseng root extract on activity of 11-HSD

Table 3. Inhibition of rat renal 11β-HSD

Compound	Mol. conc. at 50% inhibition	
	Oxidase	Reductase
CHAPS	1.4×10^{-4}	6.1×10^{-4}
Big CHAP	2.8×10^{-6}	6.0×10^{-6}
Deoxy Big CHAP	7.1×10^{-5}	$-^a$
Glycyrrhetinic acid	3.4×10^{-9}	1.2×10^{-8}
Remefa[b]	7.1×10^{-7}	1.2×10^{-6}

Substrate: corticosterone/11-dehydrocorticosterone 10^{-7} M $n = 6-12$
[a]No inhibition within range of solubility. When solubilized 11-HSD
was used instead of microsomes deoxyBigCHAP inhibited 50% of
reductase at 4.0×10^{-4} M
[b]Conc. of active principle: glycyrrhizin (From [53])

affinity to the active center of 11-HSD. Therefore, extracts of ginseng root and subsequently isolated and purified ginsenosides (kindly provided by Tsumura Co., Tokyo, Japan) were tested in vitro using, again, rat renal microsomal 11-HSD. Figure 5 shows the results of pilot experiments which demonstrate that total extract inhibits the enzyme. This is of particular interest, since the extract contains several steroidal compounds of comparable structure and thus may provide a means of testing the structural details which have a bearing upon inhibitor affinity to the enzyme. So far, only one member of the group seems to exert inhibitory effects. Obviously, the results of further experiments, which are under way, will have to be waited for. Table 3 summarizes results hitherto established in our laboratory. It is pertinent to note that glyc. acid is the most effective exogenous inhibitor so far.

Endogenous Inhibitors of 11-HSD

The observations presented above tempted us to search for the possible existence of endogenous inhibitors of 11-HSD. Bile acids were likely candidates, since they resemble CHAPS, as far as the hydrophobic tail segment is concerned, and differ only in the hydrophilic head. So far we have tested cholic acid and chenodeoxycholic acid, deoxycholic acid and lithocholic acid, as well as ursodeoxycholic acid as primary, secondary, and tertiary bile acids, respectively. Studies with conjugated bile acids are under way.

Figure 6 shows an inhibitory curve of both oxidative and reductive activity of 11-HSD, obtained with cholic acid. The experiments were carried out with renal cortical microsomes. As demonstrated, enzymatic oxidative and reductive activities are inhibited in a dose dependent manner. Table 4 lists molar bile acid concentrations which are required in order to induce a 50% inhibition under experimental conditions in vitro.

From these studies we conclude that, in principle, bile acids can act as modulators of 11-HSD and possibly of other CS-degrading enzyme systems. This is important in view of older reports which have pointed to an abnormal cortisol metabolism in liver cirrhosis, in extrahepatic biliary obstruction, and after ingestion of bile acids [47-49].

Figure 7 summarizes the sites of steroidal compounds which may be of strategic importance in controlling the fitting of an inhibitor to 11-HSD. An oxygen function

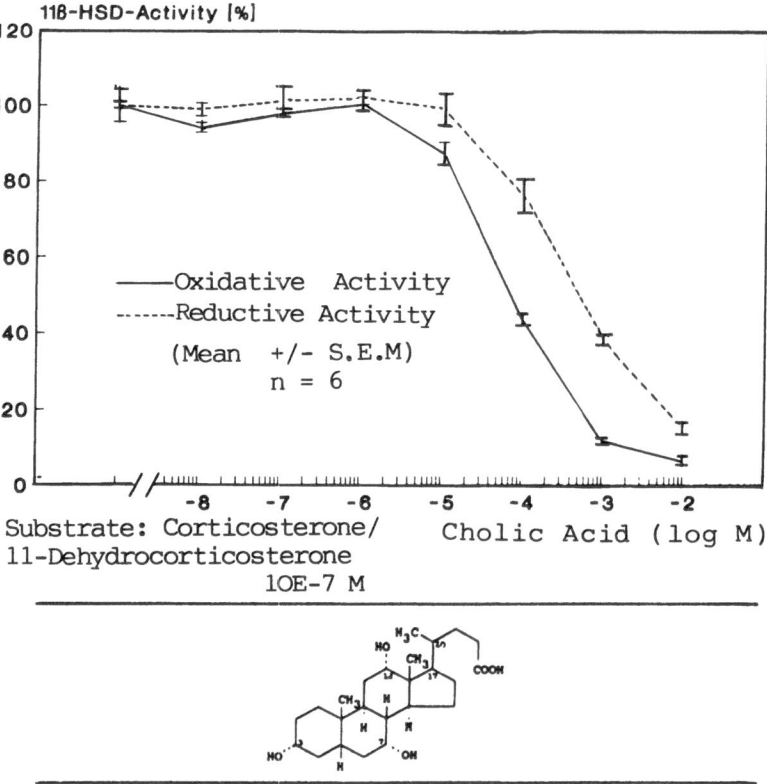

Fig. 6. Inhibition of 11-HSD by cholic acid; experiments and presentation as in Fig. 3. (Adapted from [54])

at C_3, either in the α- or β-position, is present in all inhibitors so far tested. The C_7 can carry a hydroxyl- or a keto group, or can be deoxidized as in deoxycholate; the same holds for C_{11}. The C_{12} can be hydroxylated, as in cholic acid. The hemiacetal configuration (C_{11}–C_{18}) does not prevent fitting (data not shown), but prevents metabolism of aldosterone. Glycyrrhetinic acid, the strongest inhibitor presently

Table 4. Inhibition of rat renal 11β-HSD by different bile acids

Class of bile acid	Compound	n	50% Inhibition	
			Ox.	Red.
Primary bile acids	Cholic acid	6	$7.1*10^{-5}$	$5.0*10^{-4}$
	Chenodeoxycholic acid	6	$2.1*10^{-6}$	$8.0*10^{-6}$
Secondary bile acids	Deoxycholic acid	8	$8.0*10^{-5}$	$3.1*10^{-3}$
	Lithocholic acid	6	$2.3*10^{-6}$	$3.1*10^{-5}$
Tertiary bile acid	Ursodeoxycholic acid	6	$2.3*10^{-5}$	$3.1*10^{-3}$

(From [54])

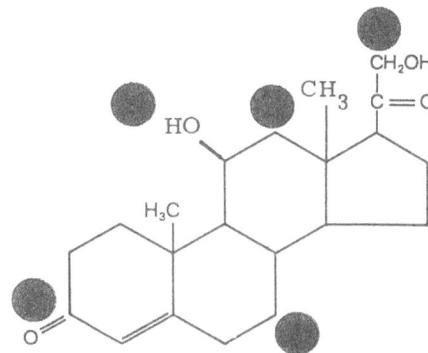

Fig. 7. Properties of inhibitors of 11-HSD

available, is characterized by a 5-ring configuration. Interestingly, large hydrophilic side chains can be tolerated, as demonstrated by the results obtained with the CHAPS-series. We realize that this is only a first overview, which needs further evaluation on the basis of three-dimensional data.

Conclusions

These experiments have demonstrated that the 11-HSD system serves several important functions. First, it effectively inactivates GCS such as F and B by oxidative degradation at C_{11}. The primary importance of the system may lie in GCS-signal inactivation; however, since 11-HSD in essence is an oxido-reductase system, it is conceivable that under certain metabolic conditions the intracellular concentrations of active GCS can be raised by conversion of cortisone to cortisol and/or 11-dehydro B to B. This would in essence constitute signal activation. Intracellular stores of inactivated GCS might, therefore, serve as a pool for active GCS and permit adjustment of local activation and inactivation of GCS, e.g., in cells like those of the proximal pars recta, which is a site of nicotinamide-adenine-dinucleotide phosphate (NADP)$^+$/H dependent enzymatic reactions [50].

More relevant for the present discussion is the notion that GCS transformation via 11-HSD may control access of CS signals to MCS receptors, as suggested by Steward et al. [32]. The situation, which is in accord with experimental data, is depicted in Fig. 8. In essence, 11-HSD constitutes a diuretic principle in preventing access of large concentrations of GCS to receptors of limited MCS- versus GCS-specificity.

Inhibition of the system, whether genetically determined, as in "apparent MCS excess syndrome" [51], or whether caused by exogenous inhibitors such as medically used glyc. acid preparations or possibly caused by endogenous inhibitors of the bile acid type, thus exerts MCS agonist effects. This is not only of theoretical value, but also of great practical importance in view of the widespread use of, e.g., glyc. acid in chronic hepatitis and AIDS or as an additive.

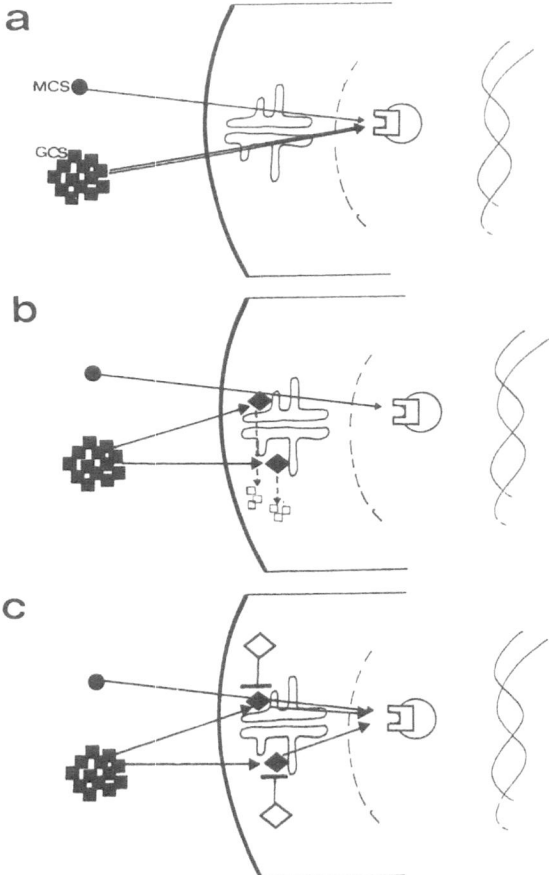

Fig. 8. Schematic presentation of different models of CS interaction with target cells: **a** due to the lack of 11-HSD, both MCS and GCS gain access to CS receptors **b** 11-HSD prevents access of 11-hydroxylated GCS by oxidative inactivation at C_{11}, **c** inhibition of 11-HSD as caused by glyc. acid, CHAPS, or bile acids converts the target cells essentially into the type shown in **a**. MCS, mineralocorticosteroids; GCS, glucocorticosteroids

Most relevant to this discussion of diuretics are recent reports that at least one inhibitor, glyc. acid, not only affects 11-HSD but induces accumulation of DH- and TH-aldosterone [35,52] and, thus, may also interfere with other CS-degrading enzymes.

Acknowledgments. KH was supported by the Deutsche Forschungsgemeinschaft Hi 97/16 1-4. Expert technical assistance of Ingrid Lichtenstein and Harald Siebe, and expert secretarial assistance of Helga Gräbener is acknowledged.

References

1. Corvol P, Claire M, Oblin ME, Geering K, Rossier B (1981) Mechanism of the antimineralocorticoid effects of spirolactones. Kidney Int 20:1–6
2. Agarwal MK (1984) An original multifaceted antihormone in vivo. Adrenal steroid antagonism. In: Proceedings of Workshop 7th International Congress Endocrinology Canada. W. De Gruyter, Berlin
3. Clark CR (1985) Intracellular localization of steroid receptors. In: Sluyser M, Horward E (eds) Interaction of steroid hormone receptors with DNA. Ellis Horwood, Chichester, pp 7–56
4. Henderson D (1987) Antiprogestational and antiglucocorticoid activities of some novel 11β-aryl substituted steroids. In: Furr BJA, Wakeling AE (eds) Pharmacology and clinical uses of inhibitors of hormone secretion and action. Bailliere Tindall, London, 184–211
5. Munck A, Holbrook NJ (1988) Cyclic, nonequilibrium models of glucocorticoid antagonism: role of activation, nuclear binding and receptor recycling. J Steroid Biochem 31 (4B):599–606
6. Kloosterboer HJ, Deckers GHJ, van der Heuvel MJ, Loozen HJJ (1988) Screening of antiprogestagens by receptor studies and bioassays. J Steroid Biochem 31 (4B):567–571
7. Teutsch G, Ojasoo T, Raynaud JP (1988) 11β-substituted steroids, an original pathway to antihormones. J Steroid Biochem 31 (4B):549–565
8. Chrousos GP, Laue L, Nieman LK, Kawai S, Udelsman RU, Brandon DD, Loriaux DL (1988) Glucocorticoids and glucocorticoid antagonists: lesson from RU 486. Kid Int 34 (Suppl 26):18–23
9. Baulieu EE (1988) Molecular mechanism of antisteroid hormones at the receptor level. Kid Int 34 (Suppl 26):2–7
10. Waeber B, Nüssberger J, Brunner HR (1988) Clinical applications of antimineralocorticoids. J Steroid Biochem 31 (4B):739–744
11. Duax WL, Griffin JF, Weeks CM, Wawrzak Z (1988) The mechanism of action of steroid antagonists: insights from crystallographic studies. J Steroid Biochem 31 (4B):481–492
12. Schmidt TJ (1989) Comparison of in vivo activation of triamcinolone acetonide- and RU 38486-receptor complexes in the CEM-C7 and IM-9 Human leukemic cell lines.[1] Cancer Res 49:4390–4395
13. Raaka BM, Finnerty M, Samuels HH (1989) The glucocorticoid antagonist 17α-methyltestosterone binds to the 10 S glucocorticoid receptor and blocks agonist-mediated dissociation of the 10 S oligomer to the 4 S deoxyribonucleic acid-binding subunit. Molecular Endocrinol 3 (2):332–341
14. Beier HM, Mootz U, Hegele-Hartung CH (1989) Studies on the establishment of mammalian pregnancy: synchronization of the maternal and the embryonic systems. Reprod Biol Med 210–223
15. Baulieu EE (1989) RU-486 as an antiprogesterone steroid. From receptor to contragestin and beyond. JAMA 262 (13):1808–1814
16. Michna H, Schneider MR, Nishino Y, El Etreby MF (1989) Antitumor activity of the antiprogestins ZK 98.299 and RU 38.486 in hormone dependent rat and mouse mammary tumors: mechanistic studies. Breast Cancer Res Treat 14:275–288
17. Schneider MR, Michna H, Nishino Y, El Etreby MF (1989) Antitumor activity of the progesterone antagonists ZK 98.299 and RU 38.486 in the hormone-dependent MXT mammary tumor model of the mouse and the DMBA- and the MNU-induced mammary tumor models of the rat. Eur J Cancer Clin Oncol 25 (4):691–701
18. Agarwal MK, Kalimi M (1989) Analysis of the mineralocorticoid receptor in rat heart with the aid of two new spirolactone derivatives. Biochem Med Metabol Biol 41:36–45
19. Brooks VL (1989) Vasporessin and ANG II in the control of ACTH secretion and arterial and atrial pressures. Am J Physiol 256:R339–R347

20. Zhu Q, Bateman A, Singh A, Solomon (1989) Isolation and biological activity of corticostatic peptides (anti-ACTH). Endocr Res Commun 15 (1,2):129-149

21. Lamberts SWJ, Bruining HA, Marzouk H, Zuiderwijk J, Uitterlinden P, Blijd JJ, Hackeng WHL, De Jong FH (1989) The new aromatase inhibitor CGS-16949A suppresses aldosterone and cortisol production by human adrenal cells in vitro. J Clin Enocrinol Metab 69 (4):896-901

22. van der Schoot P, Uilenbroek JThJ, Slappendel EJ (1990) Effect of the progesterone antagonist mifepristone on the hypothalamo-hypophysial-ovarian axis in rats. J Endocrinol 124:425-432

23. Hierholzer K, Schöneshöfer M, Siebe H, Tsiakiras D, Weskamp P (1984) Corticosteroid metabolism in isolated rat kidney in vitro I. Formation of lipid soluble metabolites from corticosterone (B) in renal tissue from male rats. Pflügers Arch 400:363-371

24. Kobayashi N, Schulz W, Hierholzer K (1987) Corticosteroid metabolism in rat kidney in vitro IV. Subcellular sites of 11β-hydroxysteroid dehydrogenase activity. Pflügers Arch 408:46-53

25. Schulz W, Lichtenstein I, Siebe H, Hierholzer K (1989) Isoelectric focusing analysis of detergent extracted renal 11β-hydroxysteroid dehydrogenase. J Steroid Biochem 32:581-590

26. l'Allemand D, Siebe H, Tsiakiras D, Hoyer GA, Vecsei P, Hierholzer K (1988) Aldosterone metabolism in rat renal tissue in vitro. Formation of lipid soluble metabolites. Pflügers Arch 411:529-539

27. Hoyer GA, Tsiakiras D, Siebe H, Hierholzer K (1984) Corticosteroid metabolism in isolated rat kidney in vitro III. Structure analysis of lipid soluble metabolites of corticosterone. Pflügers Arch 400:377-380

28. Spieth A, Hierholzer K (1987) Longitudinal heterogeneity of renal corticosterone metabolism in mouse nephron. Pflügers Arch 408:R42

29. Castello R, Schwarting R, Müller C, Hierholzer K, Lichtenstein I (1989) Immuno-histochemical localization of 11-hydroxysteroid dehydrogenase in rat kidney with a monoclonal antibody. Renal Physiol Biochem 12:320-327

30. Hierholzer K, Castello R, Kobayashi N, Fromm M (1989) Sites and significance of renal corticosteroid metabolism. In: Berliner RW, Honda N, Ullrich KJ (eds) The frontiers of nephrology, Elsevier, Amsterdam, pp 67-76

31. Hierholzer K, Siebe H, Fromm M (1990) Inhibition of 11β-hydroxysteroid dehydrogenase and its effect on epithelial sodium transport. Kidney Int 38:673-678

32. Stewart PM, Valentino R, Wallace AM, Burt D, Shackleton CHL, Edwards CRW (1987) Mineralocorticoid activity of liquorice: 11β-hydroxysteroid dehydrogenase deficiency comes of age. Lancet II:821-24

33. Edwards CRW, Stewart PM, Burt D, Brett L, McIntyre MA, Sutanto WS, De Kloet ER, Monder C (1988) Localisation of 11β-Hydroxysteroid dehydrogenase-tissue specific protector of the mineralocorticoid receptor. Lancet 29:986-989

34. Edwards CRW, Burt D, Stewart PM (1989) The specificity of the human mineralocorticoid receptor: Clinical clues to a biological conundrum. J Steroid Biochem 32 (1B):213-216

35. Morris DJ, Souness GW (1990) The 11β-OHSD inhibitor, carbenoxolone, enhances Na retention by aldosterone and 11-deoxycorticosterone. Am J Physiol 258:F756-F759

36. Funder JW, Pearce PT, Smith R, Smith AI (1988) Mineralocorticoid action: Target tissue specificity is enzyme, not receptor, mediated. Science 242:583-585

37. Molhuysen JA, Gerbrandy J, De Vries IA (1950) A liquorice extract with "deoxycortone-like" action. Lancet II:381-386

38. Epstein MT, Espiner EA, Donald RA, Hughes H (1977) Liquorice toxicity and the renin-angiotensin-aldosterone axis in man. Br Med J [Clin Res] 1:209-210

39. Ulmann A, Menard J, Corvol P (1975) Binding of glycyrrhetinic acid to kidney mineralocorticoid and glucocorticoid receptors. Endocrinology 97:46-51

40. Borst JGG, Tenholt SP, De Vries LA, Molhuysen JA (1953) Synergistic action of liquorice and cortisone in Addison's and Simmonds's disease. Lancet II:657–663
41. Epstein MT, Espiner EA, Donald RA, Hughes H, Cowles RJ, Lun S (1978) Licorice raises urinary cortisol in man. J Clin Endocrinol Metab 47:397–400
42. Salassa RM, Mattox VR, Rosevear JW (1982) Inhibition of the "mineralocorticoid" activity of licorice by spironolactone. J Clin Endocrinol Metab 22:1156–1159
43. Hoefnagels WHL, Kloppenburg PWC (1983) Antimineralocorticoid effects of dexamethasone in subjects treated with glycyrrhetinic acid. J Hypertens 1 (Suppl 2):313–315
44. Card WI, Mitchell W, Strong JA, Taylor NRW, Tompsett SL, Wilson JMG, (1953) Effects of liquorice and its derivatives on salt and water metabolism. Lancet II:663–667
45. Gaeggeler HP, Edwards CRW, Rossier BC (1989) Steroid metabolism determines mineralocorticoid specificity in the toad bladder. Am J Physiol 257:F690–F695
46. Brem AS, Matheson KL, Conca T, Morris DJ (1989) Effect of corbenoxolone on glucocorticoid metabolism and Na transport in toad bladder. Am J Physiol 257:F700–F704
47. Zumoff B, Bradlow HL, Gallagher TF, Hellamn L (1967) Cortisol metabolism in cirrhosis. J Clin Invest 46:1735–1742
48. Zumoff B, Bradlow HL, Gallagher TF (1971) Cortisol metabolism in total extrahepatic biliary obstruction. J Clin Endocrinol Metab 32:36–41
49. Gerdes H, Riemenschneider H, Littmann KP (1971) Effect of bile acids and some biliary excreted drugs on the metabolism of cortisol. Acta Endocrinol (Copenh) 173:10
50. Guder WG, Ross BD (1984) Enzyme distribution along the nephron. Kidney Int 26:101–111
51. Ulick S, Levine LS, Gunczler P, Zanconato G, Ramirez LC, Rauh W, Rösler A, Bradlow HL, New MI (1979) A syndrome of apparent mineralocorticoid excess associated with defects in the peripheral metabolism of cortisol. Endocrinol Soc 49:757–764
52. Latif SA, Conca TJ, Morris DJ (1990) The effects of the licorice derivative, glycyrrhetinic acid, on hepatic 3α- and 3β-hydroxysteroid dehydrogenases and 5α- and 5β-reductase pathways of metabolism of aldosterone in male rats. Steroids 55:52–58
53. Bühler H, Kobayashi N, Lichtenstein I, Perschel FH, Siebe H, Hierholzer K (1990) Reversible inhibition of renal 11-hydroxysteroid dehydrogenase (11-HSD) by steroids, structure-function-relationship. Nieren + Hochdruckkrankheiten 19:374
54. Perschel FH, Bühler H, Siebe H, Lichtenstein I, Hierholzer K (1990) Bile acids as endogenous inhibitors of 11β-hydroxysteroid dehydrogenase (11-HSD). Nieren + Hochdruckkrankheiten 19:406

Glomerular Cells and Extracellular Matrix

Chair: R. Bernd Sterzel (FRG)
Fujio Shimizu (Japan)

Ultrastructure of the Mesangial Matrix

Wilhelm Kriz and Marlies Elger[1]

Introduction

The glomerular mesangium and the glomerular capillaries are enclosed in a single compartment bounded by a common basement membrane. The capillary-mesangium interface consists only of a fenestrated endothelium. There is no basement membrane at this interface. Thus, a discrete hydraulic barrier is not established. Therefore, the range of hydraulic pressure in the mesangium, i.e., in the mesangial matrix, can be expected to be of the same magnitude as the range of glomerular capillary pressure. Tracer studies [1,2], which show the rapid entry of macromolecular compounds into the mesangium from the blood, support this postulate. As a result, the transmural hydraulic pressure difference across the perimesangial glomerular basement membrane (GBM) should also be of about the same magnitude as that across the capillary wall. These hydraulic pressure differences have to be counteracted to prevent capillary and mesangial expansion [3,4].

As shown by recent studies, counteraction is established by the connection of the GBM to the contractile apparatus of mesangial cells [3–5]. By these connections the GBM is pulled centrally to the axial region of the mesangium. These connections are most prominent at mesangial angles, but are found along the entire perimesangial GBM. In addition to direct attachments of mesangial cells to the GBM, the mesangial matrix has been suggested to be the connecting element [6]. In our view, the ultrastructural equivalent underlying this mechanical function is represented by a *microfibrillar network*. This review summarizes the findings on this subject.

Ultrastructure and Composition of the Mesangial Matrix

The mesangial matrix may be regarded as a specific interstitial space, filled with a matrix of relatively high electron density. Ultrastructurally, the mesangial matrix has

[1]Institut für Anatomie und Zellbiologie, Universität Heidelberg, D-6900 Heidelberg, Federal Republic of Germany

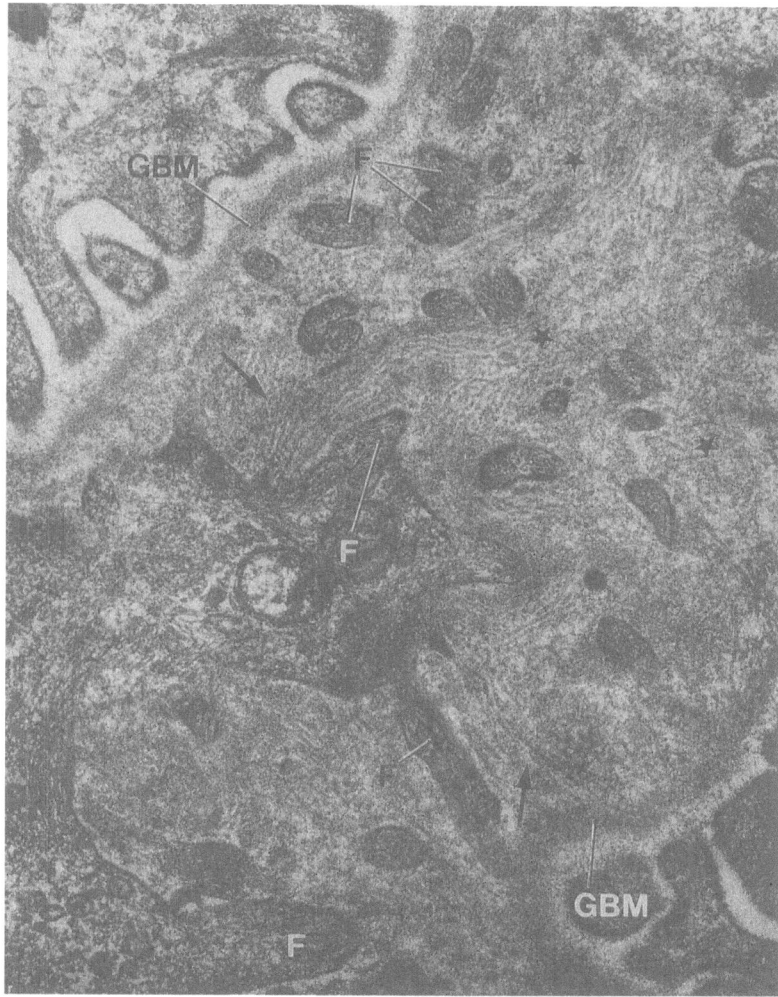

Fig. 1. Rat glomerulus; section through the mesangium, which is bounded by the glomerular basement membrane (*GBM*). The numerous processes of the mesangial cells contain microfilament bundles (*F*). In the mesangial matrix abundant microfibrils are seen, which form a network (*asterisks*) or are arranged in bundles (*arrows*). Transmission electron micrograph (*TEM*), × 37000

been described as similar to but clearly different "from the basement membrane proper by its looser texture and by the presence of small bundles of fine fibers (D = 100 Å) embedded in its feltwork of finer fibrils" [7]. Microfibrils can be identified clearly in cross section by their tubular structure. Several authors, using this criterion, have described microfibrils as a component of the mesangial matrix [8,9]. By

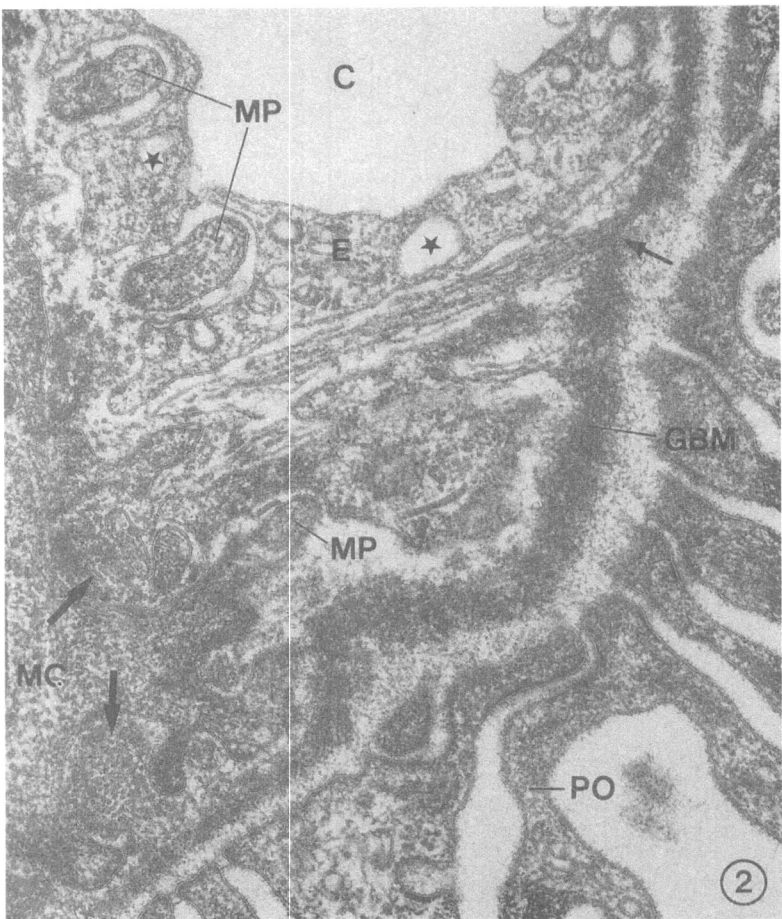

Fig. 2. Rat glomerulus; tangential section through the capillary-mesangial interface. Beneath the endothelium (*E*) a bundle of microfibrils is seen attaching to the GBM at a mesangial angle (*thin arrow*). Mesangial cell processes (*MP*) and part of a mesangial cell body (*MC*) are seen. Thick bundles of microfibrils are entrapped within invaginations of the cell body (*thick arrows*). Note that there is no basement membrane between the endothelium and the mesangium; the endothelium is fenestrated (*asterisks*). C, capillary lumen; PO, foot processes of podocytes. TEM, × 40000

combining tannic acid staining with a dehydration technique in the cold, we found that the mesangial matrix basically consists of a dense network of microfibrils [5,10] (Fig. 1).

Microfibrils represent a specific extracellular entity, characterized structurally by their typical appearance as hollow, nonbranching fibrils of undefined length. In the mesangial matrix we measured a very uniform thickness of almost exactly 15 nm

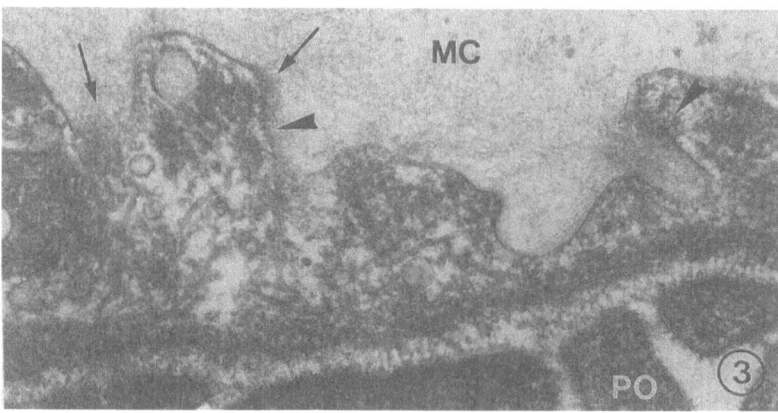

Fig. 3. Part of a mesangial cell (*MC*) with small processes running towards the GBM. The faint staining of the cell (the tissue has not been treated by OsO$_4$ and was stained with tannic acid, see [10]) allows identification of the narrow association of extracellular microfibrils (*dark stained*) and intracellular microfilaments (*faintly stained*) along the cell membrane (*arrows*). At favorable sites microfibrils are found in close relation to periodically spaced substructures on the outside of the cell membrane (*arrowheads*). PO, foot processes of podocytes. TEM, × 60000

[10]. This thickness is in good agreement with microfibril diameters measured at other sites and in other species [9,11–14].

Various elaborations of the mesangial microfibrillar network have to be considered. First, discrete microfibrillar connections are found between processes of mesangial cells and the GBM. They are most prominent at mesangial angles [3–5] (Fig. 2). In these connections, microfibrils appear to be attached to sites in the mesangial cell membrane that serve for the anchorage of intracellular actin filaments (Fig. 3). At opposite sites these bundles of microfibrils are closely associated with the GBM: at favorable sites microfibrils can clearly be recognized to penetrate into the lamina densa of the GBM (Fig. 2).

Second, in between these distinct connections, a network of interwoven microfibrils is found (Fig. 1), which attaches to the inner surface of the GBM and to the surface of mesangial cells at countless sites and is also associated with the discrete mesangial cell/GBM-connections described above.

Third, cross sections of microfibrillar bundles are regularly recognized running within bay-like cytoplasmic invaginations of mesangial cells (Fig. 2). They seem to run fairly parallel to the cell surface. They are more frequently found associated with cell bodies and larger processes than with peripheral parts of mesangial cells. Their course, their beginning, and their termination are unclear.

By means of immunocytochemistry, collagen type IV, V, and VI [15,16], fibronectin [17–19], laminin [19], and entactin [20] have been detected as components of the mesangial matrix. Among them fibronectin is the most abundant. This is in agreement with the ultrastructural observation that the mesangial matrix basically consists of a microfibrillar network, since microfibrils have been shown to be consistently associated with fibronectin [18,21]. The abundant mesangial fibronectin has been interpreted as serving for the linkage of mesangial cell surfaces to extracellular structures [2,18]. In addition, one may suggest that fibronectin interconnects the interwoven microfibrils at their crossing points, thus stabilizing the matrix net. Very recently, a 340 kDa protein, representing a major component of elastic microfibrils, has also been detected in the glomerular mesangium in the rat [22].

Functional Relevance

A function of the mesangial matrix as a connecting structure between mesangial cells and the GBM has been proposed previously, in studies in which the supposed failure of such a connection may have produced microaneurysms [23–25]. The microfibrillar network establishes a solid base of contact between mesangial cells and the GBM. In addition to direct attachments of mesangial cell processes to the GBM, microfibrils represent the connecting element between the contractile apparatus of mesangial cells and the GBM. Probably, the fundamental relevance of this system is that it counteracts the distending forces which are exerted on the GBM by high intracapillary and intramesangial pressures. The microfibrillar network of the mesangial matrix appears to be capable of balancing distending forces which act essentially in all directions.

Acknowledgments. We thank Ms Hiltraud Hosser for skillful technical assistance and Ms Ingrid Ertel for photographic work. Secretarial help was provided by Ms Helene Dehoust. Supported by Deutsche Forschungs-gemeinschaft, Kr 546/5–3, Forschergruppe "Niere," Heidelberg.

References

1. Michael AF, Keane WF, Raij L, Vernier RL, Mauer SM (1980) The glomerular mesangium. Kidney Int 17:141–154
2. Latta H, Fligiel S (1985) Mesangial fenestrations, sieving, filtration, and flow. Lab Invest 52:591–598
3. Kriz W, Elger M, Lemley K, Sakai T (1990) The structure of the glomerular mesangium: a biomechanical interpretation. Kidney Int 38 (suppl 30):52–59
4. Kriz W, Elger M, Lemley KV, Sakai T (1990) Mesangial cell-glomerular basement membrane connections counteract glomerular capillary and mesangium expansion. Am J Nephrol 10 (suppl 1):4–13
5. Sakai T, Kriz W (1987) The structural relationship between mesangial cells and basement membrane of the renal glomerulus. Anat Embryol (Berl) 176:373–386
6. Latta H, Maunsbach AB, Madden SC (1960) The centrolobular region of the renal glomerulus studied by electron microscopy. J Ultrastruct Res 4:455–472
7. Farquhar MG, Palade GE (1962) Functional evidence for the existence of a third cell type in the renal glomerulus. Phagocytosis of filtration residues by a distinctive "third" cell. J Cell Biol 13:55–87
8. Farquhar MG (1964) Glomerular permeability investigated by electron microscopy. In: Siperstein MD, Colwell AR, Meyer K (eds) Proceedings of the conference on small blood

vessel involvement in Diabetes Mellitus, 1963. Warrenton, USA. Am Inst Biol Sci, Washington, pp 31–80

9. Reale E, Luciano L, Kühn KW, Stolte H, Brod J (1981) Glomerular basement membrane and mesangial matrix. A comparative study in different vertebrates. In: Thomas S, Berlyne GM (eds) Renal physiology. Karger, Basel, pp 85–89

10. Mundel P, Elger M, Sakai T, Kriz W (1988) Microfibrils are a major component of the mesangial matrix in the glomerulus of the rat kidney. Cell Tissue Res 254:183–187

11. Ross R, Bornstein P (1969) The elastic fiber: I. The separation and partial characterization of its macromolecular components. J Cell Biol 40:366–381

12. Hsu H-C, Churg J (1979) Glomerular microfibrils in renal disease: A comparative electron microscopic study. Kidney Int 16:497–504

13. Cleary EG, Gibson MA (1983) Elastin-associated microfibrils and microfibrillar proteins. Int Rev Connect Tissue Res 10:97–209

14. Inoué S, Leblond CP (1986) The microfibrils of connective tissue: I. Ultrastructure. Am J Anat 176:121–138

15. Roll JF, Madri JA, Albert J, Futhmayr H (1980) Codistribution of collagen types IV and AB2 in basement membranes and mesangium of the kidney: an immunoferritin study of ultrathin frozen sections. J Cell Biol 85:597–616

16. Karkavelas G, Kefalides NA (1988) Comparative ultrastructural localization of collagen types III, IV, VI and laminin in rat uterus and kidney. J Ultrastruct Mol Struct Res 100:137–155

17. Oberley TD, Mosher DF, Mills MD (1979) Localization of fibronectin within the renal glomerulus and its production by cultured glomerular cells. Am J Physiol 96:651–658

18. Courtoy PJ, Kanwar YS, Hynes RO, Farquhar MG (1980) Fibronectin localization in the rat glomerulus. J Cell Biol 87:691–696

19. Madri JA, Roll FJ, Furthmayr H, Foidart J-M (1980) Ultrastructural localization of fibronectin and laminin in the basement membranes of the murine kidney. J Cell Biol 86:682–687

20. Bender BL, Jaffe R, Carlin B, Chung AE (1981) Immunolocalization of entactin, a sulfated basement membrane component in rodent tissues, and comparison with GP-2(laminin). Am J Pathol 103:419–426

21. Schwartz E, Goldfischer S, Coltoff-Schiller B, Blumenfeld OO (1985) Extracellular matrix microfibrils are composed of core proteins coated with fibronectin. J Histochem Cytochem 33:268–274

22. Gibson MA, Kumaratilake JS, Cleary EG (1989) The protein components of the 12-nanometer microfibrils of elastic and nonelastic tissues. J Biol Chem 264:4590–4598

23. Bloodworth JMB (1978) A re-evaluation of diabetic glomerulosclerosis 50 years after the discovery of insulin. Hum Pathol 9:439–453

24. Morita T, Churg J (1983) Mesangiolysis. Kidney Int 24:1–9

25. Saito Y, Kida H, Takeda S-I, Yoshimura M, Yokoyama H, Koshino Y, Hattori N (1988) Mesangiolysis in diabetic glomeruli: Its role in the formation of nodular lesions. Kidney Int 34:389–396

The Proteoglycans of Glomerular Mesangial Cells

Malcolm Davies, Gareth J. Thomas, Lorna Shewring[1],
and Roger M. Mason[2]

Introduction

Proteoglycans are located on cell membranes, in basement membranes and extracellular matrices, and are widely distributed in tissues [1]. They have many important biological roles, including cell adhesion, migration, and proliferation [2]. In the
kidney they are of particular interest, because proteoglycans in the glomerular basement membrane (GBM) form the main charge and steric exclusion barriers to trans-
capillary passage of plasma proteins [3]. Loss of anionic sites is associated with
proteinuria and has been noted in several nephropathies, including diabetic nephropathy, congenital nephrotic syndrome, and autologous immune complex disease.
The anionic sites in the glomerular filter are mainly due to the presence of heparan
sulfate proteoglycan (HSPG) [4]. Other proteoglycans, however, have been localised
in the glomerulus, including chondroitin sulfate proteoglycan (CSPG) [5-7]. This
proteoglycan is not present in the GBM in any significant amount, but does appear
to be localised in the mesangium. In this chapter, investigations on the localization,
biosynthesis, and metabolic turnover of mesangial proteoglycans from our own and
other laboratories are reviewed. A short section which speculates on the possible
role of CSPG in mesangial cell function is also included.

Chondroitin Sulphate Proteoglycans

Proteoglycans are a heterogenous and complex family of macromolecules composed
of a core protein to which a number of charged linear polysaccharides called
glycosaminoglycans (GAG) are covalently linked [1]. The GAG chains are made up

[1]Institute of Nephrology, University of Wales College of Medicine, Cardiff CF2 1SZ, Wales, UK
[2]Department of Biochemistry, Charing Cross and Westminster Hospital Medical School,
London, UK

of repeating disaccharide units of a hexuronic acid and an N-acetylhexosamine to which a sulfate group may be coupled via ester or amide linkage. At present, proteoglycans are classified according to their glycosaminoglycan chain but as more information becomes available on core proteins these components may provide a better means of classification. Five main classes have been identified: hyaluronan, keratan sulfate, heparan sulfate (including heparin), chondroitin sulfate (CS) and dermatan sulfate (DS). Of these, the latter two are the subject of this chapter. In CS-GAG the disaccharide repeat unit consists of D-glucuronic acid linked β (1–3) to N-acetyl galactosamine. The hexosamine residue carries ester-linked sulfated groups either at the C-4 position (CS-4-SO$_4$) or at C-6 (CS-6-SO$_4$). Dermatan sulfate is an epimer of chondroitin sulfate and the uronic acid residue in the repeat disaccharides is iduronic acid, i.e., L-iduronic acid linked α(1–3) to N-acetylgalactosamine. Chondroitin sulfate-GAG and DS-GAG can best be distinguished from each other by their susceptibility to fragmentation by chondroitin ABC lyase and chondroitin AC-II lyase. Chondroitin sulfate-GAG is degraded by both glycosidases to disaccharides whereas DS-GAG is degraded by chondroitin ABC lyase but is insensitive to chondroitin AC-II lyase. Since CS-GAG and DS-GAG are both resistant to deamination with nitrous acid not only is it possible to distinguish these glycosaminoglycans from each other but it is also possible to distinguish them from heparan sulfate (HS-GAG).

Localization of Proteoglycans in the Glomerular Mesangium

The proteoglycans that have been localised in the mesangium of the glomerulus are summarized in Table 1. The first evidence that the mesangium is enriched in CS-GAG was obtained by Kanwar et al. [5]. These authors used radiolabelled cationized ferritin as a probe for in situ labeling of the glomerular anionic sites. The localization of CS-GAG chains was demonstrated by a combination of enzymatic digestion with chondroitin ABC lyase and quantitative electron microscopy. Prior perfusion of the kidney with the enzyme revealed a decrease in binding of the radiolabelled probe to the anionic sits of the mesangial matrix but not in glomerular basement membrane. The presence of CS-GAG on the mesangium was confirmed by immuno-

Table 1. Mesangial proteoglycans detected by immunostaining and other procedures

Location	Method	Proteoglycan	Reference
Mesangial matrix	EM-Autoradiography	Chondroitin-dermatan	Kanwar et al. [5]
	IMS	Heparan sulfate	Miettinen et al. [8]
			Mynderse et al. [9]
			Isemura et al. [10]
	IMS	Chondroitin-4-sulfate	Couchman et al. [6]
	IMS	Basement membrane chondroitin sulfate	McCarthy et al. [7]
	Tissue culture/IMS	Basement membrane chondroitin sulfate	Shewring et al. [11]
	Tissue culture/IMS	Dermatan sulfate (PGII)	Shewring et al. [11]
Mesangial cell surface	IMS	Heparan sulfate	Farquhar et al. [3]

IMS, immunostaining

histochemical staining with monoclonal antibody against CS-4-SO$_4$ and CS-6-SO$_4$ [6]. Both these antibodies stained the mesangial matrix but not the GBM. Recently the same author [7] showed that four monoclonals with anti-CSPG specificity immunostained different rat basement membranes but not the GBM. All these macromolecules did, however, stain the kidney mesangium. The CSPG used in the preparation of these monoclonals was extracted from Reichert's membrane and characterized as a large macromolecule (Mr ~ 500 kD) with a protein core of approximately Mr 150 kD and GAG chains of Mr 15–18 kD. Identical elution profiles after treatment of the glycosaminoglycan chains with both chondroitin ABC and AC-II lyase indicated the absence of iduronic acid rich regions in the chains and identified the molecules as CS and not as DS proteoglycan. This proteoglycan has been termed a basement membrane-CSPG. A similar proteoglycan was extracted and partially purified from rat kidney [7].

Thus, immunostaining data suggest that different sub-classes of CSPG are located in the mesangial matrix.

Biosynthesis and Characterization of Mesangial Cell Proteoglycans

Investigations on the biosynthesis of glomerular proteoglycans have utilized techniques of radiolabelling in vivo, organ perfusion with medium containing ^{35}S-sulphate, or incubation of isolated glomeruli with ^{35}S-sulphate, or ^{3}H-glucosamine in vitro [12]. Based on the information included in Table 1 it has been widely accepted that newly synthesized radiolabelled CS/DS proteoglycans extracted from the glomeruli in these experiments are all derived from the biosynthetic activity of mesangial cells. However, this assumption is open to criticism. For example, the proportion of ^{35}S-proteoglycans that were accounted for as CS/DS-like molecules varied between the in vivo and in vitro studies. Kidneys perfused in situ or in vivo synthesized a comparatively low proportion of CS/DS GAG chains (~ 15% of the total ^{35}S-GAGs) whereas in vitro these molecules represented 65% of the total ^{35}S-proteoglycans. One possible explanation is that the pattern of synthesis in vitro is due to the preferential survival or activation of the mesangial cells. Another is that glomeruli in culture change their proteoglycan phenotype. These and other explanations, together with the advantages and disadvantages of the different experimental protocols, have been reviewed by us [12].

The labelled ^{35}S-proteoglycans synthesized by isolated glomeruli in vitro have been extensively characterized by Klein et al. [13]. Two major ^{35}S-DSPG were described. One (DS-tll) was extracted from the tissue eluted from DEAE-Sephacel with 0.56 M NaCl (i.e. high charge density) and by dissociative Sepharose CL-4B chromatography was estimated to have a Mr 500 kD. It was not displaced from the tissue with heparin. The second (DS-MII) was present in the medium only and was considerably smaller (Mr 200 kD) than DS-tII. In addition, a small dermatan sulfate (DS-tIA) was extracted from the glomeruli. It was a minor component and accounted for 5% of the total ^{35}S-proteoglycans compared to DS-tII and DS-IIM, which represented 29% and 32% respectively. This proteoglycan was released from the glomeruli

Table 2. ^{35}S-Proteoglycans synthesized by glomeruli[a] and mesangial cells[b] in culture

Species	Proteoglycan	Location	Mr (kD)	Core protein (kD)	Comment	Reference
Rat[a]	DSPG	Tissue extract	150	na	Displaced by heparin	Klein et al. [13]
		Tissue extract	500	na	–	
		Tissue extract	200	na	–	
Rat[b]	DSPG	Medium	220	45	Biglycan (PGI)	Border et al. [15]
		Medium	120	45	Decorin (PGII)	
Rat[b]	CSPG	Layer	230	na	Biglycan ?	Yaoita et al. [16]
		Layer	150	na	Decorin ?	
		Medium	135	na	Decorin ?	
Rat[b]	Basement membrane/ CSPG	Medium	–	na	Identified with Mab 2D6	Shewring et al. [11]
	DSPG	Medium/layer	220	na	Cell layer PG hydrophobic	
	DSPG	Medium/layer	110	na	Cell layer PG hydrophobic	
Human[b]	CS/DS-PG	Medium	na	na	–	Striker et al. [17]
Human	CSPG	Layer/ medium	>1000	400	Cell layer hydro-phobic	Davies et al. [18]
	DSPG	Layer/ medium	450	40		
		Medium	200	40		

by incubation with heparin. These findings, taken together with pulse-chase experiments, suggested that DS-tIA, once synthesized, was intercalated into cell membranes and then rapidly released into the medium. Since DS-tII required extraction with dissociative buffer it was suggested that this molecule is associated with matrix GAG binding sites. Radiolabelled DSPG similar to DS-tIA and DS-MII were separated from cultures of glomeruli labelled in vitro by Beavan et al. [14]. In addition, a large CSPG (Kav 0.3 on Sepharose CL4B) of high charge density was extracted from a GBM fraction and may be a product of mesangial cells.

Recent studies have used well established renal cell cultures to investigate proteoglycans synthesized by different glomerular cells. These studies have allowed information to determine whether particular proteoglycans are intercalated into cell membranes or are destined for export and integration with receptors for GAGs in the extracellular matrix. Proteoglycans synthesized by rat [15,16] and human [17,18] mesangial cell lines have been characterized and in general appear similar to those isolated from the in vitro experiments described above (Table 2). Moreover, these tissue culture studies indicate that the predominant GAG synthesized by mesangial cells are chondroitin and dermatan sulfate.

In human mesangial cells the majority of the proteoglycans synthesized are small DSPG which are released extracellularly. These were resolved into two sub-classes, namely DSPGI and DSPGII, in a ratio of 4:1. Both these DSPG have similar size protein cores (Mr $\sim$ 40 kD) and identical size GAG chains (Mr 25 kD). The difference in their overall molecular size (DSPGI $\sim$ 400000; DSPGII $\sim$ 200000) is most likely due to the number of GAG chains covalently linked to the protein core. Thus DSPGI and DSPGII have physical properties similar to, but not identical to, biglycan (also known as PGI) [19] and decorin (also known as PGII) [20], respectively. Furthermore DSPGII was recognized in a dot, blot assay by an antiserum raised against human fibroblast PGII (i.e., decorin).

In the cell extract DSPGI and DSPGII are also present, but as minor components. Indeed, pulse-chase experiments indicated that the majority of these proteoglycans, once synthesized, were rapidly released into the culture medium.

The prominent species in the cell extract of human mesangial cells is a high molecular weight CSPG (CSPGI Mr > 1000 kD). The GAG chains of this CSPG were totally sensitive to chondroitin ABC lyase and ACII lyase digestion. Thus CSPGI does not contain iduronic acid residues and can be classified as a chondroitin sulphate. The CSPGI in the cell layer was accessible to mild trypsin treatment, bound to octyl-Sepharose, and could be inserted into liposomes, indicating that this proteoglycan originated from cell surfaces where it is intercalated via its core protein into the cell membrane.

Two large HSPG (Mr $\sim$ 1000 and 450 kD) are synthesized by human mesangial cells in vitro [18]. They comprise about 20% of the total ^{35}S-proteoglycans. Both these proteoglycans are considerably larger than the HSPG extracted from human glomerular epithelial cells [21,22].

Chondroitin sulfate/DS proteoglycans synthesized by cultures of rat mesangial cells have also been recently characterized and found to be similar to those found in the human cultures above (Table 2). Border et al. [15] separated two DSPG from the culture medium using gradient SDS-polyacrylamide gel electrophoresis. These, on the basis of their Mr, were identified as biglycan and decorin.

In their studies Yaoita et al. [16], using cesium chloride density gradient centrifugation and column chromatography, also identified several sub-classes of small DS proteoglycans. Two of these (Mr 230 and 150 kD) may be associated with the plasma membrane, while a third (Mr 135 kD) was only present in the culture medium. Data on their core proteins were not given, but it is likely that these DS proteoglycans are related to biglycan and decorin.

We can confirm that rat mesangial cells synthesize mainly small DSPG. In addition we have used an affinity column prepared by coupling monoclonal 2D6 (which recognizes the basement membrane-CSPG from Reichert's membrane [7]) to investigate the ^{35}S-proteoglycans synthesized by rat mesangial cells [11]. Approximately 6% of the total ^{35}S-proteoglycans extracted from the medium bound to this column. The radiolabelled GAG released by alkaline-borohydride treatment of the bound material were completely susceptible to digestion with chondroitin ABC and ACII lyase. The hydrodynamic size of the intact proteoglycan was similar to the CSPG isolated from Reichert's membrane. The same monoclonal used for the affinity column also immunostained rat mesangial cells, as did the other three monoclonal antibodies described by McCarthy et al. [7].

Thus, at least four populations of CS/DS proteoglycans that differ in respect to hydrodynamic size and glycosaminoglycan composition as well as location, have been identified in mesangial cells. These proteoglycans show striking similarities to those found in aortic medial smooth muscle cells [23].

Turnover of Mesangial Cell Proteoglycans

Recently we have reported an in vivo model designed to follow the metabolism of proteoglycans in the rat glomerulus [24]. An important feature of the experimental design was that, after labelling experiments in which rats were given repeated intraperitoneal injections of ^{35}S-sulphate, the newly synthesized ^{35}S-proteoglycans were fixed in the tissue by perfusing the kidney in situ with 0.1% cetyl pyridinium chloride [14]. This approach ensured complete recovery of labelled molecules. The ^{35}S-GAGs accounted for 80% of the labelled macromolecules, the remainder being due to ^{35}S-glycoproteins. Of the ^{35}S-GAGs synthesized, 85% were HS-GAG and the remainder were CS-GAG [24]. A pulse-chase experiment was undertaken to determine the metabolic half-life of the ^{35}S-proteoglycans in the rat glomeruli. At defined times after the pulse with ^{35}S-sulphate, glomeruli were isolated and analyzed for ^{35}S-labelled macromolecules by autoradiographic and immunochemical methods, and by biochemical analysis. Together, these methods allowed the measurement of turnover times for the different proteoglycans in the glomerulus. Overall, the results showed a complex turnover pattern of ^{35}S-labelled macromolecules consisting of a rapid phase followed by a slower phase. The total population of ^{35}S-HSPG had a metabolic half-life ($t_{1/2}$) of 20 h and 60 h in the first and second phases, respectively. The turnover of basement membrane ^{35}S-HSPG was even faster and revealed $t_{1/2}$ of 5 h and 20 h, respectively. In contrast, the turnover of ^{35}S-CSPG differed from that of HSPG. Whilst it decreased initially with a $t_{1/2}$ of 20 h, the ^{35}S-CSPG pool showed little or no turnover during the second phase. One possible inference from this finding is that the turnover of mesangial cell proteoglycans is different from that of other cells of the glomerulus (endothelial and epithelial). This finding and the above discussion on the glomerular localization of CSPG suggest that mesangial cell proteoglycans may have a relatively slow turnover. Interestingly, the metabolism of ^{35}S-proteoglycans by cultured human glomerular mesangial cells is considerably slower than in human glomerular epithelial cells (Fig. 1). Thus, with mesangial cells after an 8 h chase, 70% of the initial proteoglycans remain associated with the cell layer. More detailed analysis of individual proteoglycans shows that a relatively small amount of DSPG enters the degradative pathway and that loss of proteoglycan from the cell layer is largely accounted for by release of DSPG into the medium.

Growth Factor and Mesangial Cell Proteoglycans

Studies on cultured glomerular cells indicate that enhancement of mesangial matrix synthesis is subject to modulation by cytokines. Tumor necrosis factor (TNFα) [25] and transforming growth factor (TGF-β) [15] have both been shown to be stimulators of mesangial cell proteoglycan production. The effects of the stimulatory cytokines were dose and time-dependent and were not the result of alteration in cell number. These cytokines did not alter the distribution of proteoglycans between the cell layer and culture medium, neither did they appear to have any significant effects on the quality of proteoglycans produced. These observations suggest a role for soluble DSPG in mesangial cell functions, possibly in the control of growth and proliferation. It is possible that the secreted DSPG interact with extracellular matrix com-

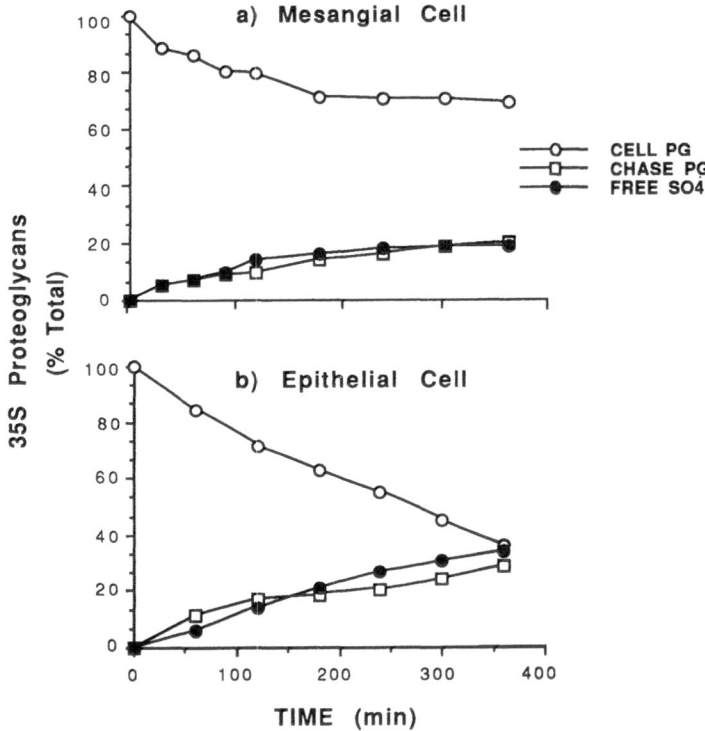

Fig. 1a,b. Pulse chase experiments with (**a**) human mesangial cells and (**b**) human glomerular epithelial cells. Cells were cultured with ^{35}S-sulfate for 24 h, the medium decanted and the cells chased for up to 6 h in fresh medium. At each time point the amount of ^{35}S-proteoglycans remaining in the cell layer (○) and released into the medium (□) was determined after chromatography on Sepharose CL-4B as well as free SO_4 (●). PG, proteoglycan

ponents such as fibronectin, with integrins, or with cytokines themselves to effect the regulation of mesangial cell growth. Such interactions have been reported in other cells [2].

Conclusions

At present it is only possible to speculate on the function of CS/DS proteoglycans in the mesangium. Table 3 contains a list of possible functions. It is possible that the basement membrane CSPG interacts, either through its protein core or GAG component, with other mesangial matrix components such as fibronectin or laminin. In this way it may serve to stabilize the architecture of the matrix. Mesangial basement membrane-CSPG co-exist with HSPG and the combined polyanionic nature of these molecules must contribute to the negative charge of the mesangium. It has been argued that proteoglycans, due to their charge, trap certain types of circulating immune complexes within the mesangium [5]. Cell surface proteoglycans possess binding sites for one or more extracellular proteins and therefore potentially link cells to matrix. Thus the large mesangial cell membrane CSPG could interact with GAG binding sites in the mesangial matrix and form part of a transmembrane cytoskeletal-matrix linkage. Such an interaction would favour cell adhesion. On the other hand, the soluble large CSPG may destabilize adhesion by "substratum conditioning," which then renders the matrix unsuitable for adhesion [26]. The small DSPG could also interact with GAG binding sites or fibronectin and interfere with cell attachment due to steric exclusion or charge repulsion [2]. Such an interaction would favour migration of cells. It is interesting to note that migration of mesangial cells into the pericapillary space between endothelium and GBM is a prominent feature in mesangio-capillary forms of glomerulonephritis [27].

Extensive research should be undertaken to shed more light on the functional and structural relationships between mesangial cell CS/DS and the other components of the mesangial matrix. In view of the known interactions of proteoglycans and fibronectin [2] and the abundance of fibronectin in the mesangial matrix, interactions between CS/DS proteoglycan may provide new insights into the function of the mesangial cell in the normal physiology of the kidney and possibly in the pathophysiology of glomerular disease. Furthermore, the observations that small DSPG are involved in cell-cell interactions and are themselves regulated by cytokines is of direct relevance to the architecture of the mesangial matrix.

Acknowledgments. Part of this work was supported by a MRC Partnership Award to MD and RMM. LS is the recipient of a Kidney Research Unit Foundation for Wales postgraduate award. The authors gratefully acknowledge Dr. John Couchman, University of Alabama at Birmingham, USA for making available Mab 2D6, 2B5, 5A3 and 4D5.

References

1. Poole AR (1986) Proteoglycans in health and disease: structure and functions. Biochem J 236:1-14
2. Ruoslahti E (1989) Proteoglycans in cell regulation. J Biol Chem 264:13369-13372
3. Farquhar MG, Lemkin MC, Stow JL (1984) Role of proteoglycans in glomerular function and pathology. In: Robinson RR (Ed) Nephrology. Springer, New York Berlin Heidelberg Tokyo, pp 580-600
4. Farquhar MG (1986) Characterisation and immunolocalization of glomerular basement membrane proteoglycans. In: Evered D, Whelan J (eds) Functions of the proteoglycans, Ciba Foundation symposium. John Wiley, Chichester, pp 223-240
5. Kanwar YS, Jakubowski ML, Rosenweig LJ (1983) Distribution of sulfated glycosaminoglycans in the glomerular basement membrane and mesangial matrix. Eur J Cell Biol 31:290-295
6. Couchman JR, Caterson B, Christner JE, Baker JR (1984) Mapping by monoclonal antibody detection of glycosaminoglycans in connective tissues. Nature 307:650-652
7. McCarthy KJ, Accavitti MA, Couchman JR (1989) Immunological characterization of a basement membrane—specific chondroitin sulfate proteoglycan. J Cell Biol 109:3187-3198

8. Miettinen A, Stow JL, Mentone S, Farquhar MG (1986) Antibodies to basement membrane heparan sulfate proteoglycans bind to the laminae rarae of the glomerular basement membrane (GBM) and induce subepithelial GBM thickening. J Exp Med 163:1064-1084

9. Mynderse LA, Hassell JR, Kleinman HK, Martin GR, Martinez-Hernandez A (1983) Loss of heparan sulfate proteoglycan from glomerular basement membrane of nephrotic rats. Lab Invest 48:292-302

10. Oomura A, Nakamura T, Arakawa M, Ooshima A, Isemura M (1989) Alterations in the extracellular matrix components in human glomerular diseases. Virchows Arch [A] 415:151-159

11. Shewring L, McCarthy K, Couchman J, Davies M (1990) Rat mesangial cells synthesize mainly chondroitin/dermatan sulphate proteoglycans. XIIth meeting of European Connective Tissue Societies, Poland.

12. Mason RM, Beavan LA, Davies M (1988) The biosynthesis and metabolic turnover of glomerular proteoglycans. In: Gubler M-C, Sternberg M (eds) Progress in basement membrane research; renal and related aspects. J Libbey, London, pp 77-89

13. Klein DJ, Brown DM, Oegema TR (1986) Partial characterization of heparan and dermatan sulfate proteoglycans synthesized by normal rat glomeruli. J Biol Chem 261:16636-16652

14. Beavan LA, Davies M, Mason RM (1988) Renal glomerular proteoglycans: An in vivo investigation of their synthesis using an in situ fixation technique. Biochem J 251:411-418

15. Border WA, Okuda S, Languino LR, Ruoslahti E (1990) Transforming growth factor-β regulates production of proteoglycans by mesangial cells. Kidney Int 37:689-695

16. Yaoita E, Oguri K, Okayama E, Kawasaki K, Koyayashi S, Kihara I, Okayama M (1990) Isolation and characterization of proteoglycans synthesized by cultured mesangial cells. J Biol Chem 265:522-531

17. Striker GE, Killen PD, Farin FM (1980) Human glomerular cells in vitro: Isolation and characterization. Transplant Proc 12:88-99

18. Davies M, Thomas GJ, Jenner L, Mason RM (1988) Human glomerular epithelial and mesangial cells produce different populations of proteoglycans. In: Gubler MC, Sternberg M (eds) Progress in basement membrane research; renal and related aspects. J Libbey, London, pp 35-42

19. Krusius T, Ruoslahti E (1986) Primary structure of an extracellular matrix proteoglycan core protein deduced from cloned cDNA. Proc Natl Acad Sci USA 83:7683-7687

20. Fisher LW, Termine JD, Young MF (1989) Deduced-protein sequence of bone small proteoglycan I (biglycan) shows homology with proteoglycan II (decorin) and several nonconnective tissues in a variety of species. J Biol Chem 264:4571-4576

21. Thomas GJ, Jenner L, Mason RM, Davies M (1990) Human glomerular epithelial cell proteoglycans. Arch Biochem Biophys 278:11-20

22. Klein DJ, Oegema TR, Fredeen TS, van der Woude F, Kim Y, Brown DM (1990) Partial characterization of proteoglycans synthesized by human glomerular epithelial cells in culture. Arch Biochem Biophys 277:389-401

23. Wight TN, Lark WL, Kinsella MG (1987) Blood vessel proteoglycans. In: Wight TN, Meacham RP (eds) Biology of extracellular matrix: Biology of proteoglycans. Academic Press, Orlando, pp 267-300

24. Beavan LA, Davies M, Couchman JR, Williams MA, Mason RM (1988) In vivo turnover of the basement and cell-associated heparan sulphate of rat glomerulus. Arch Biochem Biophys 269:576-585

25. Shewring L, Thomas GJ, Davies M (1989) Proteoglycan synthesis is stimulated by TNF in rat mesangial cells in vitro. Clin Sci 76:S20

26. Funderburg FM, Markwald RR (1986) Conditioning of native substrates by chondroitin sulphate proteoglycan during cardiac mesenchymal cell migration. J Cell Biol 103:2475-2487

27. Sterzel RB, Lovett DH, Stein HD, Kashgarian M (1982) The mesangium and glomerulonephritis. Klin Wochenschr 60:1077-1094

Cell and Matrix in Monoclonal Antibody-Induced Mesangiolysis

Fujio Shimizu[1]

Summary. In order to investigate the mutual relationship between mesangial cells and matrix, we used a monoclonal antibody (mAb) to develop an experimental model in rats, in which the rats have transient but massive proteinuria and mesangiolysis, followed by an increase in cell number and an increase of matrix size in the mesangial area.

Proteinuria was induced immediately after a single intravenous injection of mAb (IgG3), which binds, in vitro, to the limited mesangial cell surface facing endothelial cells; proteinuria peaked on day 5, with average values of over 150mg/day. Deposition of mouse IgG and rat C3 in the mesangial area, as well as infiltration of polymorphonuclear cells and degenerative signs of mesangial cells, was observed 30 minutes after mAb injection. Mesangiolytic change occurred 24 or 48 hours after mAb injection, followed by an increase in cell number (4 or 6 days after injection) and an increase in matrix size (2 or 4 weeks after injection) in the mesangial area.

Preliminary study using this model revealed some alterations in cell and mesangial matrix composition (e.g., abnormal production of type I collagen) during the course of this experiment.

We regard this model as a valuable tool for investigating, in vivo, the interrelationship between mesangial cells and matrix.

Introduction

There is increasing evidence that cell structure and function are deeply influenced by the extracellular matrix [1,2].

[1]Department of Immunology, Institute of Nephrology, Niigata University School of Medicine, Asahimachi-dori, Niigata, 951 Japan

A growing interest has been taken in the interrelationship between mesangial cells and matrix in order to better understand the mechanism of proliferation of mesangial cells and matrix leading to progressive glomerular sclerosis.

The information accumulated on this mutual relationship has been obtained mainly from in vitro studies [3].

However, it is well known that cultured mesangial cells are structurally and functionally different from those in vivo. For example, mesangial cells in vitro synthesize mainly type I collagen [4], which cannot be immunohistochemically demonstrated in the normal glomerular mesangium.

The remarkable effects of matrix on the morphology, growth rate, and proteoglycan synthesis of mesangial cells were reported by Yaoita [5]. He demonstrated that mesangial cells, cultured in E gel (prepared from EHS tumor), showed characteristics of morphology and growth rate similar to those in vivo. These findings suggested the possibility that we could partly mimic in vivo surroundings. However, even in his system, mesangial cells cultured in E gel synthesized mainly chondroitin sulphate proteoglycan. Thus, such an imitation has its limits.

In vivo models, used to examine the mutual relationship between mesangial cells and matrix, have been developed by Ishizaki et al. [6] and Yamamoto et al. [7]. According to their reports, mesangiolysis, followed by cellular and matrix increase in the mesangial area, was induced in rats with intravenous injection of anti-rat thymocyte serum. However, lesions are not so uniformly induced by polyclonal anti-thymocyte serum, especially those lesions which relate to the degree of proteinuria. If we could use an antibody which is always identical and monospecific against a limited epitope, it would be ideal for minimizing individual differences and also for further analysis of this model. A monoclonal antibody is the best tool for such purposes.

We have produced a monoclonal antibody (mAb) which also induces mesangiolysis in rats with a single intravenous injection [8]. In this paper, we describe the details of this model and the preliminary results on the alteration of cell and matrix components which were obtained during the course of this experiment.

Monoclonal Antibody-Induced Mesangial Lesions

As reported by Kawachi et al. [8], an intravenous injection of mAb 1–22–3 (IgG3) in rats can induce a massive but transient proteinuria with mesangiolysis, followed by an increase in cell number and an increase in matrix size, in the mesangial area.

This mAb reacts with the limited mesangial cell surface facing endothelial cells. Reactivity of this mAb to thymus, brain, and intestine could also be observed.

Urinary protein excretion started immediately following 500ug mAb injection and peaked on day 5, with average values of over 150mg/day; this was followed by a gradual decline and virtual normalization by day 18. Deposition of mouse IgG and rat C3 in the mesangial area and the infiltration of neutrophils and lymphocytes were observed in rats 30 minutes after mAb injection. Twenty four hours after injection, the staining intensity of IgG or rat C3 decreased.

Mesangiolytic change occurred 24 or 48 hours after mAb injection, followed by an increase in cell number (4 or 6 days after injection) and an increase in matrix size (2 or 4 weeks after injection) in the mesangial area [8].

Mesangial Area Cells in This Model

Preliminary examination with monoclonal antibodies (anti-thy-1, anti-macrophage) revealed that the cells which accumulated after mesangiolysis in this model have more characteristics of intrinsic mesangial cells.

Mesangial Matrix in This Model

Preliminary examination with polyclonal anti-laminin, anti-fibronectin and monoclonal anti-type I, type IV collagen antibodies demonstrated positive fluorescence for laminin and fibronectin in the increased matrix.

Positive staining for type I collagen was observed 2 or 4 weeks after injection.

Type I collagen, not detectable in normal rat glomeruli, may be produced by the cells which are no longer regulated by the matrix, which has disappeared or become disorganized.

We are planning to develop an ideal model for chronic progressive sclerotic lesions, varying the dose and intervals of mAb administration. Applying many advanced techniques in basic cell biology and genetics, the kinetics of cells and matrix in this model will be further examined, with special reference to the influence of cytokines.

Acknowledgments. This work was supported, in part, by a research grant from the Ministry of Education, Science, and Culture (01480163) and from the Ministry of Health and Welfare, Japan (1989).

References

1. Kashgarian M (1985) Mesangium and glomerular disease. Lab Invest 52:569–571
2. Border WA, Okuda S, Nakamura T (1989) Extracellular matrix and glomerular disease. Semin Nephrol 9:307–317
3. Lovett PH, Sterzel RB (1986) Cell culture approaches to the analysis of glomerular inflammation. Kidney Int 30:246–252
4. Haralson MA, Jacobson HR, Hoover RL (1987) Collagen polymorphism in cultured rat kidney mesangial cells. Lab Invest 57:513–519
5. Yaoita E (1989) Behavior of rat mesangial cells cultured within extracellular matrix. Lab Invest 61:410–418
6. Ishizaki M, Masuda Y, Fukuda Y, Sugisaki Y, Yamanaka N, Masugi Y (1986) Experimental mesangioproliferative glomerulonephritis in rats induced by intravenous administration of anti-thymocyte serum. Acta Pathol Jpn 36:1191–1203
7. Yamamoto T, Wilson CB (1987) Complement dependence of antibody-induced mesangial cell injury in the rat. J Immunol 138:3758–3765
8. Kawachi H, Orikasa M, Matsui K, Morioka T, Oite T, Shimizu F (1990) Induction of proteinuria and morphological change in the rat by a monoclonal antibody against mesangial cell surface (abstract). Kidney Int 37:418

Regulation of Collagen IV Expression

PAUL D. KILLEN, CYNTHIA A. DEMEESTER, ROBERT A. LONG, ERIN O'BRIEN, and JOSEPH P. GRANDE[1]

SUMMARY. Recent advances in the molecular biology of basement membrane components have resulted in new tools for the study of basement membrane metabolism during normal renal development and growth. Collagen IV, the major structural protein of basement membranes, is assembled from at least 5 distinct gene products. mRNA encoding the $\alpha 1$(IV) and $\alpha 2$(IV) chains vary in a precise temporal and spatial fashion during nephronogenesis. Inflammation, such as that observed in antiglomerular basement membrane (GBM) nephritis or in the metabolic or hemodynamic disturbances exemplified by diabetes mellitus, leads to increased steady-state levels of mRNA for these basement membrane components. Increased transcription of these genes may, in part, account for the increase. These two genes are separated by a 130 bp bidirectional promoter which is regulated by sequences contained within the genes. We have directly measured transcription of each gene by the nuclear run-on method and have correlated this with the steady-state mRNA level for each chain. The data suggest that transcriptional attenuation may play an important role in determining the ratio of $\alpha 1$(IV)/$\alpha 2$(IV) mRNA as well as the relative abundance of these mRNA in different tissues. These methods should provide new insights into the mechanism of collagen IV gene expression during renal development and in experimental disease models.

Introduction

Basement membranes play an important role during tissue morphogenesis [1]. By providing a substratum for adhesion, the basement membrane orients cells for the maintenance of cell polarity and a differentiated phenotype [2] and it acts as a template for the restoration of normal tissue architecture following injury [3]. Further,

---

[1]Department of Pathology, School of Medicine, University of Michigan, Ann Arbor, MI 48109-0602, USA

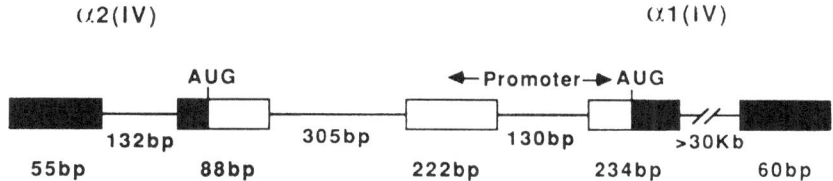

Fig. 1. Bidirectional transcription of collagen IV genes

it constitutes an important permeability barrier for the filtration of plasma to form urine [4]. Changes in the abundance or morphological appearance of glomerular matrices characterize the glomerular response to inflammatory, hemodynamic, or metabolic disorders. The deposition of this extracellular matrix is currently viewed as irreversible and inexorable, leading to diminished function or organ failure. The mechanisms regulating the synthesis of these matrix components during renal development or in response to injury are unknown.

Collagen IV occurs uniquely in basement membranes where it provides tensile strength. Each triple helical molecule is assembled from an assortment of 5 genetically distinct α chains. All basement membranes contain α1(IV) and α2(IV) collagen chains, whereas α3-5(IV) have a restricted anatomic distribution [5–7]. The abundance of the α1(IV) and α2(IV) mRNA vary widely between [8] and within tissues [9]. The molecular mechanisms regulating the steady-state levels of these MRNA are not known. The α1(IV) and α2(IV) genes are clustered with the 5′ ends of the genes, separated by a 130 bp (in the mouse) bidirectional promoter [10,11] (Fig. 1). Differential transcription of these genes could cause the observed differences in the abundance of these MRNA. In order to directly assess the transcription of these genes, we have studied transcription of the α1(IV) and α2(IV) genes by expressing and non-expressing cell types in vitro. Our results suggest that differences in transcription elongation may, in part, regulate the abundance of these mRNA.

Methods

Cell Culture

NIH-3T3 cells were obtained from the American Type Culture Collection. PF-HR9 cells were the generous gift of R. Kramer, UCSF. Cells were maintained in Dulbecco's modified Eagle's medium (DMEM) supplemented with 1 mM L-glutamine, penicillin/streptomycin (100U/1μg per ml) and 10% calf serum. In some experiments, calf serum was incubated, with stirring, with activated charcoal for 60 minutes.

Quantitation of Collagen IV mRNA

Total cellular RNA was purified from confluent cultures of NIH-3T3 cells or PF-HR9 cells as previously described [11]. Then 10 μg of denatured RNA were electrophoresed in a 2.2 M formaldehyde 1% agarose gel and the RNA was transferred to nylon

TRANSCRIPTIONAL ATTENUATION REGULATES COLLAGEN IV GENE EXPRESSION IN NIH-3T3 AND PF-HR9 CELLS

SEQUENCE	SIZE
$\alpha 2$(IV) 3' UT	600 bp
$\alpha 2$(IV) 3' TH	660 bp
$\alpha 2$(IV) 1ST EXON	380 bp
$\alpha 1$(IV) 1ST EXON	345 bp
$\alpha 1$(IV) 2ND EXON	1400 bp
$\alpha 1$(IV) 3' TH	494 bp
$\alpha 1$(IV) 3' UT	560 bp
pBLUESCRIPT	
β ACTIN	
28S rRNA*	

* 1 hour exposure

Fig. 2. Transcriptional attenuation regulates collagen IV gene expression in NIH-3T3 and PF-HR9 cells

filters by capillary blotting. Serial dilutions of RNA were directly applied to the filters with the aid of a vacuum manifold. RNA was fixed to the filters by baking in vacuo at 80°C for 2 hours. Purified fragments of the murine $\alpha 1$(IV), $\alpha 2$(IV), or β-actin cDNA [12] were labeled with α^{32}P dCTP to a specific activity of 10^9 dpm/μg [13]. Filters were hybridized and washed as previously described [8]. X-OMAT AR film (Kodak) was preflashed, and exposed to the filters at −80°C with intensifying screens. The Northern blot was intentionally overexposed. The relative abundance of the $\alpha 1$(IV) or $\alpha 2$(IV) mRNA in these cells was determined with a laser densitometer.

Nuclear Run-on Transcription

Direct assessment of $\alpha 1$(IV) gene transcription was determined by the nuclear run-on method. In brief, nuclei were isolated following cell lysis in NP-40 and incubated for 30 minutes at 30°C in 45 mM TRIS, pH 8.3, 6 mM MgCl$_2$, 150 mM KCl, 250 μM ATP, CTP, GTP and 0.33 μM α^{32}P UTP (3000 Ci/mM) essentially as described by McKnight and Palmiter [14]. The labeled RNA transcripts were precipitated, and separated from unincorporated nucleotides on mini-spin columns of G-100. The RNA was partially hydrolyzed with alkali, precipitated, and redissolved at a final concentration of 5×10^6 dpm/ml in hybridization buffer. Five μg of denatured DNA was applied to nitrocellulose with a slot blot manifold. Fragments from the 5' end of the murine α1(IV) or α2(IV) gene and from cDNAs encoding the 3' end of the triple helical domain or from the 3' untranslated region served as test sequences. Special attention was given to the potential of cross hybridization of the collagen IV transcripts. In particular, it was observed in preliminary studies that hybridization to a NCl domain encoding sequence was approximately twice the expected radiodensity for its length. Presumably, both α1 and α2 transcripts were hybridizing to this sequence due to the high homology between the NCl domain encoding sequences of the two genes. Positive and negative controls included β-actin [12], the 28S rRNA gene [15], and pBluescript KSM13+ (Stratagene, La Jolla). Filters were hybridized for 72 hours at 65°C in equal volumes of 10 mM TES, pH 7.4, 0.3 M NaCl, 10 mM EDTA, 0.2% SDS containing 1X Denhardt's solution, and 0.25 mg/ml E. Coli RNA. Filters were washed three times at 65°C in 2X SSC, 0.1% SDS, and twice in 0.1X SSC, 0.1% SDS. Autoradiograms were prepared as described above.

Results

Northern blots of total cellular RNA isolated from PF-HR9 and 3T3 cells hybridized with cDNA probes specific for the α1(IV) or α2(IV) chain demonstrated strong signals of the expected size in RNA from the PF-HR9 cells. In contrast, NIH 3T3 cells displayed a weak signal which required several days exposure to adequately visualize. No differences in the steady-state level of β-actin mRNA were observed between the two cell types. Since the cDNA probes hybridized specifically, the relative abundance of these mRNA could be determined by serial dilutions of RNA on "dot blots." Laser densitometry demonstrated that the collagen IV mRNA were more than 50-fold more abundant in the PF-HR9 cells than in the NIH 3T3 cells.

In order to directly measure the transcription of each gene, we subcloned in pBluescript, segments of the α1(IV) and α2(IV) gene which lacked repetitive sequence as assessed by hybridization with ^{32}P labeled murine genomic DNA in plasmids. In addition, fragments of cDNAs were also subcloned. Fragments of the α1(IV) gene included a 345 bp fragment containing the first exon, a 1.4 kb fragment containing the second exon, a 494 bp cDNA fragment encoding the 3' portion of the triple-helical (3'TH) domain, and a 560 bp segment of the 3' untranslated sequence (3'UT) proximal to the first polyadenylation site. Fragments of the murine α2(IV) gene included a 380 bp fragment containing the first exon, a 660 bp cDNA fragment encoding the 3'TH domain, and a 600 bp segment of the 3'UT sequence downstream from the B2 repeat but upstream from the polyadenylation site [16]. No significant hybridization was observed with the negative control, pBluescript. Hybridization to the 28S rRNA gene sequences were similar in the two cell types, indicating that the specific activity of the labeled transcripts was similar for the two filters. Furthermore, the hybridization to the β-actin cDNA was similar in the two cell types. When transcription of the two collagen IV genes was compared in the PF-HR9 cells, transcript initiation, as detected by the sequences containing the first exon, was nearly equally efficient in the α2(IV) or α1(IV) directions. However, there was a modest decrease in transcriptional efficiency along the length of the gene. Hybridization to the 3'UT sequences was significantly weaker than the first exon, and the predicted signal (assuming 100% completion of transcripts) should be greater than the first exon due to the greater length of the 3'UT sequences.

If differences in the abundance of the α1(IV) and α2(IV) mRNA were exclusively due to differences in transcription, then hybridization of these transcripts to the collagen IV gene transcripts should be more than 50-fold less than that observed with the PF-HR9 cells. Surprisingly, transcription initiation, as reflected by hybridization of transcripts to the first exon, was nearly identical in the two cell types. However, hybridization to the 3'UT sequences was virtually undetectable in NIH 3T3 cells. Thus, somewhere within the gene, there is significant attenuation of transcription. Indeed, in the case of the α1(IV) gene transcript elongation must be blocked in the first intron.

Discussion

The expression of collagen IV genes is highly regulated in both space and time. The α1(IV) and α2(IV) mRNA appear early in nephronogenesis and reach a maximal level at birth or shortly thereafter [17]. Subsequently, the abundance of these mRNA rapidly falls to a low level, which in the adult kidney, is less than 10% of maximal. In situ hybridization demonstrates these transcripts in a characteristic pattern that changes with renal development and growth [18]. Renal injury alters the abundance of these mRNA in adult animals. For instance, within 4 days of administration of anti-GBM antibody, α1(IV) mRNA are increased some 9-fold in rabbit kidney cortex [19]. Increases in collagen IV mRNA have also been noted in diabetic and spontaneously hypertensive rat kidneys (unpublished work). Whether these changes are due to changes in the transcription of the collagen IV genes or due to changes in mRNA stability is unknown.

In order to develop methods for the analysis of collagen IV gene transcription in vivo, we have studied the expression of collagen IV genes in cell lines in vitro. We compared PF-HR9 cells, which constitutively synthesize collagen IV chains, to NIH 3T3 cells, which do not synthesize these proteins. Our results indicate that differences in transcription, in part, underlie the differences in collagen IV gene expression. However, this may not be due to differences in transcript initiation by the collagen IV promoter, but rather may be due to differences in the efficiency of transcript elongation, as has been observed with other genes [20–22]. This observation may explain why the collagen IV promoter resembles promoters of "housekeeping" genes [23]. Initiation of transcripts may occur in all cells, but elongation of transcripts may occur in a cell- or tissue-specific fashion. The transcriptional block occurs in the first intron of the α1(IV) gene, as has been observed for the proto-oncogenes c-myb and c-myc [21,22]. In studies reported at this meeting [24], we have found that sequences within the first intron of the α1(IV) gene are capable of decreasing transcription of heterologous promoters in NIH 3T3 cells. These sequences bind specifically to proteins in nuclear extracts from NIH 3T3. Future studies will determine whether differences in transcription initiation and elongation regulate expression of collagen IV genes during renal development or in pathological contexts.

Acknowledgments. We gratefully acknowledge the many helpful discussions with Craig Thompson during the course of these studies and the assistance of Kimberly

Drake in the preparation of this manuscript. This work was supported in part by NIH grant, HL-31963. JPG is supported by NIH training grant, HL-07517.

References

1. Ekblom P, Vestweber D, Kemler R (1986) Cell-matrix interactions and cell adhesion during development. Annu Rev Cell Biol 2:27–47
2. Sugrue SP, Hay ED (1986) The identification of extracellular matrix (ECM) binding sites on the basal surface of embryonic corneal epithelium and the effect of ECM binding on epithelial collagen production. J Cell Biol 102:1907–1916
3. Vracko, R (1974) Basal lamina scaffold-anatomy and significance for maintenance of orderly tissue structure. Am J Pathol 77:314–346
4. Maddox DA, Brenner BM (1977) Glomerular filtration of fluid and macromolecules: the renal response to injury. Annu Rev Med 28:91–102
5. Saus J, Wieslander J, Langveld JP, Quinones S, Hudson BG (1988) Identification of the Goodpasture antigen as the $\alpha3(IV)$ chain of collagen IV. J Biol Chem 263:13374–13380
6. Kleppel MM, Santi PA, Cameron JD, Wieslander J, Michael AF (1989) Human tissue distribution of novel basement membrane collagen. Am J Pathol 134:813–825
7. Hostikka S, Eddy RL, Byers MG, Hoyhtya M, Shows TB, Tryggvason K (1990) Identification of a distinct type IV collagen alpha chain with restricted kidney distribution and assignment of its gene to the locus of X chromosome-linked Alport syndrome. Proc Natl Acad Sci USA 87:1606–1610
8. Kleinman HK, Ebihara I, Killen PD, Sasaki M, Cannon FB, Yamada Y, Martin GR (1987) Genes for basement membrane proteins are coordinately expressed in differentiating F9 cells but not in normal adult murine tissues. Dev Biol 122:373–378
9. Boot-Hanford RP, Kurkinen M, Prockop DJ (1987) Steady-state levels of mRNAs for the type IV collagen and laminin polypeptide chains of basement membranes exhibit marked tissue-specific stoichiometric variations in the rat. J Biol Chem 262:12475–12478
10. Burbelo PD, Yamada Y, Martin GR (1988) Alpha 1(IV) and alpha2(IV) collagen genes are regulated by a bidirectional promoter and a shared enhancer. Proc Natl Acad Sci USA 85:9679–9682
11. Poschl E, Pollner R, Kuhn K (1988) The genes for the alpha 1 (IV) and alpha 2(IV) chains of human basement membrane collagen IV are arranged head-to-head and separated by a bidirectional promoter of unique structure. EMBO J 7:2687–2695
12. Cleveland DW, Lopata MA, McDonald RJ, Cowan NJ, Rutter WJ (1980) Number and evolutionary conservation of α- and β-tubulin and cytoplasmic β- and γ-actin genes using specific cloned cDNA probes. Cell 20:95–105
13. Feinberg A, Vogelstein B (1982) A technique for radiolabeling DNA restriction endonuclease fragments to high specific activity. Anal Biochem 132:6–13
14. McKnight GS, Palmiter RD (1979) Transcriptional regulation of the ovalbumin and conalbumin genes by steroid hormones in chick oviduct. J Biol Chem 254:9050–9058
15. Chan YL, Olvera J, Wool IG (1983) Structure of rat 28S ribosomal ribonucleic acid inferred from the sequence of nucleotides in a gene. Nucleic Acids Res 11:7819–7831
16. Oberbaumer I, Magdolen U (1988) The 3′ untranslated region of the murine mRNA for the alpha 2 chain of type IV collagen contains a B1-like element. Nucleic Acids Res 16:7181
17. Ebihara I, Killen PD, Laurie GW, Huang T, Yamada Y, Martin GR, Brown KS (1988) Altered mRNA expression of basement membrane components in a murine model of polycystic kidney disease. Lab Invest 58:262–269
18. Laurie GW, Horikoshi S, Killen PD, Segui-Real B, Yamada Y (1989) In situ hybridization reveals temporal and spatial changes in cellular expression of mRNA for a laminin recep-

tor, laminin, and basement membrane (type IV) collagen in the developing kidney. J Cell Biol 109:1351–1362

19. Merrit S, Killen PD, Wiggins R (to be published) Analysis of α1(I) procollagen, α1(IV) collagen β and β-actin mRNA in glomeruli and cortex of rabbits with experimental anti-GBM disease. Evidence of early extraglomerular collagen biosynthesis. Lab Invest

20. Bender TP, Thompson CB, Kuehl WM (1987) Differential expression of c-*myb* mRNA in murine B lymphomas by a block to transcription elongation. Science 237:1473–1476

21. Lindstein T, June CH, Thompson CB (1988) Multiple mechanisms regulate c-*myc* expression during normal T cell activation. EMBO J 7:2787–2794

22. Lindsten T, June CH, Thompson CB, Leiden JM (1988) Regulation of 4F2 heavy-chain gene expression during normal human T-cell activation can be mediated by multiple distinct molecular mechanisms. Mol Cell Biol 8:3820–3826

23. Killen PD, Burbelo PD, Martin GR, Yamada Y (1988) Characterization of the promoter of the α1(IV) collagen gene. J Biol Chem 263:12310–12314

24. Killen PD, DeMeester CA, Long R, O'Brien E (1991) Identification of sequences which enhance or repress collagen IV gene transcription. Proceedings of the XIth International Congress of Nephrology, July 15–20 1990. Tokyo, Japan

Renal Tubular Acidosis

Chair: Robert J. Alpern (USA)
Teruo Kitagawa (Japan)

Proximal Renal Tubular Acidosis (RTA): Normal Proximal Tubule Function and Evidence of Cellular Defects

SEI SASAKI[1]

SUMMARY. During the last ten years, the mechanisms and regulation of HCO_3^-/H^+ transport across the cell membranes of proximal tubule cells, have been extensively studied. The generally accepted view is that tubular acidification is performed by H^+ secretion into the lumen. This secretion is mostly due to a luminal Na/H exchange; a small portion is mediated by an ATP-dependent H^+ pump. Most basolateral HCO_3^- exit is through a $Na-(HCO_3)_3$ cotransport; a small fraction (15%) is mediated by Na^+ coupled Cl^-/HCO_3^- exchange. The amount of passive HCO_3^- leak from the peritubular to the tubular lumen is relatively small compared to the active H^+ secretion. Based on this concept, I will discuss possible mechanisms of proximal RTA; (1) decreased luminal H^+ secretion, (2) decreased basolateral HCO_3^- exit, (3) inhibition of Na-K-ATPase pump, (4) decreased generation of ATP, and (5) increased passive permeability of HCO_3^-.

Introduction

Proximal renal tubular acidosis (RTA) is a clinical syndrome characterized by hyperchloremic metabolic acidosis, which is caused by a defect in proximal tubular acidification. Proximal tubule reabsorbs most of the filtered water and solutes. As shown in Fig. 1, the data in rat free flow micropuncture studies have shown that proximal tubule reabsorbs 85% of filtered HCO_3^-, 98% of glucose, 90% of amino acids, 50% of phosphate, and about 60% of the organic anions, such as acetate, citrate, and uric acid [1]. One important characteristic of the reabsorption of these solutes is a coupling with Na^+. For example, HCO_3^- is reabsorbed by proton secretion, mediated by luminal Na^+/H^+ exchange, into the lumen. The driving force of this exchange is an electrochemical gradient of Na^+ across the luminal membrane. Cell Na^+ is maintained at a low level by the basolateral Na-K-ATPase pump, and intracellular potential is highly negative. Following this large electrochemical gradient of Na^+ across the cell mem-

---

[1]Second Department of Internal Medicine, Tokyo Medical and Dental University, 1-5-45 Yushima, Bunkyo-ku, Tokyo, 113 Japan

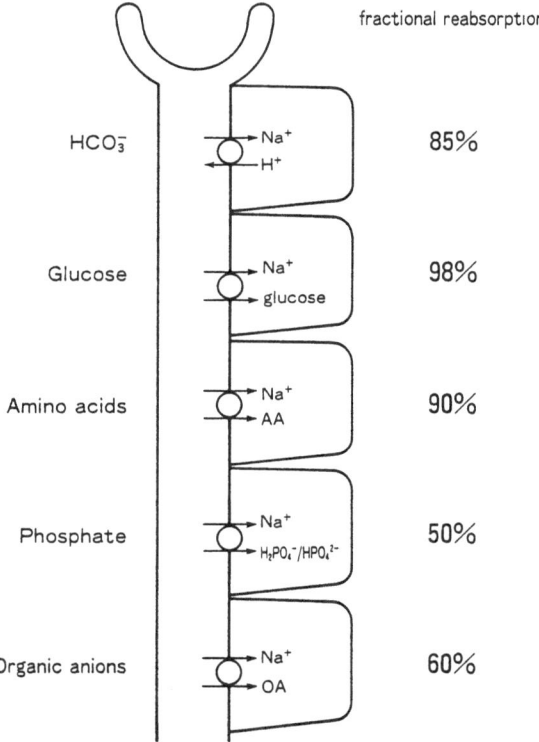

fractional reabsorption

HCO₃⁻ ... Na⁺ / H⁺ ... 85%

Glucose ... Na⁺ / glucose ... 98%

Amino acids ... Na⁺ / AA ... 90%

Phosphate ... Na⁺ / H₂PO₄⁻/HPO₄²⁻ ... 50%

Organic anions ... Na⁺ / OA ... 60%

Fig. 1. Solute reabsorption in the proximal tubules. Most glomerular filtered solutes are reabsorbed in the proximal tubules. Generalized defects of proximal reabsorption will cause inhibition of the reabsorption of these solutes. One important character of these transports is a coupling with Na. AA, amino acids; OA, organic anions

brane, Na^+ goes inside the cell and proton is extruded from the cell. Reabsorption of other solutes also uses this Na^+ electrochemical gradient. Thus, reabsorption of solutes in the proximal tubule is, in general, mediated by secondary active processes.

Proximal RTA can be divided into two forms. One form, "the Fanconi syndrome," is a proximal acidification defect which is accompanied by a generalized proximal reabsorption defect. The other form, which is rare, is a selective defect of proximal acidification. A simple expectation from Fig. 1 is that if this electrochemical gradient of Na^+ is not maintained, this lack of maintenance will cause a generalized defect of proximal solute reabsorption, i.e., the Fanconi syndrome.

Normal Proximal Acidification

During the last 10 years, mechanisms of proximal acidification have been clarified by advances in experimental techniques, such as ion selective microelectrodes, fluorescent measurements, and vesicle studies. Figure 2 shows a currently accepted

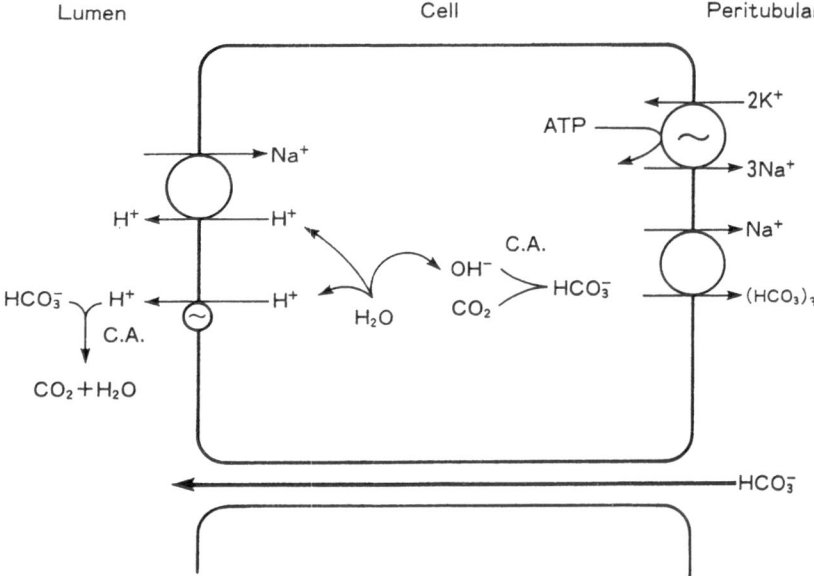

Fig. 2. Mechanisms of proximal acidification. Luminal proton secretion is mediated by Na/H exchange and ATP dependent pump. Basolateral HCO_3 exit is mainly mediated by Na-HCO_3 cotransporter. A small portion of reabsorbed HCO_3 leaks back to the lumen through a paracellular shunt pathway. C.A., carbonic anhydrase

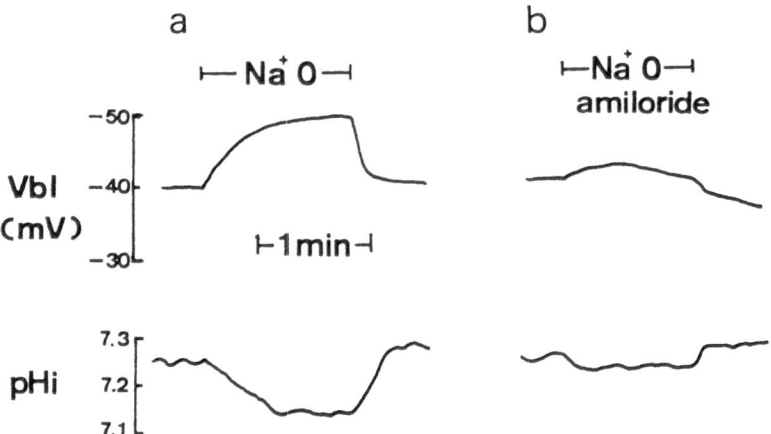

Fig. 3a,b. Luminal Na/H exchange examined by pH-selective microelectrode. In response to luminal Na removal, cell pH (*pHi*) was acidified (**a**) and this effect was inhibited by amiloride (**b**). Vbl, basolateral membrane potential. (From [4] with permission)

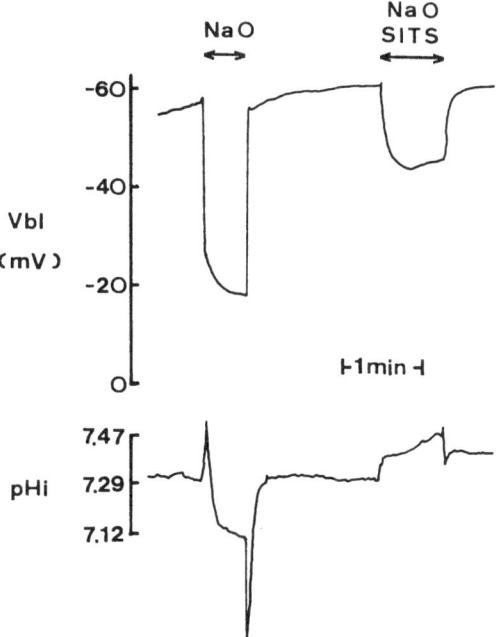

Fig. 4. Basolateral Na-HCO₃ cotransporter examined by pH electrode. Bath Na removal decreased cell pH. This cell acidification was accompanied by a large depolarization of basolateral membrane potential (*Vbl*). These effects were inhibited by the anion transport inhibitor, SITS. (Data from [4] with permission)

model of proximal acidification, in which an important step is proton secretion across the luminal membrane. Most of the proton secretion is performed by the luminal Na^+/H^+ antiporter. In addition to the antiporter, a small amount of proton is secreted by a luminal ATP-dependent H^+ pump [2]. Secreted H^+ titrates luminal HCO_3^-, making CO_2 and water in the presence of luminal carbonic anhydrase (CA). Inside the cell, OH^- is left, and this OH^- reacts with CO_2 to make HCO_3^-.

This process is also CA-dependent. Most of the generated HCO_3^- exits the basolateral membrane through the Na-$(HCO_3)_3$ cotransporter. Stoichiometry of this cotransport has been shown as 1 Na^+: 3 HCO_3^-. As already described, luminal Na^+/H^+ exchange is driven by a Na^+ electrochemical gradient, and the basolateral NaK-ATPase pump maintains this Na^+ electrochemical gradient.

Figure 3 shows our data, obtained by pH sensitive microelectrode which examined the luminal Na^+/H^+ exchange in rabbit proximal straight tubules [4]. Removal of luminal Na^+ caused a significant cell pH decrease. This cell pH decrease was partly inhibited by a high dose of amiloride, an inhibitor of Na^+/H^+ exchange, thus demonstrating the presence of a Na^+/H^+ exchange. An example of an experiment which examined the basolateral Na^+-HCO_3^- cotransport is shown in Fig. 4 [4,5]. Na^+ removal from basolateral fluid rapidly decreased cell pH. This cell acidification was accompanied by a large cell membrane depolarization, indicating the electrogenic nature of this transport. This Na^+ coupled HCO_3^- transport was inhibited by SITS, an anion transport inhibitor, indicating the presence of Na^+-HCO_3^- cotransport across the basolateral membrane. Further studies have shown that a small fraction (15%) of basolateral HCO_3^- transport is mediated by Na^+-dependent Cl^-/HCO_3^- exchange [6].

Defects of Proximal Acidification: Increased Passive Leak vs Inhibited Active Proton Secretion

Defects of proximal acidification can be caused by either of two mechanisms; increased passive leak of reabsorbed solutes and/or inhibited active reabsorption. Because proximal tubule epithelium is leaky, and because a large concentration gradient is generated between tubular lumen and peritubular cells, reabsorbed solutes can diffuse back to the tubular lumen along their chemical gradient. Therefore, increased passive permeability (presumably through the paracellular shunt), can, theoretically, cause a generalized defect in proximal solute reabsorption.

Figure 5 shows a summary of active and passive fluxes of HCO_3^- and glucose, based on kinetic analysis of rat proximal convoluted tubule. Active HCO_3^- reabsorption is 800 peq/min per single proximal convoluted tubule in normal condition. On the other hand, passive leak flux is 100, which is 13% of the value for active flux [7]. Thus, a large change in passive flux may not affect total HCO_3^- flux very much. Indeed, Alpern et al. showed that a 50% increase in passive HCO_3^- permeability did not appreciably change net HCO_3^- reabsorption [8]. In the case of glucose reabsorption, the difference between active and passive fluxes is more striking. Passive flux is only 6% of active reabsorptive flux [9]. Thus, these calculations indicate that the

HCO₃⁻

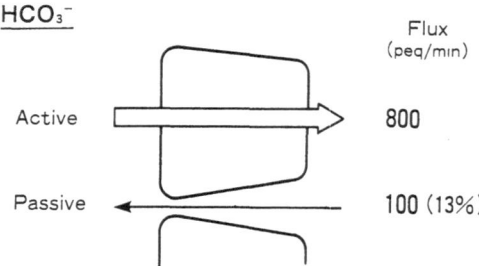

Flux
(peq/min)

Active   800

Passive   100 (13%)

Glucose

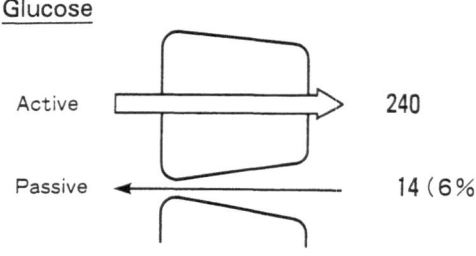

Active   240

Passive   14 (6%)

Fig. 5. Active reabsorption and passive leak in proximal solute reabsorption. Data are taken from rat micropuncture studies. In HCO_3 reabsorption, active reabsorption is 800 peq/min per single proximal convoluted tubule, whereas the value for passive leak is only 100, demonstrating the small contribution made by passive leak flux

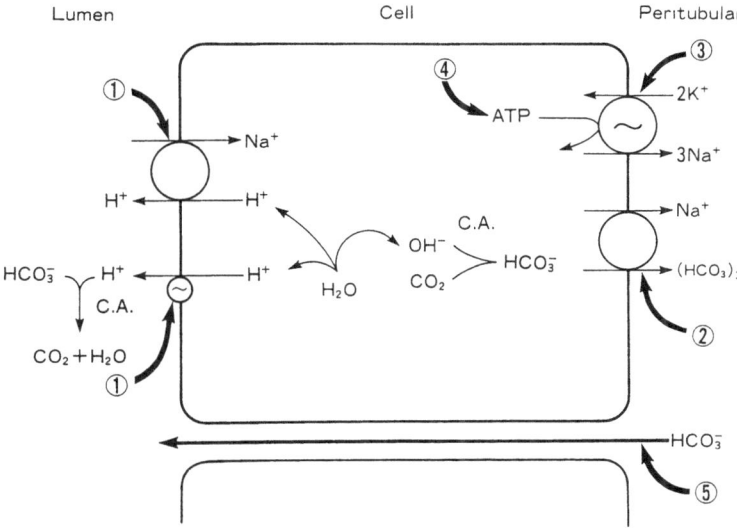

Fig. 6. Possible mechanisms of proximal RTA. See text (under heading "Pathogenesis of RTA") for details. C.A., carbonic anhydrase

contribution of increased passive fluxes of solutes to the genesis of RTA may be small. Furthermore, the existence of selective defects of passive leak may be unlikely. Defects in passive leak would accompany more generalized cell function defects, and generalized cell function defects would affect active reabsorption, which has a dominant role in net solute reabsorption.

Pathogenesis of Proximal RTA

In theory, proximal RTA can be introduced through defects in any of the H^+/HCO_3^- transporters shown in Fig. 2. Defects in the transporters are caused by many mechanisms, for example, chemical modification of transporters, such as phosphorylation; decreased numbers of transporting proteins, decreased energy supply for transporters; and decreased driving force for secondary active transporters. Figure 6 shows possible mechanisms of proximal acidification defects. 1) Decreased luminal H^+ extrusion through the Na^+/H^+ exchange and proton pump causes an acidification defect. This defect may be caused by chemical modification of these transport proteins and the decreased number of these transporters. We have recently shown that parathyroid hormone (PTH) causes an inhibition of proximal acidification, which is mediated by decreased Na^+/H^+ antiporter activity, which in turn is due to phosphorylation by cAMP dependent A-kinase. Also, lack of luminal carbonic anhydrase inhibits luminal H^+ excretion by increasing luminal H^+ concentration. An inherited syndrome which accompanies RTA has been reported to be due to a deficiency of carbonic anhydrase II [10].

2) Proximal acidification defects can be caused by inhibition of basolateral HCO_3^- exit. This may be due to inhibition of either Na^+-HCO_3^- cotransport or inhibition of Na^+-dependent Cl^-/HCO_3^- exchange. An example of this type defect is obtained by administration of carbonic anhydrase inhibitors. We have shown that acetazolamide, a carbonic anhydrase inhibitor, inhibits basolateral HCO_3^- exit by reducing intracellular HCO_3^- availability [11].

3) Inhibition of the Na-K-ATPase pump can cause a proximal acidification defect by reducing electrochemical driving force for Na^+ across the luminal membrane. It is interesting that activation of protein kinase C has been reported to inhibit NaK-ATPase in rat proximal tubules [12]. This result may indicate the possibility that stimulation of protein kinase C decreases luminal acidification. A recent study in rabbit proximal tubules supports this expectation [13].

4) Decreased supply of ATP to the pumps, NaK-ATPase and the luminal H^+ pump, decreases proximal acidification. A decreased level of ATP in renal cortical homogenate has been reported in an experimental model of Fanconi's syndrome produced by maleic acid infusion [14]. This type of defect can easily affect generalized proximal solute reabsorption. In hereditary fructose intolerance, which causes proximal RTA, intracellular accumulation of fructose-1-phosphate occurs, inducing intracellular phosphate depletion, which in turn causes a decreased generation of ATP [15].

5) Increased passive leak of reabsorbed solutes can cause Fanconi syndrome. However, as described above, the contribution of this mechanism may be small. Recent experimental data, in which the passive permeability of HCO_3^- was measured, denied the contribution of this mechanism [16,17].

References

1. Rector FC (1983) Sodium, bicarbonate, and chloride absorption by the proximal tubule. Am J Physiol 244:F461–F471
2. Preisig PA, Ives HE, Cragoe EJ, Alpern RJ, Rector FC (1987) Role of the Na/H antiporter in rat proximal tubule bicarbonate absorption. J Clin Invest 80:970–978
3. Yoshitomi K, Burckhardt B-Ch, Fromter E (1985) Rheogenic sodium-bicarbonate cotransport in the peritubular cell membrane of rat renal proximal tubule. Pflugers Arch 405:360–366
4. Sasaki S, Shiigai T, Takeuchi J (1985) Intracellular pH in the isolated perfused rabbit proximal straight tubule. Am J Physiol 249:F417–F423
5. Sasaki S, Shiigai T, Yoshiyama N, Takeuchi J (1987) Mechanism of bicarbonate exit across basolateral membrane of rabbit proximal straight tubule. Am J Physiol 252:F11–F18
6. Sasaki S, Yoshiyama N (1988) Interaction of chloride and bicarbonate transport across the basolateral membrane of rabbit proximal straight tubule. Evidence for sodium coupled chloride/bicarbonate exchange. J Clin Invest 81:1004–1011
7. Alpern RJ, Rector FC (1985) A model of proximal tubular bicarbonate absorption. Am J Physiol 248:F272–F281
8. Alpern RJ, Cogan MG, Rector FC (1983) Effects of extracellular fluid volume and plasma bicarbonate concentration on proximal acidification. J Clin Invest 71:736–746

9. Barfuss DW, Schafer JA (1981) Differences in active and passive glucose transport along the proximal nephron. Am J Physiol 241:F322–F332

10. Sly WS, Whyte MP, Sundaram V, Tashian RE, Hewett-Emmett D, Guibaud P, Vainsel M, Baluarte HJ, Gruskin A, Al-Mosawi M, Sakati N, Ohlsson A (1985) Carbonic anhydrase II deficiency in 12 families with the autosomal recessive syndrome of osteopetrosis with renal tubular acidosis and cerebral calcification. N Engl J Med 313:139–145

11. Sasaki S, Marumo F (1989) Effect of carbonic anhydrase inhibitors on basolateral base transport of rabbit proximal straight tubule. Am J Physiol 247:F947–F952

12. Bertorello A, Aperia A (1989) Na-K-ATPase is an effector protein for protein kinase C in renal proximal tubule cells. Am J Physiol 256:F370–F373

13. Baum M, Hays SR (1988) Phorbol myristate acetate and dioctanoylglycerol inhibit transport in rabbit proximal convoluted tubule. Am J Physiol 254:F9–F14

14. Kramer HJ, Gonick HC (1970) Experimental Fanconi syndrome. I. Effect of maleic acid on renal cortical Na-K-ATPase activity and ATP levels. J Lab Clin Med 76:799–808

15. Burch HB, Choi S, Dence CN, Alvey TR, Cole BR, Lowry OH (1980) Metabolic effects of large fructose loads in different parts of the rat nephron. J Biol Chem 255:8239–8244

16. Bank N, Aynedjian HS, Mutz BF (1986) Microperfusion study of proximal tubule bicarbonate transport in maleic acid-induced renal tubular acidosis. Am J Physiol 250:F476–F482

17. Salmon RJ, Baum M (1990) Intracellular cystine loading inhibits transport in the rabbit proximal convoluted tubule. J Clin Invest 85:340–344

Cellular Mechanisms of Type 2 Renal Tubular Acidosis/Fanconi Syndrome

R. Curtis Morris[1]

Introduction

As depicted in Fig. 1, impaired proximal bicarbonate reabsorption might result from a selective disorder of the acidification process affecting: 1) the Na^+/H^+ antiporter required for hydrogen ion secretion (labeled 1); 2) the Na^+/HCO_3^- symporter responsible for bicarbonate exit from the proximal tubule cell (labeled 2); 3) the carbonic anhydrases (labeled 3 and 4) or possibly luminal H^+ ATPase. An abnormality in the mechanism by which intracellular sodium concentration is maintained at a normally low level would dictate a diminished reabsorption of all solutes that depend on a Na^+-coupled transport, including not only most of bicarbonate but also glucose, amino acids, phosphate and uric acid, and hence the expression of renal tubule acidosis Type 2 (RTA-2) combined with the Fanconi syndrome (RTA2/FS) [1]. Such a global abnormality might result from several mechanisms: a large increase in cell sodium permeability (labeled 5); diminished activity of the Na^+/K^+-ATPase pump itself (labeled 6); diminished availability of phosphate/impaired metabolic generation of ATP needed to energize the pump (labeled 7); impaired membrane recycling, vacuolar transport or trafficking (labeled 8) and loss of epithelial mass.

Acute RTA2/FS

Hereditary Fructose Intolerance (HFI)

The renal tubular disorder reversibly induced within minutes by intravenous administration of fructose in patients with HFI [2] can be both a dramatic clinical cause of RTA-2/FS and, uniquely, an acute experimental model of RTA-2/FS in humans. The

[1]General Clinical Research Center, School of Medicine, Moffitt Hospital, San Francisco, CA 94143-0126, USA

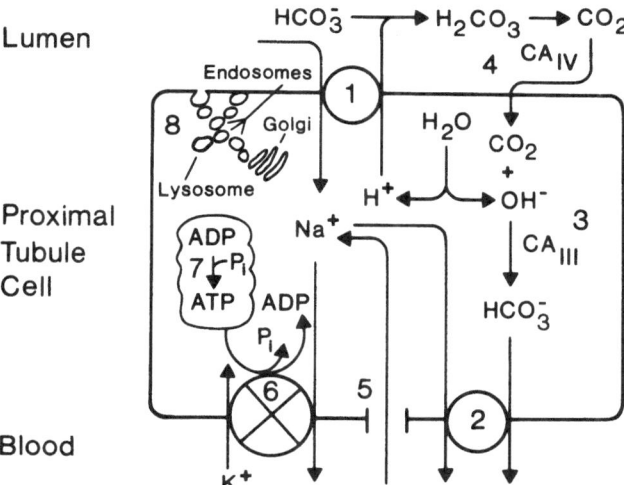

Fig. 1. Potential cellular mechanisms of proximal (Type II) RTA. Possible causes of impaired proximal acidification include defects in the luminal Na^+-H^+ antiport (*1*); the basolateral Na^+-HCO_3^- symport (*2*); the intracellular (*3*) or luminal (*4*) carbonic anhydrases (*CA*); sodium permeability (*5*); The Na-K ATPase (*6*); the intracellular generation of ATP (*7*); or membrane recycling, metabolism, or trafficking (*8*)

pathogenesis of this acute form of RTA2/FS is presumed to depend on an induced incapacity of the proximal tubule to generate the energy necessary to drive its Na^+-coupled resorptive transport processes. Aldolase B, the genetically defective enzyme in HFI, is a cytoplasmic enzyme which catalyzes the cleavage of fructose-1-phosphate. The enzyme normally occurs only in the liver, small bowel, and proximal renal tubule. When patients with HFI are acutely exposed to fructose, their enzymatic defect dictates in the cells of these tissues the near immediate occurrence of a rapid sequence of biochemical events: accumulation of F-1-P → depletion of P_i → depletion of ATP. In these tissues, the acute P_i depletion 1) triggers a massive degradation of preformed total adenine nucleotides (ATP, ADP, and AMP) by activating cytoplasmic AMP deaminase, and 2) restricts the rate at which mitochondria can regenerate ATP. In the fructose-loaded rat, prior phosphate loading largely prevents the otherwise striking reduction of ATP and total adenine nucleotides in the renal cortex despite doubling its concentration of F-1-P.

In patients with HFI given fructose experimentally, phosphate loading initiated beforehand attenuates the severity of the RTA-2/FS, as well as that of the attendant hyperuricemia and hyperinosinuria, phenomena entrained by the P_i depletion-dependent breakdown of preformed adenine nucleotides. In a woman with HFI in whom fructose was administered intravenously over two 1-hour periods, which were interrupted by a period of 100 min, phosphate loading initiated before the second period prevented the occurrence of RTA2/FS. Accordingly, and since fructose-induced depletion of hepatic adenine nucleotides in humans persists for at least 2 hours, it seems likely that phosphate loading attenuated the renal tubular dysfunc-

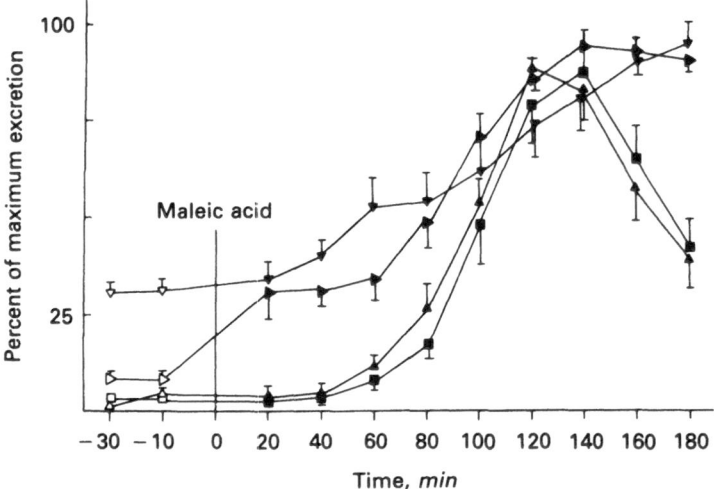

Fig. 2. Time course of the maleic acid-induced increases in urinary excretion of N-acetyl-β-glucosaminidase (NAG) (■), lysozyme (▲, alpha-amino nitrogen (▼), and sodium (►). Values are expressed as percent of the maximal excretion rates attained after administration of maleic acid

tion despite continued, severely reduced concentrations of ATP and total adenine nucleotide in the proximal renal tubule, possibly by enhancing this tissue's mitochondrial respiration and rate of regeneration of ATP.

The Experimental Model Induced by Maleic Acid (MA)

The experimental model of RTA-2/FS acutely induced by fructose in patients with HFI has striking parallels with the experimental model of RTA-2/FS acutely induced within minutes of initiating parenterally administered MA in the dog and rat [1] (Fig. 2). From clearance studies in the dog studied during water diureses, Al-Bander et al. concluded that MA induced the proximal tubule to reject greatly increased amounts of HCO_3^- (and sodium and chloride) that accounted for the maleate-induced bicarbonaturia of RTA2 [3]. On the basis of microperfusion studies of the proximal tubule in rats given maleate, Bank et al. and Reboucas et al. [4] concluded that the maleate-induced, acute reduction of net reabsorption of HCO_3^- in the proximal tubule did not result from back-flux of HCO_3^- through an abnormally leaky membrane, but rather from impaired active reabsorption of HCO_3^-, i.e., impaired H^+ secretion. In microperfusion studies of MA-induced aminoaciduria, Gunther and his coworkers concluded that MA inhibits the saturable reabsorption of amino acids along the proximal tubule; they showed that MA does not induce a greater efflux of amino acid into the lumen at distal sites of the nephron [5].

Although not occurring in nature, maleic acid is the cis isomer of fumaric acid, and like that naturally occurring metabolite of the Krebs oxidative cycle, readily metabolized by renal cortical mitochondria. At doses that induce RTA-2/FS, maleic acid induces in the proximal renal tubule striking structural abnormalities in the mitochondria, an impairment in their oxidative metabolism, and a reduced renal cortical concentration of ATP and activity of Na^+/K^+ ATPase [6]. Presumably, in part by impairing mitochondrial oxidation, maleic acid also induces in the renal cortex greatly increased rates of glucose uptake and glycolysis and increased concentrations of phosphorylated glycolytic intermediates [7]. That the increase in glycolysis induced by maleic acid might participate in the pathogenesis of its nephrotoxicity is suggested by one of Berliner's original observations [1]. Whereas maleic acid administered alone induced only transient renal dysfunction, it induced persisting renal failure when administered in combination with previously initiated glucose loading [1]. The metabolic pathogenesis of RTA 2/FS acutely induced by maleic acid could then involve a positive feedback loop in cells of the proximal renal tubule: impaired mitochondrial oxidation → increased glucose uptake → increased formation and concentration of phosphorylated glycolytic intermediates → limitation on the availability of cellular P_i → more severely impaired mitochondrial oxidative metabolism and possibly increased production of lactic acid [8]. In support of this hypothesis, Al-Bander et al. observed in the dog given maleic acid that prior phosphate loading attenuated RTA2/FS, whereas glucose loading exacerbated it, even when initiated after the dysfunction had already occurred [8]. Consistent with this hypothesis and its possible relevance to the pathogenetic mechanism of chronic clinical RTA2/FS is the recent observation by Jonas et al. that urinary excretion of lactic acid and d-glyceraldehyde is greatly increased in patients with chronic RTA2/FS in whom the plasma concentrations of lactate and d-glyceraldehyde are not increased [9]. The phenomenon was observed in a group of 16 patients affected with RTA2/FS, most of whom had cystinosis; others had cytochrome c oxidase deficiency, tyrosinosis, glycogenosis, and Lowe's syndrome, respectively, and in one disorder was judged to be idiopathic. Hyperlacticaciduria without hyperlacticacidemia in combination with "tubular" proteinuria, which included B_2 microglobin, has also been reported as the earliest finding in young children affected with an autosomal dominant renal disorder that is expressed in early childhood as RTA2/FS and sometime later as severe renal insufficiency as well. In those described with this disorder, the severity of aminoaciduria and hyperlacticaciduria has increased with age.

Lysozymuria, Lysosomal Enzymuria — Pathogenetic Implications

Whether occurring as part of either an acute experimental disorder or as a chronic clinical disorder, RTA2/FS is attended by a reduction in renal tubular reabsorption of lysozyme and other low molecular weight proteins (LMWP) readily filtered by the normal glomerulus. Normally these LMWP are almost completely reabsorbed in the proximal renal tubule by a vacuolar transport system of some selectivity [10]. Given the extensive system of clathrin coated pits located at the base of the microvilli in the proximal tubule [11], and the active participation of clathrin in the process of receptor-mediated endocytosis, it seems likely that at least some of the selective reabsorption of LMWP represents a form of receptor-mediated endocytosis [10]. The reabsorbed LMWP, which also include B_2 microglobulin, insulin, immunoglobulin L Chain, and ribonuclease, first attach to the luminal membrane, presumably in coated pits, when they are internalized in apical endocytic vesicles and subsequently conveyed through endosomes [10] to a prelysosomal compartment, and finally to lysosomes, where they are enzymatically degraded [10]. In the experimental model of FS/RTA2 induced acutely in the rat given maleic acid, Christensen and Maunsbach reported the direct histochemical demonstration of impaired renal tubular uptake and vacuolar transport of lysozyme to lysosomes, an impairment which occurred restrictively in the proximal tubule and within 20 minutes of administering maleic acid [12].

Also observed whenever sought in either experimental or clinical FS/RTA2 is the phenomenon of increased urinary excretion of lysosomal enzymes such as N-acetyl-β-Glucosaminidase (NAG) [13]. Although too large to be filtered by the normal glomerulus, these proteins normally occur in the renal tubule, predominantly segregated in lysosomes of the proximal tubule in whose cells they are synthesized in the endoplasmic reticulum. An increased urinary excretion of NAG and other lysosomal enzymes is generally inferred to reflect "damage" or "injury" to the proximal tubule, and simple leakage of lysosomal enzymes from its damaged lysosomes.

But hyperexcretion of lysosomal enzymes could reflect much more complex mechanisms. Since the process of endocytosis is dynamically coupled to that of exocytosis [14], the combined hyperexcretion of lysozyme and lysosomal enzymes in FS/RTA2 could reflect a complex proximal tubular disorder of vacuolar transport affecting both endocytosis and exocytosis. In accordance with this hypothesis, Al-Bander et al. [15] observed in the dog that minutes after the onset of maleate-induced RTA2/FS, the urinary excretion of lysosomal enzymes, N-Acetyl-β-Glucosaminidase, β-Glucuronidase and β-Galactosidase increased simultaneously with the anticipated increase in renal clearance of lysozyme (Figs. 2–3). The severities of all these enzymurias increased rapidly and in parallel, all reaching a peak some 80–100 minutes after onset, then decreasing rapidly and in parallel. Sodium phosphate loading strikingly attenuates, and glucose loading exacerbates, the severities of both the RTA2/FS and hyperexcretion of lysozyme and lysosomal enzymes [15] (Fig. 4). These observations suggest that in the RTA2/FS induced by maleic acid in the dog, a P_i-dependent disorder of carbohydrate metabolism in the cells of the proximal renal tubule underlies both its dysfunction of transepithelial solute transport and derangement of protein handling [15]. In the RTA-2/FS acutely induced by intravenously administering fructose to patients with HFI, an acute, rapidly reversible hyperexcretion of lysozyme and lysosomal enzymes also occurs.

The process of endocytosis and exocytosis are coupled such that they constitute opposing limbs of cyclic continua in which membrane fragments of endocytotic vacuoles are recycled to exocytotic vacuoles through endosomes and to the plasma membrane, the recycling occurring within minutes. The process is energy dependent, as is that of orderly clathrin assembly/disassembly. In the proximal renal tubule cells of the rat, just minutes after its receipt of maleate, large endocytic apical vacuoles accumulate, most of the apical tubules disappear [11,12], coated pits lose their clathrin coat [11], and the corresponding coated pits membrane, which normally remains restricted to the base of the microvilli during endocytosis, becomes internalized to the newly formed, large apical vacuoles [11]. The membrane incorporated into these vacuoles appears not to derive from either microvillar membranes or lysosomal membranes [11]. If, as seems likely, apical tubules function to return membrane material from the endocytic vacuoles to the luminal plasma membrane [12], the maleate-induced disappearance of these tubules would indicate altered recycling of membrane to the luminal membrane [12].

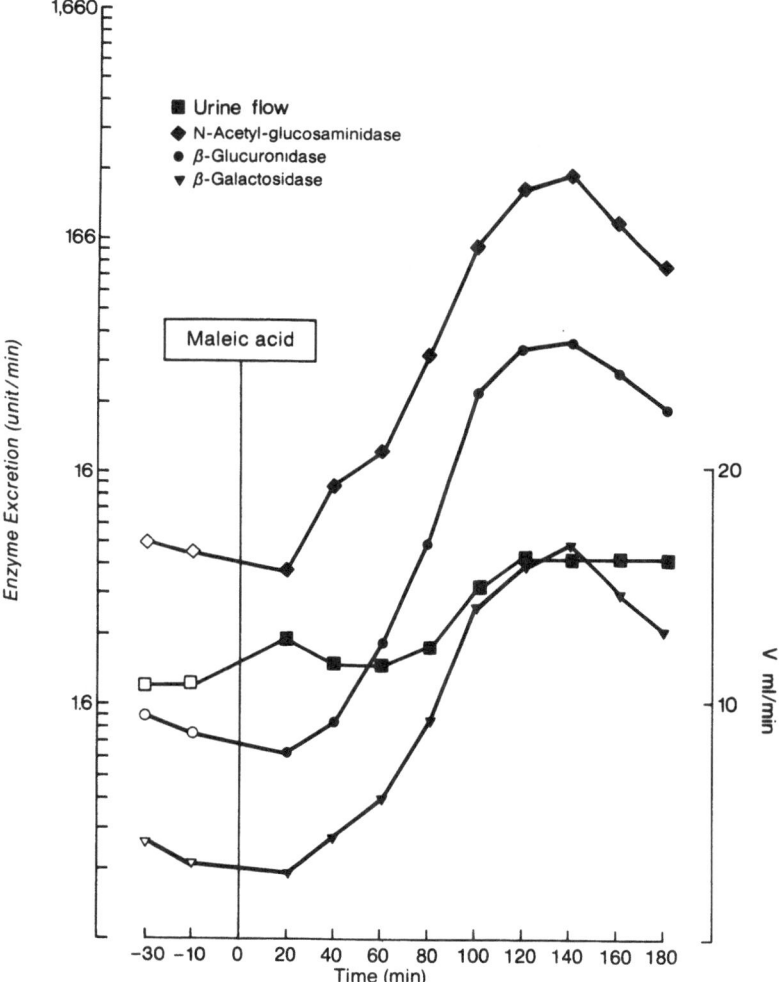

Fig. 3. Urine flow (■) and urinary excretion of N-acetyl-β-glucosaminidase (♦), β-glucuronidase (●), and β-galactosidase (▼) before (*open symbols*) and after (*closed symbols*) administration of maleic acid in 8 dogs. Values are the mean. Data are plotted on a semilog basis. Parallel lines indicate relatively constant enzyme excretion ratios

Since a variety of cells can be induced to secrete newly synthesized lysosomal enzymes with enzymatic activity, the lysosomal enzymes hyperexcreted in RTA2/FS may not be the mature, smaller enzymes normally segregated in renal lysosomes. In both acquired and genetically transmitted human disease, increased amounts of newly synthesized, larger lysosomal enzymes exit affected cells and occur in "pathological" urine [16,17]. In fact, both newly synthesized and mature lysosomal enzymes occur in the urine of normal humans, the first apparently being secreted by a non-lysosomal pathway, the second by a lysosomal pathway [16].

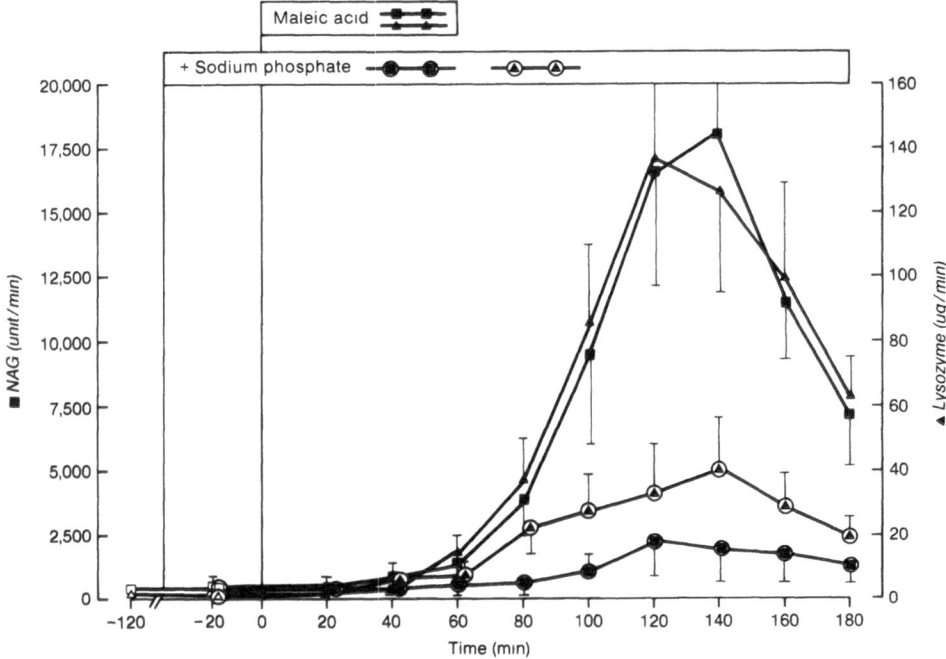

Fig. 4. Urinary excretion of lysozyme (▲ μg/min, *right scale*) and N-acetyl-β-glucosaminidase (*NAG*, ■ U/min, *left scale*) before (*open symbols*) and after (*circled symbols*) intravenous administration of maleic acid alone (8 studies) or after sodium phosphate loading (8 studies, circled symbols). Values are the mean ± SEM

After their synthesis in rough endoplasmic reticulum, enzymes destined for segregation in lysosomes traverse the Golgi complex. There, most of these proteins gain phosphomannosyl residues which bind them to mannose-6-phosphate receptors and thereby "address" them to lysosomes [18]. The ligand-receptor complexes exit the trans-Golgi network, the last station along the Golgi pathway, in clathrin-coated vesicles and proceed to a "late" endosome "prelysosomal compartment." The more acidic interior of this compartment effects the disassociation of the ligand-receptor complex, thus allowing the released enzymes to be segregated in lysosomes and the unoccupied receptors to be recycled to the Golgi apparatus and plasma membrane. In normal rat kidney cells, the prelysosomal compartments appears to be stationed on the "main endocytic route" from the plasma membrane to the lysosomes [19]. In consequence, both lysosomal enzymes bound to mannose-6-phosphate receptors in the Golgi network and proteins endocytosed by receptor mediation accumulate attached to their receptors in the prelysosomal compartment, immediately before either dissociates from its receptor and is transferred to lysosomes [19].

By rendering the "late" endosome prelysosomal compartment less acidic and thus retarding the dissociation of ligand-receptor complexes, certain weak bases like chloroquine and NH_4Cl, or genetically decreased activity of endosomal $H^+ATPase$, can restrict the recycling of unoccupied mannose-6-phosphate receptors to the Golgi apparatus. Accordingly, these bases and this enzymatic disorder can effect the constitutive secretion of immature, mannose-6-phosphate-bearing lysosomal enzymes and impair receptor-mediated endocytosis. Caplan and his colleagues recently reported that treatment of canine renal tubule cells (Mardin-Darby canine kidney cell line) with NH_4Cl induced secretion of newly synthesized cathepsin "D," a lysosomal enzyme, into both apical and basolateral media [20]. In preliminary studies chloroquine has been reported to inhibit endocytic reabsorption of protein in the isolated perfused rabbit proximal renal tubule [21]. While it remains to be demonstrated that the lysosomal enzymes hyperexcreted in RTA2/FS contain mannose-6-phosphate, Tager and his colleagues have demonstrated the occurrence in urine of normal subjects a mannose-6-phosphate-bearing immature lysosomal enzyme, α glucosidase, as well as a smaller, mature form of this enzyme that contained no mannose-6-phosphate residues [22]. In acute RTA2/FS, rapidly reversible, coordinate hyperexcretion of lysozyme and mannose-6-phosphate-bearing immature lysosomal enzymes could then result from a rapidly reversible loss of normal acidity in the late endosome prelysosomal compartment in cells of the proximal renal tubule. This loss could be caused by a reversible reduction in function of endosomal H^+-ATPase consequent to impaired metabolic generation of ATP.

Whatever the details of its character and mechanism, the fact of the coordinate, rapidly reversible lysozymuria/lysosomal enzymuria characteristic of acute RTA2/FS, in conjunction with the loss of apical tubules in cells of the proximal tubule, and the accumulation there of large apical vacuoles containing membrane normally restricted to the base of microvilli, almost certainly reflects a severe disordering of endocytosis/exocytosis and membrane recycling in the proximal tubule. This disordering could impair exocytotic replenishment of transport components of its luminal membrane and thereby entrain varied and complex disturbances of its physiological functions [1,4], somewhat as proposed by Bergeron et al. [23]. Such a disordering could impair exocytotic insertion into the luminal membrane of not only electrogenic H^+ ATPase, but possibly also the endosomal electroneutral H^+/Na^+ antiporter recently described in the proximal tubule. Impaired mitochondrial generation of ATP induced in the proximal tubule by maleic acid in animals, or by fructose in patients with HFI, might then be pathogenetically linked to RTA2/FS through diminished activity of both basolateral Na^+-K^+ ATPase and apical H^+ ATPase and consequent impairment of not only electroneutral H^+/Na^+ exchange and electrogenic H^+ secretion, but possibly also impairment of net luminal plasma membrane transport of such normally reabsorbed solutes as glucose and phosphate.

The Junk Mail Message Hypothesis

If patients with RTA-2/FS, or FS alone, hyperexcrete immature enzymes bearing mannose-6-phosphate (because these enzymes are constitutively secreted by metabolically disordered proximal tubules), the consequent occurrence of increased concentrations of these glycoproteins in the tubular lumen fluid and peritubular blood (basolateral secretion) [20] could have important pathogenetic implications. The mannose-6-phosphate receptor (cation independent) that normally ferries immature lysosomal enzymes from the Golgi (and the plasma membrane) to the prelysosomal compartment [19], is also the insulin-like growth factor (IGF)-II receptor [24]. Specifically, a single protein binds and transports mannose-6-phosphate-liganded lysosomal enzymes and IGF-II. Mannose-6-phosphate and IGF-II can modulate each others binding to this dual ligand receptor. The receptor occurs both on the brush border and basolateral membrane of the mammalian proximal renal tubule and in the glomeruli. Hammerman and his colleagues [25] have recently demonstrated that mannose-6-phosphate amplifies the biological effect of IGF-II at the basolateral membrane of the proximal renal tubule of the rat: At this site, mannose-6-phosphate amplifies the capacity of IGF-II to stimulate phospholipase C, as measured by increased production of inositol triphosphate, a reaction product of phosphoinositide hydrolysis. While the physiological consequences of this phenomenon are by no means clear, it is clear that IGF-II can evoke a number of biological phenomena, and stimulation of phospholipase C and the consequent production of inositol triphosphate (and diacylglycerol) are critical to signal transmission of a variety of hormones and growth factors. It is also clear that mannose-6-phosphate-bearing lysosomal enzymes can modulate the binding of IGF-II to the IGF-II/mannose-6-phosphate receptor [26]. Thus, in patients with RTA-2/FS the IGF-II/mannose-6-phosphate receptor might be pathologically modulated at multiple sites of the renal tubule by increased concentrations of mannose-6-phosphate-bearing lysosomal enzymes.

Chronic RTA2/FS – Cystinosis

In patients with cystinosis, the most common cause of RTA2/FS in children, "storage" of cystine in lysosomes may be a primary pathogenetic event in many tissues affected [27,28], and the occurrence of this phenomenon in the proximal renal tubule might underlie RTA2/FS. In so-called nephropathic or "infantile" cystinosis, lysosomal accumulation of cystine occurs prenatally, RTA/FS is expressed within the first 12 months of life, progressive reduction in glomerular filtration rate leads to uremia by midchildhood, and the free-cystine content of leukocytes is 80 times normal.

Cystine is the only aminoacid stored in cystinotic lysosomes. A defect in carrier mediated transport of cystine across lysosomal membrane accounts for its massive accumulation in the lysosomes of those homozygous for infantile cystinosis [28]. Lysosomal accumulation of cystine occurs throughout the kidney, particularly in the interstitium and glomerulus, and apparently also in the cells of the proximal tubule. The phenomenon of cystine "storage" would seem to be important to the pathogenesis of the glomerulopathy and progressive renal failure characteristic of cystinosis in childhood. Cysteamine depletes intracellular cystine stores. In cystinotic children, early treatment with cysteamine, which greatly reduces lysosomal cystine concentration in leukocytes, can attenuate and perhaps prevent the otherwise predictable occurrence of both the progressive reduction of GFR and the severe stunting of somatic growth characteristic of this disease. Yet, with one apparent exception, institution of cysteamine, even in the first weeks of life, has failed to either prevent the occurrence of RTA2/FS or to attenuate established RTA2/FS. This failure might reflect restricted access of cysteamine to cystine-laden lysosomes in the proximal renal tubule. It is not clear, however, that lysosomal accumulation of cystine, per se, in the proximal tubule, or whatever "destruction" such accumulation might entrain there, accounts for either the RTA2/FS of cystinosis or the massive urinary excretion of lysosomal enzymes characteristic of this disease. Portale and his associates have recently studied a young girl with RTA-2/FS, massively increased urinary excretion of N-acetylglucosaminidase, and the classic clinical characteristics of cystinosis, including photophobia and retarded growth. Yet excessive cystine was demonstrably not present in leucocytes or fibroblasts. Renal biopsy revealed no evidence of cystinosis.

It might be noted that neither RTA2/FS nor any of the other clinical features of cystinosis have been described in I cell disease, a disorder in which cystine also accumulates in lysosomes because of its impaired transport, and in which urinary excretion of newly synthesized lysosomal enzymes is also increased. In I cell disease newly synthesized lysosomal enzymes, and perhaps also component proteins of lysosomal membrane transport systems, fail to acquire the mannose-6-phosphate residues that "address" them to lysosomes and are thus diverted from their normal lysosomal destination and secreted. Lacking mannose-6-phosphate, these proteins would not be expected to modulate binding of IGF II to its receptor on the plasma membrane of the renal tubule (see above).

Recent observations with cystine dimethylester may provide a clue to the mechanism through which cystine might evoke RTA-2/FS in patients with cystinosis. Foreman, Segal, and their coworkers [29] demonstrated that parenteral administration of this substance for four days led to an increased urinary volume and excretion of phosphate, glucose and α-amino nitrogen and various amino acids. Cystine dimethylester treatment did not affect the creatinine clearance. In studies of isolated renal tubules, preincubation with cystine dimethylester greatly inhibited the uptake of lysine, glycine and α-methylglucoside. In the isolated perfused rabbit proximal renal tubule, Salmon and Baum [30] demonstrated that cystine dimethylester added to the bath induced, within 10 minutes, large reductions in J_V, bicarbonate transport (J_{TCO_2}) and glucose transport. The methylesters of leucine and tryptophan had no effect on these transport systems. Cystine dimethylester had no effect on mannitol or bicarbonate permeability. Thus, the inhibition of transport observed was due to inhibition of active transport.

Incubation of renal tubules with cystine dimethylester led to an increased tissue concentration of cystine, comparable to that measured in kidney tissue of cystinotics who had nephrectomies before renal transplantation. Additionally, there was a fivefold increase in cysteine. Intraperitoneal administration of cystine which induced features of the FS resulted in increased renal concentration of cysteine, but neither cystine nor cystine dimethylester was detected. In the isolated perfused proximal convoluted tubule, addition of cysteine methylester to the bath induced a transport impairment like that induced by cystine dimethylester, but only with four times higher concentrations. Preliminary observations by Baum and Salmon would indicate that cystine dimethylester induces an immediate 50% reduction in ATP and O_2 consumption of renal tubules. Thus, the mechanism through which cystinosis gives rise to RTA-2/FS may involve impaired mitochondrial oxidative metabolism in the proximal renal tubule. Such a mechanism has obvious parallels with that inferred in both the RTA-2/FS induced by fructose in patients with hereditary fructose intolerance and that induced by maleate in experimental animals.

References

1. Berliner RW, Kennedy TJ, Hilton JG (1950) Effect of maleic acid on renal function. Proc Soc Exp Biol Med 75:791–794

2. Morris RC Jr, Sebastian A (1983) Renal Tubular Acidosis and Fanconi Syndrome. In: Stanbury JB, Wyngaarden JB, Fredrickson DS, Goldstein JL, Brown MS (eds) The metabolic basis of inherited disease. McGraw-Hill, New York, pp 1808–1866

3. Al-Bander HA, Weiss RA, Humphreys MH, Morris RC Jr (1982) Dysfunction of the proximal tubule underlies maleic acid-induced type II renal tubular acidosis. Am J Physiol 243:F604–F611

4. Bank N, Aynedjian HS, Mutz BF (1986) Microperfusion study of proximal tubule bicarbonate transport in maleic acid-induced renal tubular acidosis. Am J Physiol 250:F476–F482

5. Gunther R, Silbernagl S, Deetjen P (1979) Maleic acid induced aminoaciduria studied by free flow micropuncture and continuous microperfusion. Pflugers Arch 382:109–114

6. Kramer HJ, Gonick HC (1970) Experimental Fanconi syndrome. I. Effect of maleic acid on renal cortical Na-K-ATPase activity and ATP levels. J Lab Clin Med 76:799–808

7. Rogulski J, Strzelecki T, Pacanis A, Kaminska E, Angielski S (1975) Effects of maleate on renal carbohydrate metabolism in vivo and in vitro. In: Angielski S, Dubach UC (eds) Biochemical aspects of renal function. Huber, Bern, pp 106–110

8. Al-Bander H, Etheredge SB, Paukert T, Humphreys MH, Morris RC Jr (1985) Phosphate loading attenuates renal tubular dysfunction induced by maleic acid in the dog. Am J Physiol 248:F513–F521

9. Jonas AJ, Lin S-N, Conley SB, Schneider JA, Williams JC, Caprioli RC (1989) Urine glyceraldehyde excretion is elevated in the renal Fanconi syndrome. Kidney Int 35:99–104

10. Wall DA, Maack T (1985) Endocytic uptake, transport, and catabolism of proteins by epithelial cells. Am J Physiol 248:C12–C20

11. Rodman JS, Seidman L, Farquhar MG (1986) The membrane composition of coated pits, microvilli, endosomes, and lysosomes is distinctive in the rat kidney proximal tubule cell. J Cell Biol 102:77–87

12. Christensen EI, Maunsbach AB (1980) Proteinuria induced by sodium maleate in rats: Effects on ultrastructure and protein handling in renal proximal tubule. Kidney Int 17:771–787

13. Kunin CM, Chesney RW, Craig WA, England AD, DeAngelis C (1978) Enzymuria as a marker of renal injury and disease: Studies of N-acetyl-beta-glucosaminidase in the general population and in patients with renal disease. Pediatrics 620:751–760

14. Steinman RM, Mellman IS, Muller WA, Cohn ZA (1983) Endocytosis and the recycling of plasma membrane. J Cell Biol 96:1–27

15. Al-Bander HA, Mock DM, Etheredge SB, Paukert TT, Humphreys MH, Morris RC Jr (1986) Coordinately increased lysozymuria and lysosomal enzymuria induced by maleic acid. Kidney Int 30:804–812

16. Kress BC, Hirani S, Freeze HH, Little L, Miller AL (1982) Mucolipidosis III B-N-acetyl-D-hexosaminidase; A purification and properties. Biochem J 207:421–428

17. Zuhlsdorf M, Imort M, Hasilik A, von Figura K (1983) Molecular forms of B-hexosaminidase and cathepsin D in serum and urine of healthy subjects and patients with elevated activity of lysosomal enzymes. Biochem J 213:733–740

18. Dahms NM, Lobel P, Kornfeld S (1989) Mannose 6-phosphate receptors and lysosomal enzyme targeting. J Biol Chem 264:12115–12118

19. Griffiths G, Hoflack B, Simons K, Mellman I, Kornfeld S (1988) The mannose 6-phosphate receptor and the biogenesis of lysosomes. Cell 52:329–341

20. Caplan MJ, Stow JL, Newman AP, Madri J, Anderson HC, Farquhar MG, Palade GE, Jamieson JD (1987) Dependence on pH of polarized sorting of secreted proteins. Nature 329:632–635

21. Park CH, Clapp WL, Madsen KM, Tisher CC (1987) Structure and function of endosomal-lysosomal (EL) system in the proximal tubule (PT) (abstract). Xth International Congress of Nephrology 589

22. Oude Elferink RPJ, Brouwer-Kelder EM, Surya I, Strijland A, Kroos M, Reuser AJJ, Tager JM (1984) Isolation and characterization of a precursor form of lysosomal alpha-glucosidase from human urine. Eur J Biochem 139:489–495
23. Bergeron M, Dubord L, Hausser C (1976) Membrane permeability as a cause of transport defects in experimental Fanconi syndrome: A new hypothesis. J Clin Invest 57:1181–1189
24. Morgan DO, Edman JC, Standring DN, Fried VA, Smith MC, Roth RA, Rutter WJ (1987) Insulin-like growth factor II receptor as a multifunctional binding protein. Nature 329:301–307
25. Hammerman MR (1989) The growth hormone-insulin-like growth factor axis in kidney. Am J Physiol 257:F503–F514
26. Kiess W, Blickenstaff GD, Sklar MM, Thomas CL, Nissley SP, Sahagian GG (1988) Biochemical evidence that the type II insulin-like growth factor receptor is identical to the cation-independent mannose 6-phosphate receptor. J Biol Chem 263:9339–9344
27. Schneider JA, Schulman JD (1983) Cystinosis. In: Stanbury JB, Wyngaarden JB, Fredrickson DS, Goldstein JL, Brown MS (eds) The metabolic basis of inherited disease. McGraw-Hill, New York, pp 1844–1866
28. Gahl WA, Renlund M, Thoene JG (1989) Lysosomal transport disorders: Cystinosis and Sialic Acid Storage. In: Scriver CR, Beaudet AL, Sly WS, Valle D (eds) The metabolic basis of inherited disease. McGraw-Hill, New York, pp 2619–2648
29. Foreman JW, Bowring MA, Lee J, States B, Segal S (1987) Effect of cystine dimethylester on renal solute handling and isolated renal tubule transport in the rat: a new model of the Fanconi syndrome. Metabolism 36:1185–1191
30. Salmon RF, Baum M (1990) Intracellular cystine loading inhibits transport in the rabbit proximal convoluted tubule. J Clin Invest 85:340–344

Mechanism of Distal Acidification: Relevance to Distal RTA

ROBERT J. ALPERN[1]

SUMMARY. Acid secretion in the distal nephron is mediated by a cell with an apical membrane ATP-coupled H pump and a basolateral membrane Cl/HCO_3 exchanger. Considering H secretion as a function of luminal pH, defects in distal acidification can be divided into three broad groups: an abnormal *leak* where net H secretion is normal in the absence of a pH gradient but becomes abnormal as luminal pH decreases; a *rate* defect where minimal urinary pH is normal but the rate of acidification is decreased at higher luminal pH; and a *voltage* defect where the rate of H secretion at all luminal pH is decreased and the minimal urinary pH is increased. The U-BPCO_2 has been used to assess the rate of H secretion in the presence of a minimal gradient for back diffusion. The presence of hyperkalemia indicates that the disease process involves the cortical collecting tubule where H and K are both secreted, or indicates an abnormality in aldosterone which stimulates H and K secretion. Lastly, the response of urinary pH and urinary K to an increase in distal Na delivery can be used to examine cortical collecting tubule function.

Normal Physiology

In considering the pathophysiologic basis of distal RTA, it is best to view this in the context of normal mechanisms of H secretion in the collecting duct. We will therefore start by defining the mechanisms of H transport in the H secreting cell of the collecting duct. This cell type has been best studied in the in vitro perfused inner stripe of the rabbit outer medullary collecting duct [1-4]. In this segment, a number of transporters have been defined, as shown in Fig. 1. The apical membrane contains an H ATPase which is most likely of the vacuolar type [3,5]. This transporter utilizes the chemical energy of ATP to transport H ions energetically uphill. In addition, data has

---

[1]Division of Nephrology, Department of Internal Medicine, University of Texas Southwestern Medical Center, 5323 Harry Hines Blvd., Dallas, TX 75235-8856, USA

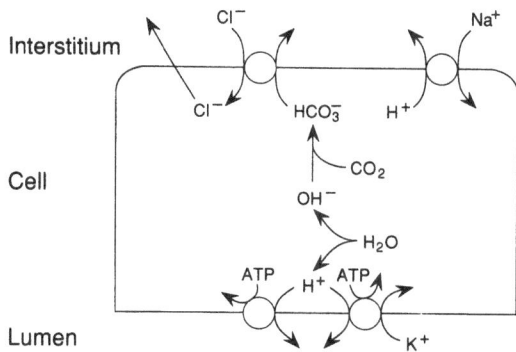

Fig. 1. Model of H secreting cell in collecting duct

been presented suggesting that during K deficiency an HK ATPase, similar to that present in gastric mucosa, is inserted into the apical membrane of these cells [4]. Hays and Alpern could not find evidence for this transporter in outer medullary collecting tubules harvested from normal animals [3]. Base, which is generated within the cell by the H pumps, then exits across the basolateral membrane on a Cl/HCO_3 exchanger. This Cl/HCO_3 exchanger appears to be similar to, but not identical to, the red cell band 3 Cl/HCO_3 exchanger. The difference resides in alternate splicing of the mRNA leading to truncation of the amino terminal portion of the exchanger in the kidney form [6,7]. Lastly, a basolateral membrane Na/H antiporter has been identified in this cell [1,2]. This transporter would not be expected to contribute to transepithelial H secretion, and in fact would decrease the rate. Most likely, this transporter serves certain housekeeping functions such as cell pH defense and cell volume defense during changes in medullary tonicity.

Also of relevance to the understanding of distal RTA is an understanding of axial heterogeneity in the distal nephron. The cortical collecting tubule possesses three cell types: a principal cell which absorbs Na and secretes K, a type A intercalated cell which secretes H, and a type B intercalated cell which secretes HCO_3. This allows the cortical collecting tubule to secrete either acid or base, in response to changes in dietary acid. In addition, this allows H secretion from the cortical collecting tubule to be regulated by changes in transepithelial voltage secondary to changes in Na transport. The medullary collecting tubule, on the other hand, appears to secrete only H ions. There is no capacity for HCO_3 secretion and there is no net Na transport. In states of chronic K deficiency, this segment is capable of absorbing K, most likely using the apical membrane HK ATPase described above [4].

Relevance to Distal RTA

The turtle urinary bladder has been used as a model to examine the regulation of H secretion by the collecting duct. Using this model, Steinmetz, Al-Awqati, and co-workers have demonstrated that the rate of H secretion is a linear function of luminal

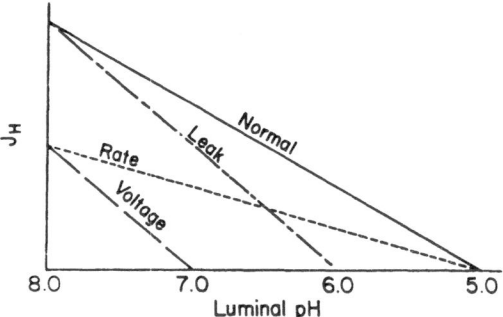

Fig. 2. Potential mechanisms for defects in distal H secretion. (From [9] with permission of McGraw Hill Inc.)

pH [8]. This is shown as the line labelled normal in Fig. 2. In addition, these investigators demonstrated that changes in luminal pH and in transepithelial voltage had similar effects on H secretion when considered as the electrochemical gradient. Thus, a tenfold pH gradient was found to be similar to a 60 mV change in voltage. Using this approach, one can consider different forms of defects in H secretion and how they would be expressed as a function of luminal pH. This then allows one to predict whether patients will be able to acidify their urine maximally in the presence of these defects.

The first defect is that of an increased leak. During normal urinary acidification, the lumen of the collecting tubule becomes markedly acidified compared to the pH of the interstitium. This sets up driving forces for leak of H, H_2CO_3 or HCO_3. As can be seen in Fig. 2, if luminal pH is similar to that of the interstitium, there is no driving force for leaks and therefore no effect on the rate of H secretion. However, as luminal fluid becomes more acid, there is increased leak and thus a greater defect in net acidification. This type of lesion has been referred to as a gradient lesion, because it is anticipated that patients would be unable to acidify their urine maximally. The best example of this lesion is the amphotericin-induced lesion.

A second category of defect is a rate defect. Here the H secreting cell is able to establish a normally acid luminal fluid, but the rate of H secretion at any luminal pH is slower than in control. Thus, if luminal flow rate is sufficiently slow, or if luminal buffer content is sufficiently low, a normally acid urine can be achieved. However, in the presence of normal rates of buffer delivery and normal tubular fluid flow rates, the slow rates of H secretion will lead to an inappropriately alkaline urine. The best example of this defect is that of aldosterone deficiency [8]. When ammoniagenesis is suppressed in these patients by hyperkalemia, they can acidify their urine normally. When hyperkalemia is corrected, ammonia synthesis is normal, and the urine is inappropriately alkaline due to the rate defect.

The last possible defect is a voltage defect. Here, the apparatus for secreting H is intact, but due to abnormalities in NaCl transport, the normal lumen-negativity of the cortical collecting tubule is not present. Because changes in voltage are additive to changes in luminal pH (see above), the line drawn in Fig. 2 is parallel to, but beneath the normal line. Thus, these patients should be unable to achieve maximally acidified urines. The best example of this phenomenon is seen in amiloride administration to experimental animals. While in theory aldosterone deficiency would also inhibit Na transport and decrease transepithelial voltage, this effect appears to be minor compared to the rate defect, as patients can normally acidify their urine in the presence of low buffer delivery.

Based on the schema presented in Fig. 2, the ability to acidify the urine normally can be extremely useful in classifying patients with distal RTA. It is also useful to measure the rate of H secretion in the distal nephron in the absence of a pH gradient. This can be done with the U-B PCO_2 (urine minus blood PCO_2). This will be described in further detail by the subsequent speakers. In general, in the presence of a HCO_3 diuresis, accumulation of carbonic acid in the lumen will lead to a high PCO_2 in the urine. As the major cause of high luminal carbonic acid concentration is H secretion, this parameter has been considered to be useful in assessing the ability of the collecting tubule to secrete H. Thus, a low U-B PCO_2 in the presence of marked bicarbonaturia can be due to decreased H secretion, back diffusion of secreted H, or back diffusion of H_2CO_3. It has been argued that back diffusion of H and H_2CO_3 would be unlikely to occur in this setting, because of the high concentration of HCO_3 in the lumen and thus an anticipated high luminal pH. However, because carbonic anhydrase is absent in the lumen of most of the collecting tubule, luminal pH is not in equilibrium with HCO_3 and is actually lower than would be predicted from the HCO_3 concentration. Thus, it remains possible that a driving force would persist for back diffusion of H and H_2CO_3.

The presence of hyperkalemia in patients with distal RTA suggests the coexistence of defects in K secretion and H secretion. This occurs in a number of clinical settings. The most common cause is aldosterone deficiency. Because aldosterone stimulates the rate of K and H secretion in the collecting tubule, aldosterone deficiency is accompanied by defects in both K and H secretion. Pseudohyperaldosteronism type I is a condition where aldosterone levels are normal, but aldosterone is unable to regulate transport in the collecting tubule (? receptor defect). Any defect in voltage in the cortical collecting tubule would also be expected to decrease H and K secretion. Lastly, any disease process which damaged the cortical collecting tubule would be expected to interfere with K and H secretion.

Some investigators have argued that the response to increased distal Na delivery is also useful in defining the mechanism of distal RTA. This will be further discussed below. In general, distal Na delivery can be increased by administration of furosemide, sodium sulfate, or sodium phosphate. If this maneuver leads to a decrease in urinary pH and an increase in urinary K, the cortical collecting tubule should be relatively intact. If increasing distal Na delivery has no effect on urine pH but increases urine K normally, there is a defect in H secretion in the cortical collecting tubule. Lastly, if increasing distal Na delivery has no effect on urine pH or on urine K, there is either a combined H and K secretory defect in the cortical collecting tubule, or there is an inability of this maneuver to alter voltage (voltage defect).

Thus, by measuring urine pH, U-B PCO_2, serum K, and the response to increased distal Na delivery, one can define the mechanisms responsible for a defect in distal acidification. In general, the urine pH and serum K are the most useful clinically. The next two chapters will further discuss the mechanisms responsible for distal RTA and the approach to the patient with distal RTA.

References

1. Hays SR, Alpern RJ (1990) Basolateral membrane Na^+-independent Cl^-/HCO_3^- exchange in the inner stripe of the rabbit outer medullary collecting tubule. J Gen Physiol 95:347–367
2. Breyer MD, Jacobson HR (1989) Regulation of rabbit medullary collecting duct cell pH by basolateral Na^+/H^+ and Cl^-/base exchange. J Clin Invest 84:996–1004
3. Hays SR, Alpern RJ (1990) Apical and basolateral membrane H^+ extrusion mechanisms in the inner stripe of the rabbit outer medullary collecting tubule. Am J Physiol 259 (Renal Fluid Electrolyte Physiol 28):F628–F635
4. Wingo CS (1989) Active proton secretion and potassium absorption in the rabbit outer medullary collecting duct. J Clin Invest 84:361–365
5. Stone DK, Xie X-S (1988) Proton translocating ATPases: Issues in structure and function. Kidney Int 33:767–774
6. Kudrycki KE, Shull GE (1989) Primary structure of the rat kidney band 3 anion exchange protein deduced from a cDNA. J Biol Chem 264:8185–8192
7. Brosius FC III, Alper SL, Garcia AM, Lodish HF (1989) The major kidney band 3 gene transcript predicts an amino-terminal truncated band 3 polypeptide. J Biol Chem 264: 7784–7787
8. Al-Awqati Q (1978) H^+ transport in urinary epithelia. Am J Physiol 235 (Renal Fluid Electrolyte Physiol 4):F77-F88
9. DuBose TD, Alpern RJ In: Metabolic basis of inherited disease, 6th edn. McGraw Hill

Pathophysiological Basis of Distal Renal Tubular Acidosis: Lessons from Animal Models

Thomas D. DuBose Jr[1]

Summary. A number of potential defects may impair acidification either directly or indirectly in segments of the distal nephron. Papillary micropuncture studies have validated the urine minus blood PCO_2 (U-B PCO_2) obtained during a bicarbonate diuresis as a reliable qualitative index of distal nephron proton pump integrity. Microelectrode determination of both PCO_2 and disequilibrium pH in the papillary collecting duct in a number of experimental models of distal renal tubular acidosis (DRTA) have demonstrated at least four types of defects: 1) The permeability or "gradient" defect is best exemplified by the amphotericin B lesion, where reduction in net acid excretion is the result of backleak of bicarbonate during excretion of an acid urine. During bicarbonate loading, the U-B PCO_2 is normal, however, demonstrating that the pump is not defective; 2) Voltage-dependent rate defects are induced by amiloride or lithium. As a result of the decrease in voltage in the cortical collecting tubule (CCT) both H^+ and K^+ secretion are reduced; 3) Nonvoltage mediated pump defects occur in the postobstructed kidney and, when corrected for voltage, are present in aldosterone deficiency; 4) Impaired buffer delivery or production compromises net acid excretion. Ammonium production is decreased in chronic hyperkalemia and with reduction of GFR. Ammonium excretion is impaired in hyperkalemia because a decrease in ammonium transport by the TALH reduces ammonium accumulation in the inner medulla and, thus, impedes transfer of ammonia into the inner medullary collecting duct. Mixed defects also exist, e.g., in aldosterone deficiency hyperkalemia impairs ammonium excretion while aldosterone deficiency compromises the capacity of the proton pump.

Introduction

The pathophysiological basis of the various types of distal renal tubular acidosis (DRTA) have not yet been described fully. Progress has been made recently, however,

[1]Division of Nephrology, Departments of Internal Medicine, Physiology, and Biophysics, University of Texas Medical Branch, Galveston, TX 77550, USA

especially with respect to the understanding of disorders involving abnormalities in "distal" nephron acidification. This presentation will review, in detail, findings from sstudies employing experimental models of DRTA which have been investigated by a number of techniques in vivo and in vitro.

Mechanism of Distal Acidification

Since most of the filtered bicarbonate is reabsorbed by the proximal tubule (90%), the distal nephron (distal convoluted tubule (DCT); cortical collecting tubule (CCT); and medullary collecting duct (MCD)) serves to reabsorb the remainder of this load, and, in addition, to secrete an additional quantity of protons which approximates the quantity of the acid load generated by metabolism [1]. Net acid excretion is facilitated, and the approach to limiting transepithelial pH gradients mitigated, by the availability of urinary buffers and by the excretion of ammonium (NH_4^+). Proton secretion mediates transepithelial bicarbonate reabsorption in the distal convoluted tubule, the cortical collecting duct, and the medullary collecting tubule, and titrates the urinary buffers as well. The cellular mechanism for this process, apical membrane secretion of hydrogen ions, appears to be similar in each of these "distal nephron" segments. Micropuncture studies which have measured the disequilibrium pH in the superficial distal tubule and inner medullary collecting duct have supported this view unequivocally [2,3]. Numerous studies have demonstrated that active proton secretion at the apical membrane is mediated by a proton-translocating, electrogenic, ATP-dependent pump [4–8].

Since the rates of net proton secretion are relatively low in these distal segments, in vitro analysis usually requires the quantitation of bicarbonate reabsorption during in vitro perfusion with bicarbonate concentrations exceeding the load delivered in vitro. A different approach has been taken to assess acidification in these terminal segments in whole kidney studies by measurement of urinary PCO_2 [9]. Micropuncture studies which have measured both acid disequilibrium pH and an elevated urinary CO_2 tension during high bicarbonate delivery to the distal tubule and medullary collecting tubule (MCT), have consistently demonstrated that the magnitude of the elevation in urinary PCO_2 (referred to as the urine-minus-blood PCO_2, or U-B PCO_2, or ΔPCO_2) is quantitatively related to distal nephron proton secretion [2]. The degree of bicarbonaturia achieved in such protocols allows the examination of distal nephron hydrogen ion secretion in the absence of blood-to-lumen bicarbonate gradients. The generation of high inner medullary and urinary CO_2 tension occurs during a bicarbonate diuresis because of the absence of luminal (or membrane-bound) carbonic anhydrase in segments of the distal nephron, and is the result of secretion of protons into bicarbonate-containing tubule fluid, with subsequent slow dehydration of carbonic acid [3].

Classification of Subtypes of DRTA

Permeability ("Leak") Defects

The best experimental model representative of a permeability defect is that induced by amphotericin-B. This antibiotic forms aqueous channels when inserted into lipid

Table 1. Pathophysiological classification of distal renal tubule acidification defects

I. Permeability or "gradient" defect
  A. Amphotericin-B
  B. Classical DRTA-(normal U-B PCO_2)
II. Rate-dependent defect
  A. Voltage-dependent
    1. Amiloride (primary impairment of Na^+ reabsorption)
    2. Lithium (secondary impairment of Na^+ reabsorption)
    *3. Postobstructed kidney
    4. Pseudohypoaldosteronism Type II (enhanced chloride shunt)
    *5. Selective aldosterone deficiency
  B. Nonvoltage-mediated pump defects
    *1. Selective aldosterone deficiency
    *2. Postobstructed kidney
    3. Carbonic anhydrase II deficiency
    4. Classical DRTA (low U-B PCO_2)
III. Reduction in ammonium excretion
    1. Chronic hyperkalemia
    *2. Selective aldosterone deficiency
    3. Tubulointerstitial disease
    *4. Nephrocalcinosis

*Denotes mixed disorders

membranes [10]. Steinmetz and associates [11] reported that amphotericin-B was associated with a reduction in net hydrogen secretion only as the pH gradient across the turtle bladder was increased, and not in the absence of a pH gradient between mucosa and serosa. Such findings are compatible with a "gradient" lesion, and indicate that an acidification defect, under such a circumstance, would be most apparent when the filtered load of bicarbonate was low and the requirement to excrete a maximally acid urine was necessary. Animals treated chronically with amphotericin-B are unable to acidify the urine maximally under control conditions, or after an acid challenge. With combined acidosis and Na_2SO_4 infusion, a maximally acid urine pH can be achieved, however [12]. In contrast, during bicarbonate-loading, the U-B PCO_2 is normal [12–14]. Microelectrode studies by our laboratory have demonstrated a normal acid disequilibrium pH during this condition in the inner medullary collecting duct (IMCD) in vivo (indicative of a normal rate of H^+ secretion) [14]. In addition, papillary PCO_2 was elevated to levels similar to that observed in controls. Thus, the features of this defect are consistent with a gradient lesion, i.e., the rate of hydrogen secretion is normal during bicarbonate loading, and the reduction in net acid excretion is most likely the result of backleak of bicarbonate, not H^+-ions, H_2CO_3, or non-bicarbonate buffers. Backleak of these latter moieties would be expected to reduce the U-B PCO_2.

Voltage-Dependent Rate Defects

Lithium administration in the rat is consistently associated with a mild metabolic acidosis and an inappropriately alkaline urine pH which does not decrease further following an acid challenge, but responds (falls below pH 5.5) after infusion of sodium sulfate [15,16]. Studies done by our laboratory in the rat receiving lithium have demonstrated, in contrast to the amphotericin-B defect, that hydrogen secretion (failure to generate an acid disequilibrium pH), was clearly impaired. Moreover, urinary and inner medullary collecting duct PCO_2 was also reduced significantly [14]. In turtle urinary bladder under open-circuited conditions, lithium impairs proton secretion by virtue of a detrimental effect on the electrical gradient, favoring H^+ secretion [17]. Since sodium sulfate infusion reduces urine pH appropriately (below pH 5.5) in lithium-induced DRTA [14–17], it is possible that lithium treatment results in a mild voltage dependent impairment by competing with sodium entry across the apical membrane. Nevertheless, potassium secretion is not impaired, since animals treated chronically do not develop hyperkalemia [14]. Since urine flow rate is an important determinant of K^+ secretion by the distal nephron, the accompanying defect in urinary concentration may maintain K^+ secretion, thus avoiding hyperkalemia.

In contrast to the findings observed during lithium treatment, the chronic administration of amiloride to rats is associated with metabolic acidosis, hyperkalemia, and an inappropriately alkaline urine pH unresponsive to infusion of sodium sulfate [18]. Moreover, net proton secretion is markedly impaired and papillary pCO_2 is reduced [14]. The amiloride model differs from the lithium-induced defect in several respects. Amiloride has no effect on H^+ secretion in turtle bladder [19] or in the CCT [20], independent of voltage. As a result of the decreased voltage, both K^+ and H^+ secretion are reduced [20]. Amiloride does not affect bicarbonate transport or voltage in the outer medullary collecting tubule [21], but reduces volume flux in the inner medullary collecting tubule [22]. Therefore, amiloride inhibits acidification predominantly through a voltage-mediated defect in the CCT. The possibility of an additional effect on proton secretion in the inner MCT is suggested, however, by the observation of obliteration, by amiloride, of the disequilibrium pH in this segment.

Non-Voltage Dependent Rate Defects

Postobstructed Kidney (POK)

Experimental studies evaluating the acidification defect occurring after 18–24 hours of unilateral ureteral obstruction have reported findings similar to those observed in the amiloride model. Similarly, we have demonstrated impaired proton secretion and an inability to generate normal papillary CO_2 tensions after bicarbonate administration in the POK [14]. Bicarbonate reabsorption and transepithelial voltage in cortical collecting tubules harvested from rabbits have also been shown to be reduced [23]. In contrast, however, a more recent in vitro study has shown by paired analysis that the medullary, not the cortical collecting tubule, exhibited a marked decrease in bicarbonate reabsorption after 2 days or more of obstruction. Transepithelial voltage in the CCT was unaffected [24]. Finally, recent preliminary studies from the same laboratory have examined $(Na^+ + K^+)$ ATPase and N-ethylmaleimide (NEM)-sensitive ATPase activities in microdissected cortical and medullary collecting tubule fragments. NEM-sensitive ATPase (H^+-ATPase activity) was most markedly reduced in the medullary collecting tubule (75%), not in the CCT (25% reduction) [25]. $(Na^+ + K^+)$ ATPase activity decreased 80% in both collecting duct segments.

Thus, the POK model may represent a combination of voltage-mediated and direct proton pump impaired defects. In this respect the POK resembles the type of defect associated with aldosterone deficiency.

Selective Aldosterone Deficiency

The CCT is responsible for reabsorption of a portion of the filtered load of sodium by an aldosterone-dependent process which increases transepithelial voltage, favoring secretion of both K^+ and H^+. Therefore, aldosterone deficiency may cause hyperkalemia and metabolic acidosis. The outer medullary collecting duct also serves as a target organ for aldosterone by increasing net proton secretory capacity independent of sodium transport [21]. Recent studies in our laboratory have demonstrated that selective aldosterone deficiency is associated with imnpaired H^+ secretion in the inner medullary collecting duct [26]. In this same study ammonia transfer into inner medullary collecting ducts was markedly impaired, so that ammonium excretion was reduced dramatically. Moreover, as a result of impaired ammonia production, ammonium delivery to the loop of Henle was also reduced. Thus, a decrease in inner medullary ammonium accumulation accounted for a portion of the reduction in ammonia transfer and inner medullary addition. Since papillary PCO_2 was reduced during bicarbonate loading [26], the rate of proton secretion also was clearly compromised. In these and other studies, when one corrects for voltage changes, it appears that the "rate" defect is quantitatively more important than the "voltage" defect in hypoaldosteronism, and thus the direct effect of aldosterone on H^+-secretion (H^+-ATPase) surpasses the indirect effects mediated through voltage changes.

Impaired Buffer Production and/or Excretion

Recent studies in our laboratory in a rat model of chronic hyperkalemia have affirmed that whole kidney ammonium excretion is reduced significantly in hyperkalemia [27]. This decrease in excretion was a result of a marked reduction in whole kidney ammonium production, which occurred even in the face of coexistent chronic metabolic acidosis. Nevertheless, chronic hyperkalemia had no effect on net transport of ammonium by the superficial proximal tubule [28]. Rather, it was demonstrated that a major nephron site of regulation of ammonium transport in response to hyperkalemia was the medullary thick ascending limb of Henle's loop [27]. Chronic hyperkalemia, by inhibition of active NH_4^+ absorption by this segment, impairs accumulation of total ammonia in the inner medulla and compromises significantly the transfer of ammonia into the inner medullary collecting duct [29].

Other disorders accompanied by chronic hyperkalemia would be expected to exhibit similar adverse effects on ammonium production and transport. Selective aldosterone deficiency could represent, therefore, a mixed model of defective acidification in which hyperkalemia impairs ammonium production and excretion, while hypoaldosteronism impairs acid secretion by the ATP-dependent proton pump. By extension of this view, it seems logical to assume that medullary interstitial disease might be associated with a defect in ammonium accumulation and transfer into the inner medulla, but it would be expected that the superficial proximal tubule would maintain intact ammonium production. Impaired ammonium production might be present in advanced renal insufficiency with metabolic acidosis (reduced functional renal mass), or in circumstances in which glutamine availability or metabolism could be compromised.

Acknowledgments. The participation in these studies by Carlton R. Caflisch and David W. Good was invaluable. I also wish to acknowledge the excellent secretarial assistance of Suzanne Rambin. Studies in the author's laboratory were supported in part by research grant DK30603 awarded by the National Institutes of Health.

References

1. Alpern RJ, Warnock DG, Rector FC Jr (1986) Renal acidification Mechanisms. In Brenner BM, Rector FC Jr (eds) The Kidney, 3rd edn. Saunders, Philadelphia, pp 206–249
2. DuBose TD Jr (1982) Hydrogen ion secretion by the collecting duct as a determinate of the urine to blood PCO_2 gradient in alkaline urine. J Clin Invest 69:145–156
3. DuBose TD Jr (1983) Application of the disequilibrium pH method to investigate the mechanism of urinary acificiation. Am J Physiol 245 (Renal Fluid Electrolyte Physiol 14):F443–F449
4. Gluck S, Al-Awqati Q (1984) An electrogenic proton-translocating adenosine triphosphatase from bovine kidney medulla. J Clin Invest 73:1704–1710
5. Stone DK, Xie XS, Racker E (1984) Comparison of the proton ATPase and chloride transporter from bovine clathrin-coated vesicles and renal medullary vesicles. Kidney Int 25:283 (A)
6. Diaz-Diaz FD, Labelle EF, Eaton DC, et al. (1986) ATP-dependent proton transport in human renal medulla. Am J Physiol 20:F297–F302
7. Kaunitz JD, Gunther RD, Sachs G (1985) Characterization of an electrogenic ATP and chloride-dependent proton translocating pump from rat renal medulla. J Biol Chem 260:11567–11571
8. Gluck S, Hirsch S, Brown D (1987) Immunocytohistochemical localization of H^+-ATPase in rat kidney. Kidney Int 31:167 (A)
9. Halperin ML, Goldstein MB, Haig A, et al. (1974) Studies on the pathogenesis of type I (distal) renal tubular acidosis as revealed by the urinary PCO_2 tension. J Clin Invest 53:669–677
10. Capasso G, Schultz H, Vickermann B, et al. (1986) Amphotericin B and amphotericin B methylester: Effect on brush border membrane permeability. Kidney Int 30:311–317
11. Steinmetz PR, Lawson LR (1970) Defect in acidification induced in vitro by amphotericin B. J Clin Invest 49:596–601
12. Garg LC (1979) Lack of effect of amphotericin-B on urine-blood $PCVO_2$ gradient in spite of urinary acidification defect. Pflugers Arch 381:137–142
13. Julka N, Arruda JAL, Kurtzman NA (1979) The mechanism of amphotericin-induced distal acidification defect in rats. Clin Sci 56:555–562
14. DuBose TD Jr, Caflisch CR (1985) Validation of the difference in urine and blood CO_2 tension during bicarbonate loading as an index of distal nephron acificiation in experimental models of distal renal tubular acidosis. J Clin Invest 75:1116–1123
15. Batlle DC, Sehy JT, Roseman MK, et al. (1981) Clinical and pathophysiologic spectrum of acquired distal renal tubular acidosis. Kidney Int 20:389–396
16. Batlle DC, Gavira M, Grupp M (1982) Distal nephron function in patients receiving chronic lithium therapy. Kidney Int 21:477–485
17. Arruda JAL, Dytko G, Mola R, et al. (1980) On the mechanism of lithium-induced distal renal tubular acidosis: Studies in the turtle bladder. Kidney Int 17:196–204
18. Arruda JAL, Subbarayudu K, Dytko G, et al. (1980) Voltage dependent distal acidification defect induced by amiloride. J Lab Clin Med 95:407–416
19. Husted RF, Steinmetz PR (1979) The effects of amiloride and ouabain on urinary acidification by turtle bladder. J Pharmacol Exp Ther 210:264–268
20. Allen GG, Barrat LJ (1979) An in vivo study of voltage-dependent renal tubular acidosis induced by amiloride. Kidney Int 35:1107–1110

21. Stone DS, Seldin DW, Kokko JP, et al. (1983) Mineralocorticoid modulation of rabbit medullary collecting duct acidification. A sodium-independent acidification. J Clin Invest 72:77–83

22. Ullrich KJ, Papavassiliou F (1979) Sodium reabsorption in the papillary collecting duct of rats. Pflugers Arch 379:49–52

23. Hanley MJ, Davidson K (1982) Isolated nephron segments from rabbit models of obstructive uropathy. J Clin Invest 69:165–174

24. Laski ME, Sabo C, Morgan VE, et al. (to be published) Site of the distal acidification defect in obstructive uropathy. Min Elect Metab

25. Sabatini S (1989) Pathophysiologic mechanisms of abnormal collecting duct function. Sem in Nephr 9:179–202

26. DuBose TD Jr, Caflisch CR (1988) Effect of selective aldosterone deficiency on acidification in nephron segments of the rat inner medulla. J Clin Invest 82:1624–1632

27. DuBose TD Jr, Caflisch CR, Good DW (1990) Effects of chronic hyperkalemia on ammonium transport in inner medulla of the rat. Kidney Int 37:535 (A)

28. DuBose TD Jr, Caflisch CR, Good DW (1989) Effects of chronic hyperkalemia on renal ammonium transport. Kidney Int 35:452 (A)

29. Good, DW (1987) Effect of potassium on ammonium transport by medullary thick ascending limb of the rat. J Clin Invest 80:1358–1365

Classification and Characterization of Types of Distal Acidification Defects in Humans

Daniel C. Batlle[1] and Taha Keilani

Introduction

The distal renal tubular acidosis (RTA) syndromes are usually characterized by the presence of a hyperchloremic type of metabolic acidosis often associated to either hypokalemia (classic RTA) or hyperkalemia (hyperkalemic types of RTA). Some patients, however, have subtle defects in urinary acidification not manifested by hyperchloremic metabolic acidosis. The identification and classification of the various types of RTA are best approached from a mechanistic point of view and should take into consideration the site of the nephron responsible for the defect in acidification.

In this article we will present a classification of distal RTA based on the deranged cellular mechanism of urinary acidification (Table 1). As discussed recently, some of the proposed mechanisms are represented by relatively well defined clinical entities whereas others are still theoretical [1].

Permeability Defects

A remarkable property of the collecting tubule is that H^+ secretion can occur against a transepithelial H^+ gradient until the H^+ concentration in the mucosal fluid is approximately 1,000 times greater than in the serosal fluid. When this large H^+ gradient is attained (collecting tubule pH $\approx$ 4.4), H^+ secretion ceases. Backleak of H^+ from mucosal fluid into the serosal site is virtually negligible. The existence of a defect in membrane permeability, however, could impair net acidification by causing either H^+ backleak or an increased HCO_3 influx into the lumen [2]. Studies in the turtle urinary bladder and in mammalian collecting tubules have shown that ampho-

[1]Northwestern University Medical School, Morton 3-615, 303 East Chicago, Chicago, IL 60611, USA

Table 1. Classification of Distal RTA subtypes

Type	Example
I. *Permeability/defects*	
a. H⁺ backleak	Amphotericin B
b. Enhanced HCO₃ secretion	Unknown
II. *Secretory/defects*	
a. Diffuse collecting tubule H⁺ pump defect	Chronic Kidney transplant rejection
b. Medullary collecting tubule H⁺ pump defect	Nephrocalcinosis (some cases)
c. Diffuse proton pump failure K⁺ secretory defect	Obstructive nephropathy
d. Medullary H⁺/K⁺ ATPase defect (?)	Endemic hypokalemic distal RTA (?)
III. *Rate-dependent/defects*	
a. Voltage-dependent defect	Amiloride
b. Enhanced chloride transport	Gordon's syndrome
c. Aldosterone deficiency	Selective Aldosterone deficiency
d. Aldosterone resistance	Pseudohypoaldosteronism
e. Reduced urinary buffer	Hyperkalemia
f. Reduced intracellular H⁺ anhydrase deficiency	Cytosolic carbonic
g. Reduced H⁺ conductance	Toluene

tericin B, applied to the mucosal site, results in H^+ backdiffusion (lumen to blood). The drug also increases potassium permeability (which may explain the occurrence of hypokalemia) but does not affect HCO_3 permeability. On the basis of these experimental findings, it has been inferred that H^+ backleak is the mechanism causing hypokalemic distal RTA in patients receiving amphotericin B [1–5].

As in most types of distal RTA, urine pH in patients treated with amphotericin B is higher than 5.5, despite acidemia. The inability to lower urine pH despite unimpaired H^+ secretion is attributable to H^+ backleak, which is more evident when the tubular urine is acidic [1–5]. Theoretically, it is conceivable that the creation of a large transtubular electrical gradient (lumen-negative) by the administration of sodium sulfate or furosemide could attenuate H^+ backleak and permit lowering of urine pH to normally low values. H^+ backleak should be minimized when the urine is made highly alkaline. That this is the case is suggested by the finding of a normal rise in urine PCO_2 when sodium bicarbonate is infused to amphotericin B-treated rats [6]. As a point of fact, this is the only known experimental model of distal RTA in which urine PCO_2 in a highly alkaline urine is normal (i.e., more than 70 mm Hg) [1]. Further, this is the only type of experimental distal RTA in which an acid disequilibrium pH in the collecting tubule has been documented during the infusion of sodium bicarbonate [6]. This finding strongly suggests that amphotericin B causes DRTA by a mechanism other than impaired collecting tubule H^+ secretion.

It must be emphasized that so far there are no patients described who displayed all of the features outlined in the amphotericin B model of experimental H^+ backleak distal RTA. At present, it seems highly unlikely that any form of hereditary or acquired distal RTA, other than that associated with amphotericin B, is caused by a H^+ backleak mechanism. Some forms of drug-induced hypokalemic distal RTA, such as that caused by toluene sniffing, originally thought to originate from H^+ backleak do not appear to cause it. This can be inferred from the finding of failure to increase urine PCO_2 after bicarbonate infusions in individuals with hypokalemic distal RTA associated with toluene sniffing [7]. Further, in turtle urinary bladders exposed to high concentrations of toluene, the rate of H^+ secretion is reduced, but unlike in amphotericin B-treated bladders, there is no discernible H^+ backleak [7].

Conceivably, a defect in collecting tubule permeability causing an increase in HCO_3 secretion could also result in a decrease in net collecting tubule acidification, thereby leading to distal RTA (Table 1). There is no experimental or clinical evidence, however, for such a defect.

Secretory Defects

Under this terminology will be considered any alteration causing an impairment of collecting tubule acidification by primarily interfering with active H^+ secretion. The collecting tubule contains a proton pump at its luminal surface. This pump, a proton translocating ATPase, secretes H^+ in an electrogenic manner (i.e., is capable of translocating a net positive charge into the lumen) and can operate independently of sodium transport and despite an unfavorable transtubular electrical gradient. The rate of sodium transport and the electrical voltage, however, importantly influence the rate of H^+ secretion. Alterations in transepithelial voltage caused by either inhibition of sodium transport or enhancement of chloride transport can reduce the rate of H^+ secretion and thereby cause distal RTA. These alterations are considered under the heading of rate-dependent defects (see below). A primary H^+ secretory defect, by definition, is limited to the proton pump.

The existence of a secretory type of distal RTA has been reasonably well characterized in patients with different diseases causing acquired distal RTA [8–10]. Derangements of collecting tubule function determined genetically (e.g., hereditary distal RTA), associated with structural abnormalities (e.g., medullary sponge kidney), immunologically mediated (e.g., chronic renal transplant rejection), or caused by impaired metabolic cell function, could all interfere with the proton pump secretory apparatus. One can envision a spectrum of secretory defects ranging from reduction in the number of proton pumps to severe proton pump dysfunction, as well as defects in the active transport pathway due to altered metabolic energy production or use. Given the variety of disease states causing distal RTA and the numerous basic mechanisms on which they could have an impact, there is no reason to believe that they all have to alter the proton secretory apparatus in the same way. There is also no a priori reason to believe that proton pump dysfunction has to involve the entire collecting tubule [10]. It is conceivable that the lesion causing proton pump dysfunction may be confined to a portion of the collecting tubule. For instance, one could anticipate from the anatomic distribution of some disease states causing distal RTA that their defect in acidification would be confined to the medullary collecting tubule [10]. The possible ways to evaluate clinically the site of abnormal H^+ secretion within the collecting tubule are discussed below.

The general features characteristic of a secretory type of distal RTA are as follows. Urine pH during spontaneous acidosis or after acid loading cannot be lowered below 5.5, and the rate of acid excretion is decreased. Ammonium excretion is reduced, a finding that can be inferred at bedside from the finding of a positive urine anion gap [11]. The urine PCO_2 measured after bicarbonate loading does not increase normally, reflecting that the rate of collecting tubule H^+ secretion is reduced [12]. This feature is useful in distinguishing a secretory from a permeability defect [7]. It is not useful, however, in differentiating a secretory from a voltage-dependent defect, which also decreases the rate of H^+ secretion (albeit indirectly). The value of measuring urine PCO_2 in a highly alkaline urine stems from its exquisite sensitivity in portraying the rate of H^+ secretion. For instance, environmental factors that reduce collecting tubule H^+ secretion, such as an alkaline diet or exposure to hypocapnia, are associated with a subnormal rise in urine PCO_2 during bicarbonate loading. Any perturbation leading to a decrease in the rate of collecting tubule H^+ secretion should thus impair the generation of a high urine PCO_2 in a highly alkaline urine. Administration of neutral sodium phosphate also stimulates distal H^+ secretion and should retard acid backleak. The rise in urinary PCO_2 normally seen after the administration of neutral sodium phosphate does not occur when H^+ secretion in the collecting tubule is impaired [8,9].

Rate-Dependent Defects

One can classify under the heading of rate-dependent defects a variety of alterations that have in common that the rate of H^+ secretion in the collecting tubule is reduced, not because of primary proton pump failure, but rather as a consequence of reduced availability of intracellular H^+ or reduced urinary buffer content or other defects (Table 1). Failure to sustain an adequate transtubular electrical gradient (voltage-dependent defects), aldosterone deficiency, and aldosterone resistance could all be viewed as rate-dependent defects (Table 1). The latter three entities will be considered separately because their clinical features are quite distinctive (see below).

A mechanism that could result in a decrease in the rate of collecting tubule H^+ secretion is reduced availability of intracellular H^+. Since an intracellular OH^- is generated for each H^+ secreted by the H^+ pump into the tubular lumen, the ability to remove OH^- is required for continued H^+ secretion. The removal of OH^- is facilitated by cytosolic carbonic anhydrase, an enzyme that catalyzes the reaction of OH^- with CO_2. Deficiency of cytosolic carbonic anhydrase in the renal intercalated cells of the collecting tubule (carbonic anhydrase type II) could, therefore, slow down the rate of H^+ secretion by interfering with intracellular OH^- disposal. Likewise, a defect in the exit step for HCO_3 (or OH^-) could reduce the rate of collecting tubule H^+. In patients with hereditary carbonic anhydrase deficiency, urine pH is higher than 5.5 during acidosis. The defect in H^+ should also impair urine PCO_2 formation after bicarbonate loading, but data on this parameter are not available.

The rate of H^+ secretion may be decreased owing to a lack of buffer in the tubular fluid. The rate of H^+ secretion by the collecting tubules is higher when the tubular fluid is alkaline (HCO_3 accepts secreted H^+) than when it is acid. In the absence of H^+ acceptors, tubular fluid is acidified rapidly, and the H^+ pump inhibits its own transport rate by the pH gradient it generates [2]. In quantitative terms, ammonia is the most important H^+ acceptor. Disease states causing decreased ammonia production, such as advanced renal insufficiency, hyperkalemia, and aldosterone deficiency —usually acting in combination—result in impaired ammonium excretion [13–15]. Delivery of ammonia to the medullary collecting tubule may be decreased, thereby limiting H^+ secretion. This situation occurs whenever the kidneys are underperfused. Phosphate depletion not only results in decreased titratable acidity from hypophosphaturia but also interferes with ammonium excretion.

In a restricted sense, the term "rate dependent" distal RTA was first introduced to designate patients with a pattern of urinary acidification characterized by failure to increase urine PCO_2 in a highly alkaline urine, but otherwise intact ability to lower urine pH during ammonium chloride-induced acidosis [16]. Since urinary pH could be lowered in the presence of mild acidosis we felt that a proton secretory defect, per se, was unlikely. Many of the patients were not acidotic but had clinical evidence of tubulointerstitial renal disease, which prompted us to initiate investigation of urinary acidification [16]. In this regard, it represents a variant of incomplete distal RTA. This pattern is also common among patients on well-controlled chronic lithium therapy [17]. The concentration of lithium in the urine of these patients ranges from 10–40 mmoles/liter, a concentration sufficient to inhibit voltage-dependent H^+ secretion in the turtle urinary bladder and in rabbit cortical collecting tubules perfused in vitro [18]. The reduced rate of collecting tubule H^+ secretion, disclosed in vivo by the failure to increase urine PCO_2 in a highly alkaline urine, has been inferred to result from failure to generate a normal transtubular voltage (lumen-negative) when lithium is present in the lumen of the cortical collecting tubule. This cation appears to compete for sodium reabsorption. The impairment in sodium reabsorption, in turn, may lessen the voltage (lumen-negative) required for optimal H^+ and K^+ secretion [18]. Hyperkalemia, however, is not a feature of lithium-treated patients, possibly because of the high urine flow (due to impaired concentrating capacity) which increases K^+ secretion.

Voltage-Dependent Renal Tubular Acidosis

Examples of voltage-dependent defects in collecting tubule acidification due to an isolated impairment of sodium transport are so far confined to lithium and to drugs that primarily block apical sodium transport, such as amiloride and triamterene. There are patients with hyperkalemic RTA in whom furosemide or sodium sulfate administration does not result in lowering of urine pH below 5.5 [10,19]. The kaliuretic response to these agents also is blunted. These findings suggest that voltage-dependent (i.e., sodium-dependent) H^+ and K^+ secretion in the cortical collecting tubule is impaired [10]. In addition to hyperkalemic hyperchloremic metabolic acidosis, one would anticipate a salt-wasting tendency, reflecting impairment of sodium transport, in such patients. Although systematic studies of sodium balance have not been performed, clinical observations of defective sodium conservation have been made on occasional patients [14]. Some of them may display sodium wastage on a normal salt diet, whereas others may manifest sodium wastage only when they are salt restricted. A consequence of salt wastage is the functional deterioration of GFR, which is reversible on fluid replacement.

Although inhibition of sodium transport in the cortical collecting tubule results in a decrease in the rate of H^+ secretion, this could be compensated by enhanced H^+ in the medullary collecting tubule, a segment with a greater capacity for urinary acidification. Unlike individuals treated with amiloride or lithium, these patients develop marked metabolic acidosis, a finding that suggests a more diffuse impairment of collecting tubule acidification. Patients with this form of hyperkalemic distal RTA probably have a proton pump secretory defect that involves the entire collecting tubule [1].

Selective Aldosterone Deficiency

Hyperkalemic metabolic acidosis associated with selective aldosterone deficiency (SAD) is the most common type of RTA in adults [13,14]. It also is the commonest cause of hyperkalemia among patients with mild to moderate insufficiency. Most of these patients have evidence of tubulointerstitial renal disease and reduced GFR. The rate of collecting tubule H^+ secretion is stimulated by aldosterone and reduced in its absence. The urine of these patients is acidic (pH 5.0–5.5) during mild metabolic acidosis. Relative to their reduced rate of ammonia excretion, however, urine pH is slightly higher than that of normal subjects made acidotic by ammonium chloride [11]. This finding reflects that the rate of collecting tubule H^+ secretion is reduced. The PCO_2 in a highly alkaline urine should be reduced, but data from patients are not available regarding this parameter. In addition to the direct stimulatory effect of aldosterone on the rate of collecting tubule H^+ secretion and its indirect effect mediated by changes in distal sodium transport, aldosterone increases ammonia production. Aldosterone deficiency is thus expected to be associated with decreased ammonia production. Further, the development of hyperkalemia causes a marked suppression of ammonium excretion.

Indeed, the main factor responsible for the acidosis of patients with SAD is a decrease in ammonium excretion. In this regard, this type of RTA could be mechanistically classified under the category of reduced concentration of urinary buffers (ammonia) (Table 1). Correction of hyperkalemia, no matter how accomplished, results in amelioration of metabolic acidosis by enhancement of ammonium excretion. Some of the patients with aldosterone deficiency also display end-organ resistance to the action of the hormone, as evidenced by the persistence of hyperkalemia despite chronic administration of large amounts of mineralocorticoid. The typical patient, however, responds reasonably well to mineralocorticoid administration. It is important to recognize that some patients have a combination of both SAD and hyperkalemic distal RTA [19]. Such patients have low ammonium excretion and low aldosterone levels and, in addition, cannot lower urinary pH below 5.5 regardless of the degree of acidosis. The clinical implication of this observation is that a patient with hyperkalemic acidosis with an inappropriately high urine pH (i.e., 5.5) has, by definition, hyperkalemic distal RTA, regardless of whether plasma aldosterone is low, normal, or high [19]. If the patient has low aldosterone and cannot lower urinary pH below 5.5 in the face of acidosis, he or she suffers from both hyperkalemic distal RTA and SAD.

Types of Renal Tubular Acidosis Associated with Aldosterone Resistance and Normal Glomerular Filtration Rate

The term "aldosterone resistance" (or pseudohypoaldosteronism) is used to designate those patients with hyperkalemic hyperchloremic metabolic acidosis in whom aldosterone deficiency clearly is not present and in whom there is no evidence of diffuse tubulointerstitial nephropathy. Two clinical pictures fit this definition: (1) the syndrome of classic pseudohypoaldosteronism of infancy, characterized by salt-wastage and hypotension and (2) a rare syndrome of aldosterone-resistant acidosis and hyperkalemia usually characterized by salt retention and hypertension (chloride shunt type of disorder).

The clinical picture of classic pseudohypoaldosteronism is characterized by dehydration and hyponatremia due to renal salt wastage, hyperkalemia, and hyperchloremic metabolic acidosis. It occurs in infants as a congenital disorder. The severity of salt wastage and potassium retention diminishes with time, but hyponatremia and hyperkalemia may recur if dietary salt is restricted. This condition appears to be a pure form of tubular aldosterone resistance not associated with discernible tubulointerstitial damage at kidney biopsy. It has been proposed that the syndrome results from a deficiency of Na^+, K^+-ATPase, because absence of this enzyme from proximal and distal nephron segments was documented in kidney biopsy material obtained from one patient with classic pseudohypoaldosteronism.

As in any state of end-organ responsiveness, the circulating levels of the hormone are greatly elevated in patients with pseudohypoaldosteronism. The features characteristic of the acidification defect associated with aldosterone resistance should be identical to those seen in states of aldosterone deficiency. Data on urinary acidification from patients with pseudohypoaldosteronism of infancy, however, are sparse. Like patients with aldosterone deficiency, those with aldosterone resistance should have a low urine pH during acidosis, but reduced rates of ammonium excretion. Whether the rate of collecting tubule H^+ secretion, assessed by the rise in urine PCO_2 in a highly alkaline urine, is diminished or not remains to be investigated.

Another aldosterone-resistant type of disorder associated with normal GFR and hyperchloremic hyperkalemic metabolic acidosis has been characterized and is referred to as type II pseudohypoaldosteronism [20]. This disorder corresponds to a similar clinical picture known as Gordon's syndrome. Evidence for aldosterone resistance in such patients is inferred from the persistence of hyperkalemia despite the administration of exogenous mineralocorticoid. In contrast, potassium excretion increases markedly after the administration of sodium sulfate or sodium bicarbonate. Hyperkalemia and metabolic acidosis can be corrected by restriction of dietary sodium or by the administration of thiazide diuretics. The primary abnormality is believed to be a tubular defect characterized by increased chloride reabsorption in the distal nephron. This results in increased NaCl reabsorption, thereby resulting in volume expansion and low-renin hypertension. Plasma aldosterone also may be suppressed and remains low relative to the prevailing hyperkalemia. Enhanced chloride transport limits the sodium-dependent and mineralocorticoid-dependent voltage driving force for potassium and hydrogen ion secretion. This defect could be classified as a voltage-dependent type of distal RTA due to enhanced chloride transport. Unlike the voltage-dependent defect caused by amiloride, the one caused by a chloride shunt type of defect does not appear to interfere with lowering of urine pH during acidosis.

Plasma Potassium and Distal RTA

Abnormalities in plasma potassium are a major feature of the various subtypes of distal RTA. The classic form of RTA is usually accompanied by hypokalemia which has been ascribed to renal K wastage [21–23]. The precise cause of hypokalemia, in our opinion, has not been completely clarified. A permeability defect, causing passive K secretion, would readily explain it but, as stated above, a permeability defect has only been shown to occur with Amphotericin B administration. It is generally held that potassium wastage occurs in the absence of abnormal collecting tubule permeability for potassium, simply because of accelerated potassium secretion in the face of impaired H^+ secretion. The enhancement in K secretion is said to be driven by secondary hyperaldosteronism which may be a feature of distal RTA [23,24]. Aldosterone oversecretion could be expected as a result of sodium wastage which has been documented in some patients with distal RTA [24]. While this may be a reasonable explanation, it is nevertheless intriguing that some patients present with striking hypokalemia whereas others do not. Further, it is unlikely that aldosterone levels would be elevated in the face of protracted potassium depletion and, indeed, few studies have reported aldosterone data from patients with hypokalemic distal RTA. It is, thus, possible that factors other than secondary hyperaldosteronism are responsible for the development of severe hypokalemia, at least in some cases of distal RTA.

A particularly attractive mechanism that could account for hypokalemia is the existence of a defect in the renal K^+/H^+ ATPase pump. Renal K excretion is determined not only by active K secretion localized largely to the distal tubule and cortical collecting tubule, but also by active K absorption localized, at least in part, to the outer medullary collecting tubule [25]. Under conditions of dietary K deprivation or extrarenal K wastage, profound K depletion would ensue unless there were a compensatory increase in K absorptive flux in more terminal nephron segments. Activation of a K conservation mechanism in the outer medullary collecting tubule could prevent further K wastage, while producing enhanced proton secretion. If the K^+/H^+ ATPase pump recently found in the medullary collecting tubule of the rabbit [25-27] were defective, one would expect the development of both hypokalemia and metabolic acidosis. Thus, the capital features of classic RTA could be readily explained by such a defective mechanism.

While the presence of a renal defect in potassium conservation does not need to be a universal defect of hypokalemic distal RTA it is a reasonable possibility, at least for those cases associated with severe hypokalemia. In some patients with distal RTA, gastric hypoactivity has been documented [28]. This suggests the existence of a defect in the H^+/K ATPase of both gastric parietal cells and renal collecting tubule cells. A partial defect in this pump could explain well the development of both hypokalemia and metabolic acidosis, especially under conditions of dietary K deprivation or enhanced extrarenal losses. In this regard, it is intriguing that the occurrence of severe hypokalemic RTA in an endemic area in the Northeastern part of Thailand peaks in the summer months [28]. Heat exposure in the summer could initiate potassium depletion, which would be aggravated by defective renal conservation owing to a K^+/H^+ ATPase defect. In this theoretical scenario we would predict that

Table 2. Theoretical distinction between collecting tubule H^+ pump defects

	H^+ ATPase defect	H^+/K^+ ATPase defect
Acidosis	$+++$	$++$
Hypokalemia	$+$	$+++$
Urine pH	>5.3	>5.3
Urine K	↑	↑↑
Correction K deficit	No effect or worsening acidosis*	Improvement of acidosis

*by removing a potent stimulus for NH_3 formation

K supplementation alone should ameliorate the metabolic acidosis by enhancing the operation of a defective K^+/H^+ pump. In contrast, a defect in the H^+ pump should not be corrected by K supplementation. In fact, the acidosis should worsen owing to correction of the hypokalemia, a potent stimulus for ammonia production. A purely theoretical list of distinctive features for the two types of defects is offered in Table 2.

Clinical Localization of Segmental Defects in Collecting Tubule H^+ Secretion

Although patients with distal RTA usually display an abnormally high urine pH during acidemia, they may or may not lower urine pH normally in response to the administration of sodium sulfate or loop diuretics. The response to the latter two maneuvers has been proposed as a way of localizing the site of the H^+ secretory defect within the collecting tubule [10]. The collecting tubule, a major site of urinary acidification within the distal nephron, displays axial heterogeneity both anatomically and functionally. In the cortical collecting tubule (CCT) active sodium reabsorption generates an electrical potential (lumen-negative) that favors the secretion of H^+ and potassium. In contrast, in outer medullary collecting tubules, H^+ secretion does not appear to be under the influence of sodium transport and is accompanied by chloride secretion. In this segment, the potential difference is oriented lumen-positive, presumably as a result of electrogenic H^+ secretion. This is in contrast with the lumen-negative electrical potential usually prevailing in the cortical segment, that is thought to be generated by active sodium reabsorption (Fig. 1). Although the relative contribution of each of these two nephron segments to net acidification in vivo has not been delineated, there is remarkable agreement from various studies, using rabbit isolated tubules perfused in vitro, showing that the rate of acidification is considerably greater in the medullary than in the cortical segment of the collecting tubule.

The clinical evaluation of the function of the collecting tubule is, to some extent, possible using maneuvers that either stimulate or inhibit proton secretion in this nephron site. A segmental approach would require a maneuver that acts selectively in each portion of the collecting tubule. The acidemic stimulus, usually provided by the administration of ammonium chloride, is not selective, because acidemia enhances acidification throughout the entire distal nephron. Because H^+ secretion in the medullary collecting tubule is sodium-dependent, one can assume that maneuvers that produce a sodium-dependent increase or decrease in H^+ secretion do not have an impact on this nephron segment. Amiloride, at low doses that inhibit apical sodium conductance but not Na^+/H^+ exchange, inhibits sodium-dependent acidification and potassium secretion in the cortical collecting tubule [10]. Loop diuretics, by blocking NaCl reabsorption in the thick ascending loop of Henle, increase Na delivery to the collecting tubule. Part of the sodium delivered to the cortical collecting tubule is reabsorbed, whereas chloride is not, resulting in the creation of a favorable transtubular voltage (lumen-negative) for H^+ and K^+ secretion. That the increase in distal Na reabsorption secondary to furosemide administration results in enhancement of voltage-dependent acidification in the cortical collecting tubule, can be inferred from the finding that the fall in urine pH and the increase in net acid excre-

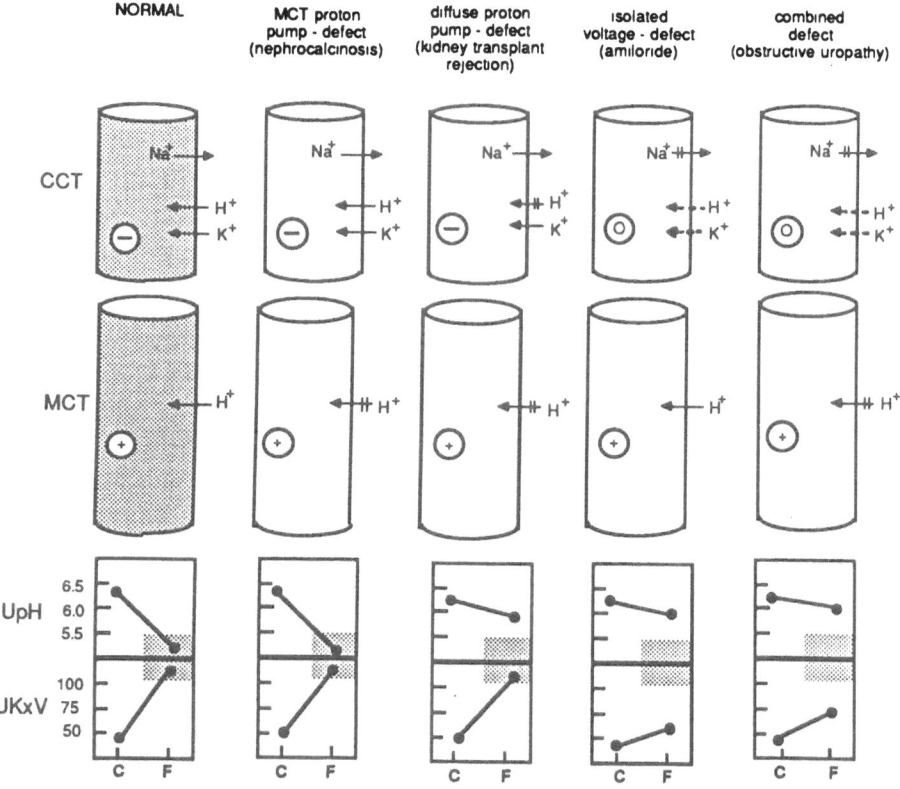

Fig. 1.

tion elicited by furosemide are obliterated by amiloride [10]. Amiloride also lessens the kaliuretic effect of furosemide, indicating that the increase in K$^+$ secretion observed when furosemide is given alone is due, in part, to an increase in transepithelial voltage. An additional effect of furosemide on renal K$^+$ excretion, independent of its indirect effect on transepithelial voltage, is apparent from the finding that K$^+$ excretion increases linearly as a function of urine flow. The difference in K$^+$ excretion observed at comparable urine flow rates when furosemide is given alone and when it is given with amiloride reflects the contribution of the amiloride-sensitive (that is, sodium-dependent) component of distal nephron H$^+$ secretion [10].

Sodium-dependent acidification also can be stimulated by the infusion of sodium sulfate. The infusion of sodium sulfate provides a poorly reabsorbable anion as well as Na load that, when reabsorbed by the cortical collecting tubule, results in an increase in transepithelial voltage. An increase in the cortical collecting tubule transepithelial voltage in response to furosemide would occur only if Na were to be reabsorbed well in excess of Cl. Both furosemide and sodium sulfate administration result in enhanced tubular reabsorption of Na, but differ in that Cl reabsorption relative to

Na is depressed after furosemide administration, because in this circumstance Cl behaves as a poorly reabsorbable anion [10].

A scheme for the interpretation of the distinctive responses to furosemide and sodium sulfate found in patients with distal RTA is presented in Fig. 1. This scheme assumes that with administration of these agents, tubular fluid pH falls below 5.3 at the level of the cortical collecting tubule as a consequence of enhanced Na-dependent H$^+$secretion. This nephron segment could be deranged in that either the number (or function) of proton pumps is reduced, or in that the ability to transport sodium and thereby generate a transepithelial voltage (lumen-negative) is impaired. The latter alteration is seen when amiloride is given to normal subjects [10]. Under these conditions, urine pH cannot be lowered below 5.3, and the kaliuretic effect of furosemide is blunted (Fig. 1). If the proton pump only were impaired, the administration of either furosemide or sodium sulfate should increase transepithelial voltage in the cortical collecting tubule. In this situation, K$^+$ excretion would increase normally, but urine pH could not be lowered maximally, owing to failure of the proton pump. According to this scheme, patients who exhibit a normal increase in K$^+$ excretion but are unable to lower urine pH below 5.3 after furosemide or sodium sulfate administration can be classified as having a proton pump defect involving the cortical collecting tubule.

In some patients with distal RTA, K$^+$ secretion increases and urine pH falls below 5.3 after either furosemide or sodium sulfate administration [19]. The fall in urine pH suggests that the cortical collecting tubule has sufficient intact proton pumps to secrete H$^+$ when a favorable transepithelial voltage is imposed by these maneuvers. By exclusion, their defect in distal acidification, uncovered by the failure to lower urine pH despite acidemia, must be located in the medullary collecting tubule and confined to this nephron segment (Fig. 1). This notion has the support of experimental work showing that acidemia causes a fall in luminal pH in the medullary collecting tubule. One could argue that normal lowering of urine pH after furosemide or sodium sulfate in some patients with distal RTA simply denoted the existence of a mild proton pump defect. Inasmuch as the response to these agents in some patients with distal RTA is similar to that observed in normal individuals, however, it seems reasonable to conclude that sodium-dependent H$^+$ secretion in the cortical collecting tubule of such patients is normal.

In some patients with hyperkalemic distal RTA, the response to sodium sulfate and furosemide is characterized by both inability to lower urine pH and a subnormal K excretion [10,19]. In patients with hyperkalemic metabolic acidosis associated with selective aldosterone deficiency, furosemide and sodium sulfate administration result in lowering of urine pH below 5.3 [13]. The pattern found in the former patients could be explained solely on the basis of an isolated voltage-dependent defect in the cortical collecting tubule, such as is seen in normal subjects given amiloride (Fig. 1). In addition to a voltage-dependent defect in the cortical collecting tubule, patients with hyperkalemic distal RTA likely have a proton pump defect affecting the entire collecting tubule (Fig. 1). Thus, these patients are best classified as having a diffuse proton pump secretory defect in the collecting tubule that is associated with impaired sodium and potassium transport in the cortical collecting tubule. This kind of structural involvement could also be anticipated from the type of renal disease (e.g., obstructive uropathy) usually associated with this form of hyperkalemic distal RTA [19].

References

1. Batlle DC (1989) Renal tubular acidosis. In: Seldin DW, Giebisch G (eds) The regulation of acid-base balance. Raven, New York, pp 353–390
2. Steinmetz PR, Lawson WJ (1970) Defect in urinary acidification induced in vitro by amphotericin B. J Clin Invest 49:596–601
3. Arruda JAL, Kurtzman NA (1980) Mechanism and classification of deranged distal urinary acidification. Am J Physiol 8:F515–523
4. Batlle DC, Kurtzman NA (1982) Distal renal tubular acidosis: Pathogenesis and classification. Am J Kidney Dis 1:128–144
5. DuBose TD Jr, Alpern RJ (1989) In: The metabolic basis of inherited disease. McGraw Hill pp 2539–2568
6. DuBose TD Jr, Calflisch CR (1985) Validation of the difference in urine and blood carbon dioxide transport during bicarbonate loading as an index of distal nephron acidification in experimental models of distal renal tubular acidosis. J Clin Invest 75:1116–1123
7. Batlle DC, Sabatini S, Kurtzman NA (1988) On the mechanism of toluene-induced renal tubular acidosis. Nephron 49:210–218
8. Batlle DC, Sehy JT, Roseman MK, Arruda JAL, Kurtzman NA (1981) Clinical and pathophysiologic spectrum of acquired distal renal tubular acidosis. Kidney Int 20:389–396
9. Batlle DC, Moses MF, Manaligod J, Arruda JAL, Kurtzman NA (1981) The pathogenesis of hyperchloremic metabolic acidosis associated with renal transplantation. Am J Med 70:786–796
10. Batlle DC (1986) Segmental characterization of defects in collecting tubule acidification. Kidney Int 30:546–553
11. Batlle DC, Hizon M, Cohen E, Gutterman C, Gupta R (1988) The use of the urinary anion gap in the diagnosis of hyperchloremic metabolic acidosis. N. Engl J Med 318:594–599
12. Halperin ML, Goldstein MB, Haig A, et al. (1974) Studies on the pathogenesis of type 1 (distal) renal tubular acidosis as revealed by the urinary pCO_2 tensions. J Clin Invest 53:669–677
13. Batlle DC (1986) Sodium-dependent urinary acidification in patients with aldosterone deficiency and adrenalectomized rats. Metabolism 35:852–860
14. Batlle DC (1981) Hyperkalemic hyperchloremic metabolic acidosis associated with selective aldosterone deficiency and distal renal tubular acidosis. Semin Nephrol 1:260–274
15. Sebastian A, Schambelan M, Lindenfeld S, et al. (1977) Amelioration of metabolic acidosis with fluorocortisone therapy in hyporeninemic hypoaldosteronism. N Engl J Med 297:576–589
16. Batlle DC, Grupp M, Gaviria M, Kurtzman NA (1982) Distal renal tubular acidosis with intact ability to lower urine pH. Am J Med 72:751–7510
17. Batlle DC, Gaviria M, Grupp M, Arruda JAL, Wynn J, Kurtzman NA (1982) Distal nephron function in patients receiving chronic lithium therapy. Kidney Int 21:477–485
18. Laski ME, Kurtzman NA (1983) Characterization of acidification in the cortical and medullary collecting tubule of the rabbit. J Clin Invest 72:2050–2059
19. Batlle DC, Arruda JAL, Kurtzman NA (1981) Hyperkalemic distal renal tubular acidosis associated with obstructive uropathy. N Engl J Med 304:373–380
20. Schambelan M, Sebastian A, Rector FC Jr (1981) Mineralocorticoid-resistant renal hyperkalemia without salt wasting (type II pseudohypoaldosteronism): Role of increased renal chloride reabsorption. Kidney Int 19:716
21. Rodriguez-Soriano J, Boichis H, Edelmann CM Jr (1967) Bicarbonate reabsorption and hydrogen ion excretion in children with renal tubular acidosis. J Pediatr 71:802–813
22. Caruana RJ, Buckalew VM Jr (1988) The syndrome of distal (Type I) renal tubular acidosis. Medicine, (Baltimore) 67:84

23. Sebastian A, McSherry E, Morris RC Jr (1971) Renal potassium wasting in renal tubular acidosis (RTA). J Clin Invest 50:667
24. Sebastian A, McSherry E, Morris RC Jr (1976) Impaired renal conservation of sodium and chloride during sustained correction of systemic acidosis in patients with Type I, classic renal tubular acidosis. J Clin Invest 58:454–469
25. Wingo CS, Straub SC (1989) Active Proton Secretion and Potassium Absorption in the Rabbit Outer Medullary Collecting Duct. J Clin Invest 84:361–365
26. Doucet A, Marsy S (1987) Characterization of K-ATPase activity in distal nephron: stimulation by potassium depletion. Am J Physiol 253 (Renal Fluid Electrolyte Physiol 22):F418–F423
27. Garg LC, Narang N (1988) Ouabain-insensitive K-adenosine triphosphatase in distal nephron segments of the rabbit. J Clin Invest 81:1204–1208
28. Nilwarangkur S, Nimmannit S, Chaovakul V, Susaengrat W, Ong-aj-yooth S, Vasuvattakul S, Pidetcha P, Malasit P (1989) Endemic Primary Distal Renal Tubular Acidosis in Thailand. Q J Med 74:275,289–301

Endothelin and the Kidney

Chair: Tomoh Masaki (Japan)
Michael J. Dunn (USA)

Endothelin in Renal Diseases

VALENTINA KON[1]

SUMMARY. Injurious stimuli can activate endothelin production and elevate circulating levels of endothelin. However, continuous elevation of endothelin is not necessary for its profound effects. Instead, local endothelin activity, which encompasses local concentration of endothelin or receptor and post-receptor mechanisms, may be of primary importance in mediating the abnormal vascular function following renal injury.

Introduction

It is well recognized that, following any of the numerous insults which lead to acute renal failure, the vascular function of the kidney is profoundly disturbed. The reduced rate of glomerular filtration, central in these disorders, is typically accompanied by decreased renal blood flow, and reflects increased vascular resistance. Even when the rate of blood flow to the kidneys normalizes or is experimentally reestablished to the normal range, the vascular responsiveness of the kidney remains aberrant, including impairment in autoregulation and paradoxical vasoconstriction [1,2]. Although some humoral and neural factors have been implicated in the persistent vasoconstriction, the mechanisms for abnormal vascular function have remained largely unresolved. It has recently been appreciated that endothelial cells are important active regulators in the complete expression of vascular dilation and constriction. Therefore, it appears likely that processes which affect endothelial cell integrity may adversely influence renal vascular function by promoting the elaboration of endothelin (also by impairing the release of other endothelium-derived substances, such as endothelium-derived relaxing factor and/or prostaglandins).

A number of pathophysiologic factors enhance endothelin production. Specifically, hypoxia, anoxia, epinephrine, thrombin, transforming growth factor (TGF)-β,

---

[1]Pediatric Nephrology, Vanderbilt University School of Medicine, Nashville, TN 37232-2584, USA

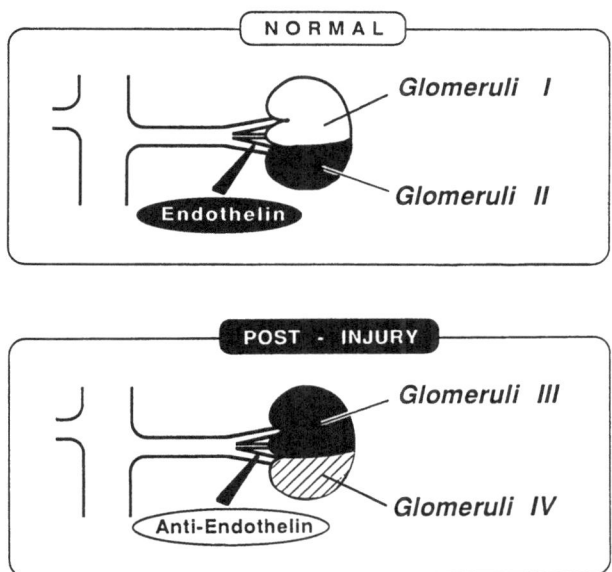

Fig. 1. Schematic illustration of infusing a branch of the main renal artery. This permits specific treatments of different populations of glomeruli within the same kidney. (*Top*) A normal kidney undergoing infusion of endothelin. Glomeruli I represent nephrons not exposed to endothelin; Glomeruli II are nephrons infused with endothelin. (*Bottom*) Kidney which has previously sustained a generalized injury to all the glomeruli. Glomeruli III reflect nephron function following the generalized injury, e.g., renal artery occlusion or intravenous infusion of cyclosporine, while Glomeruli IV represent nephron function from the same damaged kidney subsequently also exposed to anti-endothelin serum. (Reprinted from *Kidney International* with permission [18])

neuropeptide Y, interleukin-1, endotoxin, cyclosporine, and shear stress are factors known to precipitate or contribute to renal injury which can increase endothelin gene expression and/or its synthesis in vitro [3–12]. It has also been shown that the circulating level of endothelin is increased in several experimental settings and in clinical disorders, including acute renal failure, congestive heart failure, cardiogenic shock, hypertension, cyclosporine toxicity, and endotoxemia [5,13–20]. In many of these conditions, systemic hypertension and/or increased vascular resistance, which are features typically observed with exogenous infusion of endothelin, have been documented. Thus, infusion of endotoxin or cyclosporine is followed by an increased level of circulating endothelin, which is associated with systemic hypertension and vasoconstriction of renal, pulmonary, and splenic vascular beds [18,21]. While there is little doubt that injurious stimuli can enhance endothelin production in vitro and that endothelin is a circulating substance whose levels are increased in vivo in conditions where vasoconstriction prevails, it is not yet clear whether the converse is true, namely, that persistently elevated levels of circulating endothelin are necessary to maintain powerful and prolonged vasoconstriction. As will be discussed below, this appears not to be the case.

Endothelin appears to affect all vessels, although its actions on different vascular beds are not uniform. The renal circulation is particularly susceptible to endothelin's vasoconstrictory effects. Ultrasonic inter-organ assessment of blood flow in the pig reveals that the renal vasculature is ten-fold more sensitive to endothelin than the other vascular beds, including coronary, bronchial, and femoral vessels [21]. Similar results have been obtained in the squirrel monkey [22], whose vasoconstrictor response was also found to be most pronounced in the renal vessels, such that a dose of endothelin (3 μg/kg) which reduced blood flow in the heart by 46%, caused virtual cessation of blood flow in the kidney [22]. The reasons for renal susceptibility to this peptide have not been well delineated, but may be related to differences in endothelin production capability and/or differences in the binding capacity for endothelin among various tissues.

Given that the potential targets for endothelin actions include renal and nonrenal vasculature, a method was devised for administration of endothelin that achieved high concentrations but did not cause the striking systemic hemodynamic changes typical of intravenous administration of endothelin [3,22]. For this purpose, a micropipette was inserted into a first-order branch of the main renal artery of Munich-Wistar rats (Fig. 1). Through this micropipette, endothelin was infused (0.4 ng/min). In the absence of changes in systemic blood pressure or arterial hematocrit, the glomerular hemodynamics were profoundly different in glomeruli exposed *versus* those not exposed to the endothelin within the same kidney [23]. Thus, single nephron glomerular filtration rate (SNGFR) was some 35% lower in glomeruli exposed to endothelin compared with glomeruli not infused with endothelin, or with SNGFR values prior to any infusion. Similarly, the glomerular plasma flow rate was some 38% lower in the endothelin-exposed glomeruli. This hypoperfusion and hypofiltration reflected an increase in the resistances in afferent and efferent arterioles. There was no difference in the glomerular capillary ultrafiltration coefficient in these two populations of glomeruli.

Postischemic Renal Failure

In view of the previous observations that vasoconstricting substances are elaborated by the vascular endothelium in response to anoxia and hypoxia [11,24], the possibility that the vasoconstriction which characteristically follows renal ischemia depends upon endogenous endothelin was assessed in functional studies. Forty-eight hours after 25 minutes of renal artery clamping, kidneys were micropunctured while rabbit anti-porcine endothelin serum was being infused into one of the branches of the main renal artery, using the branch infusion technique shown in Fig. 1 [23]. When compared with glomeruli not exposed to the antiserum, glomeruli which were infused with the antiserum showed a remarkable amelioration in post-ischemic renal vasoconstriction, with an almost 60% increase in the SNGFR and a doubling in the glomerular plasma flow rate. Compared with non-infused glomeruli, there was also an increase in the glomerular capillary pressure and a fall in both afferent and efferent arteriolar resistances in previously ischemic glomeruli exposed to anti-endothelin serum. In this regard, Shibuota recently observed that the endothelin concentration in kidney tissues increased 20 hours following 45 minutes of bilateral renal artery occlusion [25]. Of interest, the circulating level of endothelin in these experimental animals was not different from normal controls. Treatment with a monoclonal antibody to endothelin (5 minutes before and 5 minutes, 1 and 2 hours after release of renal occlusion) lessened the accumulation of blood urea nitrogen (BUN) and creatinine, protected cells from development of renal edema and histological damage, and suppressed accumulation of calcium in necrotic tissue [25]. Taken together, ischemia appears to stimulate endothelin release which contributes to renal vascular constriction after ischemic injury.

In addition, it appears that tissue ischemia potentiates endothelin's vasoconstricting and toxic effects. Rats made hypoxemic (by lowering the ventilation volume) showed a doubling of the vasoconstrictor potency of exogenous endothelin and an increase in its myocardial toxicity [26]. It was postulated that this enhanced effect might be related to changes in the receptor characteristics or in the efficiency of coupling to effector mechanisms. In this regard, ischemia has been shown to increase endothelin-1 binding density in rat cardiac membranes [27]. In particular, 60 minutes of cardiac ischemia increased the crude plasma membrane binding density, suggesting upregulation of surface receptors, while the light membrane fraction, presumably representing the intracellular component, fell [27]. These results were taken to show that ischemia increases endothelin binding by externalizing cardiac binding sites for endothelin.

It should be noted that hypoperfusion, and therefore the potential for tissue hypoxia, is a regular feature of injuries which lead to renal dysfunction. Thus, any disorder which has *hypoperfusion* as a feature may activate and/or potentiate a pathophysiologic role for endothelin.

Endotoxemia

Endotoxin-mediated endothelial cell damage has been implicated as central in the pathogenic mechanism of endotoxic injury. Thus, in cultured endothelial cells of bovine transformed thoracic aorta, the addition of E. coli endotoxin to the culture medium increased the release of endothelin in a dose-dependent manner (Fig. 2). Intravenous injection of the endotoxin into rats was associated with a prompt (occuring in 10–15 minutes) increase in circulating endothelin: ~ 120 pg/ml compared with < 2 pg/ml in control rats [5]. In comparison studies, it was shown that while intravenous infusion of endotoxin was followed by a marked reduction in glomerular filtration rate (GFR) in both kidneys, endothelin antiserum infused into the left main renal artery ameliorated renal hypofiltration in that kidney, but not in the contralateral kidney, of the same endotoxemic animals [28].

Cyclosporine Toxicity

Cyclosporine A is an immunosuppressant which has dramatically improved graft survival of a variety of organ transplants during the last decade. Among its recognized adverse side effects, which include hepatotoxicity, hypertension, and central nervous system toxicity, nephrotoxicity is the most important and may be the inevitable consequence of cyclosporine treatment [29,30]. Early renal involvement appears to reflect intense, reversible renal vasoconstriction and has been linked to the renin-

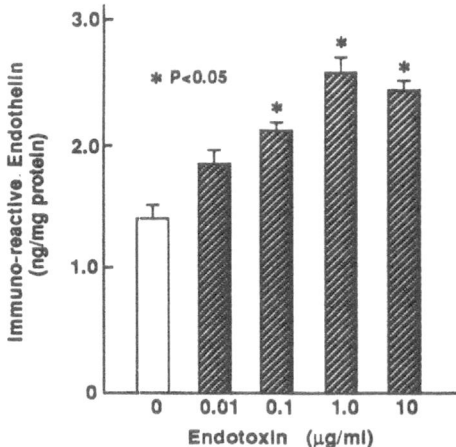

Fig. 2. Dose-dependent stimulating effect of endotoxin on endothelin secretion. Each *bar* represents the mean value in cultured endothelial cells of triplicate experiments. (Adapted from [5])

angiotensin and adrenergic systems and to vasoconstricting thromboxane (A_2). It is likely that cyclosporine-induced vasospasm, at least in part, also reflects altered vascular reactivity due to endothelial cell damage.

Cyclosporine added directly to cultured human vascular cells increases the level of endothelin in the culture medium [6]. An in vivo experimental study showed that intravenous administration of cyclosporine (20 mg/kg) caused an increase in the circulating endothelin level (43 pg/ml, as compared with < 2 pg/ml of endothelin found

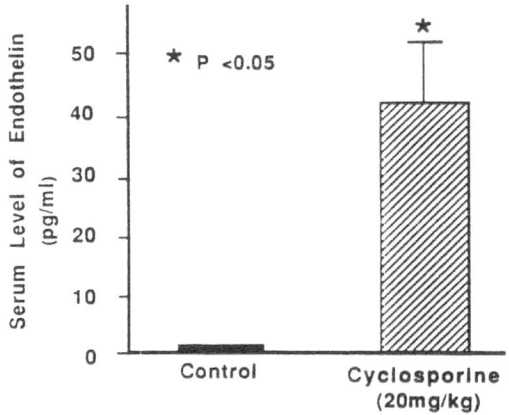

Fig. 3. Circulating levels of endothelin in cyclosporine and vehicle treated rats. (Reprinted from *Kidney International* with permission [18])

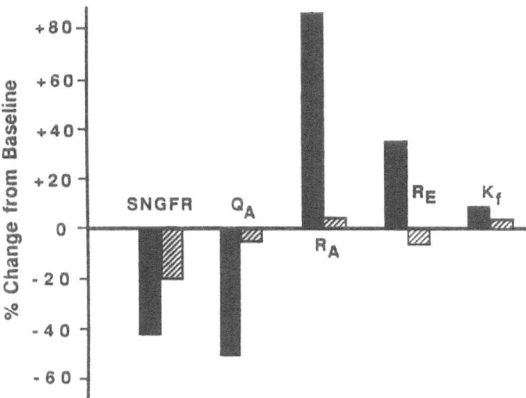

Fig. 4. Change from baseline values in microcirculatory parameters in cyclosporine treated kidneys comparing glomeruli which were not exposed (*black bars:* Glomeruli III in Fig. 1) with those which were exposed to anti-endothelin serum (*stippled bars:* Glomeruli IV in Fig. 1). (Reprinted from *Kidney International* with permission [18])

in identically instrumented rats not given cyclosporine) (Fig. 3) [18]. The elevation in endogenous circulating endothelin occurred in association with an increase in the systemic blood pressure (115 mmHg at baseline versus 133 mmHg at the time of blood collection), an observation in agreement with the well recognized pressor effect of exogenous endothelin.

In a different group of rats, the functional consequences of cyclosporine treatment on glomerular hemodynamics were examined. One hour following cyclosporine administration, rabbit anti-porcine endothelin serum was infused continuously into a first order branch of the main renal artery, whereupon the glomeruli not infused with endothelin antiserum as well as those infused with endothelin antiserum were simultaneously assessed by micropuncture (Fig. 1). A dramatically different hemodynamic pattern was seen in these two groups of nephrons (Fig. 4). The SNGFR fell by more than 40% in glomeruli after cyclosporine administration, while SNGFR in glomeruli of the same injured kidneys which were exposed to endothelin antiserum was only 20% lower than the baseline value. Amelioration of hypoperfusion in association with lower afferent and efferent arteriolar resistances was also apparent in cyclosporine-injured glomeruli infused with endothelin antiserum, when compared with glomeruli not infused with endothelin antiserum. Perico et al. also found that endothelin antiserum ameliorated renal hypoperfusion and hypofiltration following intravenous administration of cyclosporine in rats [31].

It is clear that injurious stimuli, including cyclosporine, can promptly stimulate endogenous endothelin production; however, as noted above, *persistent elevation in the circulating endothelin* level is not necessary to effect its compelling actions. That is, by sixty minutes after cyclosporine administration, at a time when glomerular hypoperfusion and hypofiltration prevail, the circulating level of endothelin is near normal. These findings correlate with the observations that, despite its short estimated half-life (< 1 minute), the biological actions of endothelin are long-lasting [3]. These findings imply persistent activation of vascular smooth muscles at the receptor or post receptor level. In this regard, the endothelin binding characteristics are strikingly different in cyclosporine-treated versus normal rats. In preliminary studies, Awazu et al. found increased endothelin binding in glomeruli of cyclosporine-treated animals [32]. This increased binding appeared specific for endothelin, since cyclosporine treatment did not alter the receptor binding characteristics for another vasoconstrictor, namely, angiotensin [32]. There was also no difference in endothelin binding in hepatic tissue between cyclosporine and control rats. Nambi et al. also showed that cyclosporine treatment (50 mg/kg intraperitoneally) for four days resulted in decreased GFR and a 60% increase in endothelin receptor density in renal tissue [33]. It appears, therefore, that cyclosporine-induced glomerular dysfunction involves upregulation of glomerular endothelin receptors and that this alteration in endothelin receptors is specific to the kidney. These findings concur with the enhanced susceptibility of renal tissue to the effects of both cyclosporine and endothelin.

References

1. Conger JD, Robinette JB, Schrier RW (1988) Smooth muscle calcium and endothelium-derived relaxing factor in the abnormal vascular responses of acute renal failure. J Clin Invest 82(2):532–537
2. Williams RH, Thomas CE, Navar LG, Evan AP (1981) Hemodynamic and single nephron function during the maintenance phase of ischemic acute renal failure in the dog. Kidney Int 19:503–515
3. Yanagisawa M, Kurihara H, Kimura S, Tomobe Y, Kobayashi M, Mitsui Y, Yazaki Y, Goto Y, Masaki T (1988) A novel potent vasoconstrictor peptide produced by vascular endothelial cells. Nature 332:411–415
4. Yoshizumi M, Kurihara H, Morita T, Yamashita T, Oh-hashi Y, Sugiyama T, Takaku F, Yanagisawa M, Masaki T, Yazaki Y (1990) Interleukin-1 increases the production of endothelin-1 by cultured endothelial cells. Biochem Biophys Res Commun 166(1):324–329
5. Sugiura M, Inagami T, Kon V (1989) Endotoxin stimulates endothelin-release in vivo and in vitro as determined by radioimmunoassay. Biochem Biophys Res Commun 161(3):1220–1227
6. Bunchman TE, Brookshire CA (1990) Cyclosporine stimulated synthesis of endothelin by human endothelial cells in tissue culture. Kidney Int 37(1):A365
7. Xuan Y-T, Whorton AR, Shearer-Poor E, Boyd J, Watkins WD (1989) Determination of immunoreactive endothelin in medium from cultured endothelial cells and human plasma. Biochem Biophys Res Commun 164(1):326–332
8. Emori T, Hirata Y, Ohta K, Shichiri M, Marumo F (1989) Secretory mechanisms of immunoreactive endothelin in cultured bovine endothelial cells. Biochem Biophys Res Commun 160(1):93–100
9. Boarder MR, Marriott DB (1989) Characterization of endothelin-1 stimulation of catecholamine release from adrenal chromaffin cells. J Cardiovasc Pharmacol 13(Suppl 5):S223–S224
10. Kohno M, Murakawa K, Yokokawa K, Yasunari K, Horio T, Kurihara N, Takeda T (1989) Production of endothelin by cultured porcine endothelial cells: modulation by adrenaline. J Hypertens 7(Suppl 6):S130–S131

11. Rubanyi GM, Vanhoutte PM (1985) Hypoxia releases a vasoconstrictor substance from the canine vascular endothelium. J Physiol 364:45–56

12. Sato M, Ohshima N (1990) Effect of wall shear rate on thrombogenesis in microvessels of the rat mesentery. Circ Res 66(4):941–949

13. Totsune K, Mouri T, Takahashi K, Ohneda M, Sone M, Saito T, Yoshinaga K (1989) Detection of immunoreactive endothelin in plasma of hemodialysis patients. FEBS Lett 249(2): 239–242

14. Koyama H, Nishzawa Y, Morii H, Tabata T, Inoue T, Yamaji T (1989) Plasma endothelin levels in patients with uraemia. Lancet I:991–992

15. Saito Y, Nakao K, Mukoyama M, Imura H (1989) Increased plasma endothelin level in patients with essential hypertension. N Engl J Med 322(3):205

16. Saliminen K, Tikkanen I, Saijonmaa O, Nieminen M, Fyhrquist F, Frick MH (1989) Modulation of coronary tone in acute myocardial infarction by endothelin. Lancet II:747

17. Nomura A, Uchida Y, Kameyama M, Saotome M, Oki K, Hasegawa S (1989) Endothelin and bronchial asthma. Lancet II:747–748

18. Kon V, Sugiura M, Inagami T, Harvie BR, Ichikawa I, Hoover RL (1990) Role of endothelin in cyclosporine-induced glomerular dysfunction. Kidney Int 37(6):1487–1491

19. Robertson RM, Susawa T, Sugiura M, Haile V, Inagami T (1990) Circulating endothelin levels: modulation by heart failure in man. Clin Res 38(2):414A

20. Tomita K, Ujiie K, Nakanishi T, Tomura S, Matsuda O, Ando K, Shichiri M, Hirata Y, Marumo F (1989) Plasma endothelin levels in patients with acute renal failure. N Engl J Med 321(16):1127

21. Pernow J, Hemsen A, Lundberg JM (1989) Increased plasma levels of endothelin-like immunoreactivity during endotoxin administration in the pig. Acta Physiol Scand 137(2):317–318

22. Clozel M, Clozel J-P (1989) Effects of endothelin on regional blood flows in squirrel monkeys. J Pharmacol Exp Ther 250(3):1125–1131

23. Kon V, Yoshioka T, Fogo A, Ichikawa I (1989) Glomerular actions of endothelin in vivo. J Clin Invest 83:1762–1767

24. DeMay JG, Vanhoutte PM (1983) Anoxia and endothelium-dependent reactivity of the canine femoral artery. J Physiol (London) 335:65–74

25. Shibouta Y, Suzuki N, Shino A, Matsumoto H, Terashita Z-I, Kondo K, Nishikawa K (1990) Pathophysiological role of endothelin in acute renal failure. Life Sci 46(22): 1611–1618

26. MacLean MR, Randall MD, Hiley CR (1989) Effects of moderate hypoxia, hypercapnia and acidosis on haemodynamic changes induced by endothelin-1 in the pithed rat. Br J Pharmacol 98:1055–1065

27. Liu J, Casley DJ, Nayler WG (1989) Ischaemia causes externalization of endothelin-1 binding sites in rat cardiac membranes. Biochem Biophys Res Commun 164(3):1220–1225

28. Kon V, Badr KF (to be published) Biologic actions and pathyphysiologic significance of endothelin in the kidney. Kidney Int

29. Myers BD (1986) Cyclosporine nephrotoxicity. Kidney Int 30(6):964–974

30. Kahan BD (1989) Medical intelligence: Cyclosporine. N Engl J Med 321(25):1725–1738

31. Perico N, Dadan J, Remuzzi G (1990) Endothlin mediates the renal vasoconstriction induced by cyclosporine in the rat. JASN 1(1):76–8332

32. Awazu M, Sugiura M, Inagami T, Kon V (1990) Cyclosporine-induced renal dysfunction involves upregulation of glomerular receptors for endothelin. Clin Res 38(2):464A

33. Nambi P, Pullen M, Contino LC, Brooks DP (1990) Upregulation of renal endothelin receptors in rats with cyclosporine A-induced nephrotoxicity. FASEB J 4(3):458A

The Cell Biology of Endothelin Peptides: Insights From Studies of Glomerular Mesangial Cells

Michael S. Simonson[1], Tomohiro Osanai[2], and Michael J. Dunn[3]

SUMMARY. Endothelins are regulatory peptides synthesized by selected endothelial and epithelial cells, and within cells of the nervous system. This ever-expanding family of peptides mediates such diverse biological processes as vasoconstriction, mitogenesis, and neurotransmission. Research efforts aimed at understanding the pathways of transmembrane signaling evoked by endothelin (ET) peptides might provide a framework for elucidating the physiological and pathophysiological roles for these peptides. Here we review recent progress towards this goal using cultured glomerular mesangial cells as a model system. Endothelin peptides evoke a phosphoinositide-based Ca^{2+} signaling system with a well-documented role mediating cell contraction. Endothelin peptides also activate alternative signaling pathways such as Na^+/H^+ exchange, prostaglandin synthesis, and *c-fos* expression, which might contribute to ET's action as a growth factor.

Introduction

Endothelins (ETs) are a family of acidic, 21-amino acid peptide hormones [1–3]. The ETs exist in at least four distinct isoforms, namely ET-1, ET-2, ET-3, and vasoactive intestinal contractor, or VIC [4–6]. Both in structure and in function ETs are closely related to sarafotoxin peptides isolated from venom of *Atractaspis engaddensis*, and it seems likely that the two peptide familes share a common evolutionary origin [7]. As shown in Fig. 1, all ET peptides and sarafotoxins share a common design including (*i*) two disulfide bonds that form a hairpin loop containing polar charged side chains and (*ii*) a hydrophobic C-terminus (residues 16–21) containing the aromatic indole side chain at Trp^{21}.

Departments of Medicine[1], Physiology[2], and Biophysics[3], School of Medicine, Case Western Reserve University, Division of Nephrology, University Hospital of Cleveland, Cleveland, OH 44106, USA

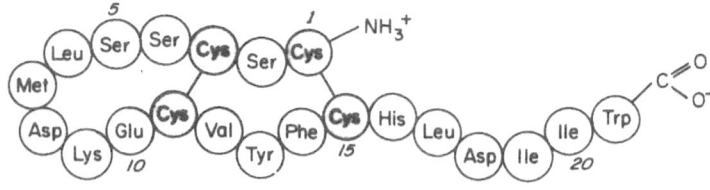

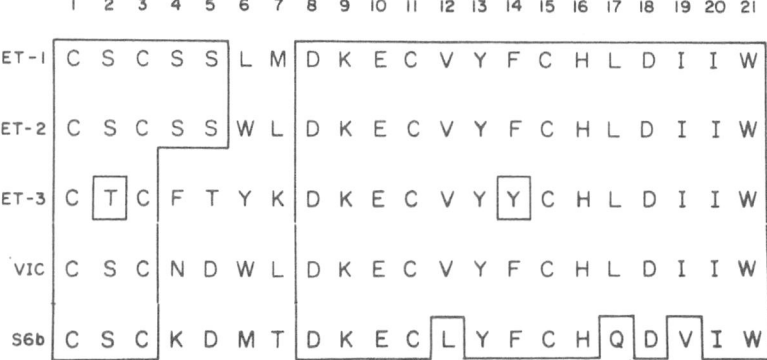

Fig. 1. The structure and sequence homologies of ET isopeptides and S6b. Homologous regions between peptide isoforms are enclosed

In a manner analogous to other peptide hormones, ETs arise via proteolytic processing of isopeptide-specific prohormones. PreproETs are large peptides (≈ 200 amino acids) that demonstrate species- and isopeptide-specific differences in amino acid sequence [1,5]. Conversion of proET to ET involves a protease with chymotrypsin-like activity and is essential for bioactivity. Although ET was first thought to be synthesized exclusively in the vascular endothelium, it is now clear that numerous extra-vascular tissues synthesize ETs. These extra-vascular sites include epithelial layers in the lung and kidney [8–10], neural tissues in the brain and spinal cord [8,11,12], and cells in the hypothalamus and posterior pituitary [13]. Release of ET requires induction of preproET gene expression. Some stimuli of ET gene expression include Ca^{2+} ionophores, phorbol esters, transforming growth factor β, and fluid-mechanical shear stress [2,14–16].

ETs are regulatory peptides with a surprisingly diverse range of biological activities. Depending on the target cell, ET can act as a vasoactive agent, growth factor, or even as a neuropeptide [2,3]. In this respect ETs are similar to other hormones, including arginine vasopressin, angiotensin II, bombesin, bradykinin, and serontonin [17]. In order to understand how ETs evoke such diverse biological actions it is necessary to define the pathways of transmembrane signaling following activation of ET receptors. Cultured mesangial cells provide a useful in vitro model for understanding the biology of ET peptides in cells of the connective tissue family [18]. Here we review our recent work analyzing the biological actions and signaling pathways of ETs in glomerular mesangial cells.

ET Peptides Have Potent Contractile and Promitogenic Actions

Contractile Activity of ET-1

At 0.1 µM ET-1 causes contraction of mesangial cells cultured on hydrated, three-dimensional collagen gels [19]. Contraction occurs along the long axis of the cell, but in many cells the cell body is also reduced. Cross-sectional area in contractile cells falls by an average of 42%, but in some cells reductions of 60–70% are common. Also induced by ET-1 are complex rearrangements of actin microfilament bundles in mesangial cells [19]; these rearrangements are consistent with an agonist-induced transition from stationary cells expressing stress fibers to motile cells elaborating a diffuse meshwork organization. The contractile state of mesangial cells in vivo is thought to be one factor regulating the glomerular ultrafiltration coefficient, and it seems possible that ET-stimulated contraction of mesangial cells might contribute to regulation of glomerular ultrafiltration. Alternatively, contraction of fibroblasts on collagen gels is thought to mimic a wound healing response, and ET might stimulate similar actions in mesangial cells and thereby contribute to the glomerular response to injury.

Promitogenic Actions of ET-1

One of the interesting biological actions of ETs is the ability to act as a mesangial growth factor [20,21]. As shown in Fig. 2, when ET-1 is added to quiescent cells they reenter G_1 and proceed to S phase 12–18 h later. The mitogenic action of ET-1 is similar to that of 2.5% fetal bovine serum. [^{3}H]Thymidine uptake in response to ET-1 is dose-dependent with a threshold at 0.1 nM, EC_{50} at 0.9 nM, and maximal stimulation at 10 nM. By itself, ET-1 is unable to stimulate mitogenesis and requires either low concentrations of fetal bovine serum (i.e., 0.5%) or a competence factor such as insulin [20]. Thus ET-1 acts as a growth factor for mesangial cells, and the promitogenic action of ET-1 has since been demonstrated in fibroblasts [22,23], vascular smooth muscle cells [24,25], and glial cells [12].

ET Peptides Evoke the Phosphoinositide Cascade

Activation of phospholipase C appears to be the initial transmembrane event following activation of ET receptors in mesangial cells [20,21]. As illustrated in Fig. 3, ET-1 causes a dose-dependent increase in phosphatidylinositol (PtdIns) turnover measured at 15 min in the presence of LiCl. Endothelin-1 stimulates greater PtdIns turnover than 0.1 µM arginine vasopression, a potent phospholipase C-linked agonist in mesangial cells [20]. Analysis of the InsP isomers reveal that both $Ins(1,4,5)P_3$ and $Ins(1,3,4,5)P_4$ are elevated by ET-1 (see Fig. 3). $Ins(1,4)P_2$ and $Ins(1,3,4)P_3$ probably result from 5-phosphomonoesterase-catalyzed dephosphorylation of $Ins(1,4,5)P_3$ and $Ins(1,3,4,5)P_4$, respectively. Activation of phospholipase C

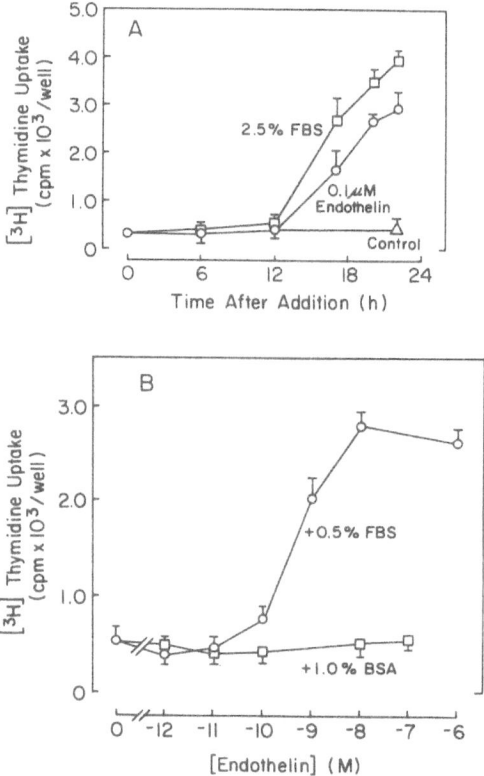

Fig. 2A,B. ET-1 stimulates mitogenesis in quiescent mesangial cells. **A** Time course of [³H]thymidine uptake in response to serum and ET-1 added to DME/F12 medium (plus 0.5% FBS) at zero time **B** Dose-response and cofactor requirements for ET-1-stimulated [³H]thymidine uptake. (From [20] with permission)

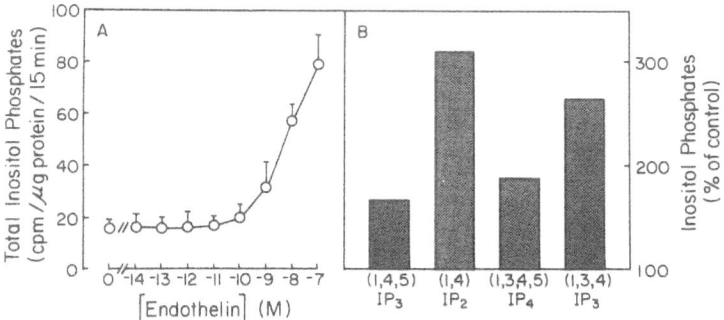

Fig. 3A,B. ET-1 activates phospholipase C to produce inositol phosphate (*InsP*) isomers. **A** Dose-dependence of total InsP turnover following addition of 0.1 μM ET-1 **B** Distribution of InsP isomers 30 sec after addition of ET-1. InsP isomers were analyzed by high pressure liquid chromatography as described in [20]. (From [18] with permission)

produces at least two second messengers: (*i*) the neutral diacylglycerol, which remains within the plane of the plasma membrane and activates protein kinase C, and (*ii*) the water-soluble Ins(1,4,5)P$_3$, which diffuses and binds to a receptor-gated Ca^{2+} channel to release Ca^{2+} from specialized stores within the endoplasmic reticulum, or calciosome [26]. Induction of the phosphoinositide cascade undoubtedly mediates many of the biological actions of ETs, and the next section discusses the complex patterns of Ca^{2+} signaling by ET peptides.

Ca^{2+} Signaling by ET Peptides

ETs and Sarafotoxin S6b Increase [Ca^{2+}]$_i$ by Two Distinct Mechanisms

We investigated Ca^{2+} signaling by ET peptides in mesangial cells loaded with the fluorescent Ca^{2+} indicator, fura-2 [20,27,28]. As shown in Fig. 4, ET isopeptides cause a biphasic increase in [Ca^{2+}]$_i$ consisting of a rapid (2–5s) spike increase followed by a lesser but sustained phase. Similar results are observed with all ET peptides and Sb6 [27]. The duration of the sustained phase was especially pronounced with ET-1 and ET-2; in some coverslips [Ca^{2+}]$_i$ returned to basal levels only after 20 min (Fig. 4). ET-1-induced Ca^{2+} signaling required conversion of proET-1 to ET-1 [27]. The peak Δ[Ca^{2+}]$_i$ was dose-dependent with ET-2 $\approx$ ET-1 > S6b > ET-3, demonstrating that ET isopeptides and S6b evoke similar elevations of [Ca^{2+}]$_i$ in mesangial cells but with dissimilar potencies and kinetics.

Two distinct but interdependent mechanisms contribute to ET-induced increments in [Ca^{2+}]$_i$. First, ET stimulates release of Ca^{2+} from intracellular stores, presumably via the action of Ins(1,4,5)P$_3$ to gate an intracellular Ca^{2+} channel in calciosomes. Second, ET increases influx of extracellular Ca^{2+} into the cytosol. ET-activated Ca^{2+} influx appears to occur through plasma membrane Ca^{2+} ion channels, which might also allow influx of other ions (see below). It is important to note, however, that these two mechanisms work in concert to produce an integrated Ca^{2+} signal. For example, the spike increase in [Ca^{2+}]$_i$ results from both intracellular release of Ca^{2+} *and* extracellular influx of Ca^{2+}, whereas the sustained phase of [Ca^{2+}]$_i$ depends on extracellular influx [27].

Mechanisms of ET-Induced Ca^{2+} Entry

Influx of Ca^{2+} from the extracellular space can occur through voltage-operated channels or through receptor-operated, voltage-independent channels [28]. Our experiments in cultured rat and human mesangial cells demonstrate that ET promotes Ca^{2+} entry via receptor-operated Ca^{2+} channels [27,28]. By using Mn^{2+} as a probe of Ca^{2+}-permeable channels [27,29], we documented rapid (<5 s) increases in Ca^{2+} influx following activation of ET receptors. Endothelin-mediated Ca^{2+} influx occurs independent of dihydropyridine- and voltage-sensitive Ca^{2+} channels and did not require prior release of intracellular Ca^{2+}. Although the biochemical mechanisms and functions of receptor-mediated Ca^{2+} entry are incompletely understood [26,28], it seems likely that receptor-mediated Ca^{2+} entry by ET contributes to rapid or localized Ca^{2+} signaling or to maintenance of the sustained elevation of [Ca^{2+}]$_i$. It is important to note that in vascular smooth muscle cells ET not only activates receptor-mediated

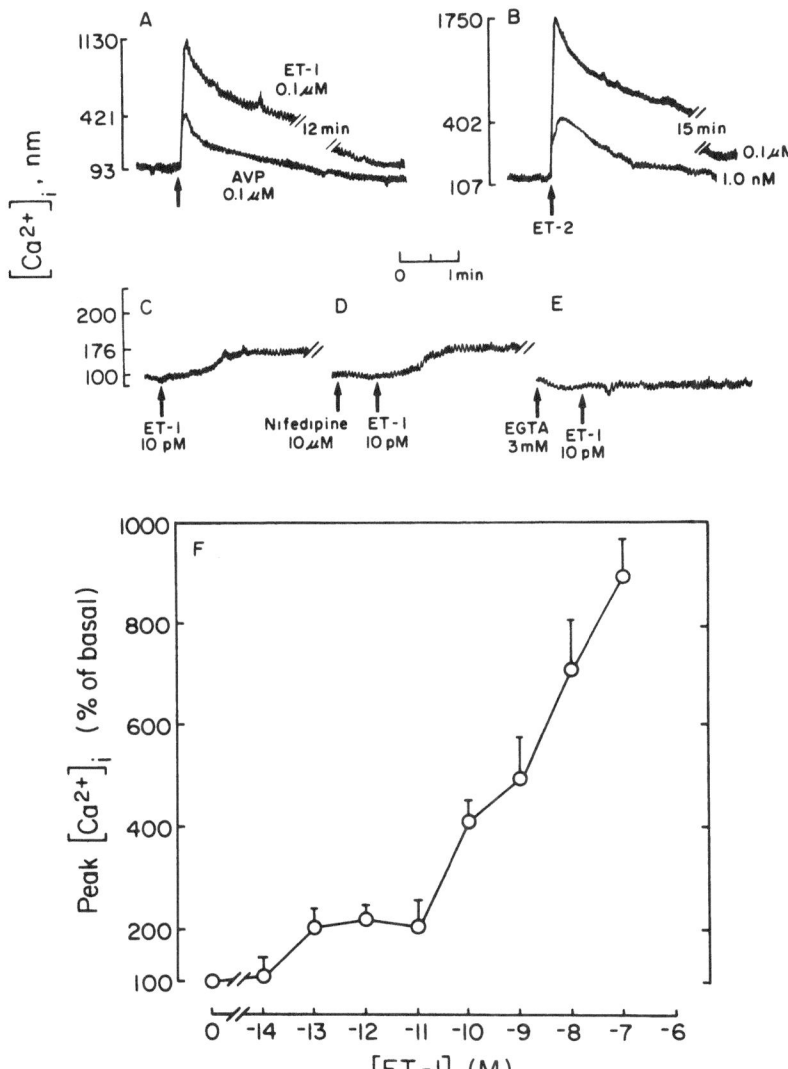

Fig. 4A-F. ET peptide evokes Ca²⁺ signaling in glomerular mesangial cells. Changes in cytosolic free [Ca²⁺]ᵢ were measured in mesangial cells loaded with the fluorescent probe, fura-2. **A,B** Biphasic increases in [Ca²⁺]ᵢ by ET-1 and ET-2 **C-E** Slow but sustained increases in [Ca²⁺]ᵢ in response to low concentrations of ET-1 **F** Dose-dependence of peak [Ca²⁺]ᵢ in response to ET-1. (From [18] with permission)

Ca^{2+} entry but also indirectly modulates the activity of L-type voltage-operated Ca^{2+} channels [30,31]. Thus, ET evokes multiple, cell-specific pathways of Ca^{2+} influx to produce diverse Ca^{2+} signals.

ET Causes Oscillations of $[Ca^{2+}]_i$ in Human Mesangial Cell Monolayers

In human mesangial cells high concentrations of ET-1 and ET-2 (0.1 μM) stimulate periodic oscillations of $[Ca^{2+}]_i$ following the spike increase [29]. These oscillations can be initiated but not sustained in the absence of extracellular Ca^{2+}. Oscillations induced by ET are especially interesting in that they occur in monolayers and represent synchronized Ca^{2+} signaling in a population of cells, as opposed to the commonly observed oscillations at a single cell level [26]. Similar results with different hormones have been observed in monolayers of ciliated tracheal epithelium [32] and cardiac trabeculae [33], and it seems likely that in human mesangial cells the ET-stimulated increment in $[Ca^{2+}]_i$ passes through gap junctions to trigger a wave of Ca^{2+} in neighboring cells. In this way ET peptides might recruit local populations of mesangial cells to function as a synctium.

ET Stimulates Contraction via Pharmacomechanical Coupling

What biological actions are triggered by ET-induced Ca^{2+} increments? Collectively, the observations that ET stimulates phospholipase C and elevates $[Ca^{2+}]_i$ suggest that ET causes contraction in mesangial cells via pharmacomechanical coupling [19]. This hypothesis is supported by the observation that contraction in response to ET occurs only at concentrations that stimulate phospholipase C. Elevation of $[Ca^{2+}]_i$ with ionomycin, to similar concentrations of $[Ca^{2+}]_i$ observed with ET, also stimulates contraction. Most important, however, ET-induced contraction is unaffected by dihydropyridine Ca^{2+} channel blockers and occurs under conditions where mesangial cells demonstrate little or no voltage-operated Ca^{2+} channel activity [19,27]. While a role for Ca^{2+} in the vasoactive properties of ET seems clear, a link between the phosphoinositide cascade and mitogenesis is less certain. Further work is necessary to evaluate alternative pathways of signal transduction in the mitogenic response to ET.

Down-Regulation of ET-Induced Ca^{2+} Signaling

The previous section discussed the mechanisms by which ET elevates $[Ca^{2+}]_i$, but, like most transduction systems, ET-mediated Ca^{2+} signaling is tightly regulated. At least three major mechanisms function as negative-feedback signals to regulate Ca^{2+} signaling by ET peptides.

Protein Kinase C (PKC)-Dependent Attenuation of Ca^{2+} Signaling

Protein Kinase C is a Ca^{2+}- and phospholipid-dependent protein kinase that modulates Ca^{2+} channel activity and Ca^{2+} signaling [26]. Phorbol esters and diacyglycerol analogs, which activate protein kinase C, fail to increase $[Ca^{2+}]_i$ in mesangial cells loaded with fura-2, suggesting that PKC does not independently increase $[Ca^{2+}]_i$ [27]. However, a 1 min preincubation with phorbol esters or diacyglycerol analogs markedly attenuates both the spike and sustained phases of Ca^{2+} signaling by ET peptides. The number and affinity of ET binding sites are unaffected by preincubation with phorbol esters (Baldi and Dunn, unpublished work). Thus, these data suggest a role for PKC in down-regulating ET-induced increments in $[Ca^{2+}]_i$. Further support for this hypothesis comes from studies in cells depleted of PKC to test the *requirement* of PKC activity in ET-activated Ca^{2+} signaling. In cells depleted of PKC, ET-1 stimulates greater increases of $[Ca^{2+}]_i$ than in concurrent controls. Because Mn^{2+} influx was similar in control and PKC-depleted cells, we conclude that activation of PKC by ET acts as a negative feedback signal to attenuate release of Ca^{2+} from intracellular stores [27]. The exact mechanism by which PKC down-regulates Ca^{2+} signaling remains unclear, but it might relate to heterologous effects on phosphoinositide metabolism [26] or it might act by inhibiting refilling of intracellular Ca^{2+} stores.

PKC-Independent Desensitization by ET Ligands

Desensitization (i.e., tachyphalyxis) induced by ligands is a common adaptive response to many hormones and neurotransmitters, including ET [27,29]. Endothelin isopeptides and S6b desensitize the increase in $[Ca^{2+}]_i$ caused by subsequent additions of the same ET agonist. In fact, preincubation with any ET isopeptide or S6b (0.1 μM) diminishes the $[Ca^{2+}]_i$ increase stimulated by the subsequent, eqimolar addition of any other isopeptide. Even low concentrations of ET-3 (10 nM), which produce only a modest increase in $[Ca^{2+}]_i$, markedly reduce the Ca^{2+} signal produced by 0.1 μM ET-2. Ligand-mediated desensitization persists in cells depleted of PKC, suggesting that this adaptive response is independent of PKC [27]. Many investigators report complex, partially irreversible binding of ET to its receptor [2,3]. Thus, continued receptor occupancy might account for some of the desensitization observed in our studies. Further experiments are necessary to define the exact mechanisms involved.

ET-Dependent Ca^{2+} Efflux Pathway(s)

In preliminary experiments we have used an inhibitor of the endoplasmic reticular Ca^{2+}-ATPase — 2,5-Di-(tert-buty)-1,4-benzohydroquinone (tBuBHQ) — to identify a Ca^{2+} efflux pathway stimulated by ET [27]. In diverse cell types tBuBHQ causes a sustained increase in $[Ca^{2+}]_i$ by preventing reuptake into the intracellular stores [34]. When ET is added to mesangial cells during the tBuBHQ-stimulated increase in $[Ca^{2+}]_i$ it causes a steady decline in $[Ca^{2+}]_i$ to basal levels [27]. That ET-stimulated Ca^{2+} influx is unaffected by tBuBHQ is confirmed by measurements of Mn^{2+} influx. Taken together, these data demonstrate that ET-stimulated Ca^{2+} signaling is attenuated by a ligand-mediated Ca^{2+} efflux pathway independent of Ca^{2+} reuptake into the microsomal pool. This pathway might constitute a mechanism whereby ET terminates its own Ca^{2+} signal. Similar results have been observed by Kass et al. [34] for other Ca^{2+}-mobilizing hormones.

Other Pathways of Signal Transducation

Studies in mesangial cells show that an increase in $[Ca^{2+}]_i$ following activation of ET receptors is only one of several possible pathways of transmembrane signaling for ET peptides. Although the increase in $[Ca^{2+}]_i$ undoubtedly mediates some short-term actions of ET peptides such as secretion and contraction [2,3,19,35], other potential pathways have been described. In mesangial [19] and other cells [2,3] ET fails to stimulate adenylate cyclase. However, ET-1 can potentiate β-adrenergic-stimulated cAMP accumulation via a mechanism involving PGE_2 [19]. Endothelin-1 is also a potent stimulus for phospholipase A_2 [19], which increases the free concentration of arachidonate to provide substrate for the cyclooxygenase and lipoxygenase pathways. Endothelin also stimulates phospholipase D activity to increase the intracellular concentration of phosphatidic acid (Kester et al., unpublished work). The increase in phosphatidic acid might contribute to the sustained increase in $[Ca^{2+}]_i$ following addition of ET peptides. Given the mitogenic action of ET in some target cells, it is interesting to note that ET stimulates electroneutral Na^+/H^+ exchange in mesangial cells [20]. In addition, the finding that ET is a mitogen for mesangial cells [20] demonstrates that ET differentially regulates gene expression to produce long-lasting response as well. In this vein it is worth noting that ET induces the gene for *c-fos* [20]. *c-Fos* is the prototype for a group of inducible genes (i.e., "immediate-early" genes) that convert short-term transmembrane signals into long-term responses requiring transcriptional regulation of target genes (See [36]). Thus activation of the "immediate-early" genes by ET peptides could play an important role in altering cell plasticity and in regulating long-term adaptive responses.

Conclusions

Cultured mesangial cells provide a useful model for investigating the cell biology of ET peptides. Although our knowledge of many components is incomplete, the outline of ET-activated pathways of signal transduction is clear and bears striking resemblance to phosphoinositide-linked signaling systems activated by other regulatory peptides. It is well-documented that ET peptides evoke complex patterns of Ca^{2+} signaling, mediating contractile and/or motile responses, but evidence regarding the role of other transduction systems remains meager. Further research into the mechanisms of cellular signaling employed by ET peptides should reveal how these peptides elicit such diverse biological events in target cells.

Acknowledgments. We gratefully acknowledge the advice and collaboration of our colleagues Drs. George Dubyak, Antonio Scarpa, Elizabetta Baldi, Mark Kester, Paolo Mene', John Sedor, and Shianq Wann. The original work, from the authors' laboratory, presented in this review was supported by National Institutes of Health Grants HL-22563 and HL-37117 to M.J.D.

References

1. Yanagisawa M, Kurihara H, Kimura S, Tombe Y, Kobayashi M, Mitsui Y, Yazaki Y, Goto K, Masaki T (1988) A novel potent vasoconstrictor peptide produced by vascular endothelial cells. Nature 332:411–415

2. Yanagisawa M, Masaki T (1989) Endothelin, a novel endothelium-derived peptide. Biochem Pharmacol 38:1877-1883
3. Simonson MS, Dunn MJ (1990) Cellular signaling by peptides of the endothelin gene family. FASEB J 4:2989-3000
4. Yanagisawa M, Akihiro I, Ishikawa T, Kasuya Y, Kimura S, Kumagaye SH, Nakajima K, Watanabe T, Sakakibara S, Goto K, Masaki T (1988) Primary structure, synthesis and biological activity of rat endothelin, and endothelium-derived vasoconstrictor peptide. Proc Natl Acad Sci USA 85:6964-6967
5. Inoue A, Yanagisawa M, Kimura S, Kasuya Y, Miyauchi T, Goto K, Masaki T (1989) The human endothelin family: Three structurally and pharmacologically distinct isopeptides predicted by three separate genes. Proc Natl Acad Sci USA 86:2863-2867
6. Saida K, Mitsui Y, Ishida N (1989) A novel peptide, vasoactive intestinal constrictor, of a new (endothelin) peptide family. J Biol Chem 264:14613-14616
7. Kloog Y, Sokolovsky M (1989) Similarities in mode and sites of action of sarafotoxins and endothelins. Trends Pharmacol Sci 10:212-214
8. MacCumber MW, Ross CA, Glaser BM, Synder SH (1989) Endothelin: Visualization of mRNAs by in situ hybridization provides evidence for local action. Proc Natl Acad Sci USA 86:7285-7289
9. Kosaka T, Suzuki N, Matasumoto H, Itoh Y, Yasuhara T, Onda H, Fujino M (1989) Synthesis of the vascoconstrictor peptide endothelin in kidney cells. FEBS Lett 249:42-46
10. Shichiri M, Hirata Y, Emori T, Ohta K, Nakajima T, Sato K, Sato A, Marumo F (1989) Secretion of endothelin and related peptides from renal epithelial cell lines. FEBS Lett 253:203-206
11. Giaid A, Gibson SJ, Ibrahim N, Legon S, Bloom SR, Yanagisawa M, Masaki T, Varndell IM, Polak JM (1989) Endothelin 1, an endothelium-derived peptide, is expressed in neurons of the human spinal cord and dorsal root ganglia. Proc Natl Acad Sci USA 86:7634-7638
12. MacCumber MW, Ross CA, Snyder SH (1990) Endothelin in brain: Receptors, mitogenesis, and biosynthesis in glial cells. Proc Natl Acad Sci USA 87:2359-2363
13. Yoshizawa T, Shinmi O, Giaid A, Yanagisawa M, Gibson SJ, Kimura S, Uchiyama Y, Polak JM, Masaki T, Kanazawa I (1990) Endothelin: A novel peptide in the posterior pituitary system. Science 247:462-464
14. Kurihara H, Yoshizumi M, Sugiyama T, Takaku F, Yanagisawa M, Masaki T, Hamaoki M, Kato H, Yazaki Y (1989) Transforming growth factor-b stimulates the expression of endothelin mRNA by vascular endothelial cells. Biochem Biophys Res Commun 159:1435-1440
15. Yoshizuma M, Kurihara H, Sugiyama T, Takaku F, Yanagisawa M, Masaki T, Yazaki Y (1989) Hemodynamic shear stress stimulates endothelin production by cultured endothelial cells. Biochem Biophys Res Commun 161:859-864
16. Schini VB, Hendrickson H, Heublein DM, Burnett JC, Vanhoutte PM (1989) Thrombin enhances the release of endothelin from cultured porcine aortic endothelial cells. Eur J Pharmacol 165:2-3
17. Seuwen K, Pouyssegur J (1990) Serotonin as a growth factor. Biochem Pharmacol 39:985-990
18. Simonson MS, Dunn MJ (1990) Endothelin: Pathways of transmembrane signaling. Hypertension 15(Suppl 1):I5-I12
19. Simonson MS, Dunn MJ (1990) Endothelin-1 stimulates contraction of rat glomerular mesangial cells and potentiates b-adrenergic-mediated cyclic adenosine monophosphate accumulation. J Clin Invest 85:790-797
20. Simonson MS, Wann S, Mene P, Dubyak G, Kester M, Nakazato Y, Sedor JR, Dunn MJ (1989) Endothelin stimulates phospholipase C, Na^+/H^+ exchange, c-fos expression, and mitogenesis in rat mesangial cells. J Clin Invest 83:708-712

21. Badr KF, Murray JJ, Breyer MD, Takahashi K, Inagami T, Harris RC (1989) Mesangial cell, glomerular, and renal vascular responses to endothelin in the kidney. J Clin Invest 83:336–342

22. Takuwa N, Takuwa Y, Yanagisawa M, Yamashita K, Masaki T (1989) A novel vasoactive peptide endothelin stimulates mitogenesis through inositol lipid turnover in Swiss 3T3 fibroblasts. J Biol Chem 264:7856–7861

23. Brown KD, Littlewood CJ (1989) Endothelin stimulates DNA synthesis in Swiss 3T3 cells. Synergy with polypeptide growth factors. Biochem J 263:977–980

24. Komuro I, Kurihara H, Sugiyama T, Takaku F, Yazaki Y (1988) Endothelin stimulates c-fos and c-myc expression and proliferation of vascular smooth muscle cells. FEBS Lett 238:249–252

25. Dubin D, Pratt RE, Cooke JP, Dzau VJ (1989) Endothelin, a potent vasoconstrictor, is a vascular smooth muscle mitogen. J Vasc Med Biol 1:150–154

26. Berridge MJ, Irvine RF (1990) Inositol phosphates and cell signaling. Nature 341:197–205

27. Simonson MS, Dunn MJ (to be published) Ca^{2+} signaling by distinct endothelin peptides in glomerular mesangial cells. Exp Cell Res

28. Hallam TJ, Rink TJ (1989) Receptor-mediated Ca^{2+} entry: diversity of function and mechanism. Trends Pharmacol Sci 10:8–10

29. Simonson MS, Osnai T, Dunn MJ (to be published) Endothelin isopeptides evoke Ca^{2+} signaling and oscillations of cytosolic free $[Ca^{2+}]$ in human mesangial cells. Biochim Biophys Acta

30. Silberberg SD, Poder TC, Lacerda AE (1989) Endothelin increases single-channel calcium currents in coronary arterial smooth muscle cells. FEBS Lett 247:68–72

31. Inoue Y, Oike M, Nakao K, Kitamura K, Kuriyama H (1990) Endothelin augments unitary calcium channel currents on the smooth muscle cell membrane of guinea-pig portal vein. J Physiol (Lond) 423:171–191

32. Sanderson MJ, Chow I, Dirksen ER (1988) Intercellular communication between ciliated cells in culture. Am J Physiol 254:C63–C74

33. Mulder BJM, deTombe PP, terKeurs HE (1989) Spontaneous and propagated contractions in rat cardiac trabeculae. J Gen Physiol 93:943–961

34. Kass GEN, Duddy SK, Moore GA, Orrenius S (1989) 2,5-Di-(tert-butyl)-1,4-benzohydroquinone rapidly elevates cytosolic Ca^{2+} concentration by mobilizing the inositol 1,4,5-trisphosphate-sensitive Ca^{2+} pool. J Biol Chem 264:15192–15198

35. Stojilkovic SS, Merelli F, Iida T, Krsmanovic LZ, Catt KJ (1990) Endothelin stimulation of cytosolic calcium and gonadotropin secretion in anterior pituitary cells. Science 248:1663–1666

36. Sassone-Corsi P, Lamph WW, Verma IM (1988) Regulation of proto-oncogene fos: A paradigm for early response genes. Cold Spring Harbor Symp Quant Biol 53:749–760

Endothelin Action and Production in Renal Tubular Cells

SHUNYA UCHIDA, MASAHIRO NARUSE, SHINYA KANAME, MITSUKO HORIE,
ETSURO OGATA[1], KIYOSHI KUROKAWA[2], MASASHI YANAGISAWA,
and TOMOH MASAKI[3]

SUMMARY. Recent studies suggest that the renal tubule is not only a target of endothelin-1 (ET-1) but is also a possible source of endothelin. Thus, we attempted to detect specific preproET-1 messenger RNA (mRNA) as well as immunoreactive ET-1 secretion in renal epithelial cell lines. Madin-Darby canine kidney (MDCK) cells expressed a single 2.3 kb preproET-1 mRNA. In medium conditioned by MDCK for 24 hours there was a significant amount of immunoreactive ET-1 detected by sandwich type immunoassay. Both mRNA expression and mature ET-1 secretion were stimulated by an addition of transforming growth factor (TGF)-β to the basolateral side in a time-dependent manner, but the increase in peptide secretion lagged behind ET-1 mRNA expression by several hours. The basal secretion of ET-1 was polarized, with 2.3-fold greater secretion into the basolateral side over the apical side, while the difference was augmented to 7.5-fold by TGF-β. In contrast, LLC-PK$_1$ (pig kidney) cells secreted little ET-1 associated with a lower level of ET-1 mRNA expression. Regarding the effect of ET-1, it elicited [Ca^{2+}]$_i$ transients in LLC-PK$_1$, but not in MDCK. These data clearly show that renal tubules can express preproET-1 mRNA, synthesize mature ET-1, and secrete it preferentially to the basolateral side of the tubule cells, all of which are enhanced by TGF-β. The data suggest that ET-1 produced by the renal tubule may function as a paracrine hormone in regulating tubular functions.

Introduction

Direct renal tubular action of endothelin has been documented recently and it has been found that endothelin may play possible important roles in the renal tubules.

[1]Fourth and [2]First Departments of Internal Medicine, University of Tokyo School of Medicine, 3-28-6 Mejirodai, Bunkyo-ku, Tokyo, 112 Japan
[3]Department of Pharmacology, Institute of Basic Medical Sciences, University of Tsukuba, Ibaraki, 112 Japan

Endothelin tubular action was first speculated by others and ourselves, based on hemodynamic data, using in vivo perfusion studies [1-3]. Thus it has been shown that despite falls in glomerular filtration rate (GFR) and renal plasma flow (RPF), (FE_{Na}) did not decline. This finding implied possible inhibition by endothelin of Na reabsorption in the terminal segment of the tubule. Also, a binding study of endothelin in the whole kidney revealed intensive binding to inner medulla in addition to glomeruli. The direct action of endothelin was demonstrated by Zeidel and his colleagues [4]. They found that ET may inhibit ouabain-sensitive Na^+-K^+-ATPase in inner medullary collecting duct (IMCD) cells, since it inhibited oxygen consumption. More recently Tomita et al., using rat intact tubules, found that ET inhibits vasopressin-stimulated cAMP production in the same nephron segments [5]. These data indicate that ET acts directly on renal tubules, especially in the collecting ducts.

Since ET was originally identified in endothelial cells by Yanagisawa and his colleagues [6], many cell types were found to be capable of producing it. Regarding ET production in the kidney, ET-like immunoreactivity was first extracted, by high-performance liquid chromatography (HPLC), from the inner medulla of pig and rat kidney [7]. This finding, however, suggests two possibilities; production and/or strong binding of ET in inner medulla. Using cultured cells, Kosaka, Suzuki, and their colleagues demonstrated that several epithelial cell lines, including renal tubular epithelial cell line MDCK, could produce ET-1 [8,9]. Similar results were reported by Shichiri et al. using another renal epithelial line, LLC-PK$_1$ [10]. Thus, it is possible that renal tubules, probably collecting duct cells, are not only a target of ET-1, but also a possible site of ET-1 production.

Therefore, we first examined the direct action of ET-1 on the tubules by monitoring cell calcium in response to ET-1, because the 2nd messenger of ET signal transduction in many cell types is now widely accepted to be an increase in cell calcium.

Furthermore, we examined ET-1 gene expression in MDCK cells as a renal tubular cell model. We used a cultured cell line because it is impossible to obtain a sufficient amount of mRNA for Northern hybridization from microdissected nephron segments.

Methods

Isolation of Individual Nephron Segments

Kidney slices from 4-6 week old male mice were incubated at 37°C for 10min in HHM (Hanks buffer containing Eagle's minimum essential medium (MEM), amino acids and vitamins, 10mM HEPES, 0.1% bovine serum albumin (BSA) and 0.1% collagenase. Dissection and identification of individual nephron segments were performed under a stereomicroscope in ice-cold HHM-BSA buffer within 40 min of sacrifice of the animal. A few pieces of 0.5-1.0mm long tubules were transferred onto thin glass slips and were kept on ice until use.

Cell Culture

MDCK (ATCC CCL34) and LLC-PK$_1$ cell lines (ATCC CL101) were cultivated in standard Dulbecco's modified Eagle's medium supplemented with 10% fetal calf serum (FCS) (regular DMEM) under humidified 5% CO_2/95% air.

Measurements of Intracellular Free Calcium Concentration

Isolated tubules or cultured cells, both attached on glass slips, were incubated with 10mM fura-2/AM (Dojin Biochemical, Kumamoto, Japan) at 37°C for 30–60min. The glass slip was then superfused on the microscope stage at 37°C with a solution containing 137 NaCl, 6 KCl, 1.2 $CaCl_2$, 1.0 $MgCl_2$, 5.5 glucose, and 20 HEPES (in mM) at pH 7.4. Cells were excited at 340 and 380 nm and emission was monitored at 500nm using a photon detector—CAM-220 (Nippon Bunko, Tokyo). $[Ca^{2+}]_i$ was calculated using the formula described by Grynkiewicz et al. [11].

Isolation of Total RNA and Purification of Poly(A)⁺ RNA from MDCK and Cultured Mesangial Cells

At the end of the experimental incubation, cells were harvested for total RNA extraction by means of guanidine thiocyanate/CsCl cushion centrifuge at 25000 rpm for 18h at 20°C. Poly(A)⁺ RNA was purified using oligo-dT column chromatography.

Northern Blots

Five µg of poly(A)⁺ RNA was size fractionated on a 1% agarose, 2.2M formaldehyde denaturing gel, and transferred by capillary blotting to Biodyne Transfer Membrane. For detecting preproET-1 mRNA, we used 1.8kb EcoR1 fragments of a full length cDNA for preproET-1 cloned from porcine aorta endothelial cells [6]. In order to normalize the preproET-1 signals for loaded amounts and transfer efficiencies, β-actin mRNA levels were used [12]. PreproET-1 and β-actin cDNA probes were nick-translated using a kit (Amersham, Buckinghamshire, U.K.) and [α-³²P]dCTP (10mCi/ml, New England Nuclear, Wilmington, Del).

Prehybridization was carried out at 42°C for 3–4 hours, and hybridization was carried out at 42°C overnight (usually > 12h). Washes were conducted with 1x SSC, 0.1% SDS, five times at room temperature; and with 0.1x SSC, 0.1% SDS, at 42°C for 30min. Autoradiography exposures were carried out for several days with two intensifying screens at −80°C.

Assay for Immunoreactive Endothelin-1 and Big-Endothelin-1

After 24 hours of incubation the medium was collected for assay. Cell proteins lysed in 0.5ml 1N NaOH were measured using a kit (Bio-Rad, Richmond, Calif.) with γ-globulin as standard. Enzyme-linked immunoassays (EIA) for ET-1 and big-ET-1 were essentially the same as reported elsewhere [9,13]. Cross reactivities of ET-1 EIA for ET-3, big-ET-1, and so-called ET-related peptides, and those of big-ET-1 EIA for ET-1, ET-3, and ET-related peptides were all less than 0.5% [9].

Polarity of Endothelin Secretion

To examine from which side of the cells ET-1 might be secreted, MDCK cells were grown to confluence on collagen (rat tail, type I, Collaborative Research, Boston, Mass.) coated Millicell-CM (Millipore Products Division, Bedford, Mass.). Each bath contained 2ml culture medium to equal the levels of both media. Permeability of the monolayers was ascertained by lack of leakiness of creatinine, where 0.4mM creatinine was placed only in the basolateral bath. In some experiments, 200pM TGF-β (TGF-β1; human platelets, R & D Systems, Minneapolis, Minn.) was added to either the apical or the basolateral bath.

Analysis of Data and Statistics

Each experiment consisted of at least three separate experiments. Data are presented as mean ± SD, and were analyzed using paired or unpaired t-tests as appropriate. P values less than 0.05 were considered significant.

Results

ET-1 Evoked Ca^{2+} Transients in Mouse Collecting Ducts

Using isolated tubules we found that ET-1 elicited Ca^{2+} transients in cortical, outer medullary, and inner medullary collecting ducts microdissected from mouse kidneys. Other tubule segments failed to increase cell Ca^{2+}. Cell Ca^{2+} increase was biphasic, with an initial peak and second sustained phase, and the response was dose-dependent between $10^{-9}M$ and $10^{-6}M$ ET-1. By removing extracellular Ca^{2+} in concert with addition of 0.5mM EDTA to the superfusate, cell Ca^{2+} increase was markedly abolished.

We previously demonstrated that arginine vasopressin (AVP) elicited Ca^{2+} transients in the cortical collecting ducts through both V_1 and V_2 receptors [14]. The effect of ET-1 on a rise in cell Ca^{2+} was independent of that of AVP. There was no additive activity regarding the effects of ET-1 and AVP. Moreover the second challenge of ET-1 failed to evoke Ca^{2+} increase, data consistent with the notion that ET does not easily dissociate from the receptors once it is bound. Thus, we speculate that these two peptide hormones increase cell Ca^{2+} by distinct mechanisms. Since ET-1 inhibits AVP-stimulated cAMP production in collecting ducts, these two peptides may act on the same cell type, probably on principal cells.

PreproET-1 mRNA Expression and ET-1 Secretion

A single 2.3kb preproET-1 mRNA was clearly expressed at the basal state in MDCK cells. This size was compatible with the one expressed in endothelial cells. TGF-β (200pM), one of the known stimulators for preproET-1 mRNA in endothelial cells, markedly upregulated this mRNA level by several-fold in 6 hours.

An increased mRNA level following 100pM TGF-β was observed as early as 30min, the earliest time point tested. TGF-β increased preproET-1 mRNA dose-dependently in 6 hours, the maximal effect appearing at 20pM and a half maximal effect at 10pM. This is regarded as a physiological concentration.

In fact, MDCK secreted mature ET-1 into the medium. TGF-β increased this secretion 2–3 times at 24 hours. It is of interest that TGF-β had no effect within 6 hours, despite dramatic upregulation of ET-1 mRNA. Thus, there seems to be a time lag of some several hours between the mRNA level and mature ET-1 secretion.

The rate of ET-1 secretion was also examined. Secretion rate was virtually unchanged until 6–12 hours after TGF-β addition, when it began to rise steeply; the rate remained several-fold greater than the basal level for up to 4 days, unless TGF-β was removed. The peak response occurred at around 2 days.

The mechanism whereby TGF-β increases mRNA level is generally thought to be a transcriptional regulation. However, since the half life of preproET-1 mRNA is quite short, actually 15 min, degradation of the transcripts may also be regulated. We investigated the change in half life of preproET-1 mRNA after TGF-β treatment.

PreproET-1 mRNA declined after addition of 10μg/ml actinomycin D to MDCK cells with or without TGF-β. However, preproET-1 mRNA was less degraded in TGF-β treated cells than in control cells. Apparent half lives were 15 min in the basal condition and longer than 30 min in the TGF-β treated condition. Similar mechanisms have been shown in other cell types for procollagen mRNA upregulation by TGF-β.

Effects of TPA on PreproET-1 mRNA and Peptides

Phorbol esters, stimulators of protein kinase C, upregulate preproET-1 mRNA rapidly and dramatically in endothelial cells [15]. Therefore, we examined the effect of TPA, one of the phorbol esters, on the mRNA levels in MDCK.

At as early as 15–30min, 0.5μM TPA increased the preproET-1 mRNA level, which reached a maximum at 45min, and then decreased below control level. No messages were found between 2 and 6 hours. These results are consistent with results reported previously using endothelial cells [15]. We next examined whether this rapid and short increase in preproET-1 mRNA was associated with actual secretion of mature peptides. ET-1 and big-ET-1 secretion from MDCK treated with TPA increased by as early as 1 hour and then by 6 hours it reached the maximum. Although peptide secretion lagged behind mRNA expression, the time courses of ET-1 and big-ET-1 secretion agree well with the profile of the mRNA time course obtained in phorbol ester experiments. The transient increases in mRNA and mature peptide secretion induced by TPA are probably due to a depletion of protein kinase C substrates.

ET-1 Secretion Was Polarized in MDCK Monolayers

One of the characteristics of epithelial cells is that they form cell polarity. Thus, we were interested in seeing to which side of the cells ET-1 secreted. To this end we utilized permeable filter chambers, which allow the separate collection of two compartments, apical baths and basolateral baths. At basal state ET-1 was released to the basolateral side twice as much as to the apical bath. Then 200pM TGF-β was added either to the apical or to the basolateral bath and cells were incubated for 24 hours; media were collected after the last 6 hours. When TGF-β was added to the apical bath, no changes were observed. However, when it was added to the basolateral bath, the amount of ET-1 secreted to the basolateral side of the monolayers increased 3–4-fold, whereas the amount in the apical bath did not increase. Thus, a stimulus like TGF-β may increase ET-1 secretion exclusively to the basolateral or to the capillary side of epithelial cells. The data also suggest that MDCK cells may have TGF-β receptors at the basolateral membranes.

ET-1 Evoked Ca²⁺ Transients in LLC-PK₁ Cells

The pattern of Ca^{2+} rise was quite similar to the patterns seen in intact collecting ducts. Again, ET-elicited Ca^{2+} transient was independent of AVP-evoked Ca^{2+} increase. Furthermore there was no additive activity of these two agonists. In contrast, MDCK cells, which produce substantial amounts of ET-1, failed to respond to ET-1. However, despite a lack of response to ET-1, MDCK cells dramatically increased cell Ca^{2+} when bradykinin was used as a positive control.

Discussion

The results of the present study clearly indicate that MDCK cells, a cell line of canine renal tubular origin, clearly express ET-1 mRNA and are capable of producing and secreting mature ET-1. The mRNA we detected was ~2.3 kb, a size compatible with preproET-1 mRNA [6]. Recent studies have shown that the kidney may express mRNAs for both ET-1 and ET-3 and that the sizes of these mRNAs were ~2.3 kb and ~3.7 kb, respectively ([16], M. Yanagisawa, unpublished work). The cDNA probe used in the present study is specific to ET-1 mRNA, and does not hybridize 3.7 kb transcripts of ET-3. Therefore, the present results do not exclude the possibility of ET-3 mRNA expression in MDCK.

The results achieved by using a specific enzyme-immunoassay for ET-1 clearly demonstrate that MDCK cells secrete mature ET-1, data consistent with an earlier report by Kosaka et al. [8]. Our present EIA system is specific to ET-1 and ET-2, and does not detect ET-3. Taken together with the mRNA data, our present findings show specific production of ET-1 by MDCK cells, but do not exclude a possible production of ET-3 by these cells.

The mRNA expression of ET-1 and secretion of ET-1 by MDCK cells increased in response to TGF-β in a time-dependent manner. Recent observations of ET-1 production and secretion have shown that ET-1 is released in response to stimuli such as thrombin, catecholamine, and TGF-β, and is not stored in the intracellular organelles such as secretory granules. Rather, ET-1 secretion occurs constitutively, so that mRNA level is a predominant determinant of ET-1 production and secretion. Our present findings in MDCK cells are consistent with this current notion of ET-1 production and secretion.

Using a specific device which allows examination of the polarized function of epithelial cells, we found that MDCK cells secrete ET-1 predominantly to the basolateral side of the cells under the basal, unstimulated condition, as well as in response to stimulation by TGF-β. At the basal state, the ratio of ET-1 secreted into the basolateral side of the cells to that secreted into the apical side was 2:3. In response to TGF-β, ET-1 mRNA level increased several-fold in 6 hours and polarized ET-1 secretion into the basolateral bath was 7.5-fold that into the apical bath between 18 and 24 hours. These data demonstrate that increased ET-1 mRNA expression with TGF-β is associated with almost exclusive increase in ET-1 secretion to the basolateral side of the epithelia with little increase in its secretion to the apical side. These data thus suggest that, in addition to the constitutive secretory process present both in the apical and in the basolateral membranes, there must exist a specific mechanism which, following certain stimuli, augments ET-1 secretion

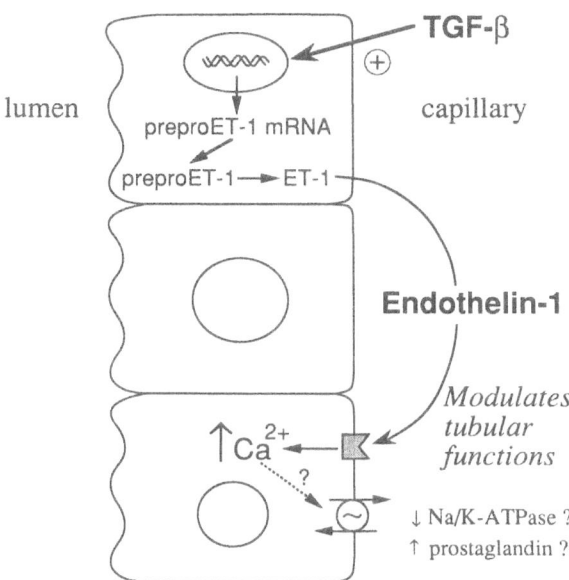

Fig. 1. Schematic model of ET-1 synthesis and secretion, and its paracrine function in the renal tubules. ET-1 can be synthesized in a tubular cell type at the basal state. TGF-β is capable of stimulating preproET-1 mRNA level, both at transcriptional steps and by inhibiting preproET-1 mRNA degradation. Mature ET-1 processed from preproET-1 is secreted by a constitutive pathway, with two-fold greater secretion through basolateral membranes, while the enhanced secretion of ET-1 by TGF-β is more polarized, leading newly produced ET-1 to enter the blood stream. Downstream, ET-1 may act on another tubule cell type, via increase in $[Ca^{2+}]_i$, as a paracrine hormone which modulates water and electrolyte transport, cell metabolism, and cell function, possibly including proliferation

preferentially into the basolateral side of the tubular cells. A mechanism which renders de novo ET that enters capillary blood flow seems physiologically tenable, in view of the fact that ET-1 secreted from apical membranes has no chance of exerting its biological effects, since ET-1 appears to act only from the basolateral side of intact renal tubules (M. Naruse, unpublished work).

Stimulation by TGF-β of ET-1 mRNA levels and ET-1 secretion in MDCK cells is similar to the stimulation reported in endothelial cells [17]. Moreover, the effects of TGF-β could be shown only when this growth factor was added to the basolateral side of MDCK cells, indicating the presence of putative TGF-β receptors on this side of the tubular cells.

TGF-β is a unique growth factor, in that this peptide inhibits the cell growth of certain cell types, including renal tubules [18] and mesangial cells [19]. Most recently we found that cultured rat mesangial cells expressed TGF-β mRNA and that this level was stimulated by fetal calf serum and phorbol ester, suggesting its protein kinase C-dependent activation mechanism [20]. Thus, mesangial cells may be one of the intrarenal sources of TGF-β, which may have access to the collecting duct system via the intrarenal circulation. The physiological implications of the axis of TGF-β-ET-1-

collecting duct system await further investigation. However, it is speculated that this system may play some role in tubular growth and fibrosis.

Regarding the action of ET-1, it evoked a transient rise in $[Ca^{2+}]_i$ in LLC-PK$_1$ cells, but not in MDCK cells, data indicating that LLC-PK$_1$ cells are a target of ET-1. Moreover, an absence of any effect of additive activity between ET-1 and AVP clearly indicates that these two peptides evoke rises in $[Ca^{2+}]_i$ through different mechanisms. Recent studies have demonstrated massive ET-1 binding in inner medulla as well as in glomeruli [21,22] and have shown direct action of ET-1 on the renal tubules. Indeed, ET-1 has been shown to inhibit Na$^+$,K$^+$-ATPase, and thus Na$^+$ transport, of the inner medullary collecting ducts, through mechanisms dependent on prostaglandin production [4]. The present findings of ET-1-elicited $[Ca^{2+}]_i$ increase in LLC-PK$_1$ cells support the presence of a direct tubular action of ET-1. More studies are required in order to elucidate the mechanisms of ET-1 action and the effects of ET-1 on specific segments of the nephron.

Our demonstration of the production and preferential, polarized secretion of ET-1, as well as its action on distinct renal tubular cell lines, clearly suggests the possibility that ET-1 produced by the renal tubules may be secreted into the basolateral side of the tubules, thence reaching another tubular segment downstream of the local blood flow, and modulating the function thereof (Fig. 1). Such a scheme suggests possible roles of ET-1 as an intrarenal paracrine hormone regulating renal tubular functions.

References

1. King AJ, Brenner BM, Anderson S (1989) Endothelin: a potent renal and systemic vasoconstrictor peptide. Am J Physiol 256:F1051–F1058
2. Kon V, Yoshioka T, Fogo A, Ichikawa I (1989) Glomerular actions of endothelin in vivo. J Clin Invest 83:1762–1767
3. Katoh T, Chang H, Uchida S, Okuda T, Kurokawa K (1990) Direct effects of endothelin in the rat kidney. Am J Physiol 258:F397–F402
4. Zeidel ML, Brady HR, Kone BC, Gullans SR, Brenner BM (1989) Endothelin, a peptide inhibitor of Na$^+$-K$^+$-ATPase in intact renal tubular epithelial cells. Am J Physiol 257:C1101–C1107
5. Tomita K, Nonoguchi H, Marumo F (1990) Effects of endothelin on peptide-dependent cyclic adenosine monophosphate accumulation along the nephron segments of the rat. J Clin Invest 85:2014–2018
6. Yanagisawa M, Kurihara H, Kimura S, Tomobe Y, Kobayashi M, Mitsui Y, Yazaki Y, Goto K, Masaki T (1988) A novel potent vasoconstrictor peptide produced by vascular endothelial cells. Nature 332:411–415
7. Kitamura K, Tanaka T, Kato J, Eto T, Tanaka K (1989) Regional distribution of immunoreactive endothelin in porcine tissue: abundance in inner medulla of kidney. Biochem Biophys Res Commun 161:348–352
8. Kosaka T, Suzuki N, Matsumoto H, Itoh Y, Yasuhara T, Onda H, Fujino M (1989) Synthesis of the vasoconstrictor peptide endothelin in kidney cells. FEBS Lett 249:42–46
9. Suzuki N, Matsumoto H, Kitada C, Kimura S, Fujino M (1989) Production of endothelin-1 and big-endothelin-1 by tumor cells with epithelial-like morphology. J Biochem (Tokyo) 106:736–741
10. Shichiri M, Hirata Y, Emori T, Ohta K, Nakajima T, Sato K, Sato A, Marumo F (1989) Secretion of endothelin and related peptides from renal epithelial cell lines. FEBS Lett 253:203–206

11. Grynkiewicz G, Poenie M, Tsien RY (1985) A new generation of Ca^{2+} indicators with greatly improved fluorescence properties. J Biol Chem 260:3440–3450

12. Nakajima-Iijima S, Hamada H, Reddy P, Kakunaga T (1985) Molecular structure of the human cytoplasmic b-actin gene: Interspecies homology of sequences in the introns. Proc Natl Acad Sci USA 82:6133–6137

13. Suzuki N, Matsumoto H, Kitada C, Masaki T, Fujino (1989) A sensitive sandwich-enzyme immunoassay for human endothelin. J Immunol Methods 118:245–250

14. Naruse M, Uchida S, Ogata E, Kurokawa K (1990) Vasopressin increases intracellular free Ca by stimulating Ca entry via V_2 receptor in cAMP independent manner in mouse cortical, outer and inner medullary collecting tubule cells. Kidney Int 37:362

15. Yanagisawa M, Inoue A, Takuwa Y, Mitsui Y, Kobayashi M, Masaki T (1989) The human preproendothelin-1 gene: possible regulation by endothelial phosphoinositide turnover signaling. J Cardiovasc Pharmacol 13:S13–S17

16. MacCumber MW, Ross CA, Glaser BM, Snyder SH (1989) Endothelin: Visualization of mRNAs by in situ hybridization provides evidence for local action. Proc Natl Acad Sci USA 86:7285–7289

17. Kurihara H, Yoshizumi M, Sugiyama T, Takaku F, Yanagisawa M, Masaki T, Hamaoki M, Kato H, Yazaki Y (1989) Transforming growth factor-β stimulates the expression of endothelin mRNA by vascular endothelial cells. Biochem Biophys Res Commun 159:1435–1440

18. Fine LG, Holley RW, Nasri H, Badie-Dezfooly B (1985) BSC-1 growth inhibitor transforms a mitogenic stimulus into a hypertrophic stimulus for renal proximal tubular cells: Relationship to Na^+/H^+ antiport activity Proc Natl Acad Sci USA 82:6163–6166

19. MacKay K, Striker LJ, Stauffer JW, Doi T, Agodoa LY, Striker GE (1989) Transforming growth factor-β. J Clin Invest 83:1160–1167

20. Kaname S, Uchida S, Ogata E, Kurokawa K (1990) Transforming growth factor-beta (TGF-β) gene expression in cultured rat mesangial cells. Kidney Int 37:197

21. Koseki C, Imai M, Hirata Y, Yanagisawa M, Masaki T (1989) Autoradiographic distribution in rat tissues of binding sites for endothelin: A neuropeptide? Am J Physiol 256:R858–R866

22. Kohzuki M, Johnson CI, Chai SY, Casley DJ, Mendelsohn FAO (1989) Localization of endothelin receptors in rat kidney. Eur J Pharmacol 160:193–194

Transplantation

Chair: Kazuo Ota (Japan)
Henri Kreis (France)

A Novel Immunosuppressive Agent, Deoxyspergualin

KOTA TAKAHASHI and KAZUO OTA

SUMMARY. A new immunosuppressive agent, deoxyspergualin (DSG), has been reported elsewhere to prolong survival of xenografts in animal models and was effective in the treatment of hyperacute rejection in our previous report of ABO-incompatible kidney transplantation, which was thought to be similar to xenograft transplantation.

A new administration modality of DSG, its prophylactic use for the prevention of acute rejection in patients with kidney transplantation from ABO-incompatible or preformed antibody-positive donors, was tried, and satisfactory clinical results were obtained.

The evidence showed that DSG was very effective in the prevention of acute rejection in patients with kidney transplantation from ABO-incompatible or preformed antibody-positive living related donors, and that DSG was also very effective in the treatment of rejection in kidney transplantation.

Introduction

Although immunosuppressive agents are indispensable in organ transplantations, at present fewer than ten agents are in clinical use. The need for new agents for clinical use is therefore very high.

Following mizoribine, deoxyspergualin (DSG) is the second immunosuppressive agent to be developed and clinically applied in Japan. It has become the focus of much attention as efforts are being made to confirm its effectiveness.

This paper summarizes our findings concerning the effectiveness of DSG in the prevention and treatment of acute rejection in kidney transplantation.

[1]Department of Urology, Tokyo Women's Medical College, 8-1, Kawada-cho, Shinjuku-ku, Tokyo, 162 Japan

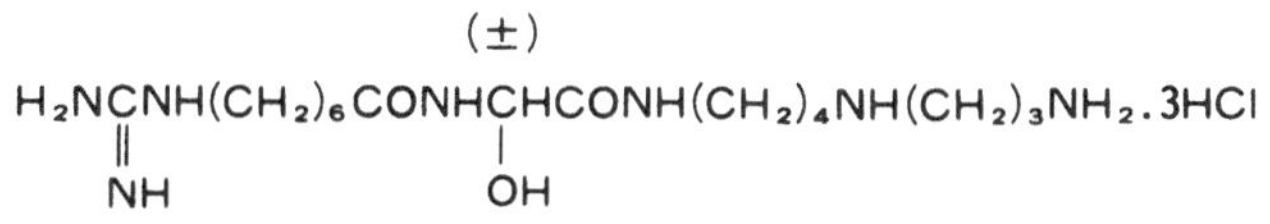

$$(\pm)$$

$$\underset{\underset{\text{NH}}{\|}}{\text{H}_2\text{NCNH(CH}_2)_6}\text{CONH}\underset{\underset{\text{OH}}{|}}{\text{CHCONH(CH}_2)_4}\text{NH(CH}_2)_3\text{NH}_2.3\text{HCl}$$

M.W. 497

Fig. 1. Structural formula of DSG

Description of Deoxyspergualin

In 1981, Takeuchi et al. isolated a new antibiotic, which was given the name spergualin from its chemical structure, from the culture filtrate of a bacillus. This antibiotic demonstrated an anti-tumor and immunosuppressive effect, and led to the synthesis of a number of derivatives, of which deoxyspergualin, or DSG, was singled out for further development.

Deoxyspergualin has a molecular weight of 497 and is characterized by the removal of a hydroxide group from spergualin, at the 15-position, as shown in Fig. 1. It comes in the form of lumpy white powder and is highly hygroscopic and deliquescent. It is easily dissolved in water, methanol, and formic acid.

At present, DSG is supplied for intravenous injection only, and is, unfortunately, not yet available in oral form, due to absorption problems. The development of an oral form is, however, expected in the near future.

Immunosuppressive Effects

Figure 2 shows the most probable mechanism for the immunosuppressive effects of DSG, based on our current knowledge of DSG characteristics described in the previous section. Possibly, DSG suppresses clonal amplification of cytotoxic T lymphocytes (CTL) through direct action on these cells, by which the functions of the suppressor T-lymphocytes are relatively enhanced. Subsequent direct action on B-lymphocytes causes the suppression of antibody production through suppression of the amplification of B-lymphocytes and plasma cells.

As described above, one of the characteristic of DSG is the suppression of antibody production by direct action on the B-cell system.

DSG was used in the induction phase to prevent kidney transplant rejections, those due to ABO-incompatibility closely related with humoral antibodies, and rejections due to preformed antibodies. The results of these efforts, as well as the use of DSG in the post-transplant treatment of rejections, are described in the following sections.

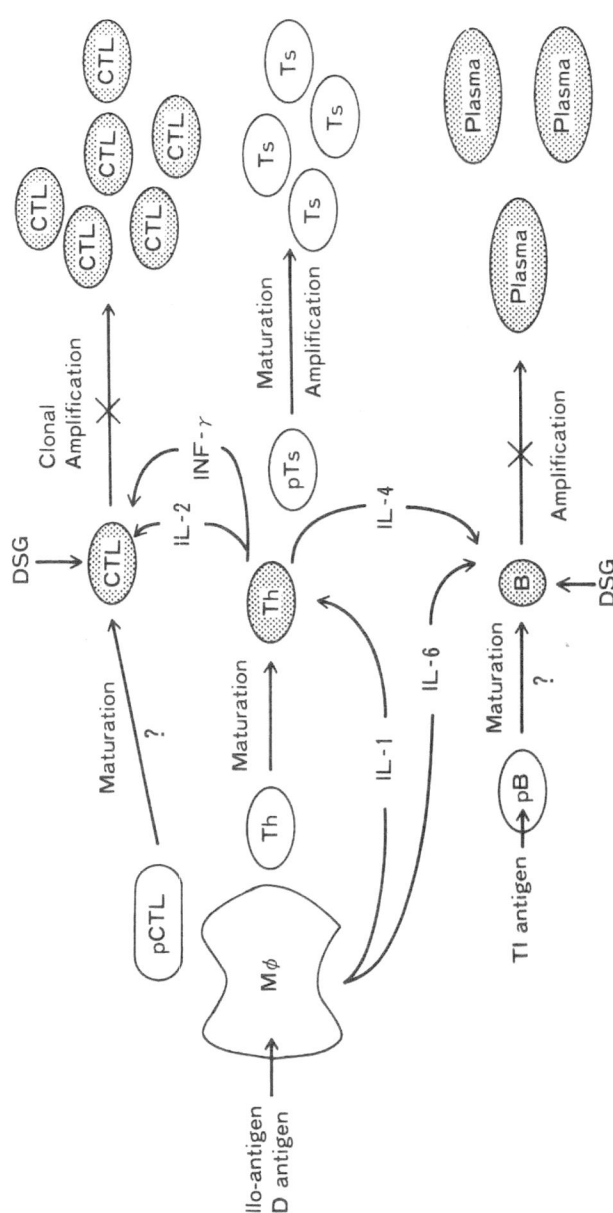

Fig. 2. Immunosuppressive mechanism of DSG

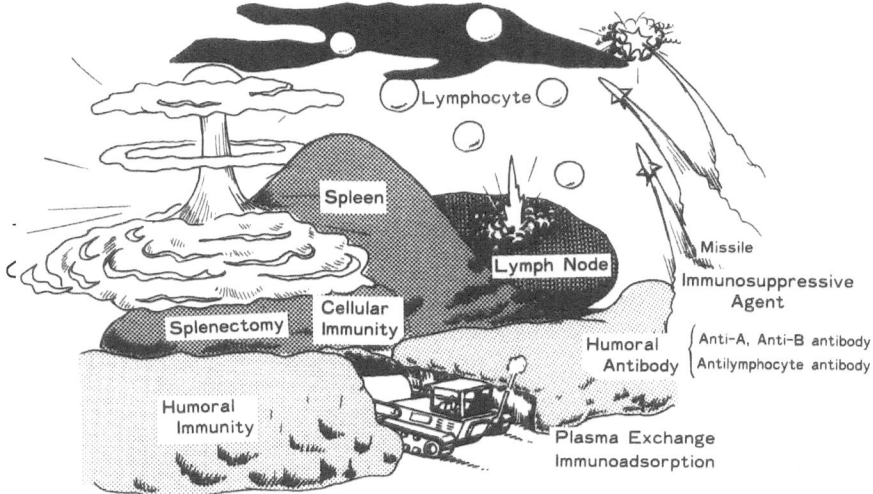

Fig. 3. ABO-incompatible and preformed antibody-positive kidney transplantation

Prophylactic Use of DSG in Kidney Transplantation from ABO-Incompatible and Preformed Antibody-Positive Donors (Fig. 3)

Patients

The patients studied were immunological high responders, consisting of 13 ABO-incompatible kidney transplant recipients and 3 preformed antibody-positive kidney transplant recipients (Table 1). In order to suppress antibody production, DSG was administered to all of these patients.

Methods

ABO-Incompatible Kidney Transplantation

Prior to surgery, anti-A or anti-B antibodies were removed from the recipients by means of double filtration plasmapheresis and immunoadsorption (using a Biosysorb column), thus lowering their anti-A and anti-B antibody titers to 1:8 or less.

In Case 1, an immunosuppressive regimen, consisting of methylprednisolone (MP), cyclosporin (CYA), azathioprine (AZ), and antilymphocyte globulin (ALG), resulted in decreased urinary output three hours after the transplantation. Due to a diagnosis of hyperacute rejection, the patient was given DSG, which resulted in increased urinary output that indicated a recovery of renal function. Based on our observation of Case 1, DSG and the same four-drug regimen were administered in cases 2–13.

Administration of MP started on the day of the transplantation, at a dose of 500 mg/day, which was reduced to a maintenance dose of 8 mg/day in the 4th month.

Table 1. ABO-incompatible kidney transplantation

Case	Sex	Age	Original disease	ABO blood type Donor→Recipient	HLA-A, B, DR mismatch No.	MLC (1way S.I.)	Rejection HAR 2	Rejection AR	Serum Cr. mg/dl (1day, 1W, 2W, 1M, 2M, 3M, 6M, 1Y)	Anti A, Anti B antibody (1W, 1M, 2M, 3M, 6M, 9M, 1Y)	Complication
1 M.N.	M	27	Chronic nephritis	B→0	3	75.0	HAR 2	(−)	6.8 2.4 1.4 1.6 4.4 2.1 2.2 Death	IgM 2 2 4 8 8 IgG 4 4 16 8 8	CMV infection, Malignant B cell lymphoma
2 T.S.	M	28	Chronic nephritis	B→0	3	68.5	(−)	1	4.3 1.3 1.3 1.7 1.7 1.5 1.5 1.5	IgM 1 32 16 8 8 4 4 IgG 1 4 8 2 2 2 2	CMV infection
3 Y.Y.	M	42	Chronic nephritis	B→A1	0	1.0	(−)	(−)	4.7 1.3 1.3 1.4 1.4 1.4 1.5	IgM 0 2 2 2 2 IgG 1 2 2 4 4	(−)
4 T.F.	M	13	Chronic nephritis	A1B→A1	3	1.7	(−)	1	2.0 0.8 0.8 1.1 1.0 1.0 0.7	IgM 0 1 1 1 1 IgG 0 0 1 1 1	UTI
5 T.S.	M	27	Chronic nephritis	A1→0	1	15.2	(−)	4	5.9 2.2 4.0 3.5 3.2 2.8 3.0	IgM 4 8 8 8 8 IgG 4 8 8 8 8	(−)
6 N.I.	F	17	Chronic nephritis	A1B→B	1	12.2	(−)	(−)	2.4 0.9 1.0 1.3 1.2 1.1 1.1	IgM 16 32 8 8 8 IgG 8 4 4 8 8	CMV infection
7 E.S.	M	27	Chronic nephritis	B→0	2	16.4	(−)	(−)	2.9 1.1 1.2 1.3 1.2 1.2 1.2	IgM 1 1 4 4 4 IgG 1 1 2 2 2	(−)
8 E.H.	F	32	Chronic nephritis	B→0	2	3.6	(−)	4	2.9 1.0 0.9 1.2 7.8 2.3 2.2	IgM 2 4 16 16 16 IgG 2 8 16 16 16	(−)
9 T.K.	M	31	Chronic nephritis	A1→0	1	35.6	(−)	(−)	4.9 1.1 1.1 1.4 1.4 1.4	IgM 2 8 16 IgG 4 16 32	Adenovirus Hemorrhagic cystitis
10 H.T.	M	23	Chronic nephritis	A1→0	4	11.2	(−)	1	7.1 1.7 1.6 1.8 1.6 1.6	IgM 2 8 16 IgG 4 4 16	(−)
11 S.S.	M	55	Chronic nephritis	A1→0	3	25.7	(−)	1	1.1 1.1 1.2 AR Graftloss Death	IgM 1 128 32 IgG 1 128 32	Cerebral haemorrhage
12 S.K.	F	58	Chronic nephritis	A1→0	5	16.4	(−)	(−)	1.4 1.3 1.3 1.3 1.3 1.3	Ig 4 4 IgG 4 4	(−)
13 Y.S.	M	53	Polycystic kidney	A1B→0	5	4.1	(−)	(−)	5.5 2.2 2.0 2.0	A IgM 4 4 4 4 IgG 4 4 4 4 B IgM 4 4 4 4 IgG 4 4 4 4	(−)

Oral administration of CYA, at a dose of 8–10 mg/kg per day, started 2 days before the transplantation; drip infusion of CYA, at a dose of 3 mg/kg per day, was administered on the day of the transplantation. Administration of CYA was then adjusted to maintain a CYA through-level in whole blood of between 150 and 200 mg/ml for a duration of 1 or 2 months after the transplantation and a CYA through-level of between 80 and 150 ng/ml thereafter.

Administration of AZ, at a dose of 2 mg/kg per day, was started 2 days before the transplantation and was continued for a period of 1 week, after which the dose was reduced to 1 mg/kg per day and adjusted according to the patient's peripheral white blood cell count.

Administration of ALG, at a dose of 30 mg/kg per day, was begun 2 days before the transplantation and, basically, continued for 14 days. Administration of ALG was discontinued when the platelet count decreased to 50,000/cmm or less. Then DSG was administered, at a dose of 5 mg/kg per day, for 5 days, starting from the day of the transplantation; local X-ray irradiation was performed, at a dose of 150 rad, on the 1st, 3rd, and 5th day after the transplantation. Kidney transplantation surgery was performed according to Murray's method, and, in all cases, a splenectomy was performed at the time of transplantation.

In the treatment of acute rejection episodes, a basic dose of 500 mg of MP was administered for 2 days. When no remission occurred, muromonab CD3 (OKT3), at a dose of 5mg/kg per day, was administered for 10 days, or DSG, at a dose of 5 mg/kg per day, was administered for 5 days. Before the administration of DSG, which remains an experimental drug, prior written consent was obtained from the patients.

Preformed Antibody-Positive Kidney Transplantation

From among the preformed antibody-positive kidney transplant patients, we selected three whose T-cell antibody counts had not become negative 6 months or more after the pre-transplant cross match tests had been carried out. In these cases, double filtration plasmapheresis was conducted a total of two to four times and transplantation was performed following the disappearance of the T-cell antibodies.

In those cases in which T-cell antibodies did not disappear after 6 months, an immunosuppressive regimen, consisting of CYA, at a dose of 2 mg/kg per day, MP, at a dose of 8 mg/day, and MZ, at a dose of 1 mg/kg per day, was administered three times per week following hemodialysis, until the time of the transplantation. After the transplantation, the same immunosuppressive regimen as that employed in ABO-incompatible cases was used. None of the three cases, however, underwent splenectomy.

Table 2 shows the maximum values of the results of cross match tests conducted prior to transplantation.

Results

ABO-Incompatible Kidney Transplantation

Of the ABO-incompatible kidney transplant cases, rejection did not occur in 4 cases, hyperacute rejection occurred once in 1 case, accelerated acute rejection occurred 2 times in 2 cases, and acute rejection occurred 12 times in 6 cases (i.e., four times

Table 2. Preformed antibody-positive kidney transplantation (Tx)

Patient	Age	Sex	Blood type	Original disease	HLA, A, B. DR mismatch No.	Cause of Senitization	Crossmatch test		
							T	BW	BC%
1 F.S.	32	F	O/O	Purpura nephritis	12.5	Pregnancy ? Blood transfusion	30	100	0
2 S.T.	40	M	O/B	Chronic nephritis	12.7	Blood transfusion	20	90	90
3 K.O.	44	F	A/A	Chronic nephritis	12.8	DST	100	100	100

Patient	Treatment before Tx		Immunosuppression		Serum Cr. value	Rejection				Complication
	Immunosupp	Plasma exchange	Induction phase	Maintenance		HR	AAR	AR	CR	
1 F.S.	CYA, MP MZ	DFPP 2	CYA, MP AZ, DSG, ALG	MP CYA, AZ	1.1mg/dℓ 1Y1M	(—)	(—)	(—)	(—)	(—)
2 S.T.	CYA, MP MZ	DFPP 3	CYA, MP AZ, DSG, ALG	MP CYA, AZ	1.5mg/dℓ 1Y	(—)	(—)	(—)	(—)	(—)
3 K.O.	CYA, MP MZ	DFPP 6	CYA, MP AZ, DSG, ALG	MP CYA, AZ	1.6mg/dℓ 3M	(—)	1	(—)	(—)	(—)

in 2 cases and once in 4 cases). Graft loss caused by rejection occurred in only 1 of the 13 cases.

Regarding anti-A or anti-B titers after transplantation, both IgM and IgG levels were maintained at 1:32 in all cases except patient 11, whose anti-A antibody titers rose to 1:128. In this case, immunoadsorption was performed four times, combined with DSG administration. Although the titer level decreased to 1:32, the rejection led to graft loss.

Complications included three cases of cytomegalovirus (CMV) infection and one case each of urinary tract infection and hemorrhagic cystitis caused by adenovirus type 11.

CMV infection was treated with ganciclovir and CMV high-titer gamma-globulin, while hemorrhagic cystitis was treated with glycyrrhizin.

There were two deaths. One patient died of malignant B cell lymphoma in the 8th month, with the causal relationship between the fatal disease and Epstein-Barr virus infection remaining unclear. The other patient died of cerebral hemorrhage in the 2nd month after transplantation.

Clinical Course

This section describes a typical post-operative course.

Case 2 consisted of a 28-year-old male with type O blood and an original diagnosis of chronic nephritis. The patient received a kidney from his living elder brother, whose blood type was B.

To lower the patient's serum antibody titers, one session of double filtration plasmapheresis (DFPP) and four sessions of immunoadsorption were performed before the transplantation, reducing his serum anti-B IgM and IgG levels to 1:4, or less, immediately before the operation. The kidney transplantation was preceded by splenectomy and the immunosuppressive regimen was carried out according to the method described above (Fig. 4).

After the transplantation, anti-B IgM and IgG titers of up to 1:32 and 1:8, respectively, were maintained. The patient suffered one acute reaction (AR), but recovered fully through MP pulse therapy. At present, 1 year after the transplantation, the patient shows a serum creatinine level of 1.6 mg/dl, which indicates satisfactory functioning of the transplanted kidney.

Preformed Antibody-Positive Kidney Transplantation

The survival rate for patients and grafts ranged from two months to a year after the transplantation, with all cases showing satisfactory functioning of the transplanted kidney and a serum creatinine level of 1.1–1.6 mg/dl.

One patient experienced an AR episode, but recovered through MP pulse therapy.

Clinical Course

The clinical course of a recent case follows:

Case 3 was a 44-year-old female with type A blood and an original diagnosis of chronic nephritis. The patient showed poor histocompatibility with her 64-year-old

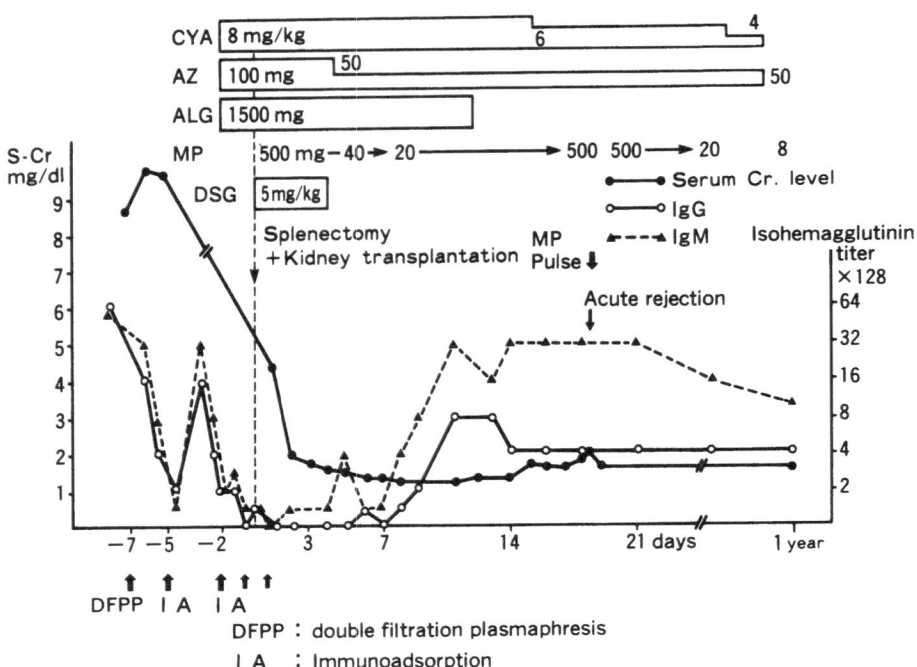

Fig. 4. ABO-incompatible kidney transplantation No. 2. T.S. 28-year-old male (B⁺→O⁺)

mother (i.e., HLA-A, B, DR 3 mismatches and an MLC 1 way S.I. 23). Prior to the transplantation, the patient received a 200-ml donor-specific blood transfusion (DST).

In a crossmatch test performed five months after the DST, the patient showed a 100% T-cell level and was B-cell antibody positive. The patient remained 100% antibody positive in later crossmatch tests over the 6-month clinical course observation which followed. Doses of CYA, at 2 mg/kg per day, were therefore administered three times a week after hemodialysis. Six months later, T-cell antibodies had decreased to 20% and warm and cold B-cell antibodies had decreased to 80%. The patient was then admitted to the hospital and underwent double filtration plasmapheresis four times over a period of 10 days. As a result, T-cell and B-cell antibodies became negative, and the transplantation was then performed. On the 6th day after the transplantation, the patient developed accelerated acute rejection, but recovered through MP pulse therapy. At present, 2 months after the transplantation, the patient shows a serum creatinine level of 1.3 mg/dl, which indicates satisfactory functioning of the transplanted kidney.

The efficacy of DSG against rejection after transplantations, previously detailed at the IVth Congress of the European Society for Organ Transplantation in 1989, is briefly described.

Efficacy of DSG in Treating Rejection Reactions After Kidney Transplantation

We used DSG in 52 rejection episodes which occurred in 44 kidney transplant cases. The 52 rejection episodes consisted of nine accelerated acute rejections (AAR), 24 acute rejections (AR), 11 late acute rejections (LAR), and 8 acute on chronic rejections (AOCR).

DSG was administered by drip infusion, in doses of 3, 5, or 7 mg/kg per day, and the efficacy of DSG against rejection reactions was evaluated on the basis of decreases in the serum creatinine level.

DSG was effective in 38 (73%) of the 52 rejection episodes. In terms of rejection type, DSG was effective in 6/9 (67%) of the cases of AAR, in 20/24 (83%) of the cases of AR, in 10/11 (91%) of the cases of LAR, and in 2/8 (25%) of the cases of AOCR (Table 3).

In cases in which remission was achieved, the serum creatinine level showed a gradual decrease, which, in most cases, started after DSG administration had been completed.

Side effects included leukopenia, which developed 14 times (or in 27% of the rejections) and thrombocytopenia, which developed 4 times (or in 8% of the rejections). There were also two cases of abdominal distension and one case each of lip numbness and facial suffusion. The severity of all side effects was slight, and no complications were observed.

Conclusions

Based on the results of our study, we arrived at the following conclusions:

1) DSG is effective in prophylactic use and in the treatment of rejection in kidney transplantation.
2) Compared to OKT3, DSG has a weaker effect on severe rejection reactions.
3) Compared to steroid pulse therapy, the effect of DSG is slowly manifested; i.e., DSG lowers serum creatinine levels gradually over a period of 3–5 days.
4) DSG has a stronger effect on late acute rejection than does OKT3 or methylprednisolone.
5) DSG suppresses the B-cell system, and therefore antibody production, and is thus effective in ABO-incompatible kidney transplantation involving humoral immunity, and in preformed antibody-positive kidney transplantation.
6) Regarding side effects, DSG slightly suppresses bone marrow function, thus leading to leukopenia and thrombocytopenia. However, granulocyte colony stimulating factor (CSF) proved to be effective in the treatment of leukopenia.
7) DSG causes fewer complications than OKT3 and steroid agents, especially in regard to infectious diseases.

References

1. Amemiya H, Suzuki S, Ota K, Takahashi K, Sonoda T, Ishibashi M, Omoto R, Koyama I, Dohi K, Fukuda Y, Fukao K (1990) A novel rescue drug, 15-deoxyspergualin. Transplantation 19:337–343

2. Takahashi K, Ota K, Tanabe K, Oba S, Teraoka S, Toma H, Agishi T, Kawaguchi H, Ito K (1990) Effect of a novel immunosuppressive agent, deoxyspergualin, on rejection in kidney transplant recipients. Transplant Proc 22:1606–1612

Therapeutic Use of Monoclonal Antibodies in Renal Transplantation

H. KREIS, C. LEGENDRE, and L. CHATENOUD[1]

Introduction

A wide variety of antilymphocyte monoclonal antibodies (MoAb) is now available for therapeutic use (Table 1). The majority of them, produced in mice and in rats, are directed against lymphocyte membrane antigens and/or receptors which are categorized in cluster of differentiation (CD). Each lymphocyte subset can be recognized according to the various CD expressed on their surface

One of the major advantages of MoAb is their homogeneous specificity and properties [1]. Monoclonal-induced immunosuppression has, therefore, greater selectivity, as each MoAb recognizes only one epitope of its target molecule. Therefore, the therapeutic use of MoAb allows: (1) more selective immunosuppression leading to decreased infectious risks, (2) a reduced rate of serum sickness because of the small amount of immunoglobulin needed, (3) blocking of the immune response at a selected level according to the role of the target molecule.

Combination of various MoAb, either simultaneously or consecutively, will probably allow better immunosuppression with risks lower than those of polyclonal antibodies and/or nonspecific chemical immunosuppressive agents.

A wide range of MoAb is already available for human use. They can be classified into three groups according to the function of the target antigen.

MoAb Directed Against the TCR/CD3 Complex

The TCR/CD3 complex allows T lymphocytes to recognize alloantigens in association with either MHC Class I or Class II molecules, and to be further activated [2]. The TCR/CD3 complex has two major parts (Fig. 1). One, devoted to antigen recognition, is made of two chains, an α chain and a β chain and represents the TCR. The

---

[1]Service de Transplantation and INSERSM U25 Hôpital Necker, Paris 75015, France

Table 1. Major monoclonal antibodies for therapeutic use

Anti CD$_2$	T11-2	(IgG$_1$)	E Rosette receptor
	T11-3	(IgG$_2$ a)	
Anti CD$_3$	OKT$_3$	(IgG$_2$ a)	T$_1$ (TCR)
	BMA	(IgG$_2$ b)	TCR $\alpha\beta$
Anti CD$_4$	OKT$_4$	(IgG$_2$ b)	T$_4$
	OKT$_4$ a	(IgG$_2$ a)	
Anti CD$_7$	RFT$_2$	(IgG$_2$ a)	T-Lymphoblasts
	CHH 380	(H-IgG$_1$ + M-IgG$_2$ a)	
Anti CD$_8$	OKT$_8$	(IgG$_1$)	T$_8$
Anti CD$_{25}$	33B3.1	(IgG$_2$ a)	
	Anti TAC		RIL-2 (a)
	CAMPATH-6		

other, the CD3 molecule allows the transduction of the activation signal produced by the recognition of the alloantigen. It is made of three chains, γ, δ, and ϵ. The specificity for an antigen is determined by the variable and constant parts of TCR. Blocking either the TCR or the CD3 will prevent lymphocyte activation and further proliferation and differentiation toward cytotoxic lymphocytes.

Anti-CD3 Monoclonal Antibodies

Anti-CD3 antibodies were the first to be used in the treatment of allograft rejection by Cosimi et al. [3,4]. Based on the very encouraging results reported in a small

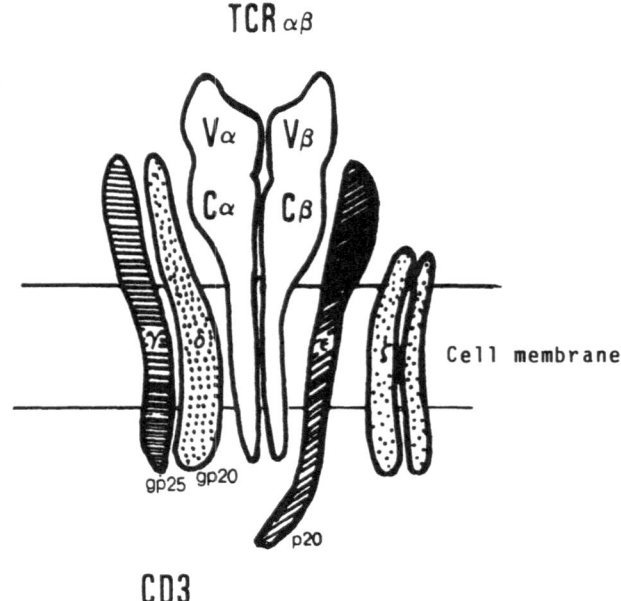

Fig. 1. The TCR/CD3 complex

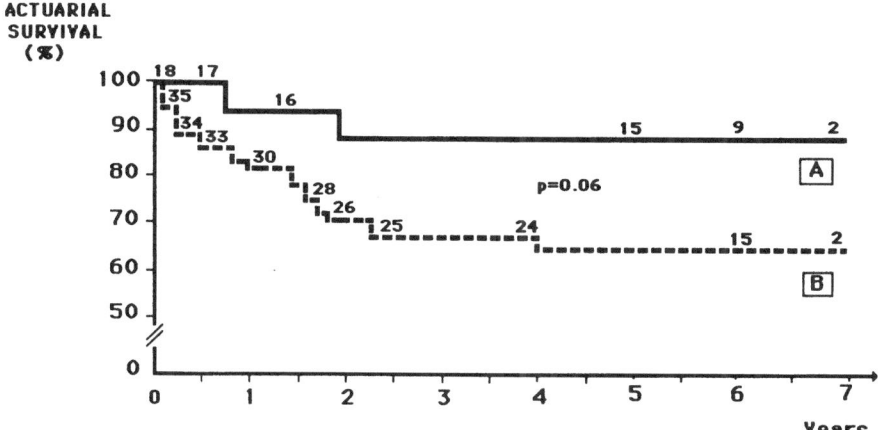

Fig. 2. Actuarial graft survival of OKT3-treated patients versus conventionally treated patients. All patients had at least 5 years of follow-up as of January 1, 1990

series of patients, a multicenter trial was performed in the United States, which demonstrated the efficacy of OKT3 used in first-line treatment of the first acute rejection episode occurring in renal transplantations, as compared with conventional high-dose steroids [5].

It was shown thereafter that OKT3 was also effective in the rescue treatment of patients undergoing rejection, who were resistant to conventional high-dose steroids and/or antithymocyte globulins [6,7]. Our group was the first to prove the efficacy (Fig. 2) of OKT3 when used as a prophylactic agent in association with conventional immunosuppressive agents which were useful in decreasing anti-OKT3 response [8–10]. Using a slightly different protocol, a multicenter trial in the United States confirmed that prophylactic OKT3 gave better results than cyclosporine A (personal communication). We have recently reported [11] that using OKT3 prophylactically was probably more effective than using it to treat ongoing acute rejection episodes (Fig. 3). OKT3 is now generally recognized as major immunosuppressive agent. However, it must not be used without knowledge of the following points.

Treatment Protocols

When used to treat acute rejection episodes, 5 mg i.v. OKT3 is usually given during a 7–10 day period without increasing or adding other immunosuppressive agents. A similar protocol is used to rescue steroid- and ATG-resistant rejection episodes [7]. However, it has recently been shown by our group that inflammatory cells infiltrating rejecting grafts were not completely cleared after 10 days of OKT3 treatment [12]. It is probable, but not yet demonstrated, that a combination treatment of OKT3 and steroids would be more effective than OKT3 used alone.

Used prophylactically, OKT3 has been administered according to two different protocols.

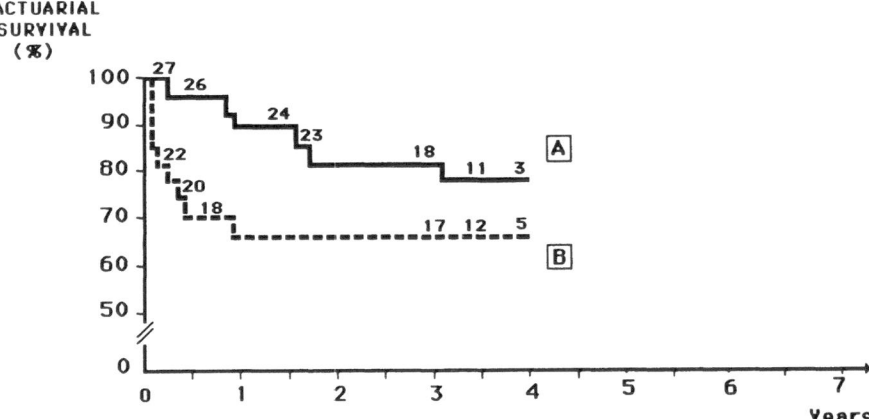

Fig. 3. Actuarial graft survival of patients receiving prophylactic treatment with OKT3 versus patients receiving OKT3 for the treatment of acute rejection episodes only

In our group [9], OKT3 is given during a maximum 30-day-period, in combination with 2–3 mg/kg per day Azathioprine and low doses of steroids. At the end of the one-month treatment period, OKT3 is withdrawn without adding any new immunosuppressive agents. It is thus possible to obtain results similar to those reported with cyclosporine A but without using that drug.

In other prophylactic protocols, OKT3 is used with either simultaneous or sequential cyclosporine A. In the latter case, cyclosporine A is started a few days before discontinuing OKT3, in order to get effective cyclosporine blood levels after MoAb withdrawal (personal communication).

Whatever the protocol, the daily dose in adults is always 5 mg per day. Attempts to decrease this dosage have always led to a higher degree of anti-OKT3 immunization and therefore to a lower activity of the MoAb (unpublished data). In contrast, increasing the daily dose to 10 or 15 mg in patients developing anti-OKT3 immunization allows the maintenance of effective OKT3 blood levels in about 50% of patients, without significantly increasing the so-called "first dose" syndrome [11].

In fact, no real attempts were made in adult patients to use drug dosage per body weight as is frequently done in children. This would probably be more appropriate than the use of reduced drugs.

Monitoring MoAb Treatment

As early as 1 hour after the first injection OKT3 MoAb induces a dramatic and concomitant decrease in T3+, T4+ and T8+ cells [4,10]. However, the impact of the MoAb on lymphocytes within the reticuloendothelial system is not well known. In mice, with similar dosages of an anti-CD3 antibody, partial T3+ cell depletion was observed in spleen and lymph nodes [13].

It is well known that after 3–5 days a significant proportion of T3−, T4+ and T3−, T8+ cells reappears in the circulation, indicating the presence of T3 modulating lymphocytes [14].

Similarly, noncirculating T lymphocytes can also demonstrate modulation of the CD3 molecule. CD3 modulating T lymphocytes were thus observed on sequential transplant biopsies performed in OKT3-treated patients [12]. It is highly probable, but not yet clearly demonstrated, that increasing the treatment dose will lead to a higher percentage of CD3 modulating cells within the lymphoreticularendothelial system, and will thus induce a more profound immunosuppression with an increased risk of infectious or mitogenic complications.

As the CD3 molecule is closely associated with the TCR, OKT3-induced antigenic modulation leads, in fact, to the modulation of the whole TCR/CD3 complex. Therefore, these cells are immunoincompetent. However, a few hours after OKT3 discontinuation, OKT3 blood levels drop below the level of efficacy and a rapidly growing number of T lymphocytes exhibiting the TCR/CD3 complex reappear. This can be observed not only in the blood, but also in the graft, where CD3 modulating lymphocytes, which have not all been cleared, reexpress the TCR/CD3 complex, making them immunocompetent again.

Therefore, monitoring the number of circulating CD3+ cells at least 3 times a week in OKT3-treated patients is mandatory. As soon as more than 10% of circulating CD3 lymphocytes are present, OKT3 must be either discontinued or increased [11]. Monitoring OKT3 blood levels and/or appearance of anti-OKT3 IgG has no clinical use. However, it will help to understand any unusual situation.

Anti-CD3 Side Effects

Among the various side effects that can be induced by OKT3 MoAb, the first-dose syndrome [8,9], induced by a transient T cell activation [15], is directly related to the drug itself. Another side effect, anti-MoAb immunization [10,16–18] appears as a consequence of a xenoprotein and is observed with all xenogeneic MoAb. The last side effect, the risk induced by overimmunosuppression, that is, infectious and mitogenic complications, is shared by all potent immunosuppressive agents, and more especially by all combinations of potent immunosuppressive agents.

The First-Dose Syndrome

Immediately following the first OKT3 injection, a clinical syndrome composed of high fever, chills, headache, diarrhea, and vomiting can be observed [8]. Fever at least is always present, attesting to the efficacy of the MoAb. Dyspnea, tachycardia, hypotension, skin rash, arthralgia, and psychiatric behavior are seldom observed. Respiratory distress with pulmonary edema does not usually occur when the patient has no fluid overload before the first OKT3 injection [4,5,9,19]. Most of these symptoms generally disappear after 2–3 days. Nevertheless, they can last throughout the treatment period in transplant recipients of HLA identical kidneys (unpublished data). This first-dose syndrome is not observed, at least with similar intensity, with other anti-T cell MoAbs. It has been shown by our group [15,20], as well as by others [21], that due to OKT3-induced monocyte activation a number of cytokines are released in the blood immediately after the first OKT3 injection. Among them are tumor necrosis factor (TNF), interferon γ (IFNγ), interleukin-2 (IL-2), IL-3, and IL-6. Cytokine levels were back to normal after 24 hours despite persistent OKT3 treatment.

Although other anti-T lymphocyte MoAb can induce T cell opsonization and depletion, only OKT3 has been held responsible for the cytokine release syndrome [22–24]. In our group [25], it has been possible to reproduce in mice a similar first-dose syndrome using an anti-CD3 MoAb. In this study, pathological studies demonstrated that organs such as liver and lung exhibited major changes. These observations could, at least partially, explain the increased incidence of transient renal failure sometimes observed after the first OKT3 injection. High doses of MoAb were correlated with significant mortality.

It is now well established that high-dose steroids, administered at least 1 hour before OKT3 injection, can drastically reduce the release of cytokines that follows the first injection of OKT3 [26–28,30] (L. Chatenoud et al., unpublished data). Clinical symptoms that follow OKT3 injection are significantly less severe in mice when steroids are administered 30–60 minutes before the MoAb [25]. In man, however, the first-dose syndrome does not seem to have decreased intensity, whether steroids are given 1 hour before, or simultaneously with OKT3 injection (L. Chatenoud et al., unpublished data).

The severity of the first-dose syndrome in kidney graft recipients is probably related to: (1) the number of activated T lymphocytes already present at the time of the first OKT3 injection and (2) the lack of steroid therapy before and during OKT3 treatment. Thus, more severe reactions were observed in recipients of an HLA-identical kidney who were treated by Azathioprine and prophylactic OKT3 without steroids, than in treatment of acute rejection episodes or in the prophylactic treatment of cadaveric kidney recipients.

Corticosteroids are not only anti-inflammatory agents, but also exhibit an inhibitory effect on cytokine production.

Anti-MoAb Immunization

Monoclonal antibodies available today are produced in animals (mice or rats). Therefore, xenogeneic immunization is one of the major side effects which can limit all MoAb utilization. When OKT3 is used as the sole immunosuppressive regimen, almost all patients develop anti-OKT3 antibodies within a short time (usually before the end of a 10-day period) [8,10,16,17,18]. We have shown [9,17] that combining OKT3 with conventional immunosuppression (Azathioprine 2–3 mg/kg per day and low doses of steroids) or cyclosporine A can drastically reduce both the frequency and the intensity of anti-OKT3 immunization and can delay its occurrence. A very small number of patients will develop anti-OKT3 immunization in a 10- to 14-day treatment course, and we observed [11] IgG anti-OKT3 antibodies in only 50% of kidney graft recipients treated prophylactically for 30 days. In fact, 32% of the patients thus treated developed anti-MoAb IgG during the treatment period, whereas in the other 18% they appeared after OKT3 discontinuation. However, there is no close correlation between the occurrence of IgG and blood repopulation by T3 + cells, as in some patients having a low antibody response, OKT3 can still be in excess although at non-effective levels as compared to the amount of IgG. This explains why monitoring cells exhibiting CD3 is more important than monitoring IgG levels.

Anti-OKT3 response is usually composed of IgM and IgG, but only the latter are neutralizing for OKT3 [10,17]. It has been shown by Baudrihaye et al. [16] and Chatenoud et al. [31] that anti-OKT3 antibodies have a very restricted specificity, as only anti-isotypic IgG2a and anti-idiotypic (F(ab), F(ab') 2) were demonstrated. Anti-idiotypic antibodies neutralize OKT3 immunosuppressive activity by preventing its linkage with T lymphocytes.

We also observed [11] that about half of our patients exhibited an early and strong anti-OKT3 immune response, whereas in the other half the response occurred later with a much lower intensity. In this latter group of patients, increasing the daily dose of OKT3 to 10–15 mg allowed restoration of the percentage of T3+ cells to 0, whereas in the early responders this percentage was not influenced by increasing the OKT3 dose to 15 mg.

It has recently been shown (personal communication) that previous anti-OKT3 immunization did not preclude the re-use of OKT3 for the treatment of a second rejection episode (or a first one, when immunization occurred during a prophylactic course), even though mild levels of anti-OKT3 were still present at the time of retreatment. This is a very strong argument in favor of using OKT3, either as prophylactic treatment or as first-line for the treatment of acute rejection.

Anti-TCR Monoclonal Antibodies

The only MoAb directed against the constant part of TCR which is so far available for human use is BMA 031, a mouse IgG2b [32,33]. Its mode of action differs from that of OKT3 in many ways: (1) There is only partial T cell depletion after BMA injection, ranging from 5 to 50 mg/day; (2) If modulation of the TCR/CD3 complex is also observed with BMA, not all T cells are modulating, and BMA coated cells are always present [32], which, in particular, is never observed with OKT3.

In addition, anti-BMA immunization always occurred rapidly and with a high intensity. This high immunogenicity is probably related to a lower immunosuppressive capacity, as compated with OKT3.

As a matter of fact, the prophylactic use of BMA in our hands (unpublished data), either at 5 or 20 mg/day has never been associated with good graft results. Almost all patients developed relatively severe graft dysfunction after only a few days, either due to rejection because of neutralization of BMA by anti-BMA antibodies or because of serum sickness related to high production of BMA anti-BMA complexes (Table 2).

However, it has been suggested by the Munich group [34] that short prophylactic treatment consisting of two boluses of 50 mg BMA each at days 0 and 2 could significantly improve the results of kidney grafts. This is in the process of being confirmed by a multicenter trial. On the other hand, it must be said that the tolerance of BMA is far better than that of OKT3 and with BMA the first-dose syndrome is either not observed or is seen on a very mild basis which consists of low fever after the first BMA injection [34]. After the first injection, only TNF were increased, without any

Table 2. Rejection episodes in cadaveric kidney recipients treated by a prophylactic course of either 20 mg/day (*I*) or 5 mg/day (*II*) of BI 51 013 (*BMA*) monoclonal antibody

Protocol	No. of patients	Rejection episodes	Reversible rejection	Mean time of onset
I	5	4	3	11 ± 2 d
II	3	3	2	9 ± 3 d

increase in IFNγ or in IL-2 [32,35]. This is in agreement with the low in vitro mitogenic capacity of BMA.

Monoclonal Antibodies Directed Against Cytokine Receptors

A wide variety of cytokines appear as important mediators during the immune response process [36,37]. Cytokines usually act through a specific receptor which is present on the surface membrane of target cells. So far the only MoAb anti cytokine receptors which are available for human use are directed against the IL-2 receptor. This receptor is present only on activated T cells [38], which explains the interest in MoAb able either to destroy this specific T cell subset or to block its function without modifying T cell subsets which are not involved in an immune process. High affinity RIL-2 is composed of two chains, an α chain and a β chain, each chain representing a low affinity receptor. So far the only anti-RIL-2 MoAbs which are available for human use are directed against the α chain of the receptor, which has a molecular weight of 55 kDa (p55) and expresses the Tac or CD25 antigen.

Kirkman et al. [39] were the first to demonstrate better survival of cardiac allografts in mice receiving an anti-CD25 MoAb. Only MoAb able to block IL-2 linkage with the IL-2 receptor have an immunosuppressive effect.

In human renal transplantation, Soulillou in Nantes [24], using the 33B3.1 MoAb directed against the α chain of RIL-2 and Strom in Boston [40], using the anti-Tac MoAb were able to prevent the occurrence of acute rejection episodes. In their hands, these two MoAbs gave results similar to those obtained with polyclonal antilymphocyte globulins, but with a lower incidence of side effects. Cyclosporine A seems to be a necessary adjunct for the anti-Tac MoAb but not for the 33B3.1.

The first attempts made with these MoAb in the treatment of acute rejection episodes were disappointing, although a large number of activated T cells expressing the IL-2 receptor were present. The fact that these MoAb are directed only against the low affinity receptor may explain these poor results.

A multicenter study using the 33B3.1 MoAb, which is in progress, will be necessary to confirm the good results already obtained in single center trials.

Monoclonal Antibodies Directed Against Cell Adhesion Molecules

Various molecules present on T cell membranes allow better adhesion between T lymphocytes and antigen-presenting cells. Among them are LFA1 (Fig. 4), CD2, CD4, and CD8 molecules and their ligand, ICAM-1 and LFA3 molecules and MHC Class II and I, respectively. Monoclonal antibodies directed against these molecules can prevent, or at least decrease, the adhesion capacity of T cells during the process of alloantigen recognition, and can therefore minimize its consequences.

Today, only anti-LFA1 MoAb have been studied in man and have allowed good survival rates of nonrelated bone marrow grafts. It is still too early to know whether anti-LFA1 MoAb will also be helpful in organ transplantation, in combination with

Fig. 4. Adhesion molecules involved in the process of alloantigen recognition by T lymphocytes

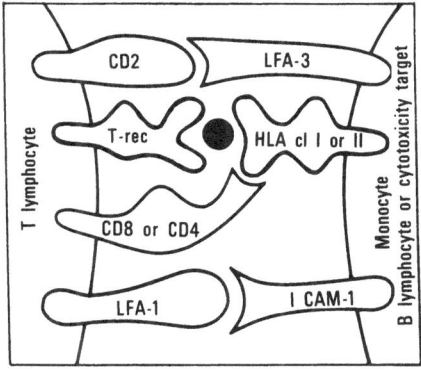

conventional immunosuppression, or in combination with other MoAb such as those directed against the TCR/CD3 complex.

CD4-bearing lymphocytes recognize MHC Class II restricted alloantigens [41]. Therefore, it can be postulated that anti-CD4 MoAb could prevent the recognition of alloantigens by CD4 + T lymphocytes and thus block the immune response process.

This immunosuppressive capacity of anti-CD4 MoAb has been shown in a number of animal experiments concerning either the prevention or the treatment of various autoimmune diseases [42–45]. Interestingly, it seems that anti-CD4 MoAb are able to induce immune tolerance for various antigens. Such tolerance can be observed without CD4 lymphocyte depletion and can be maintained indefinitely, provided antigen injection is periodically repeated [46–48]. The latter effect appears especially interesting in organ transplantation.

As human anti-CD4 MoAb also recognize primate T cells, the first experiments with anti-CD4 MoAb were performed in monkeys. These experiments were performed both by Cosimi [49] and by Jonker [50,51]. Using isolated OKT4A, or a combination of OKT4 and OKT4A, they were able to significantly prolong kidney allografts in Rhesus or Cynomolgus monkeys. Human studies using anti-CD4 MoAb are only starting. According to Chatenoud et al. [35], it seems that another anti-CD4 MoAb, BL4, led to only partial and transient CD4 + cell depletion, but that all CD4 + T cells were coated with the MoAb without any observed antigenic modulation of the CD4 molecule. In addition, none of the patients thus treated had increased cytokine levels and none presented any side effects other than xenoimmunization. A protocol using OKT4A prophylactic treatment of renal grafts in man is now in progress in Boston. MoAb directed against other cell adhesion molecules have not yet been used in organ transplantation.

However, in the years to come, a wide variety of monoclonal antibodies will be available in man, allowing, by their selectivity, and by their combined administration, either consecutively or simultaneously as "poly-monoclonal" sera, a more specific type of immunosuppression. Antixenogeneic immunization will probably be avoided by humanized constructs of MoAb, such as the anti-CD7 (SDZ CHH 380), which is in the process of being studied in man. We are still only at the dawn of immunosuppression in organ transplantation, but monoclonal antibodies are certain to constitute a fundamental new step toward specific tolerance.

References

1. Kohler G, Milstein C (1975) Continuous cultures of fused cells secreting antibody of predefined specificity. Nature 256:495–497
2. Kronenberg M, Siu G, Hood LE, Shastri N (1986) The molecular genetics of the T-cell antigen recognition. Annu Rev Immunol 4:529–591
3. Cosimi AB, Colvin RB, Burton RC, Rubin RH, Godstein G, Kung PC, Hansen WP, Delmonico FL, Russel PS (1981) Use of monoclonal antibodies to T-cell subsets for immunologic monitoring and treatment in recipients of renal allograft. N Engl J Med 305:308–314
4. Cosimi AB, Burton RC, Colvin B, Goldstein G, Delmonico FL, Laquaglia MP, Tolkoff-Rubin N, Rubin RH, Herrin JT, Russel PS (1981) Treatment of acute renal allograft rejection with OKT3 monoclonal antibody. Transplantation 32:535–539
5. Ortho multicenter transplant study group (1985) A randomized clinical trial of OKT3 monoclonal antibody for acute rejection of cadaveric renal transplant. N Engl J Med 313:337–342
6. Goldstein G, Norman DJ, Shield CF, Kreis H, Burdick J, Flye MW, Rivolta E, Starzl T, Monaco A (1986) OKT3 monoclonal antibody reversal of acute renal allograft rejection unresponsive to conventional immunosuppressive treatments. In: Meryman HT (ed) Transplantation approaches to graft rejection. Alan R. Liss, New York, pp 239–249
7. Norman DJ, Barry JM, Bennett WM, Leone M, Henell K, Funnell B, Hubert B (1988) The use of OKT3 in cadaveric renal transplantation for rejection that is unresponsive to conventional anti rejection therapy. Am J Kidney Dis 11:90–93
8. Vigeral P, Chkoff N, Chatenoud L, Campos H, Lacombe M, Droz D, Goldstein G, Bach JF, Kreis H (1986) Prophylactic use of OKT3 monoclonal antibody in cadaver kidney recipients. Utilization of OKT3 as the sole immunosuppressive agent. Transplantation 41:730–733
9. Debure A, Chkoff N, Chatenoud L, Lacombe M, Campos H, Noël LH, Goldstein G, Bach JF, Kreis H (1988) One-month prophylactic use of OKT3 in cadaver kidney transplant recipients. Transplantation 45:546–553
10. Chatenoud L, Baudrihaye MF, Chkoff N, Kreis H, Bach JF (1983) Immunologic follow up of renal allograft recipients treated prophylactically by OKT3 alone. Transplant Proc 15:643–645
11. Kreis H, Chkoff N, Chatenoud L, Debure A, Lacombe M, Chrétien Y, Legendre C, Caillat S, Bach JF (1989) A randomized trial comparing the efficacy of OKT3 used to prevent or to treat rejection. Transplant Proc 21:3–6
12. Caillat-Zucman S, Blumenfeld N, Legendre C, Noël LH, Bach JF, Kreis H, Chatenoud L (to be published) Human in vivo antigenic modulation induced by the anti-T cell OKT3 monoclonal antibody. Transplantation
13. Hirsch R, Eckhaus M, Auchincloss H, Sachs DH, Bluestone JA (1988) Effects of in vivo administration of anti-T3 monoclonal antibody on T cell function in mice: immunosuppression of transplantation response. J Immunol 140:3766–3772
14. Chatenoud L, Baudrihaye MF, Schindler J, Kreis H, Goldstein G, Bach JF (1982) Human in vivo antigenic modulation induced by the anti-T cell OKT3 monoclonal antibody. Eur J Immunol 12:979–982
15. Chatenoud L, Ferran C, Legendre C, Thouard I, Reuter A, Gevaert Y, Kreis H, Franchimont P, Bach JF (to be published) In vivo cell activation following OKT3 administration: systemic cytokine release and modulation by corticosteroids. Transplantation
16. Baudrihaye MF, Chatenoud L, Kreis H, Goldstein G, Bach JF (1984) Unusually restricted anti-isotype human immune response to OKT3 monoclonal antibody. Eur J Immunol 14:686–691
17. Chatenoud L (1986) The immune response against therapeutic monoclonal antibodies. Immunol Today 7:367–368

18. Chatenoud L, Jonker M, Villemain F, Goldstein G, Bach JF (1986) The human immune response to the OKT3 monoclonal antibody is oligoclonal. Science 232:1406–1408

19. Thistlethwaite JR, Gaber AO, Haag BW, Aronson AJ, Broelsh CE, Suart JK, Stuart FP (1987) OKT3 treatment of steroid-resistant renal allograft rejection. Transplantation 43:176–184

20. Chatenoud L, Ferran C, Reuter A, Legendre C, Gevaert Y, Kreis H, Franchimont P, Bach JF (1989) Systemic reaction to the anti-T-cell monoclonal antibody OKT3 in relation to serum levels of tumor necrosis factor and interferon γ. New Engl J Med 320:1420–1421

21. Abramowicz D, Schandenne L, Goldman M, Crusiaux A, Vereerstraeten O, De Pauw L, Wybran J, Kinneart P, Dupont E, Toussaint C (1989) Release of tumor necrosis factor, interleukin 2 and gamma-interferon in serum after injection of OKT3 monoclonal antibody in kidney transplant recipients. Transplantation 47:606–608

22. Kirkman RL, Araujo JL, Brush GF, Carpenter CB, Milford EL, Reinherz EL, Schlossman SF, Strom TB, Tilney NL (1983) Treatment of acute renal allograft rejection with monoclonal anti-T12 antibody. Transplantation 36:620–626

23. Jonker M, Goldstein G, Balner H (1983) Effects of in vivo administration of monoclonal antibodies specific for human T cell subpopulations on the immune system in a Rhesus monkey model. Transplantation 35:521–529

24. Soulillou JP, Peyronnel P, Le Mauff B, Hourmant M, Olive D, Mawas C, Delaage M, Hirn M, Jacques Y (1987) Prevention of rejection of kidney transplants by monoclonal antibody directed against interleukin-2 receptor. Lancet I:1339–1342

25. Ferran C, Sheehan K, Dy M, Schreiber R, Landais P, Noël LH, Grau G, Bluestone J, Bach JF, Chatenoud L (to be published) Cytokine related syndrome following injection of anti-CD3 monoclonal antibody: further evidence for transient in vivo T cell activation. Eur J Immunol

26. Gyure PM, Girard MT, Morganelli PM, Manganiello PD (1988) Glucocorticoid effects on the production and actions of immune cytokines. J Steroid Biochem 30:89–93

27. Kern JA, Lamb RJ, Reed JC, Daniele RP, Nowell PC (1988) Dexamethasone inhibition of interleukin 1 beta production by human monocytes. Posttranscriptional Mechanisms. J Clin Invest 81:237–244

28. Reed JC, Abidi AH, Alpers JD, Hoover RG, Robb RJ, Nowell PC (1986) Effect of cyclosporin A and dexamethasone on interleukin 2 receptor gene expression. J Immunol 137:150–154

29. Sariban E, Imamura K, Luebbers R, Kufe D (1988) Transcriptional and posttranscriptional regulation of tumor necrosis factor gene expression in human monocytes. J Clin Invest 81:1506–1510

30. Waage A, Bakke O (1987) Glucocorticoids suppress the production of tumour necrosis factor by lipopolysaccharide-stimulated human monocytes. Immunology 63:299–302

31. Chatenoud L, Baudrihaye MF, Chkoff N, Kreis H, Goldstein G, Bach JF (1986) Restriction of the human in vivo immune response against the mouse monoclonal antibody OKT3. J Imunol 137:830–838

32. Chatenoud L, Ferran C, Legendre C, Kurrle R, Kreis H, Bach JF (to be published) Immunological follow-up of renal allograft recipients treated with the BMA 031 (anti-TCR) monoclonal antibody. Transplant Proc

33. Nashan B, Wonigeit K, Schwinzer R, Schlitt HJ, Kurrle R, Pichlmayr R (1987) Fine specificity of a panel of antibodies against the TCR/CD3 complex. Transplant Proc 19:4270–4272

34. Hillebrand G, Rothang E, Hammer C, Illner WD, Schleibner S, Racenberg J, Gurland HJ, Land W (1989) Experience with a new monoclonal antibody in clinical kidney. Transplantation 21:1776–1777

35. Chatenoud L, Ferran C, Bach JF (1990) Utilisation clinique des anticorps anti-lymphocytes T. In: Flammarion (ed) Actualitées Néphrologiques, Hôpital Necker, Paris, pp 183–203

36. Balkwill F (1988) Cytokinea-soluble factors in immune responses. Curr Opin Immunol 1:241–249

37. Balkwill FR, Burke F (1989) The cytokine network. Immunol Today 10:299–301

38. Waldmann TA (1988) The multichain interleukin-2 receptor: A target for immunotherapy of patients with adult T cell leukemia, autoimmune disorders and individuals receiving allografts. J Autoimmunity 1:641–653

39. Kirkman RL, Barett LV, Gaulton GN, Kelley VE, Ythier A, Strom TB (1985) Administration of anti-interleukin 2 receptor monoclonal antibody prolongs cardiac allograft survival in mice. J Exp Med 162:358–362

40. Shapiro MD, Kirkman RL, Carpenter CB, Milford EL, Tilney NL, Waldmann TA, Zimmerman CE, Ramos EL, Strom TB (1988) Initial trials of the anti-human IL-2 receptor monoclonal antibody anti-Tac in clinical renal transplantation. Transplant Proc 21:1766–1768

41. Swain SL (1983) T cell subsets and the recognition of MHC class. Immunol Rev 74:129–142

42. Wofsy D, Ledbetter JA, Hendler PL, Seaman WE (1985) Treatment of murine lupus with monoclonal anti T-cell antibody. J Immunol 134:852–857

43. Shizuru MA, Tayloedwards C, Bank BA, Gregory AK, Fathman CG (1985) Immunotherapy of the non-obese diabetic mouse: treatment with an antibody to T helper lymphocytes. Science 240:659–661

44. Waldor MK, Sriram S, Hardy R, Herzenberg LA, Lamer L, Lim M, Steinman L (1985) Reversal of experimental allergic encephalomyelitis with monoclonal antibody to a T-cell subset marker. Science 227:415–417

45. Ranges GE, Sriram S, Copper SM (1985) Prevention of type II collagen-induced arthritis by in vivo treatment with anti-L3T4. J Exp Med 162:1105–1110

46. Benjamin RJ, Waldmann H (1986) Induction of tolerance of monoclonal antibody therapy. Nature 320:449–451

47. Benjamin RJ, Qin S, Wise MP (1988) Monoclonal antibodies for tolerance induction: a possible role for the CD4 (L3T4) and CD11a (LFA-1) molecules in self-nonself discrimination. Eur J Immunol 18:1079–1088

48. Gutstein NL, Seaman WE, Scott JH, Wofsy D (1986) Induction of immune tolerance by administration of monoclonal antibody to L3T4. J Immunol 137:1127–1132

49. Cosimi AB, Burton RC, Kung RC, Colvin R, Goldstein G, Lifter H, Rhodes W, Russel PS (1981) Evaluation in primate renal allograft recipients of monoclonal antibody to human T-cell subclasses. Transplant Proc 13:499–503

50. Jonker M, Neuhaus P, Zurcher C, Fucello A, Goldstein G (1985) OKT4 and OKT4A antibody treatment as immunosuppression for kidney transplantation in rhesus monkeys. Transplantation 39:247–253

51. Jonker M, Nooij FJM, Chatenoud L (1986) Immunosuppression by monoclonal anti-T cell antibodies. Transplant Proc 18:1287–1290

Long-Term Follow-Up of Renal Transplantation – Chronic Rejection and Recurrence of Nephritis

RICHARD N. FINE[1]

SUMMARY. Graft loss in long-term (> 10 years) surviving recipients occurs at a rate of 3%–5% annually. The most frequent cause of graft loss is chronic rejection. Unfortunately, no current therapeutic intervention is uniformly successful in forestalling the inevitable decline in graft function. The proposal that hyperfiltration is a significant factor contributing to nephron loss in long-term surviving grafts is interesting; however, controlled clinical trials of protein restricted diets, with concomitant accurate serial measurements of graft function are required before such an approach can be recommended.

Acute rejection and non-compliance with the immunosuppressive medications should be considered with abrupt declines in graft function in long-term recipients. Since such reduction in graft function is often asymptomatic, it is important that surveillance be continued in long-term recipients.

Recurrence of the original disease in the graft contributes minimally to graft loss in long-term surviving grafts. However, the incidence of recurrence causing graft failure during the second decade of function is < 5%. Recurrence of diabetic nephropathy may take > 20 years to become clinically manifest. The simultaneous transplantation of both the pancreas and kidney may ultimately arrest the recurrence of diabetic nephropathy.

Introduction

In the 21 reports [1] between 1974 and 1988 detailing long-term (> 10 years) patient and graft survival following renal transplantation the mortality rate was 3–5% per annum after 10 years. For patients alive after 10 years, 72–85% survived an additional 5 years. Graft loss after 10 years paralleled patient mortality, with 71–90% of the grafts still functioning at 15 years. Therefore, deterioration of graft function in

---

[1]Department of Pediatrics, School of Medicine, State University of New York at Stony Brook, Stony Brook, NY 11794-8111, USA

long-term (> 10 years) surviving renal allograft recipients is not an unusual occurrence. The potential causes of declining graft function are: (1) chronic rejection, (2) non-immunological phenomenon, (3) acute rejection, (4) recurrence of the primary disease in the graft, (5) non-compliance with immunosuppressive drugs, (6) de novo glomerulonephritis, (7) nephrotoxic drugs, (8) renal artery stenosis, (9) hypertension, (10) concomitant infection, and (11) volume depletion. Although all of the above phenomena require consideration anytime there are perturbations of renal function in a long-term surviving renal allograft recipient, I will discuss only the first five entities in any detail in this manuscript.

Results and Discussion

Chronic Rejection

The *clinical manifestations* of chronic rejection are: (1) a progressive deterioration of graft function which ultimately results in graft loss, (2) proteinuria which frequently is associated with the nephrotic syndrome, and (3) hypertension [2]. The *histological manifestations* of chronic rejection are: (1) *Transplant glomerulopathy* with splitting and reduplication of the glomerular basement membrane without evidence of immune complex deposition by either immunofluorescence or electron microscopy; and (2) *Vascular rejection* manifested by nephron loss with interstitial fibrosis and tubular atrophy [3].

The incidence of graft loss from chronic rejection in grafts surviving > 10 years has been variable; however, it is the most common cause of graft loss in long-term functioning grafts [1]. In 6 series from centers in the United States, Europe, and Australia which were reported between 1982 and 1989 the incidence has varied from 8%–24% (Table 1) with 5 of the 6 centers indicating an incidence between 8% and 11% [4–9].

Once chronic rejection is present no treatment has been uniformly successful in changing the clinical course of inevitable decline in graft function with ultimate graft loss. Feehally et al. [10] state that "no immune-modulating maneuver is consistently successful once chronic rejection is established with histopathological evidence of nephron loss and mesangial sclerosis." These authors further state that "no treatment has yet been shown to change the rate of decline in renal function in recipients with chronic rejection." Consequently, once the diagnosis of chronic rejection is established, treatment should be directed toward optimizing the conservative management of chronic renal failure. The admonition against the use of additional corticosteroid

Table 1. Incidence of chronic rejection in grafts surviving > 10 years

Report	Center	Year	% Chronic rejection
Mahoney et al. [4]	Sydney	1982	8
Gueco et al. [5]	Cambridge	1985	24
Grapin et al. [6]	Paris/Tenon	1987	9
Lee et al. [7]	Richmond	1987	8
LeFrançois et al. [8]	Lyon	1987	11
Rao et al. [9]	Minneapolis	1989	9

treatment in a setting of chronic rejection is emphasized by Kirkman et al. [11] who note that "increased dosages of corticosteroids may have contributed to the deaths of 2 of 22 patients" with chronic rejection who were treated with increased dosages on one or more occasions.

Non-Immunologic Phenomenon

Feehally et al. [10] hypothesized that chronic renal transplant failure was primarily related to non-immune mechanisms. These authors postulated that hyperfiltration of the remnant nephrons of the graft was the dominant factor leading to the unrelenting decline of graft function. In order to test this hypothesis the authors prescribed a low protein (0.6 gm/kg per day) diet to 5 recipients with chronic renal transplant failure. Following initiation of the diet there was a significant decrease in the slope of the 1/serum creatinine curve for a period of 2–12 months. This hypothesis was further supported by Schmidt [12] who discontinued azathioprine in 5 recipients with chronic rejection and noted that the rate of loss of graft function, as indicated by the slope of 1/serum creatinine, did not change. From these data he concluded "that immunologic mechanisms do not play a major role in the predictable loss of graft function" from chronic rejection. Although this hypothesis is interesting, it is obvious that more detailed studies, on a larger number of recipients, are required before the concept receives additional support. Controlled clinical trials utilizing precise measurements of glomerular filtration rate may be indicated in the future.

Acute Rejection

Acute rejection in the early post-transplant period is well described; however, there is a paucity of information detailing acute rejection episodes in recipients surviving a second decade with a functioning graft. Rao et al. [9] analyzed the incidence, clinical and histological data, and outcome of 69 recipients who survived > 10 years with a functioning graft. During the second decade of graft function, 15 recipients developed 20 acute rejection episodes. *Clinical manifestations* — proteinuria (0.7–6.3 gm), hypertension, fluid retention, and congestive heart failure — were present in only 8 of the 20 (40%) episodes of acute rejection, whereas in 12 of the 20 (60%) episodes the recipients were asymptomatic. *Histologic manifestations* were interstitial edema and interstitial mononuclear cell infiltrate without involvement of the glomeruli and blood vessels. These histologic changes were at times superimposed upon evidence of chronic rejection. Thirteen of the acute rejection episodes in 8 recipients were treated with intravenous corticosteroids. The response to treatment was as follows: complete response, 6 out of 13 (46%); partial response, 4 out of 13 (31%); and no response, 3 out of 13 (23%). Of the 8 recipients 2 died of septic complications within one month of treatment and 2 recipients resumed dialysis at 6 and 12 months following corticosteroid treatment. These authors concluded that: (1) long-term surveillance of recipients with long-term surviving renal allografts is required, because the majority of recipients who manifested acute rejection during the second decade of graft function were asymptomatic, (2) the potential response of a late occurring acute rejection episode to intravenous corticosteroids is excellent, and (3) a precise diagnosis is imperative in order to avoid unnecessary corticosteroid treatment of chronic rejection without any potential salutary effect.

Non-Compliance

In a recent report by Schweizer et al. [13] the *incidence* of non-compliance with immunosuppressive therapy following renal transplantation was determined, both prospectively and retrospectively. Between 1971 and 1984 the incidence of non-compliance was determined retrospectively and was found to be 18% (47 out of 269), whereas in the prospective analysis from 1984–1987 the incidence was 15% (30 out of 196). Didlake et al. [14] noted an incidence of non-compliance of 4.7% (25 out of 531) between 1980 and 1986, and stated that all graft losses after 36 months occurred in patients with documented non-compliance. The latter data are from patients transplanted in the cyclosporine era, and therefore the contribution of non-compliance to long-term (> 10 years) graft dysfunction could not be determined. Potter et al. [15] described the course of 29 pediatric recipients who had a functioning graft for > 10 years and a serum creatinine level of < 2.0 mg/dl. During the second post-transplant decade 2 recipients, of whom one was non-compliant, each lost their graft and 5 recipients, 2 of whom were non-compliant, had an increase in the serum creatinine level of > 1.0 mg/dl. Therefore, non-compliance can contribute to both *early* and *late graft dysfunction*. In the report of Schweizer et al. [13] rejection and/or death occurred in 91% of the non-compliant recipients in the retrospective analysis and in 37% of the recipients in the prospective study. Early identification of the non-compliant recipient, with subsequent treatment of the acute rejection episode, followed by reinstitution of the maintenance immunosuppressive regimen may be effective in sustaining long-term graft function in the non-compliant recipient.

Recurrence of Primary Disease

Recurrence of either a metabolic or a glomerular primary disease accounts for < 2% of all graft failures, whereas the overall incidence of recurrence is probably 5–10 times more common [16]. Most recurrence occurs in the early post-transplant period; only rarely does recurrence from such primary renal diseases as membranoproliferative glomerulonephritis types I and II, IgA nephropathy, and focal glomerulosclerosis contribute to late graft failure [16].

Starzl et al. [17] in 1974, reporting on a decade of follow-up in early cases of renal transplantation, noted "transmission glomerulonephritis" in 8 of 35 graft biopsies obtained at 2 years post-transplant. Seven of the 8 grafts failed at 27–77 months following transplantation. The precise definition of "transmission glomerulonephritis" was not provided. In 1982, Kirkman et al. [11] reported that biopsy proven recurrent glomerulonephritis was evident at 10–11 years post-transplant in 3 out of 32 (9%) grafts which were lost > 5 years post-transplant. Of the 21 reports [1] detailing the outcome of long-term (> 10 years) surviving renal allografts, only 4 [6,8,18,19] mention recurrent disease as a cause of late graft failure. In these 4 reports the incidence of graft failure from recurrence was < 5% and no specific data was provided regarding the type of primary disease (Table 2).

The incidence of recurrent disease in diabetic recipients is currently underestimated because, from recurrence of the diabetic lesion, a mean time of about 20 years for graft failure to occur seems likely [16]. However, there is the possibility that combined pancreas and kidney transplantation may protect the kidney from recurrence of the diabetic lesion. Bohman et al. [20] noted that the glomerular basement

Table 2. Recurrence in long-term (> 10 years) functioning renal allografts

Report	Year	No. of patients	No. of recurrences	
			< 10 Years	> 10 Years
Vanrenterghem et al. [18]	1987	93	2	1
Grapin et al. [6]	1987	90		1
LeFrançois et al. [8]	1987	64		3
McGeown et al. [19]	1988	62	4	

membrane thickening and mesangial expansion typical of diabetic nephropathy in all kidneys >2 years post-transplant were not seen in diabetic recipients who received simultaneous pancreas and kidney transplants.

References

1. Mahony JF (1989) Long term results and complications of transplantation: The kidney. Transplant Proc 21:1433–1434
2. Kreis H (1981) Transplanted kidney: Natural history. In: Hamburger J, Crosnier J, Bach J, Kreis H (eds) Renal transplantation theory and practice. Williams and Wilkins, London, pp 177–231
3. Zhang P, Rao RV, Anderson WR (1988) An ultra-structural study of the memranoproliferative variant of transplant glomerulopathy. Ultrastruct Pathol 12:185
4. Mahony JF, Savdie E, Caterson RJ, Furlong T, Storey BG, Stewart JH, Sheil AGR (1986) The natural history of cadaveric renal allografts beyond ten years. Transplant Proc 18:135–137
5. Gueco IP, Evans DB, Calne RY (1985) Prolonged survival after renal transplantation: A study of 54 patients who lived ten or more years after operation with functioning allografts. Transplant Proc 17:108–109
6. Grapin C, Michel F, Charpentier B, Frantz F, Fries D, Kuss R, Legrain M, Luciani H, Mohamedi D, Poisson J, Thibault P, Sraer JD (1987) Long-term prognosis of renal transplantation: A retrospective study of 90 patients living more than 10 years with a functioning allograft. Transplant Proc 19:3765–3766
7. Lee HM, Mendez-Picon G, Goldman MH, Mohanakumar T, Posner MP (1985) The course of long-term survival in kidney transplantation: One center's experience. Transplant Proc 17:106–107
8. LeFrançois N, Elmghabbar N, Chossegros P, Betuel H, Faure JL, Revillard JP, Traeger J, Dubernard JM, Touraine JL (1987) Long-term results in kidney transplantation: Patient and graft survival, causes of graft failure and mortality, renal function and complications after 10 years. Transplant Proc 19:3767–3768
9. Rao KV, Kasiske BL, Bloom PM (1989) Acute graft rejection in the late survivors of renal transplantation: Clinical and histological observations in the second decade. Transplantation 47:290–292
10. Feehally J, Harris KPG, Bennett SE, Walls J (1986) Is chronic renal transplant rejection a non-immunological phenomenon? Lancet II:486–488
11. Kirkman RL, Strom TB, Weir MR, Tilney NL (1982) Late mortality and morbidity in recipients of long-term renal allografts. Transplantation 34:347–351
12. Schmidt P (1986) Is chronic renal transplant rejection a non-immunological phenomenon? Lancet II:693
13. Schweizer RT, Rovelli M, Palmeri D, Vossler E, Hull D, Bartus S (1990) Noncompliance in organ transplant recipients. Transplantation 49:374–377

14. Didlake RH, Dreyfus K, Kerman RH, Van Buren CTm, Kahan BD (1988) Patient noncompliance: A major cause of late graft failure in cyclosporine-treated renal transplants. Transplant Proc 20:63–69
15. Potter D, Feduska N, Melzer J, Garovoy M, Hopper S, Duca R, Salvatierra O (1986) Twenty years of renal transplantation in children. Pediatrics 77:465–470
16. Mathew TH (1988) Recurrence of disease following renal transplantation. Am J Kidney Dis 12:85–96
17. Starzl TE, Porter KA, Halgrimson CG, Husberg BS, Penn I, Putnam CW (1974) A decade follow-up in early cases of renal homotransplantation. Ann Surg 180:606–617
18. Vanrenterghem Y, Roels L, Lerut T, Waer M, Gruwez J, Michielsen P (1987) Long-term prognosis after cadaveric kidney transplantation. Transplant Proc 19:3762–3764
19. McGeown MG, Douglas JF, Donaldson RA, Hill CM, Kennedy JA, Loughridge WGG, Middleton D (1988) Ten-year results of renal transplantation with azathioprine and prednisone as only immunosuppression. Lancet I:983–985
20. Bohman SO, Wilczek H, Tyden G, et al. (1987) Recurrent diabetic nephropathy in renal allografts placed in diabetic patients and protective effect of simultaneous pancreatic transplantation. Transplant Proc 19:2290–2293

Advances in Managements of Vasculitis and Lupus Nephritis

Chair: D. Keith Peters (UK)
Pao-Hsii Feng (Singapore)

The Specificity of the Autoimmune Response in Vasculitis

L.A. van Es, M.R. Daha, C. Halma, F.J. van der Woude[1],
J.W. Cohen Tervaert, C.G.M. Kallenberg[2], A.E.G.Kr van dem Borne,
and R. Goldschmeding[3]

Introduction

Systemic vasculitis is one of the most elusive subjects of human pathology. The vasculitides differ in pathology, and in the caliber and localization of the affected blood vessels. The definition and classification of vasculitides is still a matter of debate. The most acceptable classification distinguishes the so-called leukocytoclastic vasculitides, or small vessel vasculitides, the polyarteritis group (polyarteritis nodosa, overlap syndromes, microscopic polyarteritis, and Kawasaki's disease), and the group of granulomatous vasculitides (Wegener's granulomatosis, relapsing polychondritis, Churg-Strauss syndrome, lymphatoid granulomatosis, giant cell arteritis, and Takayasu's disease). To the group of leukocytoclastic vasculitides belong allergic vasculitis, anaphylactoid purpura (Henoch-Schoenlein purpura), hypocomplementemic urticarial vasculitis, postinfectious vasculitis, rheumatoid vasculitis, and vasculitis in systemic lupus erythematosus (SLE) and in Sjögren's syndrome, and in mixed cryoglobulinemia.

As a result of the diversity of clinical presentation of systemic vasculitides, a wide variety of clinical specialists are involved in the management of this relatively rare group of patients. Only few clinical centers have the opportunity to study sufficiently large groups of patients in each category of vasculitis. Therefore, for further progress, national and international collaboration is essential. Most of the data presented

[1]Department of Nephrology, Academish Ziekenhuis Leiden, University Hospital Postbus 9600, 2300 Leiden, The Netherlands
[2]Department of Clinical Immunology, University Hospital, Groningen, The Netherlands
[3]Department of Immunohaematology, Central Laboratory of Bloodtransfusion Service, Amsterdam, The Netherlands

in this review are the result of collaboration between three groups of investigators in the Netherlands.

The Pathogenetic Significance of Autoimmune Antibodies in Vasculitis

Since the detection of antinuclear antibodies in patients with SLE, autoimmune phenomena have received great attention. It is now clear that antinuclear antibodies (ANA) are not specific for SLE. They occur in many other disorders, including infectious diseases. The most useful application of the ANA-test is to exclude the possibility that a patient has SLE. The level of ANA does not correlate with the severity of the disease. A correlation between the level of anti-double stranded DNA (dsDNA) and the severity of lupus nephritis has been claimed by some, but has not been confirmed by others.

Several criteria can be used to demonstrate the pathogenetic significance of autoimmune antibodies. These antibodies should recognize autoantigens in those tissues that are affected by the disease process (the so called target organ). Secondly, disease activity should fluctuate with antibody levels. Artificial removal of antibodies by plasma exchange should result in improvement. On the other hand, transplacental passive transfer of the antibodies to a newborn child should induce the disease manifestations, as has been demonstrated for several autoimmune diseases. Finally, the pathogenetic effect of the antibodies should be reproducible in experimental animals. Except for anti-glomerular basement membrane (GBM) disease, which fulfils most of these criteria, no other auto-antibodies associated with systemic vasculitis meet these criteria. Most of these autoantibodies are considered to be autoimmune phenomena without a causal relationship to the disease process. An important exception to this rule could be made for the so called anti-neutrophil cytoplasmic antibodies (ANCA). These antibodies were first described by Davies in 1982, in patients with crescentic glomerulonephritis possibly caused by arbovirus [1]. In 1984 Hall et al. described these antibodies in patients with vasculitis and glomerulonephritis [2]. In 1985 we described the diagnostic significance of ANCA in patients with Wegener's granulomatosis [3]. The level of these antibodies also correlated with the activity of the disease. In 1988 Falk and Jenette described two types of ANCA: the cytoplasmic type, or c-ANCA, and the perinuclear type, or p-ANCA [4]. The latter frequently, but not always, represent autoantibodies directed against myeloperoxidase (MPO).

The Specificity of c-ANCA

ANCA was discovered by applying patients's serum onto the fixed granulocytes of healthy donors. Fixation by formaldehyde or absolute alcohol influences the immunofluorescence pattern of p-ANCA [4]. Using the indirect immunofluorescence technique it could be demonstrated that ANC detects an antigen present in the polymorphonuclear (PMN) leukocytes and monocytes of humans and chimpanzees but not in lower animals (Goldschmeding, unpublished work). The antigen can first be detected at the stage of differentiation of promyelocyte and promonocyte. Interestingly, it can also bind an antigen in the HL60 cell line that does not contain specific granules or alkaline phosphatase [5]. The antigen cannot be demonstrated in lymphocytes, erythrocytes, or platelets.

Several groups of investigators have attempted to isolate the antigen recognized by c-ANCA in order to develop radioimmunoassays or enzyme-linked immunosorbent assays (ELISA) for objective detection and accurate quantification of ANCA. Lockwood et al. have used an acid extract of sonicated neutrophil cytoplasmic components [6]. After purification by gel filtration and high performance liquid chromatography (HPLC), Wegener's granulomatosis (WG) sera bound to 100, 6.2, and 1.8 kDa components. The 100 kDa component shared epitopes with alkaline phosphatase. Daha et al. [7] isolated, by ion exchange chromatography and gel filtration, a protein that migrated on SDS-PAGE analysis as a 91 kDa protein and on HPLC gel filtration had a molecular weight of 68 kDa. A monoclonal antibody was raised against this antigen. The antigen was found to react with the cytoplasmic area of PMN leukocytes and it recognized, on immunoblots, the 29 kDa triplet isolated by Goldschmeding et al. [8]. Goldschmeding and colleagues used nitrogen bomb cavitation and subcellular fractionation of PMN leukocytes by Percoll density gradient centrifugation. With the use of marker proteins they could demonstrate, by Western blot analysis, that sera from patients with Wegener's granulomatosis (WG) bound to a 29 kDa protein in the α-fraction, representing azurophilic or primary granules [8]. By extraction in a buffer containing 3.5 M urea and 1 M KCl, followed by radioiodination and immunoprecipitation, it could be shown that the ANCA antigen migrates as a triplet of bands with M_r 29000, 30500, and 32000. All 12 c-ANCA-positive WG sera, but not the 23 ANCA-negative control sera, specifically precipitated the 29 kDa antigen. Sera with high ANCA titers precipitated two additional bands at M_r 30500 and 32000. The c-ANCA antigen was found to be a saline-soluble triplet present in azurophilic granules of normal neutrophils [8]. Using ^{3}H-labeled diisopropylfluorophosphate (DFP), it could be shown that ^{3}H-DFP was coprecipitated by WG serum together with the radioionated c-ANCA antigen. The binding of DFP indicates that the ANCA antigen is a serine protease. Using polyclonal antibodies to elastase and cathepsin G, it could be demonstrated by sequential immunoprecipitation that the c-ANCA antigen is not identical to elastase or to cathepsin [8]. Recently, a third serine protease (protease 3) has been described in azurophilic granules [9]. Lüdeman et al. [10] have purified the ANCA-antigen from the supernatant of stimulted PMN by immunoaffinity chromatography, using purified IgG from an ANCA-positive serum. The characteristics of this antigen are very similar to the described properties of protease 3 [9]. Lüdeman et al. have determined the [17] NH$_2$-terminal amino acid sequence of the c-ANCA antigen [10].

They found it to be:

$$I-V-G-G-H-E-A-Q-P-H-I-R-P-I-Y-M-A.$$

A similar study by Niles et al. [11] revealed a similar, but not identical, amino acid sequence:

$$I-V-G-G-H-E-A-Q-P-H-S-X-P-Y-M-A-S-L-Q-M$$

These N-terminal sequences show a striking homology with other serine proteases [11].

Table 1. Stimulation of peripheral blood lymphocytes from five healthy donors (*HD*) and four patients with Wegener's granulomatosis (*WG*)

Donor	Proliferative response (pm × 10⁻³)			
	Medium	91 kDa	29 kDa	PWM
HD-1	1.3	1.0	1.2	17.5
HD-2	1.4	0.9	1.3	18.2
HD-3	1.0	1.2	1.1	31.5
HD-4	1.6	1.3	1.5	18.6
HD-5	1.2	0.5	1.4	24.3
WG-1	1.2	13.3	12.1	18.7
WG-2	1.5	14.7	13.8	19.3
WG-3	1.3	16.9	16.9	20.9
WH-4	1.4	2.3	4.1	23.7

PWM, pokeweed mitogen

Specificity of the Cellular Response in WG

In preliminary experiments, we exposed peripheral blood lymphocytes from five healthy donors and four WG patients to the 91 kDa sputum antigen isolated by Daha and to the 29 kDa antigen isolated by Goldschmeding (Table 1). The proliferative responses of the normal controls in the presence of these two specific antigens did not differ from the proliferation in medium alone (Daha, unpublished work). Peripheral blood lymphocytes from the four WG patients showed a significantly higher proliferative response in the presence of either the 91 kDa or the 29 kDa antigen. The two groups did not differ in their response to pokeweed mitogen. These data indicate that patients with WG not only develop a humoral autoimmune response against 91 kDa and 29 kDa, but also a cellular autoimmune response against these neutrophil antigens.

Specificity of p-ANCA

The specificity of p-ANCA is less clear than the specificity of c-ANCA. First of all, alcohol fixation may not only lead to perinuclear staining, but also to nuclear staining. This artefact is caused by solubilization of nucleophilic constituents of the azurophilic granules which diffuse and bind to the nuclei [12].

In a prospective study, it was found that not only patients with WG, but also patients with microscopic polyarteritis (MPA) have ANCA [13]. MPA has been defined as a primary systemic vasculitis with segmental necrotizing glomerulonephritis [14]. In practice, this definition also includes patients with leukocytoclastic vasculitis (i.e., venulitis). The majority of these patients have crescent formation in their glomeruli. Later ANCA was also detected in sera of patients with primary or idiopathic crescentic glomerulonephritis [4]. In contrast to WG sera, these sera frequently show a p-ANCA. Most, but not all, of these p-ANCA could be explained by a specificity for myeloperoxidase (MPO), another constituent of the azurophilic granules of PMN leukocytes [4].

At Groningen University Hospital, of 42 biopsies taken from patients with crescentic glomerulonephritis, 35 showed no or scanty immune deposits in the glomeruli [15]. All patients with biopsy proven WG ($n=9$) had c-ANCA. Of patients who were suspected to have WG, two-thirds ($n=10$) had c-ANCA and one third ($n=5$) had p-ANCA [15]. Of 8 patients with idiopathic crescentic glomerulonephritis (GN), only 2 had c-ANCA and the remaining 6 patients had p-ANCA. All patients with p-ANCA also had autoimmune antibodies to MPO, as first described by Falk and Jenette [4].

In a few cases, p-ANCA can be based on autoimmune antibodies directed against elastase. However, the p-ANCA observed in SLE patients usually do not have a specificity for MPO or for elastase. The perinuclear and nuclear staining pattern of p-ANCA is indistinguishable from a staining pattern described earlier by Wiik [16] for granulocyte-specific antinuclear antibodies (GS-ANA). These antibodies were originally described in a patient with Felty's syndrome. They are found in 75% of patients with active rheumatoid arthritis, especially in cases having autoimmune neutropenia [17].

References

1. Davies DJ, Moran JE, Nial JF, Ryan GB (1982) Segmental necrotising glomerulonephritis with antineutrophil antibody: possible arbovirus aetiology? Br Med J [Clin Res] 285:606
2. Hall JB, Waldham BMcN, Wood CJ, Ashton V, Adam WR (1984) Vasculitis and glomerulonephritis: a subgroup with an antineutrophil cytoplasmic antibody. Aust NZ J Med 14:277–278
3. Van der Woude FJ, Rasmussen N, Lobatto S, Wiik A, Permin H, Van Es LA, Van der Giessen M, Van der Hem GK, The TH (1985) Autoantibodies against neutrophils and monocytes: tool for diagnosis and marker of disease activity in Wegener's granulomatosis. Lancet I:425–429
4. Falk RJ, Jenette JC (1988) Anti-neutrophil cytoplasmic autoantibodies with specificity for myeloperoxidase in patients with systemic vasculitis and idiopathic necrotizing and crescentic glomerulonephritis. N Engl J Med 318:1651–1657
5. Charles LA, Falk RJ, Jenette JG (1989) Reactivity of anti-neutrophil cytoplasmic autoantibodies with HL-60 cells. Clin Immunol Immunopathol 53:243–253
6. Lockwood CM, Bakes D, Jones S, Whitaker KB, Moss DW, Savage COS (1987) Association of alkaline phosphatase with an autoantigen recognized by circulating anti-neutrophil antibodies in systemic vasculitis. Lancet I:716–720
7. Daha MR, Leusen J, Kramps JA, Schrama E, Van Es LA, Van der Woude FJ (1990) Isolation from purulent sputum of an antigen reactive with antibodies in serum of patients with Wegener's granulomatosis. Neth J Med 36:117–120
8. Goldschmeding R, Van der Schoot CE, Ten Bokkel Huinink D, Hack CE, Van den Ende ME, Kallenberg CGM, Von dem Borne AEGKr (1989) Wegener's granulomatosis antibodies identify a novel diisopropylfluorophosphate-binding protein in the lysosomes of normal human neutrophils. J Clin Invest 84:1577–1587
9. Kao RC, Wehner NG, Skubitz KM, Gray BH, Hoidal JR (1988) Proteinase 3. A distinct human polymorphonuclear leukocyte proteinase that produces emphysema in hamsters. J Clin Invest 82:1963–1973
10. Lüdeman J, Utecht B, Gross WL (1990) Anti-neutrophil cytoplasm antibodies in Wegener's granulomatosis recognize an elastinolytic enzyme. J Exp Med 171:357–362

11. Niles JL, McCluskey RT, Ahmad MF, Arnaout MA (1989) Wegener's granulomatosis autoantigen is a novel neutrophil serine protease. Blood 74:1888–1893
12. Falk RJ, Hogan S, Wilkman AS, Terrell RS, Lautizen S, Charles LA, Jenette JC (1990) Myeloperoxidase specific anti-neutrophil cytoplasmic autoantibodies (MPO-ANCA). Neth J Med 36:121–125
13. Savage LOS, Winearls CG, Jones S, Marshall PD, Lockwood CM (1987) Prospective study of radioimmunoassay for antibodies against neutrophil cytoplasm in diagnosis of systemic vasculitis. Lancet I:1389–1393
14. Savage LOS, Winearls CG, Evans DJ, Rees AJ, Lockwood M (1985) Microscopic polyarteritis: presentation, pathology and prognosis. Q J Med 56:467–483
15. Cohen Tevaert JW, Goldschmeding R, Elema JD, Van der Giessen M, Huitema MG, Van der Hem GK, The TH, Von dem Borne AEGKr, Kallenberg CGM (1990) Autoantibodies against myeloid lysosomal enzymes in crescentic glomerulonephritis. Kidney Int 37:799–806
16. Wiik A (1987) The value of specific ANA determination in rheumatology. Allergy 42:241–261
17. Wiik A (1980) Granulocyte-specific antinuclear antibodies? Possible significance for the pathogenesis, clinical features and diagnosis of rheumatoid arthritis. Allergy 35:362–389

New Perspectives on Systemic Vasculitis: Implications for Diagnosis and Treatment

C. Martin Lockwood[1]

Introduction

There is now growing evidence that autoimmune mechanisms play an important role in the systemic vasculitides: their demonstration forms the basis of the first diagnostic laboratory test for this group of diseases and their manipulation constitutes the first advance towards specific immunotherapy for their treatment [1,2]. The systemic vasculitides form a loosely associated group which have as their pathological basis a chronic necrotizing inflammation which affects vessels of varying sizes at varying sites throughout the body. There are primary and secondary forms, primary, which involve blood vessels exclusively and which are the subject of this article, and secondary, which arise in association with disease elsewhere, for example, vasculitis secondary to Crohn's disease. Some primary forms are associated with granulomata, for example, Takayasu's disease and Wegener's granulomatosis. Because so little is known of their pathogenesis, a morphological approach has been adopted toward their classification, see Table 1. Because of the same uncertainty, the evolution of a treatment strategy has been mainly empirical, driven by the high morbidity and mortality rates if no therapy was given. Thus, until recently, the best evidence that autoimmune processes played an important role in the systemic vasculitides came from evidence that powerful immunosuppressive agents were beneficial, [3] and that these might be humoral mechanisms was supported by the finding that additional plasma exchange was useful in the management of severe forms of these diseases, particularly rapidly progressive nephritis [4].

In 1982, Davies et al. reported that patients with polyarteritis and renal vasculitis had circulating autoantibodies which reacted with the cytoplasm of normal granulocytes [5]. A similar report in 1985 by Van der Woude et al. documented the same phenomenon occurring in patients with Wegener's granulomatosis [6]. These auto-

[1]Department of Medicine, University of Cambridge School of Clinical Medicine, Addenbrooke's Hospital, Cambridge, CB2 2QQ, UK

Table 1. Morphological classification of systemic vasculitides

| Vessel size | Granulomata | |
	Present	Absent
Large	Takayasu's[a]	Giant cell arteritis
Medium	Churg-Strauss[a]	Polyarteritis nodosa
Small	Wegener's granulomatosis[a]	Microscopic polyarteritis[a]
		Kawasaki disease[a]
		Henoch-Schönlein purpura[a]

[a]Denote vasculitides in which anti-neutrophil cytoplasm antibodies have been reported

antibodies were detected by indirect immunofluorescence techniques which were subjective and relatively insensitive. The development of solid phase immunoradiometric assays obviated both problems and showed that detection of autoantibodies to neutrophil cytoplasm antigens (ANCA) by these techniques provided both sensitive and specific means for diagnosis of the common primary vasculitides [7]. That these autoimmune mechanisms operate in systemic vasculitis has provided new perspectives on these diseases, with consequent implications for diagnosis and treatment.

ANCA and Disease Activity

The close association of ANCA with the development of certain vasculitides indicated that serial measurements might reflect disease activity, which could be useful not only in managing treatment, but also in predicting disease relapse. Van der Woude showed that by indirect immunofluorescence assays ANCA levels correlated with disease activity [6] and we also used this test in a retrospective study of patients' progress after discharge from hospital. We monitored 18 patients over a period of three years. Eight had become ANCA negative during their initial inpatient treatment but 10 still had detectable ANCA at the beginning of the study. No relapses occurred in the ANCA negative group, but eight relapses occurred in the ANCA positive group. In six of the eight who relapsed, relapses seemed to occur in relation to reductions in immunosuppressive therapy. This underlined the connection between ANCA and active disease. However, there were some patients who remained ANCA positive without symptomatology. In such patients further studies showed the importance of other factors in promoting disease expression, for example, ANCA isotype (see below).

This early experience led us to adopt a treatment strategy aimed at inducing both clinical and serological remission. We then tested the assay's predictive performance in a prospective fashion by assessing patients' progress at regular intervals both clinically and serologically. We have now studied 20 patients who were in clinical and serological remission at the beginning of the study, for a mean of 48 patient weeks. The patients were assessed clinically at monthly intervals. ANCA seroconversion was taken to indicate serological relapse and the Creative protein (CRP) level was used as a nonspecific indicator either of this or other inflammatory events (such as intercurrent infection). We observed 11 relapses in 9 patients. A rise in ANCA preceded relapse in eight and occurred at the same time in two; no seroconversion could be detected in one relapse. On two occasions ANCA tests became positive, but disease did not follow.

Only on one occasion did a rise in CRP precede relapse. Thus, although a rise in CRP was not a good predictive test, ANCA seroconversion was useful. Furthermore, since the mean time to relapse after seroconversion was one month, this raised the prospect that monthly patient follow-up might be carried out remote from specialist centers, with recall if ANCA titers rose.

Class and Subclass of ANCA

In Wegener's disease and microscopic polyarteritis, ANCA are usually of IgG isotype. Rarely, patients with a polyarteritis pulmonary-renal syndrome have been identified where ANCA are restricted to IgM isotype [8]. These patients have severe disease, readily responsive to plasma exchange, an appropriate treatment since IgM is predominantly confined to the intravascular compartment. With treatment a late isotype switch (to IgG) has been documented in three patients as the disease remitted, and ANCA of both IgM and IgG isotypes have been eluted from the kidneys of one patient at autopsy. This suggested that the IgM autoantibody might not only have determined the pattern of organ involvement, but also the severity of disease activity. A similar relationship of disease to isotype has been reported for Henoch-Schonlein purpura in adults (who have IgA ANCA) [9].

We have also studied the ANCA IgG subclass in patients at presentation and again in remission (yet still ANCA positive). Initially there was a predominance of ANCA of IgG3 isotype, but this later switched to IgG2 [10]. This is interesting, since IgG3 antibodies can fix complement and engage macrophages through receptors which IgG2 antibodies lack (complement and macrophages can substantially augment the inflammatory response once activated). Thus, these findings might explain why some patients in remission continue to have raised ANCA levels yet little disease activity.

Incidence of ANCA Positive Systemic Vasculitis

For the first time ANCA assays have provided a powerful diagnostic tool for the systemic vasculitides, which is not dependent on clinical interpretation. Our laboratory acts as a reference center for the population of East Anglia and this has allowed the incidence of ANCA positive disease to be estimated at 1:2,000, a level greater than for SLE and as high as that for rheumatoid arthritis. No doubt the tendency for vasculitis to present under any medical discipline, and the lack of a diagnostic laboratory test, has served to diminish estimates of its incidence.

Pathophysiological Role of ANCA

Whether ANCA fulfill a pathogenetic role is yet undecided. Levels of ANCA correlate with disease activity [6] and ANCA immunoglobulin can be eluted from vasculitic lesions and will bind to appropriate cells cultured in vitro [8,11]. Attempts to transfer disease to an experimental model have been frustrated by lack of a suitable recipient species (cross-reactive antigens are present only in baboons) and by the short time available, since serum sickness lesions, themselves vasculitic, develop from day 7 on. In a pilot study in baboons we did find a striking neutropenia in recipients given ANCA-rich immunoglobulin (C.M. Lockwood and C.B. Wilson, unpublished work).

This turned attention to in vitro effects of ANCA on neutrophil function, and on signal transduction in particular. We found that preincubation with ANCA markedly inhibited neutrophil activation brought about by agents such as phorbol myristate acetate (PMA), probably because ANCA can lead to sustained activation of polymorphs [12]. This is particularly interesting, since systemic vasculitis is hallmarked histologically by evidence of chronic polymorph activation, and argues for a direct role of ANCA in the disease process.

ANCA and Network Control of Immune Responses

If autoantibodies in patients with systemic vasculitis can mediate disease, then study of the regulation of these autoimmune responses may help to guide new strategies for treatment. The best understood immunological regulatory mechanisms involve control by way of a "network" of idiotypic anti-idiotypic reactions predicted by the "network theory" [13]. Idiotypic determinants have been characterized on autoantibodies occurring in different autoimmune diseases, and heterologous anti-idiotypic antibodies to those have been shown to have a regulatory effect in vitro [14]. The possibility that natural homeostatic mechanisms operate within the network framework has been supported by the finding that "normal" B cells possess the necessary genetic information to manufacture autoantibodies [15] and, that within the population of normal immunoglobulins, there exists a range of "natural" anti-idiotypic antibodies [16]. This has been exploited therapeutically for the treatment of a number of autoimmune diseases, best exemplified by spontaneous anti-factor VIII disease, where control of autoantibody formation has been shown to be explainable by idiotypic anti-idiotypic regulation [17]. It is of note that the treatment of choice for Kawasaki disease, an ANCA positive childhood vasculitis, is the administration of pooled normal immunoglobulin intravenously [18].

This has led us to study the properties of pooled immunoglobulins on ANCA reactions [19]. We have shown that F(ab)₂ of normal pooled immunoglobulin can inhibit binding of ANCA in vitro. The degree of inhibition ranged from 0%–100%, with up to 75% of a panel of 21 pretreatment ANCA positive sera being substantially inhibited by a single F(ab)₂ preparation of pooled immunoglobulin. Inhibitory reactivity was also found in remission sera, which were ANCA negative, including sera from patients whose remission occurred spontaneously. That this inhibition of binding fulfilled the criteria of idiotypic anti-idiotypic reactions was demonstrated by showing that the F(ab)₂ of affinity purified immunoglobulin reacted with, and was inhibited in its specific binding by, IgG from normal immunoglobulin. These experimental data have encouraged pilot studies of the use of pooled immunoglobulin for treatment of certain patients with systemic vasculitis.

Treatment of Systemic Vasculitis with Intravenous Immunoglobulin (IVIg)

We have treated four patients with pooled normal immunoglobulin given by intravenous infusion (Sandoglobulin, Sandoz, UK). All had ANCA positive vasculitis: for two this was the only treatment given, for the other two IVIg was given after failure

Table 2. Clinical and laboratory features of four patients treated with IVIg

Patient no.	Age	Sex	Diagnosis	Other treatment	Disease activity pre/post	CRP pre/post	Follow-ups (months)
1	62	F	WG	CP	2/0	148/10	6
2	57	M	WG	0	1/0	18/N	4
3	73	M	MP	0	1/0	N/N	11
4	61	M	MP	CP	1/0	N/N	5

C, cyclophosphamide; P, prednisolone; N, Normal (>6mg/100ml); CRP, C reactive protein; WG, Wegener's granulomatosis; MP, microscopic polyarteris

of conventional immunosuppressive drugs. The four patients were observed for a mean of three months before and six months after therapy. Clinical disease activity was recorded using a 2,1,0 scale (2, active disease requiring hospital or home care; 1, still symptomatic but institutionally independent; 0, remission); levels of ANCA (by radio-immunoassay) and C reactive protein (CRP) were measured serially. The potential efficacy of the Sandoglobulin was assessed by an in vitro test of inhibition of ANCA-binding activity. The clinical and laboratory data are shown in Table 2.

Clinical improvement was seen in all four patients, including the two resistant to standard therapy. After the IVIg, ANCA levels rose initially in all four patients, but in three then fell to levels substantially lower than pretreatment values, becoming undetectable in the fourth. Low levels of ANCA continued to be detectable, without overt evidence of disease, during follow-up in these three patients.

The numbers of patients studied so far is small but some points of interest emerge already. Firstly, clinical improvement occurred in all the patients treated and was maintained for periods of follow up ranging from four to eleven months (mean, six). Secondly, after the IVIg infusion ANCA levels rose transiently in all the patients, and remained detectable in three, without deleterious effect on the clinical outcome. The initial rise may have been due to displacement of ANCA from tissue-bound sites, since competitive inhibition of binding was demonstrated between the intravenous immunoglobulin (F(ab)$_2$ preparations) and the autoantibodies in each of the patients treated. It is equally possible that the persisting ANCA were from populations of autoantibodies bearing idiotypes not recognized by the normal pooled IgG and possibly not pathogenetically important. Thirdly, in the two untreated patients, in vitro tests of ANCA producing B cell activity indicated that in both patients this was abrogated after IVIg infusion, suggesting an immediate down regulation of autoantibody synthesis had been achieved (Mathieson et al., work in progress).

A Role for Plasma Exchange?

The balance of idiotypic and anti-idiotypic reactions appears symmetrical, but if ascendancy of one component could be promoted, then new strategies for therapy could be encouraged. Recently we have found that there is a difference in the isotype of the anti-idiotypic antibodies: a substantial proportion are IgM. IgM synthesis rates are markedly faster than those of IgG. Thus, depletion of all circulatory immunoglobulins by plasmapheresis might allow this desired alteration in homeostasis by virtue of the greater synthetic rate of IgM. In this context it is of interest that plasmapheresis has been shown to have an intrinsic benefit in treatment of patients with severe renal and systemic vasculitis (as tested in a randomized prospective controlled trial) [4].

Conclusions

It is now evident that autoimmune mechanisms may play an important role in systemic vasculitis, and their identification is useful for diagnosis and management of these disorders. Their further study may allow an understanding of the pathogenesis of these disorders and open up the prospects of new strategies for treatment. At the present time, one such strategy we are exploring involves a combination of treatment by plasma exchange followed by intravenous immunoglobulin infusion therapy.

References

1. Savage COS and Lockwood CM (1989) Autoantibodies in primary systemic vasculitis. In: Stollerman GH (ed) Advances in internal medicine, vol 35. Year Book Medical, Chicago, pp 73–92
2. Van der Woude FJ, Daha MR, Van Es LA (1989) The current status of neutrophil cytoplasmic antibodies. Clin Exp Immunol 78, 143–148
3. Katz P, Fauci AS (1981) Treatment of immune complex mediated diseases: corticosteroids and cytotoxic agents. In: Fauci AS (ed) Clinics in immunology, 1981. Saunders, Eastbourne, pp 415–431
4. Pusey CD, Lockwood CM (1985) Plasma exchange for glomerular disease. In: Robinson RR (ed) Nephrology, 1985. Springer, New York, pp 1474–1486
5. Davies DJ, Moran JE, Niall JF, Ryan GB (1982) Segmental necrotizing glomerulonephritis with antineutrophil antibody: possible arbovirus aetiology? Br Med J [Clin Res] 285:606
6. Van der Woude FJ, Rasmussen N, Lobatto S, Wiik A, Permin H, Van Es LA, Van der Giessen M, Van der Hem GK, The TH (1985) Autoantibodies against neutrophils and monocytes: tool for diagnosis and marker for disease activity in Wegener's granulomatosis. Lancet I:425–429
7. Savage COS, Winearls CG, Jones S, Marshall PD, Lockwood CM (1987) Prospective study of radioimmunoassay for antibodies against neutrophil cytoplasm in diagnosis of systemic vasculitis. Lancet I:1389–1393
8. Jayne DRW, Jones SJ, Severn A, Shaumack S, Murphy J, Lockwood CM (1989) Severe pulmonary haemorrhage and systemic vasculitis in association with circulating anti-neutrophil antibodies of IgM class only. Clin Nephrol 32:101–106
9. Van den Wall Bake AWL, Lobatto S, Jonges L, Daha MR, Van Es LA (1987) IgA antibodies directed against cytoplasmic antigens of polymorphonuclear leucocytes in patients with Henoch-Schonlein purpura. In: Mestecky J, et al. (eds) Recent advances in mucosal immunity: Part B, 1987. Plenum, London, p 1593
10. Jayne DRW, Lockwood CM (to be published) Subclass specificity of autoantibodies to neutrophil cytoplasm antigens in systemic vasculitis
11. Abbott F, Jones SJ, Lockwood CM, Rees AJ (1989) Autoantibodies to glomerular antigens in patients with Wegener's granulomatosis. Nephrol Dial Transpl 4:1–8
12. Lai KN, Lockwood CM (to be published) Down-regulation of signal transduction in human neutrophils by anti-neutrophil cytoplasm antibodies

13. Jerne NK (1974) Towards a network theory of the immune response. Ann Immunol (Paris) 125:373–389

14. Lockwood CM, Pye RJ (1990) Basic mechanisms in autoimmunity. In: Champion RH, Pye RJ (eds) Adv in dermatology, vol 8. Churchill Livingstone, Edinburgh, pp 71–84

15. Painter C, Monestier M, Bonin B, Bing CA (1986) Functional and molecular studies of V genes expressed in autoantibodies. Immunol Rev 94:75–98

16. Rossi F, Jayne DRW, Lockwood CM, Kazatchkine MD (to be published) Anti-idiotypes against anti-neutrophil cytoplasm antibodies in normal human polyspecific IgG for therapeutic use and in the serum of patients with systemic vasculitis in remission

17. Sultan Y, Rossi F, Kazatchkine MD (1987) Recovery from anti-VIII:C (anti-haemophilic factor) autoimmune disease dependent on generation of anti-idiotypes against anti-VIII:C autoantibodies. PNAS 84:828–830

18. Leung DYM, Burns JC, Neuburger M, Geha RS (1987) Reversal of lymphocyte activation in vivo in the Kawasaki syndrome by intravenous gamma globulin. J Clin Invest 79:468–472

19. Rossi F, Jayne DRW, Lockwood CM, Kazatchkine MD (to be published) Anti-idiotypes against anti-neutrophil cytoplasmic antigen (ANCA) autoantibodies in normal human polyspecific IgG for therapeutic use and in the remission sera of patients with systemic vasculitis. Clin Exp Immunol

Therapeutic Trials in Lupus Nephritis

JAMES E. BALOW[1]

SUMMARY. Corticosteroids have had a profound effect on survival of patients with systemic lupus erythematosus. The salutary effects of these agents on lupus nephritis have been less satisfactory, from the perspective of both efficacy and long-term toxicity. Initial investigations of cytotoxic drugs in human lupus nephritis have been mostly contentious, while studies in murine lupus have demonstrated unequivocal advantages of cyclophosphamide over corticosteroids; increased longevity of the mice has been primarily due to control of nephritis by cyclophosphamide. The advantages of intermittent over continuous cyclophosphamide have been evident in the murine experiments and from experience in clinical oncology.

Controlled trials of corticosteroids, azathioprine and cyclophosphamide have demonstrated the best short-term control of the clinical signs of proliferative lupus nephritis in subjects under cyclophosphamide treatment. Studies of sustained treatment have documented long-term advantage of cyclophosphamide over prednisone in reducing clinical evidence of active nephritis, pathologic evidence of renal progression and the risk of developing end stage renal failure. Intermittent pulse cyclophosphamide has been demonstrated to have a better therapeutic index than conventional daily therapy.

Introduction

Among the numerous therapeutic advances in medicine and surgery achieved during the mid-twentieth century, corticosteroids played a key role in improved management of many of the critical components and complications of systemic lupus erythematosus. As longevity of lupus patients increased, nephritis became a central component of this disease. Lupus nephritis remains a pre-occupying concern of clinicians because its prevention is uncertain and treatment is controversial, usually com-

[1]National Institute of Health, Building 10, Room 9N222, Bethesda, MD 20892, USA

plicated, and often unsuccessful [1,2]. Moreover, patients who reach end stage renal failure as the result of lupus nephritis continue to have decreased longevity as a consequence of numerous systemic complications of lupus [3]. In the context of this historical background and of the therapeutic inadequacies, the rationale for continued pursuit of better techniques for management of lupus nephritis is self-evident.

Conventional Management of Lupus

The beneficial effects of corticosteroids on many of the systemic components of lupus have been so striking that controlled clinical trials have, by consensus, been considered superfluous. Although intellectually provocative, it is unlikely that prospective trials will ever be performed to document rigorously the superiority of corticosteroids over no immunosuppressive or anti-inflammatory treatment. Neither did knowledge of the short-term advantage of corticosteroids on the proliferative forms of lupus nephritis derive from prospective, controlled trials. The seminal observations of Pollak [4] and Baldwin [5] of the salutary effects of high-dose corticosteroids set the standards for therapy of lupus nephritis for several decades. Nonetheless, dissatisfaction with efficacy in many cases and with unacceptable toxicities in most cases fueled controversy about the use of prolonged high-dose corticosteroids and intensified the search for alternative treatments.

Experimental Aspects of Lupus

Lupus nephritis is the prototypical immune complex disease of the kidney. Lymphoid hyperplasia and spontaneous in vivo overactivity are nearly invariable and account for the exuberant production of polyclonal autoantibodies and immune complexes. Although a host of immunoregulatory disturbances surround the B lymphocyte excess, primary and secondary relationships among these immune system perturbations are nebulous [2]. Corticosteroids were shown experimentally to have a modest effect on B lymphocyte responses [6]. The search for agents which would more effectively suppress the excessive immune responses of lupus led investigators to the cytotoxic agents used in oncology. Among the chemotherapeutic drugs, cyclophosphamide was recognized to have a preferential effect on B lymphocyte responses [7].

Inbred stains of mice which exhibited immunological and clinical similarities to human lupus and which predictably succumbed from renal failure became invaluable resources for pilot studies of the effectiveness of cytotoxic drugs in lupus nephritis. Numerous controlled studies documented dramatic extensions of the longevity of these mice when treated with cytotoxic drugs [2,8]. Cyclophosphamide was among the most effective and high-dose intermittent pulse therapy appeared to have the highest therapeutic index [2].

Therapeutic Trials of Cytotoxic Drugs in Human Lupus Nephritis

Despite the encouraging results of treatment in the animal models of lupus nephritis, skepticism about their relevance to human disease prevailed. This was fueled by observations of serious drug-related morbidity in early (and often overzealous) clinical applications of cytotoxic drugs [9]. As clinical and laboratory experience accumulated, it appeared that a therapeutic window of efficacy and toxicity could be realized.

Controlled trials of cytotoxic drugs in patients with lupus nephritis were initiated around 1970. Azathioprine was shown in several early studies to have little advantage over corticosteroids alone [10,11,12]. Subsequent efforts began to focus on cyclophosphamide.

Studies at the Mayo Clinic [13] were designed to analyze the benefit of adding a brief course of daily oral cyclophosphamide to prednisone, while studies at the National Institutes of Health were designed to evaluate the effects of long-term cytotoxic drug therapy [14]. In the latter study, comparisons were made among patients treated with prednisone alone or prednisone plus azathioprine, cyclophosphamide, combined low-dose azathioprine and cyclophosphamide, or intermittent pulse cyclophosphamide. Both centers reported that the highest probabilities of stabilizing or improving clinical and laboratory signs of renal disease were observed in patients receiving cyclophosphamide in addition to prednisone. Follow-up renal biopsies obtained from patients in the National Institutes of Health studies showed that cytotoxic drug treatment protected against progressive renal damage more effectively than prednisone alone [15]. However, in the studies from both institutions, renal failure events were infrequent and no differences in risk of end stage renal failure among the treatment groups were discernible through the first five years of follow-up [13,14]. Understandably, the results of these studies provoked debate and controversy; the advantages of cyclophosphamide seemed modest and were of uncertain long-term value and the magnitude of delayed side-effects was unknown.

Extended follow-up of the patients in the Mayo Clinic trial failed to show a reduction of late renal failure events in patients who had received the initial short-course of cyclophosphamide [16]. On the other hand, after a median follow-up of seven years for the patients receiving long-term treatment in the National Institutes of Health studies, the risk of developing end stage renal failure was higher with prednisone alone than with intermittent pulse cyclophosphamide [14]. Also, treatment with daily oral cyclophosphamide or with daily low-dose combined cyclophosphamide and azathioprine has subsequently been shown to be more efficacious than prednisone, but consideration of high rates of side-effects of daily cytotoxic drugs led us to discontinue these therapeutic options despite their apparent efficacy. Intermittent pulse cyclophosphamide clearly had the highest therapeutic index among the options tested. Toxicity of the various regimens used in the studies at the National Institutes of Health has recently been reviewed [2,9]. Several recent reports have confirmed the efficacy of intermittent pulse cyclophosphamide for treatment of lupus nephritis [17,18] and of other systemic complications of lupus [19].

Other Therapeutic Options

Pulse methylprednisolone has been reported to be effective in management of lupus nephritis [20]. In a controlled trial currently being conducted at the National Institutes of Health, the hypothesis that intermittent pulse methylprednisolone is as efficacious as intermittent pulse cyclophosphamide is being tested in patients with severe proliferative lupus nephritis. In this study, 24 patients received monthly pulse methylprednisolone, 21 patients received monthly pulse cyclophosphamide for six months only, and 19 patients received monthly pulse cyclophosphamide for six months followed by quarterly pulse cyclophosphamide for an additional two years. Preliminary results show that patients receiving pulse methylprednisolone have the highest trend in risk of doubling their serum creatinine and of progressing to end stage renal failure. Long-term follow-up is in progress to provide valid statistically significant analysis.

Cyclosporine [21,22] and total lymphoid irradiation [23] have proven efficacious in lupus nephritis. No controlled clinical trials of these agents have been reported for treatment of human lupus nephritis.

Plasma exchange therapy has been utilized for a number of systemic complications of lupus. Controlled studies to date have not supported the benefit of plasma exchange therapy. In a double-blind study from the National Institutes of Health of real or sham procedure in patients with mild systemic lupus, little objective benefit of plasma exchange was found [24]. In a subsequent multi-centered study of patients with severe proliferative lupus nephritis, no difference in the rate of progression of renal disease was observed between the group of patients receiving immunosuppression alone and that receiving immunosuppression and adjunctive plasma exchange [25].

Novel Therapeutic Approaches to Lupus Nephritis

Controlled studies in murine lupus nephritis offer the promise of new and alternative approaches to the treatment of human disease. Monoclonal antibodies to subsets of T lymphocytes have been shown to prevent renal failure and prolong survival in animal models [26,27]. Similarly, exciting prospects for the use of biologic response modifiers, such as recombinant cytokines, appear to be ready for testing. Recombinant tumor necrosis factor has produced a salutary effect on murine lupus nephritis [28]. Preliminary data from human studies suggest that defective production of tumor necrosis factor may be genetically related to the predisposition for lupus [29].

Continued acquisition of insights into the multiplicity of immunologic disturbances contributing to the lupus syndrome may, in turn, lead to additional novel therapeutic options for management of patients with lupus nephritis.

References

1. Balow JE (1986) Lupus nephritis: natural history, prognosis and treatment. Clin Immunol Allergy 6:391–404
2. Balow JE, Austin HA III, Tsokos GC, Antonovych TT, Steinberg AD, Klippel JH (1987) Lupus nephritis. Ann Intern Med 106:79–94
3. Rosansky S, Eggers P (1987) Trends in the US end stage renal disease population: 1973–1983 Am J Kidney Dis 9:91–97
4. Pollak VE, Pirani CL, Kark RM (1961) Effect of large doses of prednisone on the renal lesions and life span of patients with lupus glomerulonephritis. J Lab Clin Med 57:495–511
5. Baldwin DS, Gluck MC, Lowenstein J, Gallo G (1977) Lupus nephritis: clinical course as related to morphologic forms and their transitions. Am J Med 62:12–30

6. Bach JF, Strom TB (1985) The mode of action of immunosuppressive agents. Elsevier, Amsterdam

7. Zhu LP, Cupps TR, Whalen G, Fauci AS (1987) Selective effects of cyclophosphamide therapy on activation, proliferation and differentiation of human B cells. J Clin Invest 79:1082–1090

8. Appleby P, Webber DG, Bowen JG (1989) Murine chronic graft-versus-host disease as a model of systemic lupus erythematosus: effect of immunosuppressive drugs on disease development. Clin Exp Immunol 78:449–453

9. Klippel JH (1990) Systemic lupus erythematosus: treatment-related complications superimposed on chronic disease. JAMA 263:1812–1815

10. Donadio JV Jr, Holley HE, Wagoner RD, Ferguson RH, McDuffie FC (1972) Treatment of lupus nephritis with prednisone and combined prednisone and azathioprine. Ann Intern Med 77:829–835

11. Decker JL, Klippel JH, Plotz PH, Steinberg AD (1975) Cyclophosphamide or azathioprine in lupus glomerulonephritis: a controlled trial: results at 28 months. Ann Intern Med 83:606–615

12. Hahn BH, Kantor, OS, Osterland CK (1975) Azathioprine plus prednisone compared with prednisone alone in the treatment of systemic lupus erythematosus. Ann Intern Med 83:597–605

13. Donadio JV Jr, Holley KE, Ferguson RH, Ilstrup DM (1978) Treatment of diffuse proliferative lupus nephritis with prednisone and combined prednisone and cyclophosphamide. N Engl J Med 299:1151–1155

14. Austin HA III, Klippel JH, Balow JE, leRiche NGH, Steinberg AD, Plotz PH, Decker JL (1986) Therapy of lupus nephritis: controlled trial of prednisone and cytotoxic drugs. N Engl J Med 314:614–619

15. Balow JE, Austin HA III, Muenz LR, Joyce KM, Antonovych TT, Klippel JH, Steinberg AD, Plotz PH, Decker JL (1984) Effect of treatment on the evolution of renal abnormalities in lupus nephritis. N Engl J Med 311:491–495

16. Donadio JV Jr, Holley KE, Ilstrup DN (1981) Adrenocorticoid and cyclophosphamide drug treatment of lupus nephropathy. In: Proc 8th Int Congress Nephrology, S. Karger, Basel, pp 643–648

17. McCune WJ, Golbus J, Zeldes W, Bohlke P, Dunne R, Fox DA (1988) Clinical and immunologic effects of monthly administration of intravenous cyclophosphamide in severe systemic lupus erythematosus. N Engl J Med 318:1423–1431

18. Lehman TJA, Sherry DD, Wagner-Weiner L, McCurdy DK, Emery HM, Magilavy DB, Kovalesky A (1989) Intermittent intravenous cyclophosphamide for lupus nephritis. J Pediatr 114:1055–1060

19. Boumpas DT, Barez S, Klippel JH, Balow JE (1990) Intermittent cyclophosphamide for the treatment of autoimmune thrombocytopenia in systemic lupus erythematosus. Ann Intern Med 112:674–677

20. Ponticelli C, Zucchelli P, Moroni G, Cagnoli L, Banfi G, Pascuali S (1987) Long-term prognosis of diffuse lupus nephritis. Clin Nephrol 28:263–271

21. Feutren G, Querin S, Tron F, Noel LH, Chatenoud L, Lesavre P, Bach JF (1986) The effects of cyclosporine in patients with systemic lupus. Transplant Proc 18:643–644

22. Mountz JD, Smith HR, Wilder RL (1987) CS-A therapy in MRL-lpr/lpr mice: amelioration of immunopathology despite autoantibody production. J Immunol 138:157–163

23. Strober S, Farinas MC, Field EH, Solovera JJ, Kiberd BA, Myers BD, Hoppe RT (1987) Lupus nephritis after total lymphoid irradiation: persistent improvement and reduction of steroid therapy. Ann Intern Med 107:689–690

24. Wei N, Klippel JH, Huston DP, Hall RP, Lawley TJ, Balow JE, Steinberg AD, Decker JL (1983) Randomized trial of plasma exchange in mild systemic lupus erythematosus. Lancet I:17–22

25. Lewis E, Lachin J (1987) Primary outcomes in the controlled trial of plasmapheresis therapy (PPT) in severe lupus nephritis (abstract). Kidney Int 31:208
26. Wofsy D, Seamon WE (1987) Reversal of advanced murine lupus in NZB/NZW F1 mice by treatment with monoclonal antibody to L3T4. J Immunol 138:3247–3253
27. Kelley VE, Gaulton GN, Ikegami H, Eisenbarth G, Strom TB (1988) Anti-interleukin 2 receptor antibody suppresses murine diabetic insulitis and lupus nephritis. J Immunol 140:59–61
28. Jacob CO, McDevitt HO (1988) Tumour necrosis factor-alpha in murine autoimmune lupus nephritis. Nature 331:356–358
29. Jacob CO, Fronek Z, Koo M, Hansen JA, McDevitt HO (1990) Heritable major histocompatibility complex class II-associated differences in production of tumor necrosis factor alpha: relevance to genetic predisposition to systemic lupus erythematosus. Proc Natl Acad Sci USA 87:1233–1237

Current Strategy of Management for Lupus Nephritis and Renal Vasculitis

Toshihiko Nagasawa[1]

Summary. Current strategy of management for lupus nephritis and renal vasculitis has been considered from clinical, morphologic, and immunologic points of view. In the immunologically active and rapidly progressive type of lupus nephritis, short-term intensive immunosuppressive therapy is recommended. However, in chronically ill patients with no flare-up of immunologic activity, long term corticosteroid administration is not recommended, especially in those patients with WHO type 5 histology. In rapidly progressive lupus nephritis, early initiation of hemodialysis is recommended, together with intensive immunosuppressive therapy, including plasma exchange. In patients on chronic hemodialysis without flare-up of immunologic activity (burning out systemic lupus erythematosus (SLE)), renal transplantation is indicated.

For the monitoring of immunosuppressive therapy in renal vasculitis, serial quantitative measurements of anti-neutrophil cytoplasmic antibodies are needed.

Introduction

Modern advances in intensive immunosuppressive therapy have remarkably prolonged the survival rates in patients with lupus nephritis (LN) and renal vasculitis (RV). However, associated with potent immunosuppressive therapy given for considerably long periods an increased number of patients with these diseases have lost their lives or have lost their ability to carry out daily life activities. Based on these facts, immunosuppressive therapy for LN and RV has been reconsidered from clinical, morphologic, and immunologic points of view. Also, modern management of end-stage renal failure in LN has been considered.

[1]The First Department of Internal Medicine, Kyorin University School of Medicine, 6-20-2 Shinkawa, Mitaka, Tokyo, 181 Japan

Type I : **Rapidly Progressive Type** : 77 cases (22.4%)

Type II : **Acute Exacerbation Type** : 154 cases (43.4%)

Type III : **Slowly Progressive Type** : 121 cases (34.2%)

Onset of LN

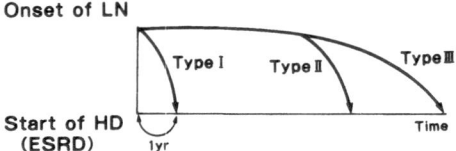

Start of HD
(ESRD)

Fig. 1. Clinical courses to end-stage renal disease (*ESRD*) in patients with systemic lupus erythematosus (*SLE*) (*n*=352)

Clinical Studies of Lupus Nephritis

The clinical courses to end-stage renal disease (ESRD) of 352 patients with LN who began hemodialysis procedure (HD) were analyzed retrospectively. As shown in Fig. 1, the clinical courses to ESRD could be classified into 3 types. Within 1 year at most after the onset of LN 77 patients (22.4%) progressed very rapidly to ESRD (Type 1 LN). Suddenly, several years after the onset of LN 154 patients (43.4%) shifted to type 1 LN (Type 2 LN). In types 1 and 2 LN, extremely strong immunologic SLE activity appeared, together with rapidly progressive glomerulonephritis (RPGN). In addition to the immunologic activity, patients showed marked thrombocytopenia, which was found to be directly related to the causes of death, as shown in Table I. Types 1 and 2 LN are essentially the same except for the time difference in the occurrence of RPGN. In order to save lives, aggressive immunosuppressive therapy is indicated in these 2 types. In contrast to the patients with Types 1 and 2 LN, in 121 other patients (34.2%) the course to ESRD was very slow, without flare-up of clinical and immunologic SLE activities (Type 3 LN). In this type, long term corticosteroid (CS) administration and large doses of CS should be avoided to prevent the further progression of glomerular sclerosis due to the effects of CS.

Table 1. Lupus nephritis with Type I clinical course (*n*=10)

Case	Age/sex	Interval between the onset of LN to HD (Mo)	Thr ×10⁴	CH_{50} (U/ml)	a-DNA Ab (U/ml)	Outcome
1	16 F	3	5.6	<12	96	† (Cerebral bleeding)
2	17 F	3	9.0	<12	90	† (Sepsis)
3	23 F	2	4.5	12	100	† (Pulm. bleeding)
4	30 F	3	6.0	12	162	† (GI bleeding)
5	31 F	3	5.5	24	130	† (GI bleeding)
6	35 F	6	2.4	12	150	Maintenance HD
7	35 F	8	1.2	12	94	† (Cerebral bleeding)
8	37 F	3	2.6	12	110	Off HD
9	43 M	3	5.1	<12	113	† (GI bleeding)
10	44 F	6	9.6	<12	150	† (Sepsis)

Table 2. Survival rate of patients with lupus nephritis in whom progress to end-stage renal failure was regarded as "end point"

	5 Years	10 Years
WHO other types	100 ⌐	91.7±8.0 ⌐
	$P<0.05$	$P<0.05$
WHO type 4	75.8± 9.0⌐	41.3±20.0⌐
Act-Sc<3.0	98.2± 2.0⌐	91.9± 6.0⌐
	$P<0.05$	$P<0.05$
Act-Sc≥3.0	73.9±11.0⌐	46.2±17.0⌐
Chr-Sc<1.7	98.0± 2.0⌐	89.5± 8.0⌐
	NS	NS
Chr-Sc≥1.7	81.2± 9.0⌐	54.2±17.0⌐
TI-Sc<1.8	93.5± 4.0⌐	75.3±10.0⌐
	NS	NS
TI-Sc≥1.8	98.1± 4.0⌐	58.9±15.0⌐

Act-Sc, activity score; Chr-Sc, chronicity score; TI-Sc, tubulointer-stitial score

Morphologic Studies of Lupus Nephritis

One hundred and eighty-nine patients with LN were biopsied. Their types of WHO classification were as follows: type 1; 14 cases (7.4%), type 2; 40 cases (21.1%), type 3; 13 cases (6.9%), type 4; 67 cases (35.4%), and type 5; 55 cases (29.1%).

Survival rates 5 and 10 years after the biopsy are shown in Table 2. Significant differences were observed between WHO type 4 and the other types, and also between patients whose activity scores were less than and more than 3.0. These results indicate that WHO type 4 LN patients with activity scores over 3.0 should be carefully treated with relatively large doses of CS in order to avoid the transition from type 2 to type 1 LN. Also, the relationship between CS therapy and the sites of glomerular immune deposits was found to be important. As shown schematically in Fig. 2, it was possible to eliminate mesangial and subendothelial immune deposits by administration of large doses of CS over a relatively short period. However, it was not possible

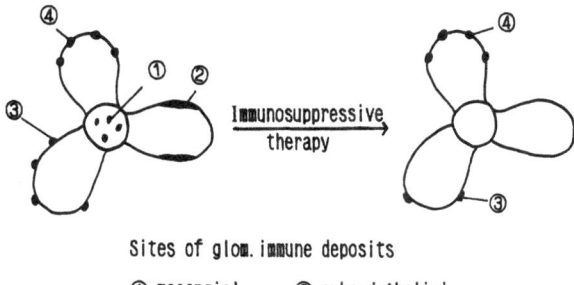

Sites of glom. immune deposits

① mesangial   ② subendothelial
③ subepithelial   ④ intramembranous

Fig. 2. Sites of glomerular immune deposits and immunosuppressive therapy

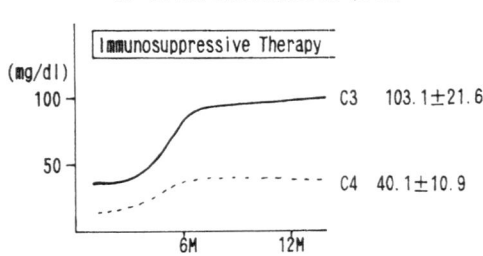

C3·C4 non dissociated LN (n=62)

Fig. 3. Clinical course of lupus nephritis and complement (*n*=88)

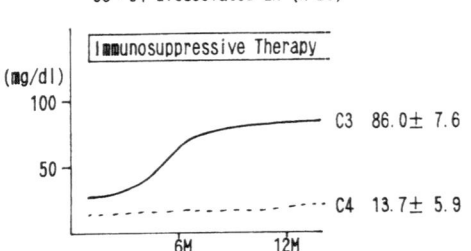

C3·C4 dissociated LN (n=26)

to eliminate subepithelial and/or intramembranous immune deposits by administration of large doses of CS and/or by long-term CS administration. These results indicate that electron microscopic observation of renal biopsied sections is important not only for the diagnosis of WHO type classification and activity scores, but also in order to be able to judge whether or not large doses of CS and/or long term CS administration are indicated.

Immunologic Studies on Lupus Nephritis

When strong immunosuppressive therapy was given to patients with LN who had low serum levels of C3 and C4 before the start of therapy, levels returned to normal in considerable numbers of cases. However, there were some cases whose C3 levels returned to normal, while their C4 levels still remained low (Fig. 3). Renal involvement was compared in these 2 groups. As shown in Table 3, nephropathy occurred nearly equally in both groups. However, interestingly, there were no cases who developed RPGN (Types 1 or 2 LN) or chronic renal failure (CRF) (Type 3 LN)

Table 3. Dissociation of C3·C4 and lupus nephritis (*n*=88)

C3·C4 Dissociation	Presence (*n*=26)	Absence (*n*=62)
Nephropathy	20 (76.9%)	46 (74.2%)
Transition to RPGN	0	9 (14.5%)
Transition to CRF	0	12 (19.4%)
Death	0	7 (11.3%)

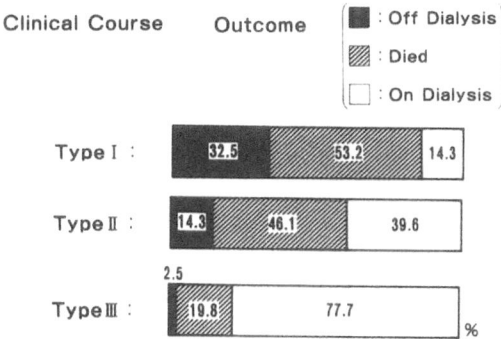

Fig. 4. Clinical courses to ESRD and outcome of hemodialysis (*HD*)

among the C3 and C4 dissociated patients. Also, there were no cases with WHO type 4 in this group, nor any with HLA DR 5. although the HLA-A, B, and C loci were not different in the 2 groups. These studies indicate that chronically ill LN patients with both C3 and C4 simultaneously normalized might still be at risk of transit from type 2 to type 1 LN, so they must be carefully followed-up.

Management of ESRD in LN

The outcome of 352 patients on HD is shown in Fig. 4. In type 1 LN, half of the patients died and one-third of the patients were able to come off HD. Plasma exchange and CS pulse therapy had excellent effects on "off dialysis," indicating that aggressive immunosuppressive therapy is still needed in type 1 LN in order to achieve "off dialysis" and to enable patients to return to type 3 LN (Table 4). The three main causes of death on HD were infections, bleeding, and heart failure. In those patients

Table 4. Treatment of systemic lupus erythematosus (SLE) at the start of hemodialysis (HD) and outcome of dialysis patients

	Outcome		
Treatment	Off dialysis	Died	On dialysis
Corticosteroids High dose oral	88.7	93.2	94.0
		NS	
Corticosteroid pulse	69 8	36.1	27.5
		***	
Immunosuppressants	22.6	19.0	9.0
		NS	
Plasma exchange	28.3	15.0	5.4
		*	

(*P<0.05 ***P<0.001) %: NS, not significant

Table 5. ANCA titer and renal injury in Wegener's granulomatosis (WG)

Cases	ANCA titer (ELISA U/ml)	Proteinuria (mg/dl) Hematuria (1hpf)	S-Cr (mg/dl)	Renal histology
1. 51 ♂	860	260/Many	18.5	Cres. GN
2. 42 ♂	760	560/Many	0.6	Cres. GN
3. 29 ♂	750	70/Many	0.8	Seg. Necrot. GN
4. 38 ♀	730	160/10–20	1.3	Seg. Necrot. GN
5. 36 ♂	460	200/20–30	4.9	Cres. GN
6. 36 ♂	180	100/10–20	1.1	n.d.
7. 30 ♂	93	300/50–60	1.1	n.d.
8. 62 ♀	72	Negative	0.6	n.d.
9. 35 ♀	70	Negative	0.6	n.d.
10. 42 ♀	58	Negative	0.8	n.d.
11. 31 ♀	Negative	Negative	0.6	n.d.

ANCA, anti-neutrophil cytoplasmic antibody

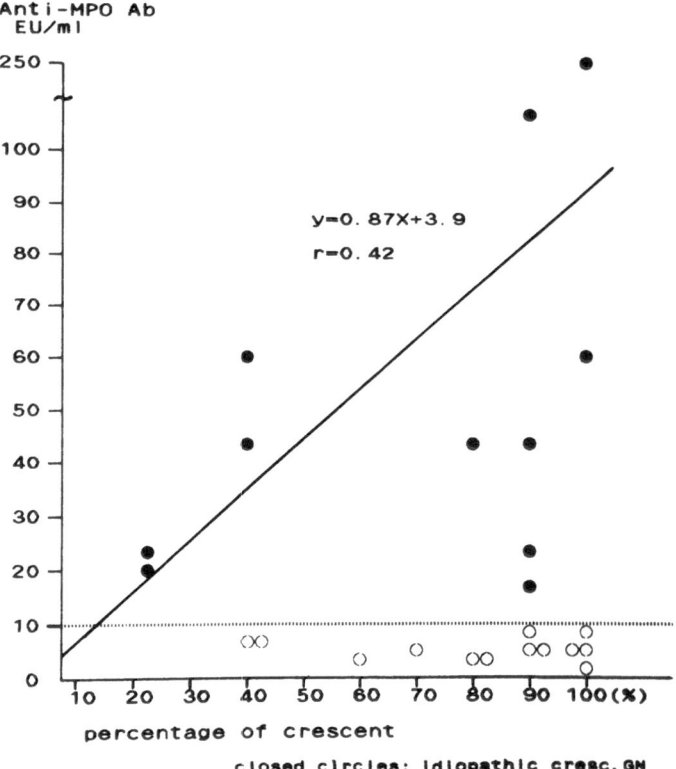

Fig. 5. Relationship between titers of anti-MPO antibodies and percentage of crescent formation

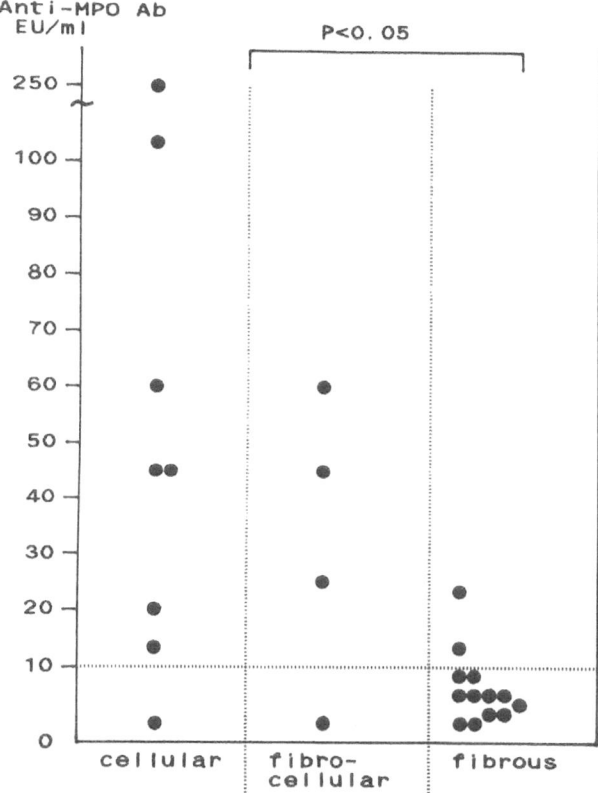

Fig. 6. Titers of anti-MPO antibodies and stage of crescent idiopathic crescentic GN

who had been on HD for less than 1 year, bleeding and heart failure had a high incidence. In type 1 LN patients especially, acute bleeding should be strictly controlled, since in these patients thrombocytopenia, as well as the influence of uremia, is the cause of bleeding.

In type 3 LN, the prognosis of patients on chronic HD was excellent. In nearly all of them immunologic and clinical SLE activities were burned out several years after beginning HD, suggesting that they were excellent candidates for renal transplantation. In fact, in Japan, a smaller number of patients received renal transplantation than in Western countries. However, these patients' long term prognosis, without LN relapse in the transplanted kidneys, are good.

Anti-Neutrophil Cytoplasmic Antibody (ANCA) and Renal Vasculitis

It is already well established that cytoplasmic ANCA is specific for Wegener's granulomatosis (WG) and that myeloperoxidase (MPO)-ANCA is specific for idiopathic crescentic glomerulonephritis (GN). Therefore, WG and idiopathic crescentic GN in Japan were examined for the presence of ANCA. As shown in Table 5, C-ANCA, examined by sandwich enzyme-linked immunoadsorbent assay (ELISA), was specifically positive in WG and its titer showed close correlation with the severity of renal injury. The same was true for anti-MPO antibody and idiopathic crescentic GN. As shown in Figs. 5 and 6, the percentages of the numbers of crescentic glomeruli and the stages of crescentic GN had close correlation with the titer of anti-MPO antibody. These results indicate that C- and MPO-ANCA should be used for monitoring WG and idiopathic crescentic GN immunosuppressive therapy.

In conclusion, when immunosuppressive therapy, especially CS therapy, is chosen for LN and RV patients the balance between its benefits and risks should be considered, utilizing new therapeutic indices, as described in this paper.